Food enrichment with omega-3 fatty acids

Related titles:

Encapsulation technologies and delivery systems for food ingredients and nutraceuticals
(ISBN 978-0-85709-124-6)

Reducing saturated fats in foods
(ISBN 978-1-84569-740-2)

Functional foods
(ISBN 978-1-84569-690-0)

Details of these books and a complete list of titles from Woodhead Publishing can be obtained by:

- visiting our web site at www.woodheadpublishing.com
- contacting Customer Services (e-mail: sales@woodheadpublishing.com; fax: +44 (0) 1223 832819; tel.: +44 (0) 1223 499140 ext. 130; address: Woodhead Publishing Limited, 80 High Street, Sawston, Cambridge CB22 3HJ, UK)
- in North America, contacting our US office (e-mail: usmarketing@ woodheadpublishing.com; tel.: (215) 928 9112; address: Woodhead Publishing, 1518 Walnut Street, Suite 1100, Philadelphia, PA 19102-3406, USA)

If you would like e-versions of our content, please visit our online platform: www.woodheadpublishingonline.com. Please recommend it to your librarian so that everyone in your institution can benefit from the wealth of content on the site.

We are always happy to receive suggestions for new books from potential editors. To enquire about contributing to our Food Science, Technology and Nutrition series, please send your name, contact address and details of the topic/s you are interested in to nell.holden@woodheadpublishing.com. We look forward to hearing from you.

The team responsible for publishing this book:

Commissioning Editor: Nell Holden
Publications Coordinator: Emily Cole
Project Editor: Kate Hardcastle
Editorial and Production Manager: Mary Campbell
Production Editor: Adam Hooper
Copyeditor: Helen MacFadyen
Proofreader: Janice Gordon
Cover Designer: Terry Callanan

Woodhead Publishing Series in Food Science, Technology and Nutrition:
Number 252

Food enrichment with omega-3 fatty acids

Edited by
Charlotte Jacobsen, Nina Skall Nielsen,
Anna Frisenfeldt Horn and
Ann-Dorit Moltke Sørensen

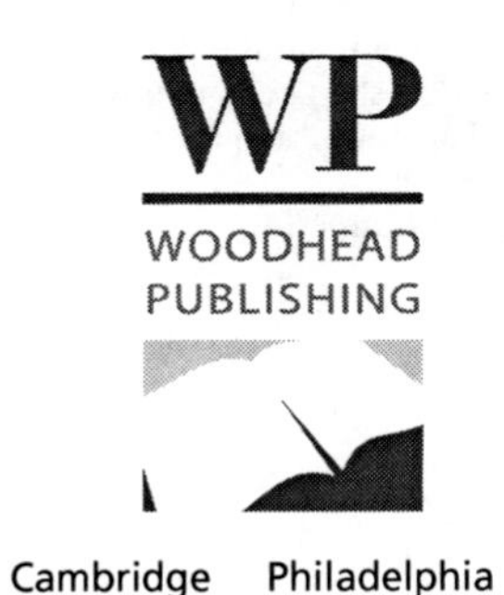

Oxford Cambridge Philadelphia New Delhi

Published by Woodhead Publishing Limited,
80 High Street, Sawston, Cambridge CB22 3HJ, UK
www.woodheadpublishing.com
www.woodheadpublishingonline.com

Woodhead Publishing, 1518 Walnut Street, Suite 1100, Philadelphia, PA 19102-3406, USA

Woodhead Publishing India Private Limited, 303 Vardaan House, 7/28 Ansari Road, Daryaganj, New Delhi – 110002, India
www.woodheadpublishingindia.com

First published 2013, Woodhead Publishing Limited

British Library Cataloguing in Publication Data
A catalogue record for this book is available from the British Library.

Library of Congress Control Number: 2013936412

ISBN 978-0-85709-428-5 (print)
ISBN 978-0-85709-886-3 (online)
ISSN 2042-8049 Woodhead Publishing Series in Food Science, Technology and Nutrition (print)
ISSN 2042-8057 Woodhead Publishing Series in Food Science, Technology and Nutrition (online)

The publisher's policy is to use permanent paper from mills that operate a sustainable forestry policy, and which has been manufactured from pulp which is processed using acid-free and elemental chlorine-free practices. Furthermore, the publisher ensures that the text paper and cover board used have met acceptable environmental accreditation standards.

Typeset by Toppan Best-set Premedia Limited
Printed by Lightning Source

Contents

Contributor contact details

(* = main contact)

Editors

Professor Charlotte Jacobsen*, Dr Nina Skall Nielsen, Dr Anna Frisenfeldt Horn and Dr Ann-Dorit Moltke Sørensen
Division of Industrial Food Research
National Food Institute
Technical University of Denmark
B. 221, Søltofts Plads, DTU
DK-2800 Kgs. Lyngby
Denmark

E-mail: chja@food.dtu.dk; nsni@food.dtu.dk; afho@food.dtu.dk; adms@food.dtu.dk

Chapter 1

Professor Philip C. Calder
Institute of Human Nutrition
Faculty of Medicine
University of Southampton
MP887 Southampton General Hospital
Tremona Road
Southampton
SO16 6YD
UK

E-mail: pcc@soton.ac.uk

Chapter 2

Anthony P. Bimbo
Technical Consultant
International Fisheries Technology
P. O. Box 1606
55 Cedar Lane
Kilmarnock
VA 22482
USA

E-mail: apbimbo@verizon.net

Chapter 3

Dr Åge Oterhals*
Division of Fisheries, Industry and Market
Marine Biotechnology
Norwegian Institute of Food, Fisheries and Aquaculture Research
Kjerreidviken 16
NO-5141 Fyllingsdalen
Norway

E-mail: aage.oterhals@nofima.no

Gjermund Vogt
Division of Food Science
Food and Health
Norwegian Institute of Food, Fisheries and Aquaculture Research
Osloveien 1
NO-1430 Ås
Norway

E-mail: gjermund.vogt@nofima.no

Chapter 4

Professor Charlotte Jacobsen*, Dr Ann-Dorit Moltke Sørensen and Dr Nina Skall Nielsen
Division of Industrial Food Research
National Food Institute
Technical University of Denmark
B. 221, Søltofts Plads, DTU
DK-2800 Kgs. Lyngby
Denmark

E-mail: chja@food.dtu.dk; adms@food.dtu.dk; nsni@food.dtu.dk

Chapter 5

Dr Claude Genot*, Tin-Hinan Kabri and Dr Anne Meynier
INRA, UR1268 Biopolymères Interactions Assemblages
Rue de la Géraudière
BP71627
F-44316 Nantes cedex
France

E-mail: claude.genot@nantes.inra.fr; tin-hinan.kabri@nantes.inra.fr; anne.meynier@nantes.inra.fr

Chapter 6

Professor Colin J. Barrow* and Dr Bo Wang
Centre for Chemistry and Biotechnology
Deakin University
Geelong, VIC 3217
Australia

E-mail: colin.barrow@deakin.edu.au; bo.wang@deakin.edu.au

Professor Benu Adhikari and Dr Huihua Liu
School of Science and Engineering
University of Ballarat
Mount Helen, VIC 3350
Australia

E-mail: b.adhikari@ballarat.edu.au; h.liu@ballarat.edu.au

Chapter 7

Professor Jonathan M. Curtis* and Brenna A. Black
Lipid Chemistry Group
Department of Agricultural, Food and Nutritional Science
University of Alberta
Edmonton
Alberta T6G 2P5
Canada

E-mail: jonathan.curtis@ualberta.ca; bblack@ualberta.ca

Chapter 8

Dr Richard J. Dewhurst* and Dr Aidan P. Moloney
Teagasc, Animal & Grassland Research and Innovation Centre
Grange
Dunsany
County Meath
Ireland

E-mail: richard.dewhurst@teagasc.ie; aidan.moloney@teagasc.ie

Chapter 9

Dr Gita Cherian
Department of Animal and Rangeland Sciences
Oregon State University
122 Withycombe Hall
Corvallis
OR 97331
USA

E-mail: gita.cherian@oregonstate.edu

Chapter 10

Dr Diana Ansorena* and Dr Iciar Astiasarán
Department of Nutrition, Food Science and Physiology
Faculty of Pharmacy
Universidad de Navarra
Irunlarrea sn 31008
Pamplona (Navarra)
Spain

E-mail: dansorena@unav.es; iastiasa@unav.es

Chapters 11 and 15

Dr Ernesto M. Hernandez
Omega Protein, Inc.
OmegaPure Technology and Innovation Center
6961 Brookhollow W Drive, Ste. 190
Houston
TX 77040
USA

E-mail: ehernandez@OmegaPure.com

Chapter 12

Professor Charlotte Jacobsen*, Dr Anna Frisenfeldt Horn and Dr Nina Skall Nielsen
Division of Industrial Food Research
National Food Institute
Technical University of Denmark
B. 221, Søltofts Plads, DTU
DK-2800 Kgs. Lyngby
Denmark

E-mail: chja@food.dtu.dk; afho@food.dtu.dk; nsni@food.dtu.dk

Chapter 13

Dr Connye N. Kuratko*,
J. Ruben Abril, James P. Hoffman and Norman Salem, Jr
Nutrition Science & Advocacy
DSM Nutritional Products
6480 Dobbin Road
Columbia
MD 21045
USA

E-mail: connye.kuratko@dsm.com; ruben.abril@dsm.com; james.hoffman@dsm.com; norman.salem@dsm.com

Chapter 14

Dr Robert J. Winwood
DSM Nutritional Products (UK) Ltd
Delves Road
Heanor Gate Industrial Estate
Heanor
Derbyshire
DE75 7SG
UK

E-mail: rob.winwood@dsm.com

Woodhead Publishing Series in Food Science, Technology and Nutrition

1. **Chilled foods: A comprehensive guide** *Edited by C. Dennis and M. Stringer*
2. **Yoghurt: Science and technology** *A. Y. Tamime and R. K. Robinson*
3. **Food processing technology: Principles and practice** *P. J. Fellows*
4. **Bender's dictionary of nutrition and food technology Sixth edition** *D. A. Bender*
5. **Determination of veterinary residues in food** *Edited by N. T. Crosby*
6. **Food contaminants: Sources and surveillance** *Edited by C. Creaser and R. Purchase*
7. **Nitrates and nitrites in food and water** *Edited by M. J. Hill*
8. **Pesticide chemistry and bioscience: The food-environment challenge** *Edited by G. T. Brooks and T. Roberts*
9. **Pesticides: Developments, impacts and controls** *Edited by G. A. Best and A. D. Ruthven*
10. **Dietary fibre: Chemical and biological aspects** *Edited by D. A. T. Southgate, K. W. Waldron, I. T. Johnson and G. R. Fenwick*
11. **Vitamins and minerals in health and nutrition** *M. Tolonen*
12. **Technology of biscuits, crackers and cookies Second edition** *D. Manley*
13. **Instrumentation and sensors for the food industry** *Edited by E. Kress-Rogers*
14. **Food and cancer prevention: Chemical and biological aspects** *Edited by K. W. Waldron, I. T. Johnson and G. R. Fenwick*
15. **Food colloids: Proteins, lipids and polysaccharides** *Edited by E. Dickinson and B. Bergenstahl*
16. **Food emulsions and foams** *Edited by E. Dickinson*
17. **Maillard reactions in chemistry, food and health** *Edited by T. P. Labuza, V. Monnier, J. Baynes and J. O'Brien*
18. **The Maillard reaction in foods and medicine** *Edited by J. O'Brien, H. E. Nursten, M. J. Crabbe and J. M. Ames*

19 **Encapsulation and controlled release** *Edited by D. R. Karsa and R. A. Stephenson*
20 **Flavours and fragrances** *Edited by A. D. Swift*
21 **Feta and related cheeses** *Edited by A. Y. Tamime and R. K. Robinson*
22 **Biochemistry of milk products** *Edited by A. T. Andrews and J. R. Varley*
23 **Physical properties of foods and food processing systems** *M. J. Lewis*
24 **Food irradiation: A reference guide** *V. M. Wilkinson and G. Gould*
25 **Kent's technology of cereals: An introduction for students of food science and agriculture Fourth edition** *N. L. Kent and A. D. Evers*
26 **Biosensors for food analysis** *Edited by A. O. Scott*
27 **Separation processes in the food and biotechnology industries: Principles and applications** *Edited by A. S. Grandison and M. J. Lewis*
28 **Handbook of indices of food quality and authenticity** *R. S. Singhal, P. K. Kulkarni and D. V. Rege*
29 **Principles and practices for the safe processing of foods** *D. A. Shapton and N. F. Shapton*
30 **Biscuit, cookie and cracker manufacturing manuals Volume 1: Ingredients** *D. Manley*
31 **Biscuit, cookie and cracker manufacturing manuals Volume 2: Biscuit doughs** *D. Manley*
32 **Biscuit, cookie and cracker manufacturing manuals Volume 3: Biscuit dough piece forming** *D. Manley*
33 **Biscuit, cookie and cracker manufacturing manuals Volume 4: Baking and cooling of biscuits** *D. Manley*
34 **Biscuit, cookie and cracker manufacturing manuals Volume 5: Secondary processing in biscuit manufacturing** *D. Manley*
35 **Biscuit, cookie and cracker manufacturing manuals Volume 6: Biscuit packaging and storage** *D. Manley*
36 **Practical dehydration Second edition** *M. Greensmith*
37 **Lawrie's meat science Sixth edition** *R. A. Lawrie*
38 **Yoghurt: Science and technology Second edition** *A. Y. Tamime and R. K. Robinson*
39 **New ingredients in food processing: Biochemistry and agriculture** *G. Linden and D. Lorient*
40 **Benders' dictionary of nutrition and food technology Seventh edition** *D. A. Bender and A. E. Bender*
41 **Technology of biscuits, crackers and cookies Third edition** *D. Manley*
42 **Food processing technology: Principles and practice Second edition** *P. J. Fellows*
43 **Managing frozen foods** *Edited by C. J. Kennedy*
44 **Handbook of hydrocolloids** *Edited by G. O. Phillips and P. A. Williams*
45 **Food labelling** *Edited by J. R. Blanchfield*
46 **Cereal biotechnology** *Edited by P. C. Morris and J. H. Bryce*
47 **Food intolerance and the food industry** *Edited by T. Dean*
48 **The stability and shelf-life of food** *Edited by D. Kilcast and P. Subramaniam*
49 **Functional foods: Concept to product** *Edited by G. R. Gibson and C. M. Williams*
50 **Chilled foods: A comprehensive guide Second edition** *Edited by M. Stringer and C. Dennis*

51 **HACCP in the meat industry** *Edited by M. Brown*
52 **Biscuit, cracker and cookie recipes for the food industry** *D. Manley*
53 **Cereals processing technology** *Edited by G. Owens*
54 **Baking problems solved** *S. P. Cauvain and L. S. Young*
55 **Thermal technologies in food processing** *Edited by P. Richardson*
56 **Frying: Improving quality** *Edited by J. B. Rossell*
57 **Food chemical safety Volume 1: Contaminants** *Edited by D. Watson*
58 **Making the most of HACCP: Learning from others' experience** *Edited by T. Mayes and S. Mortimore*
59 **Food process modelling** *Edited by L. M. M. Tijskens, M. L. A. T. M. Hertog and B. M. Nicolaï*
60 **EU food law: A practical guide** *Edited by K. Goodburn*
61 **Extrusion cooking: Technologies and applications** *Edited by R. Guy*
62 **Auditing in the food industry: From safety and quality to environmental and other audits** *Edited by M. Dillon and C. Griffith*
63 **Handbook of herbs and spices Volume 1** *Edited by K. V. Peter*
64 **Food product development: Maximising success** *M. Earle, R. Earle and A. Anderson*
65 **Instrumentation and sensors for the food industry Second edition** *Edited by E. Kress-Rogers and C. J. B. Brimelow*
66 **Food chemical safety Volume 2: Additives** *Edited by D. Watson*
67 **Fruit and vegetable biotechnology** *Edited by V. Valpuesta*
68 **Foodborne pathogens: Hazards, risk analysis and control** *Edited by C. de W. Blackburn and P. J. McClure*
69 **Meat refrigeration** *S. J. James and C. James*
70 **Lockhart and Wiseman's crop husbandry Eighth edition** *H. J. S. Finch, A. M. Samuel and G. P. F. Lane*
71 **Safety and quality issues in fish processing** *Edited by H. A. Bremner*
72 **Minimal processing technologies in the food industries** *Edited by T. Ohlsson and N. Bengtsson*
73 **Fruit and vegetable processing: Improving quality** *Edited by W. Jongen*
74 **The nutrition handbook for food processors** *Edited by C. J. K. Henry and C. Chapman*
75 **Colour in food: Improving quality** *Edited by D. MacDougall*
76 **Meat processing: Improving quality** *Edited by J. P. Kerry, J. F. Kerry and D. A. Ledward*
77 **Microbiological risk assessment in food processing** *Edited by M. Brown and M. Stringer*
78 **Performance functional foods** *Edited by D. Watson*
79 **Functional dairy products Volume 1** *Edited by T. Mattila-Sandholm and M. Saarela*
80 **Taints and off-flavours in foods** *Edited by B. Baigrie*
81 **Yeasts in food** *Edited by T. Boekhout and V. Robert*
82 **Phytochemical functional foods** *Edited by I. T. Johnson and G. Williamson*
83 **Novel food packaging techniques** *Edited by R. Ahvenainen*
84 **Detecting pathogens in food** *Edited by T. A. McMeekin*
85 **Natural antimicrobials for the minimal processing of foods** *Edited by S. Roller*
86 **Texture in food Volume 1: Semi-solid foods** *Edited by B. M. McKenna*

122 **Food spoilage microorganisms** *Edited by C. de W. Blackburn*
123 **Emerging foodborne pathogens** *Edited by Y. Motarjemi and M. Adams*
124 **Benders' dictionary of nutrition and food technology Eighth edition** *D. A. Bender*
125 **Optimising sweet taste in foods** *Edited by W. J. Spillane*
126 **Brewing: New technologies** *Edited by C. Bamforth*
127 **Handbook of herbs and spices Volume 3** *Edited by K. V. Peter*
128 **Lawrie's meat science Seventh edition** *R. A. Lawrie in collaboration with D. A. Ledward*
129 **Modifying lipids for use in food** *Edited by F. Gunstone*
130 **Meat products handbook: Practical science and technology** *G. Feiner*
131 **Food consumption and disease risk: Consumer–pathogen interactions** *Edited by M. Potter*
132 **Acrylamide and other hazardous compounds in heat-treated foods** *Edited by K. Skog and J. Alexander*
133 **Managing allergens in food** *Edited by C. Mills, H. Wichers and K. Hoffman-Sommergruber*
134 **Microbiological analysis of red meat, poultry and eggs** *Edited by G. Mead*
135 **Maximising the value of marine by-products** *Edited by F. Shahidi*
136 **Chemical migration and food contact materials** *Edited by K. Barnes, R. Sinclair and D. Watson*
137 **Understanding consumers of food products** *Edited by L. Frewer and H. van Trijp*
138 **Reducing salt in foods: Practical strategies** *Edited by D. Kilcast and F. Angus*
139 **Modelling microorganisms in food** *Edited by S. Brul, S. Van Gerwen and M. Zwietering*
140 **Tamime and Robinson's Yoghurt: Science and technology Third edition** *A. Y. Tamime and R. K. Robinson*
141 **Handbook of waste management and co-product recovery in food processing Volume 1** *Edited by K. W. Waldron*
142 **Improving the flavour of cheese** *Edited by B. Weimer*
143 **Novel food ingredients for weight control** *Edited by C. J. K. Henry*
144 **Consumer-led food product development** *Edited by H. MacFie*
145 **Functional dairy products Volume 2** *Edited by M. Saarela*
146 **Modifying flavour in food** *Edited by A. J. Taylor and J. Hort*
147 **Cheese problems solved** *Edited by P. L. H. McSweeney*
148 **Handbook of organic food safety and quality** *Edited by J. Cooper, C. Leifert and U. Niggli*
149 **Understanding and controlling the microstructure of complex foods** *Edited by D. J. McClements*
150 **Novel enzyme technology for food applications** *Edited by R. Rastall*
151 **Food preservation by pulsed electric fields: From research to application** *Edited by H. L. M. Lelieveld and S. W. H. de Haan*
152 **Technology of functional cereal products** *Edited by B. R. Hamaker*
153 **Case studies in food product development** *Edited by M. Earle and R. Earle*
154 **Delivery and controlled release of bioactives in foods and nutraceuticals** *Edited by N. Garti*
155 **Fruit and vegetable flavour: Recent advances and future prospects** *Edited by B. Brückner and S. G. Wyllie*

156 **Food fortification and supplementation: Technological, safety and regulatory aspects** *Edited by P. Berry Ottaway*
157 **Improving the health-promoting properties of fruit and vegetable products** *Edited by F. A. Tomás-Barberán and M. I. Gil*
158 **Improving seafood products for the consumer** *Edited by T. Børresen*
159 **In-pack processed foods: Improving quality** *Edited by P. Richardson*
160 **Handbook of water and energy management in food processing** *Edited by J. Klemeš, R. Smith and J.-K. Kim*
161 **Environmentally compatible food packaging** *Edited by E. Chiellini*
162 **Improving farmed fish quality and safety** *Edited by Ø. Lie*
163 **Carbohydrate-active enzymes** *Edited by K.-H. Park*
164 **Chilled foods: A comprehensive guide Third edition** *Edited by M. Brown*
165 **Food for the ageing population** *Edited by M. M. Raats, C. P. G. M. de Groot and W. A Van Staveren*
166 **Improving the sensory and nutritional quality of fresh meat** *Edited by J. P. Kerry and D. A. Ledward*
167 **Shellfish safety and quality** *Edited by S. E. Shumway and G. E. Rodrick*
168 **Functional and speciality beverage technology** *Edited by P. Paquin*
169 **Functional foods: Principles and technology** *M. Guo*
170 **Endocrine-disrupting chemicals in food** *Edited by I. Shaw*
171 **Meals in science and practice: Interdisciplinary research and business applications** *Edited by H. L. Meiselman*
172 **Food constituents and oral health: Current status and future prospects** *Edited by M. Wilson*
173 **Handbook of hydrocolloids Second edition** *Edited by G. O. Phillips and P. A. Williams*
174 **Food processing technology: Principles and practice Third edition** *P. J. Fellows*
175 **Science and technology of enrobed and filled chocolate, confectionery and bakery products** *Edited by G. Talbot*
176 **Foodborne pathogens: Hazards, risk analysis and control Second edition** *Edited by C. de W. Blackburn and P. J. McClure*
177 **Designing functional foods: Measuring and controlling food structure breakdown and absorption** *Edited by D. J. McClements and E. A. Decker*
178 **New technologies in aquaculture: Improving production efficiency, quality and environmental management** *Edited by G. Burnell and G. Allan*
179 **More baking problems solved** *S. P. Cauvain and L. S. Young*
180 **Soft drink and fruit juice problems solved** *P. Ashurst and R. Hargitt*
181 **Biofilms in the food and beverage industries** *Edited by P. M. Fratamico, B. A. Annous and N. W. Gunther*
182 **Dairy-derived ingredients: Food and neutraceutical uses** *Edited by M. Corredig*
183 **Handbook of waste management and co-product recovery in food processing Volume 2** *Edited by K. W. Waldron*
184 **Innovations in food labelling** *Edited by J. Albert*
185 **Delivering performance in food supply chains** *Edited by C. Mena and G. Stevens*
186 **Chemical deterioration and physical instability of food and beverages** *Edited by L. H. Skibsted, J. Risbo and M. L. Andersen*

187 **Managing wine quality Volume 1: Viticulture and wine quality** *Edited by A. G. Reynolds*
188 **Improving the safety and quality of milk Volume 1: Milk production and processing** *Edited by M. Griffiths*
189 **Improving the safety and quality of milk Volume 2: Improving quality in milk products** *Edited by M. Griffiths*
190 **Cereal grains: Assessing and managing quality** *Edited by C. Wrigley and I. Batey*
191 **Sensory analysis for food and beverage quality control: A practical guide** *Edited by D. Kilcast*
192 **Managing wine quality Volume 2: Oenology and wine quality** *Edited by A. G. Reynolds*
193 **Winemaking problems solved** *Edited by C. E. Butzke*
194 **Environmental assessment and management in the food industry** *Edited by U. Sonesson, J. Berlin and F. Ziegler*
195 **Consumer-driven innovation in food and personal care products** *Edited by S. R. Jaeger and H. MacFie*
196 **Tracing pathogens in the food chain** *Edited by S. Brul, P. M. Fratamico and T. A. McMeekin*
197 **Case studies in novel food processing technologies: Innovations in processing, packaging, and predictive modelling** *Edited by C. J. Doona, K. Kustin and F. E. Feeherry*
198 **Freeze-drying of pharmaceutical and food products** *T.-C. Hua, B.-L. Liu and H. Zhang*
199 **Oxidation in foods and beverages and antioxidant applications Volume 1: Understanding mechanisms of oxidation and antioxidant activity** *Edited by E. A. Decker, R. J. Elias and D. J. McClements*
200 **Oxidation in foods and beverages and antioxidant applications Volume 2: Management in different industry sectors** *Edited by E. A. Decker, R. J. Elias and D. J. McClements*
201 **Protective cultures, antimicrobial metabolites and bacteriophages for food and beverage biopreservation** *Edited by C. Lacroix*
202 **Separation, extraction and concentration processes in the food, beverage and nutraceutical industries** *Edited by S. S. H. Rizvi*
203 **Determining mycotoxins and mycotoxigenic fungi in food and feed** *Edited by S. De Saeger*
204 **Developing children's food products** *Edited by D. Kilcast and F. Angus*
205 **Functional foods: Concept to product Second edition** *Edited by M. Saarela*
206 **Postharvest biology and technology of tropical and subtropical fruits Volume 1: Fundamental issues** *Edited by E. M. Yahia*
207 **Postharvest biology and technology of tropical and subtropical fruits Volume 2: Açai to citrus** *Edited by E. M. Yahia*
208 **Postharvest biology and technology of tropical and subtropical fruits Volume 3: Cocona to mango** *Edited by E. M. Yahia*
209 **Postharvest biology and technology of tropical and subtropical fruits Volume 4: Mangosteen to white sapote** *Edited by E. M. Yahia*
210 **Food and beverage stability and shelf life** *Edited by D. Kilcast and P. Subramaniam*

211 **Processed Meats: Improving safety, nutrition and quality** *Edited by J. P. Kerry and J. F. Kerry*
212 **Food chain integrity: A holistic approach to food traceability, safety, quality and authenticity** *Edited by J. Hoorfar, K. Jordan, F. Butler and R. Prugger*
213 **Improving the safety and quality of eggs and egg products Volume 1** *Edited by Y. Nys, M. Bain and F. Van Immerseel*
214 **Improving the safety and quality of eggs and egg products Volume 2** *Edited by F. Van Immerseel, Y. Nys and M. Bain*
215 **Animal feed contamination: Effects on livestock and food safety** *Edited by J. Fink-Gremmels*
216 **Hygienic design of food factories** *Edited by J. Holah and H. L. M. Lelieveld*
217 **Manley's technology of biscuits, crackers and cookies Fourth edition** *Edited by D. Manley*
218 **Nanotechnology in the food, beverage and nutraceutical industries** *Edited by Q. Huang*
219 **Rice quality: A guide to rice properties and analysis** *K. R. Bhattacharya*
220 **Advances in meat, poultry and seafood packaging** *Edited by J. P. Kerry*
221 **Reducing saturated fats in foods** *Edited by G. Talbot*
222 **Handbook of food proteins** *Edited by G. O. Phillips and P. A. Williams*
223 **Lifetime nutritional influences on cognition, behaviour and psychiatric illness** *Edited by D. Benton*
224 **Food machinery for the production of cereal foods, snack foods and confectionery** *L.-M. Cheng*
225 **Alcoholic beverages: Sensory evaluation and consumer research** *Edited by J. Piggott*
226 **Extrusion problems solved: Food, pet food and feed** *M. N. Riaz and G. J. Rokey*
227 **Handbook of herbs and spices Second edition Volume 1** *Edited by K. V. Peter*
228 **Handbook of herbs and spices Second edition Volume 2** *Edited by K. V. Peter*
229 **Breadmaking: Improving quality Second edition** *Edited by S. P. Cauvain*
230 **Emerging food packaging technologies: Principles and practice** *Edited by K. L. Yam and D. S. Lee*
231 **Infectious disease in aquaculture: Prevention and control** *Edited by B. Austin*
232 **Diet, immunity and inflammation** *Edited by P. C. Calder and P. Yaqoob*
233 **Natural food additives, ingredients and flavourings** *Edited by D. Baines and R. Seal*
234 **Microbial decontamination in the food industry: Novel methods and applications** *Edited by A. Demirci and M.O. Ngadi*
235 **Chemical contaminants and residues in foods** *Edited by D. Schrenk*
236 **Robotics and automation in the food industry: Current and future technologies** *Edited by D. G. Caldwell*
237 **Fibre-rich and wholegrain foods: Improving quality** *Edited by J. A. Delcour and K. Poutanen*
238 **Computer vision technology in the food and beverage industries** *Edited by D.-W. Sun*

239 **Encapsulation technologies and delivery systems for food ingredients and nutraceuticals** *Edited by N. Garti and D. J. McClements*
240 **Case studies in food safety and authenticity** *Edited by J. Hoorfar*
241 **Heat treatment for insect control: Developments and applications** *D. Hammond*
242 **Advances in aquaculture hatchery technology** *Edited by G. Allan and G. Burnell*
243 **Open innovation in the food and beverage industry** *Edited by M. Garcia Martinez*
244 **Trends in packaging of food, beverages and other fast-moving consumer goods (FMCG)** *Edited by Neil Farmer*
245 **New analytical approaches for verifying the origin of food** *Edited by P. Brereton*
246 **Microbial production of food ingredients, enzymes and nutraceuticals** *Edited by B. McNeil, D. Archer, I. Giavasis and L. Harvey*
247 **Persistent organic pollutants and toxic metals in foods** *Edited by M. Rose and A. Fernandes*
248 **Cereal grains for the food and beverage industries** *E. Arendt and E. Zannini*
249 **Viruses in food and water: Risks, surveillance and control** *Edited by N. Cook*
250 **Improving the safety and quality of nuts** *Edited by L. J. Harris*
251 **Metabolomics in food and nutrition** *Edited by B. C. Weimer and C. Slupsky*
252 **Food enrichment with omega-3 fatty acids** *Edited by C. Jacobsen, N. S. Nielsen, A. F. Horn and A.-D. M. Sørensen*
253 **Instrumental assessment of food sensory quality: A practical guide** *Edited by D. Kilcast*
254 **Food microstructures: Microscopy, measurement and modelling** *Edited by V. J. Morris and K. Groves*
255 **Handbook of food powders: Processes and properties** *Edited by B. R. Bhandari, N. Bansal, M. Zhang and P. Schuck*
256 **Functional ingredients from algae for foods and nutraceuticals** *Edited by H. Domínguez*
257 **Satiation, satiety and the control of food intake: Theory and practice** *Edited by J. E. Blundell and F. Bellisle*
258 **Hygiene in food processing: Principles and practice Second edition** *Edited by H. L. M. Lelieveld, J. Holah and D. Napper*
259 **Advances in microbial food safety Volume 1** *Edited by J. Sofos*
260 **Global safety of fresh produce: A handbook of best practice, innovative commercial solutions and case studies** *Edited by J. Hoorfar*
261 **Human milk biochemistry and infant formula manufacturing technology** *Edited by M. Guo*
262 **High throughput screening for food safety assessment: Biosensor technologies, hyperspectral imaging and practical applications** *Edited by A. K. Bhunia, M. S. Kim and C. R. Taitt*
263 **Foods, nutrients and food ingredients with authorised EU health claims** *Edited by M. J. Sadler*
264 **Handbook of food allergen detection and control** *Edited by S. Flanagan*
265 **Advances in fermented foods and beverages: Improving quality, technologies and health benefits** *Edited by W. Holzapfel*

266 **Metabolomics as a tool in nutritional research** *Edited by J.-L. Sebedio and L. Brennan*
267 **Dietary supplements: Safety, efficacy and quality** *Edited by K. Berginc and S. Kreft*
268 **Grapevine breeding programs for the wine industry: Traditional and molecular technologies** *Edited by A. G. Reynolds*
269 **Handbook of natural antimicrobials for food safety and quality** *Edited by M. Taylor*
270 **Managing and preventing obesity: Behavioural factors and dietary interventions** *Edited by T. Gill*
271 **Electron beam pasteurization and complementary food processing technologies** *Edited by S. Pillai and S. Shayanfar*
272 **Advances in food and beverage labelling: Information and regulations** *Edited by P. Berryman*
273 **Flavour development, analysis and perception in food and beverages** *Edited by J. K. Parker, S. Elmore and L. Methven*
274 **Rapid sensory profiling techniques and related methods: Applications in new product development and consumer research**, *Edited by J. Delarue, B. Lawlor and M. Rogeaux*
275 **Advances in microbial food safety: Volume 2** *Edited by J. Sofos*
276 **Handbook of antioxidants in food preservation** *Edited by F. Shahidi*
277 **Lockhart and Wiseman's crop husbandry including grassland: Ninth edition** *H. J. S. Finch, A. M. Samuel and G. P. F. Lane*
278 **Global legislation for food contact materials: Processing, storage and packaging** *Edited by J. S. Baughan*
279 **Colour additives for food and beverages: Development, safety and applications** *Edited by M. Scotter*

Preface

Seafood and seafood products are rich in the long chain highly unsaturated omega-3 fatty acids eicosapentaenoic acid (EPA) and docosahexaenoic acid (DHA). Fatty fish such as salmon and mackerel in particular have a high natural content of these two fatty acids, but the livers of lean fish are also rich sources. In the 1970s, Bang and Dyerberg discovered that Greenland Inuits, who consume large amounts of seafood (including seal and whale meat) as part of their native lifestyle, had a much lower cardiovascular mortality (10–30%) compared to the Danes, who consume much less seafood. This difference in mortality was ascribed to the high content of marine omega-3 fatty acids in the diet of the Inuits. These discoveries subsequently led to new studies on the role of marine omega-3 fatty acids in cardiovascular disease. Results from such studies have demonstrated that omega-3 fatty acids beneficially alter a range of cardiovascular disease risk factors, which suggests that they are able to reduce the atherosclerotic process. This may explain their preventative effect on cardiovascular mortality; however, the mechanisms of this process are still not fully understood. Since the 1990s, the number of studies on the effect of marine omega-3 fatty acids on other lifestyle-related diseases has increased significantly. Data from these studies suggest that marine omega-3 fatty acids may also play an important role in brain development in the infant, in maintaining normal eye and brain function (reducing depressions, dementia, etc.) in adults, in alleviating the symptoms of rheumatoid arthritis and perhaps also in the prevention of certain forms of cancer. This research has spurred industrial interest in exploiting the health benefits of omega-3 fatty acids for the production of dietary supplements and functional foods. To develop such products, a number of challenges must be overcome, such as the development of gentle technologies for the extraction of omega-3 oils and the subsequent removal of undesirable substances, the development of new technologies to maintain oil quality and the communication of the benefits of the omega-3 fatty acids to the consumer. This book aims to provide the reader with a comprehensive overview of current research on the entire chain, from production and refining of omega-3 oils to their applications in different foods, including the possible health benefits.

The current state of knowledge about the role of marine omega-3 fatty acids in human nutrition is covered in Chapter 1, which also discusses the effects of omega-3 fatty acids from plant oils. Plant oils do not contain EPA and DHA, but only the shorter chain omega-3 fatty acid α-linolenic acid (ALA), which do not have the same nutritional effects as EPA and DHA.

An increasing proportion of global fish consumption is supplied by farmed fish. Feed for cultured fish has traditionally been produced from fish oil and fish meal. However, the sources of fish used to produce fish oil and fish meal are stagnating. At the same time, the demand for fish oil for direct human consumption (either via dietary supplements or functional foods) is increasing due to increased awareness of the health benefits of marine omega-3 fatty acids. The current sources of fish oil are not able to cover the increasing demand for omega-3 fatty acids for use in aquaculture and direct human consumption. Novel sources of omega-3 fatty acids are therefore needed. Chapter 2 discusses the possibilities for increasing the utilization of by-products from the fish industry for the production of fish oil, as well as providing an overview of other novel sources of omega-3 fatty acids. One such novel source is algal oil, and the production of omega-3 fatty acids from microalgae is discussed in Chapter 14.

Fish oils for feed production are used without any further refining, but fish oils for human consumption have to undergo a refining and deodorization process to remove undesirable substances, including contaminants and lipid oxidation products. Moreover, for many dietary supplements the fish oil is further concentrated, for example to 70 % EPA and DHA. State-of-the-art processes for concentrating, refining and deodorizing fish oils are summarized in Chapter 3.

One major challenge when using marine omega-3 fatty acids for human consumption is their high susceptibility to lipid oxidation, which results in undesirable off-flavours and can lead to formation of potentially harmful compounds. Therefore, precautions must be taken to avoid or minimize lipid oxidation. Different strategies are available for this purpose, including the addition of antioxidants, emulsification and microencapsulation of omega-3 oils. Chapters 4, 5 and 6 provide an overview of the current state of the art in these areas.

It is possible to enrich foods with omega-3 fatty acids by adding marine or plant omega-3 fatty acids to animal diets, which are then transferred to humans upon intake of meat, dairy products or eggs. Challenges associated with such enrichment, including protection against oxidation, are discussed in chapters 8, 9 and 10. An alternative strategy for enriching foods with omega-3 fatty acids is the direct addition of omega-3 oils to foods such as bread, margarine, mayonnaise and infant formula. Special precautions have to be taken when enriching these products to avoid lipid oxidation, for example by optimizing the processing conditions and packaging technologies. These issues are addressed in chapters 11, 12 and 13.

Although many consumers are aware of the health benefits of omega-3 fatty acids, it is still necessary to provide information on food packaging regarding nutritional facts and possible health claims. This issue is much debated and different regulations are in place in different parts of the world. Chapter 15 provides an overview of the current status on health claims and labeling of omega-3 fatty acids. In order for manufacturers of omega-3 products to correctly label the omega-3 fatty acid content, they need to implement accurate methods for determining the content of omega-3 fatty acids in their product. Chapter 7 discusses the advantages and pitfalls of the different methods available.

This book should be of interest to both scientists with a research interest in omega-3 fatty acids and industry professionals working in the fish oil producing industry, the food industry, analytical laboratories, nutrition and health care systems, and legislation.

C. Jacobsen

Part I

Background to omega-3 food enrichment

1

Nutritional benefits of omega-3 fatty acids

P. C. Calder, University of Southampton, UK

DOI: 10.1533/9780857098863.1.3

Abstract: This chapter describes nutritional and biochemical aspects of omega-3 (ω-3) fatty acids, their effects on outcomes related to human health and disease, and the underlying mechanisms of action. Both marine- and plant-derived omega-3 fatty acids are described. The chapter ends with a discussion of future trends for research in this area.

Key words: fish, fish oil, eicosapentaenoic acid, docosahexaenoic acid, cardiovascular disease, omega-3 fatty acids.

1.1 Introduction

This chapter describes nutritional and biochemical aspects of omega-3 (ω-3) fatty acids, their effects on outcomes related to human health and disease, and the underlying mechanisms of action. The chapter begins with a description of the structure, naming and metabolic relationships of the various omega-3 fatty acids. This is followed by an examination of the dietary sources of the major plant-derived omega-3 fatty acid, α-linolenic acid, and of the more biologically active fish-derived omega-3 fatty acids eicosapentaenoic acid (EPA) and docosahexaenoic acid (DHA), and of typical intakes of these fatty acids. The manner in which EPA and DHA are handled within the body is described as are the resulting concentrations in various sites. The impact of consuming preformed EPA and DHA (e.g. from fish oil supplements) on the contents of these fatty acids in various blood plasma and cell fractions is considered, followed by coverage of the main mechanisms by which these fatty acids can influence cellular behaviour and organ physiology. Next, the benefits of EPA and DHA to human development and health through the life cycle are described, leading to a discussion of current recommendations for intake of EPA and DHA. Then, the health effects of α-linolenic acid are reviewed briefly as is the evidence for

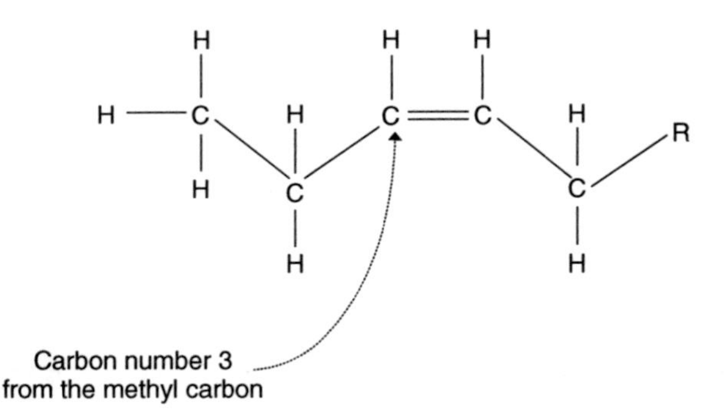

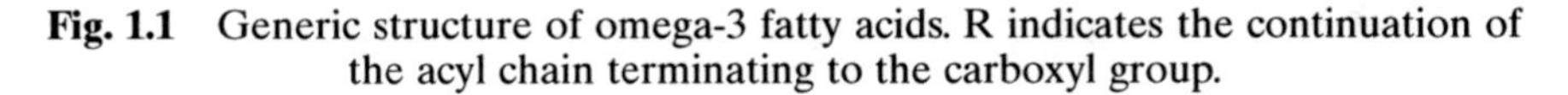

Fig. 1.1 Generic structure of omega-3 fatty acids. R indicates the continuation of the acyl chain terminating to the carboxyl group.

conversion of α-linolenic acid to EPA and DHA in humans. The chapter ends with a summary and conclusions section followed by a discussion of future trends.

1.1.1 Structure, naming and metabolic relationships of omega-3 fatty acids

The term omega-3 (also notated as ω-3 or n-3) is a structural descriptor for a family of polyunsaturated fatty acids (PUFA): it denotes the position of the double bond that is closest to the methyl terminus of the acyl chain of the fatty acid. All omega-3 fatty acids have this double bond on carbon 3, counting the methyl carbon as carbon 1 (Fig. 1.1). In common with all fatty acids, omega-3 fatty acids have systematic and common names (Table 1.1). However, they are also referred to by a shorthand nomenclature that denotes the number of carbon atoms in the chain, the number of double bonds and the position of the first double bond relative to the methyl carbon (Table 1.1). Thus α-linolenic acid (18:3 ω-3) is the simplest omega-3 fatty acid. α-Linolenic acid is synthesised from linoleic acid (18:2 ω-6) by desaturation, catalysed by Δ^{15} desaturase (the desaturase enzymes are named according to the first carbon carrying the newly inserted double bond and counting the carboxyl carbon as carbon number one). Like other animals, humans do not possess the Δ^{15} desaturase enzyme and so cannot synthesise α-linolenic acid *de novo*. It is for this reason that α-linolenic acid is considered to be an essential fatty acid. The other classically essential fatty acid is linoleic acid. Because plants possess Δ^{15} desaturase they can synthesise α-linolenic acid (Fig. 1.2). Although they cannot synthesise α-linolenic acid, animals can metabolise it by further desaturation and elongation; desaturation occurs at carbon atoms below carbon number 9 (counting from the carboxyl carbon) and mainly occurs in the liver. Through this pathway, α-linolenic acid is converted to stearidonic acid (18:4 ω-3) by Δ^{6} desaturase and then stearidonic acid is elongated to

Table 1.1 The omega-3 polyunsaturated fatty acid family

Systematic name	Common name	Shorthand nomenclature
all-cis-9,12, 15-Octadecatrienoic acid	α-Linolenic acid	18:3 ω-3
all-cis-6,9,12, 15-Octadecatetraenoic acid	Stearidonic acid	18:4 ω-3
all-cis-8,11,14, 17-Eicosatetraenoic acid	Eicosatetraenoic acid	20:4 ω-3
all-cis-5,8,11,14, 17-Eicosapentaenoic acid	Eicosapentaenoic acid	20:5 ω-3
all-cis-7,10,13,16, 19-Docosapentaenoic acid	Docosapentaenoic acid; also clupanodonic acid	22:5 ω-3
all-cis-4,7,10,13,16, 19-Docosahexaenoic acid	Docosahexaenoic acid	22:6 ω-3

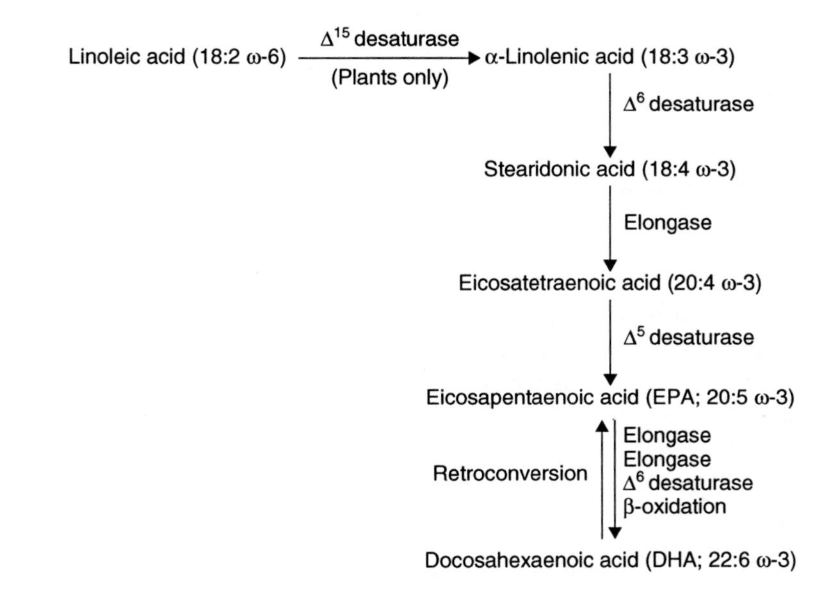

Fig. 1.2 Pathway of conversion of linoleic acid to α-linolenic acid and of α-linolenic acid to longer chain, more unsaturated omega-3 fatty acids.

eicosatetraenoic acid (20:4 ω-3), which is further desaturated by Δ^5 desaturase to yield EPA (20:5 ω-3) (Fig. 1.2). It is important to note that this pathway of conversion of α-linolenic acid to EPA is in direct competition with the conversion of linoleic acid to arachidonic acid (20:4 ω-6) since the same enzymes are used. The Δ^6 desaturase reaction is the rate-limiting step in this pathway and, because linoleic acid is much more prevalent in most human diets than α-linolenic acid, metabolism of omega-6 fatty acids is quantitatively the more important.

There is a pathway for conversion of EPA to DHA (22:6 ω-3) (Fig. 1.2). This rather complex pathway involves addition of two carbons to form docosapentaenoic acid (DPA) (22:5 ω-3), addition of two further carbons to produce 24:5 ω-3, desaturation at the Δ^6 position to form 24:6 ω-3, translocation of 24:6 ω-3 from the endoplasmic reticulum to peroxisomes where two carbons are removed by limited β-oxidation to yield DHA (Fig. 1.2). It is not clear why the pathway of EPA conversion to DHA is so complex, but this perhaps aids in close regulation of the EPA to DHA conversion process. The extent to which this pathway is active in humans has been examined in short-term studies by using stable isotopically-labelled α-linolenic acid and in long-term studies using significantly increased intakes of α-linolenic acid. Both approaches have produced the same finding, that the conversion of α-linolenic acid to EPA, DPA and DHA is generally poor in humans, with very limited conversion all the way to DHA being observed (Arterburn *et al.*, 2006; Burdge and Calder, 2006; see Section 1.4 on health effects of α-linolenic acid). EPA and DPA can also be synthesised from DHA by retro-conversion due to limited peroxisomal β-oxidation (Fig. 1.2). In this chapter, EPA, DPA and DHA are collectively referred to as marine omega-3 PUFA to denote their origin in seafood (see Section 1.2.1).

1.2 Dietary sources and typical intakes of omega-3 fatty acids

1.2.1 Dietary sources

α-Linolenic acid from plant sources

α-Linolenic acid makes a significant contribution to the fatty acids within green leafy tissues of plants, typically comprising over 50 % of the fatty acids present. This is because α-linolenic acid is a key component of the membranes of thylakoids within chloroplasts. However, green leaves are not rich sources of fat so they are not major dietary sources of fatty acids including α-linolenic acid. α-Linolenic acid is found in significant amounts in several seeds, seed oils and nuts. Linseeds (also called flaxseeds) and their oil typically contain 45–55 % of fatty acids as α-linolenic acid. Soybean oil, rapeseed oil and walnuts contain 5–10 % of fatty acids as α-linolenic acid. In contrast, corn oil, sunflower oil and safflower oil, which are rich in linoleic acid, contain little α-linolenic acid. Typical intakes of α-linolenic acid among Western adults are between 0.5 and 2 g/day (BNF, 1999; Burdge and Calder, 2006). In most Western diets, the main PUFA is the omega-6 fatty acid linoleic acid which is typically consumed in 5–20-fold greater amounts than α-linolenic acid (BNF, 1999; Burdge and Calder, 2006).

EPA, DPA and DHA from seafood

Lean fish (e.g. cod) store lipid in the liver while fatty (sometimes called oily) fish (e.g. mackerel, herring, salmon, tuna and sardines) store lipid in the flesh. Compared with other foodstuffs, fish and other seafood are good sources of the very long chain, highly unsaturated omega-3 fatty acids EPA, DPA and DHA (BNF, 1999). Different types of fish contain different amounts of these fatty acids and different ratios of EPA to DHA. The different amounts and ratios of EPA and DHA occur because of the different metabolic characteristics of the fish and differences in their diet, and the water temperature, season, etc. A single lean fish meal, such as one serving of cod, could provide about 0.2–0.3 g of marine omega-3 fatty acids. A single oily fish meal, such as one serving of salmon or mackerel, could provide 1.5–3.0 g of these fatty acids. In most Western populations, more lean fish than oily fish is consumed, and overall fish intake is fairly low. Consequently, average (mean) intakes of marine omega-3 fatty acids among adults in the UK, in other Northern and in Eastern European, North American and Australasian countries are quoted to be about 0.1–0.2 g/day (Meyer *et al.*, 2003; Scientific Advisory Committee on Nutrition and Committee on Toxicity, 2004). However, this average represents that of two sub-groups of the population, one that consumes oily fish regularly and one that does not. The former sub-group is frequently in the minority. Australian researchers carefully evaluated marine omega-3 fatty acid intake among a small group of healthy adults. They identified a mean intake of about 0.19 g/day, in agreement with other estimates. However, the median intake of EPA+DPA+DHA was only about 0.03 g/day (Meyer *et al.*, 2003). This would indicate that 50 % of the adult population is consuming 30 mg or less of marine omega-3 fatty acids each day. Those populations where oily fish is consumed more regularly and in greater amounts than in most Western populations (e.g. the Japanese) have a greater average intake of marine omega-3 fatty acids.

Fish oils

The oil obtained from the flesh of oily fish or from the livers of lean fish is generically termed 'fish oil'. Fish oil contains EPA and DHA. In a typical 1 g fish oil capsule EPA and DHA comprise about 30 % of the fatty acids present. Thus, a 1 g capsule of a standard fish oil would provide about 0.3 g of EPA+DHA. However, because the absolute and relative amounts of EPA and DHA vary among fish, they vary among fish oils. Most standard fish oils contain EPA and DHA in a ratio of 1.5:1. In contrast, tuna oil is richer in DHA than EPA. More concentrated oil preparations are available commercially. Different chemical formulations of marine omega-3 fatty acids are also available. In most fish oils the fatty acids are present in the form of triacylglycerols. However, it is now possible to obtain capsules where the omega-3 fatty acids are present partly as phospholipids, for example in krill oil, or as free fatty acids. Furthermore, ethyl ester preparations of omega-3 fatty acids are available, such as in the highly concentrated pharmaceutical preparation Omacor, also known as Lovaza® in North America. Clearly capsules could make a significant contribution to marine omega-3 fatty acid intake.

Algal oils

Some algal oils are particularly rich in DHA which may comprise as much as 45 % of fatty acids present. Such oils are used in infant formulas where provision of DHA is particularly desired.

1.2.2 Handling and distribution of dietary omega-3 fatty acids

Orally consumed omega-3 fatty acids are handled in the same way as other dietary fatty acids: they are hydrolysed from the parent complex lipid, most often triacylglycerol, absorbed into enterocytes, re-esterified back into triacylglycerols which are assembled into lipoproteins known as chylomicrons, and then released into the lymphatic circulation, later entering the bloodstream (Gurr *et al.*, 2002). Fatty acids from chylomicron triacylglycerols are targeted towards storage in adipose tissue, with those remaining in the remnant particle being cleared by the liver. Once in the liver, omega-3 fatty acids may be oxidised, metabolised to other omega-3 fatty acids, or re-secreted into the bloodstream as a component of liver-derived lipoproteins. There is on-going interest in whether marine omega-3 fatty acids are more available from fish than from fish oil supplements (Visioli *et al.*, 2003; Arterburn *et al.*, 2008) and whether they are more available from some chemical forms, such as phospholipids, than from others, such as triacylglycerols (Schuchardt *et al.*, 2011). So far these questions are not completely answered.

Lipoproteins form a vehicle for transport of omega-3 fatty acids between tissues (Fig. 1.3). Omega-3 fatty acids within cell membranes have a number of functional roles (Miles and Calder, 1998). Thus, it is possible to identify storage, transport and functional pools of fatty acids including omega-3 fatty acids (Fig. 1.3). Different plasma lipid pools, cells and tissues have different, characteristic, fatty acid compositions. These compositions are influenced by the availability of different fatty acids but also by the metabolic characteristics and functional requirements of the particular pool, cell or tissue. The EPA and DHA contents differ amongst these pools, although the EPA content is typically below 1 % of total fatty acids (Table 1.2). The DHA content is usually higher than that of EPA, and there are some sites where DHA is present in high amounts (Table 1.2). For example, high DHA contents are seen in parts of the brain and eye, suggesting an important role for DHA at those sites.

1.2.3 Increased intake of marine omega-3 fatty acids results in an increase in EPA and DHA in plasma lipids, cells and tissues in humans

Modification of fatty acid profiles has been widely reported after supplementation of the diet with fish oil capsules; such supplementation results in increased amounts of EPA and DHA in plasma lipids, platelets,

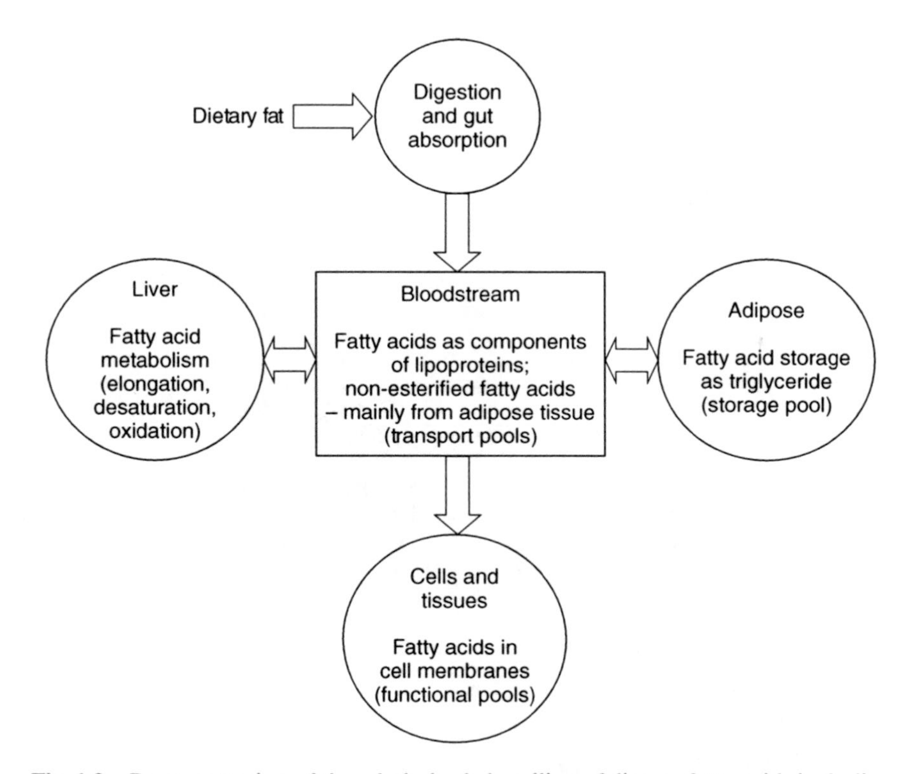

Fig. 1.3 Representation of the whole-body handling of dietary fatty acids including marine omega-3 fatty acids.

Table 1.2 Typical marine omega-3 fatty acid content (% of total fatty acids) of various sites in humans

Site	EPA content	DHA content
Plasma phosphatidylcholine	0.75	3.0
Plasma cholesteryl esters	0.75	0.5
Plasma triglycerides	0.75	0.5
Platelet phosphatidylcholine	0.2	1.0
Platelet phosphatidylethanolamine	0.5	6.0
Mononuclear cell phospholipid	0.75	2.5
Neutrophil phospholipid	0.5	1.5
Erythrocyte phospholipid	0.75	3.5
Liver phosphatidylethanolamine	1.5	7.5
Cardiac atrium phosphatidylcholine	0.75	3.5
Cardiac atrium phosphatidylethanolamine	1.5	12
Brain grey matter phosphatidylethanolamine	<0.1	25
Brain grey matter phosphatidylserine	<0.1	35
Brain grey matter phosphatidylcholine	<0.1	3.0
Brain white matter phosphatidylethanolamine	<0.1	3.5
Retina phosphatidylcholine	<0.1	22
Retina phosphatidylethanolamine	<0.1	18
Testis total lipid	<0.1	8.5
White adipose tissue	0.1	0.2

Source: Burdge and Calder, 2006.

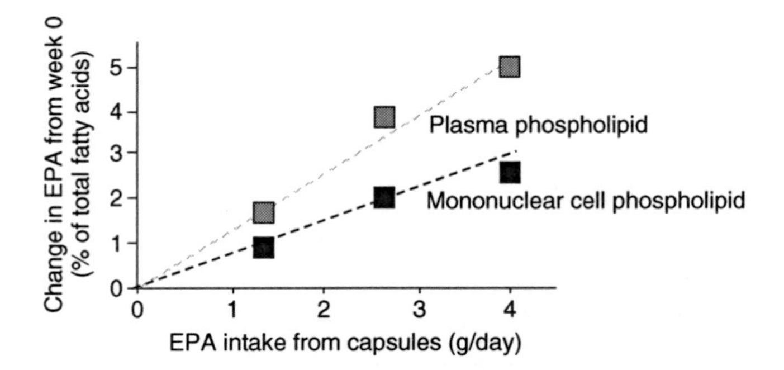

Fig. 1.4 Dose-dependent incorporation of EPA into human plasma phospholipids and blood mononuclear cell phospholipids. Healthy young males supplemented their diet with differing amounts of an EPA-rich oil for a period of 12 weeks. Plasma and blood mononuclear cell phospholipids were isolated and their fatty acid composition determined by gas chromatography. Data are mean from 23 or 24 subjects per group and are expressed as change in EPA from week 0 (study entry). Data are from Rees *et al.* (2006).

erythrocytes, leukocytes, colon tissue, cardiac tissue and, most likely, in many other cell and tissue types. The incorporation of EPA and DHA from fish oil capsules is partly at the expense of omega-6 fatty acids, like arachidonic acid, and occurs in a dose–response fashion. For example, studies using a range of EPA+DHA intakes from 1–6 g/day report near linear relationships between EPA and DHA intake and the resulting EPA and DHA contents of plasma phospholipids (Blonk *et al.*, 1990; Harris *et al.*, 1991; Marsen *et al.*, 1992) and of platelet phospholipids (Sanders and Roshanai, 1983). In other studies, incorporation of EPA and DHA into blood neutrophils (Healy *et al.*, 2000) and of EPA into plasma phospholipids and blood immune cells (Rees *et al.*, 2006) occurred in a linear dose–response manner (Fig. 1.4). A study combining dose–response and time course over 12 months in older male subjects confirmed that EPA and DHA are incorporated into circulating lipid pools and into erythrocytes when their intakes are increased and showed that there was also incorporation into adipose tissue, a storage pool (Katan *et al.*, 1997). This study also clearly showed that incorporation of EPA and DHA into different pools occurs at different rates and to differing extents; there was near-maximal incorporation of EPA and DHA into serum cholesteryl esters within 30 days of beginning supplementation, while maximal incorporation into erythrocytes did not occur until some time between 56 and 182 days.

Yaqoob *et al.* (2000) found that incorporation of both EPA and DHA into blood immune cells was near-maximal after four weeks of fish oil supplementation (Fig. 1.5). A recent study suggests that this near-maximal incorporation is achieved after one week (Faber *et al.*, 2011). Upon cessation of fish oil supplementation, EPA in blood immune cells returned to starting levels within eight weeks, while the cells appeared to retain DHA

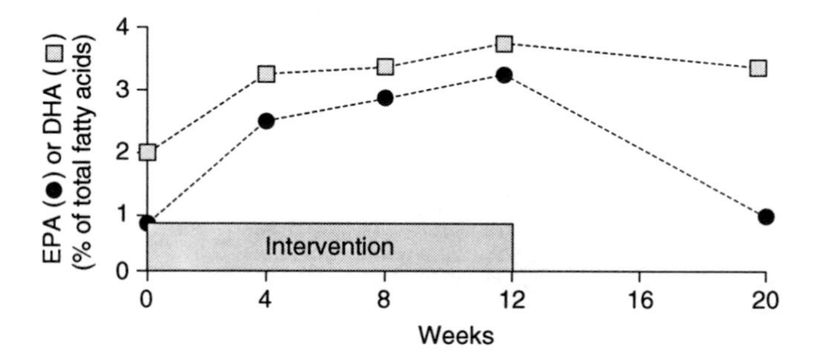

Fig. 1.5 Time course of changes in EPA and DHA contents of human blood mononuclear cells in subjects consuming fish oil. Healthy subjects supplemented their diet with fish oil capsules providing 2.1 g EPA plus 1.1 g DHA per day for a period of 12 weeks (indicated by the grey area). Blood mononuclear cell phospholipids were isolated at 0, 4, 8, 12 and 20 weeks and their fatty acid composition determined by gas chromatography. Data are mean from eight subjects and are from Yaqoob *et al.* (2000).

(Fig. 1.5)(Yaqoob *et al.*, 2000). The same observations of rapid loss of EPA and selective retention of DHA upon cessation of fish oil supplementation have been made for erthrocytes (Popp-Snijders *et al.*, 1986) and platelets (von Schacky *et al.*, 1985). These changes most likely reflect differences in turnover of EPA and DHA once incorporated into cell membranes, although they may also indicate net conversion of EPA to DHA once the oral supply has been diminished.

1.3 Marine omega-3 fatty acids

1.3.1 Mechanisms by which marine omega-3 fatty acids can influence cell function

Increased cell and tissue omega-3 fatty acid content can influence cell and tissue function through a variety of mechanisms as shown in Fig. 1.6 (Calder, 2012a).

Alterations in membrane structure and function

Increased EPA and DHA content of membrane phospholipids can lead to modifications of the physical properties of the membrane, such as membrane order (how liquid or 'fluid' the membrane is), and of the structure of membrane regions termed rafts. Rafts are membrane microdomains with a particular lipid and fatty acid makeup and which play a role as platforms for receptor action and for the initiation of intracellular signalling pathways. In turn, changes in membrane order and in raft structure can influence the activity of membrane proteins including receptors, transporters, ion channels and signalling enzymes (Miles and Calder, 1998; Yaqoob, 2009). As a result of these effects, intracellular signal transduction and transcription

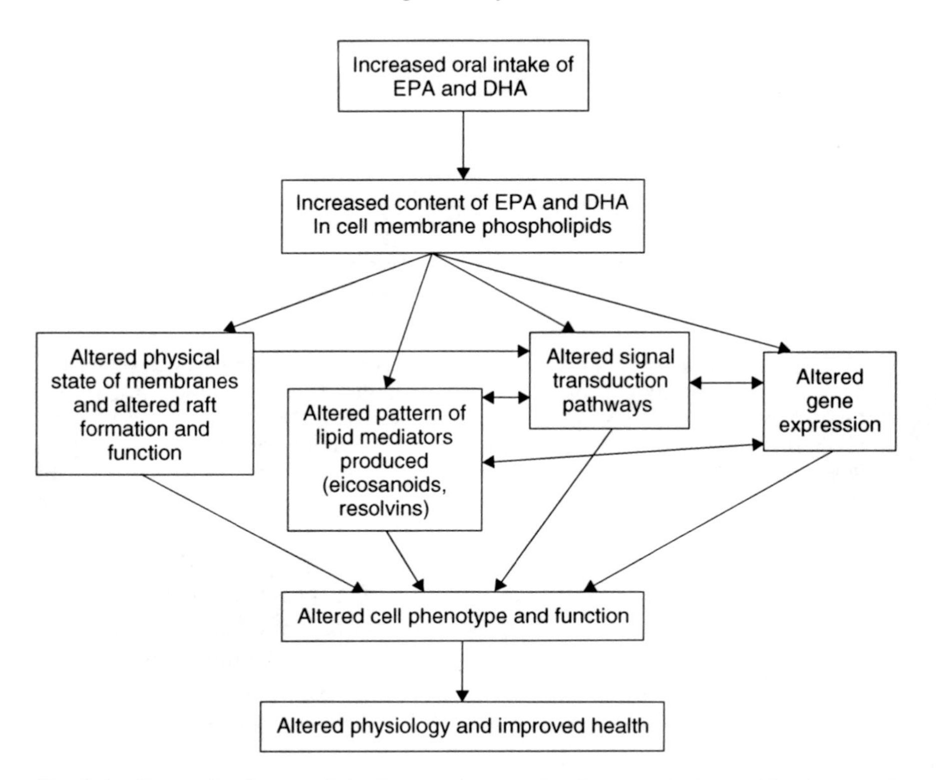

Fig. 1.6 General scheme of the interacting mechanisms whereby marine omega-3 fatty acids can influence cell function.

factor activation may be altered and gene expression modified. Transcription factors reported to be modified by the presence of marine omega-3 PUFA include nuclear factor κB (important in regulating inflammatory processes), peroxisome proliferator-activated receptor-α (important in regulating lipid metabolism) and -γ (important in regulating lipid metabolism, adipocyte differentiation, insulin sensitivity and inflammatory processes), and the sterol regulatory element binding proteins (important in regulating lipid metabolism) (Jump, 2002, 2008; Clarke, 2004; Lapillonne *et al.*, 2004; Deckelbaum *et al.*, 2006). Thus, alterations to cell membrane fatty acid composition are intimately linked with changes to membrane function, intracellular signalling cascades, and gene expression.

Effects on lipid mediators

Eicosanoids are potent chemical messengers that have well-established roles in regulation of inflammation, immunity, platelet aggregation, smooth muscle contraction and renal function (Nicolaou and Kafatos, 2004). They include prostaglandins, thromboxanes and leukotrienes and are usually produced from the omega-6 fatty acid arachidonic acid. The enzymes involved in synthesis of eicosanoids are usually the cyclo-oxygenases (COX), that lead to the prostaglandin pathway, or the lipoxygenases, which lead to the leukotriene pathway, although there are other routes for eicosanoid synthesis. Excess or inappropriate production of these eicosanoids is associated with disease processes. For example cysteinyl-leukotrienes play an important role in asthma. A range of drugs of varying specificity are used clinically to suppress the production of eicosanoids from arachidonic acid. These drugs include aspirin, ibuprofen, several corticosteroids and specific COX inhibitors. Marine omega-3 fatty acids are also able to decrease the production of eicosanoids from arachidonic acid and so can impact on the actions regulated by those mediators, such as inflammation (Calder, 2008a). The decreased production of eicosanoids brought about by marine omega-3 fatty acids may occur as the result of two separate effects. Firstly, as indicated earlier, EPA incorporation into cell membranes is partly at the expense of arachidonic acid and so increased EPA is associated with a decreased availability of the eicosanoid substrate arachidonic acid in cell membranes. Secondly, EPA and DHA are inhibitors of arachidonic acid metabolism by COX enzymes (Ringbom *et al.*, 2001). EPA is also a substrate for the COX and lipoxygenase enzymes leading to the synthesis of alternative eicosanoids, which are typically less potent than those produced from arachidonic acid (Calder, 2008a). Thus, the presence of marine omega-3 fatty acids alters the eicosanoid milieu from one which promotes inflammation, platelet aggregation and vasoconstriction to one which is less inflammatory, less thrombotic and more vaso-relaxed.

Relatively recently a new family of lipid mediators, termed resolvins, synthesised from both EPA (E-series resolvins) and DHA (D-series resolvins) have been described. These mediators have been demonstrated in cell culture and animal feeding studies to be potently anti-inflammatory, inflammation resolving and immunomodulatory (Serhan *et al.*, 2000a, b). Protectin D1, produced from DHA, appears to have an important role in protecting tissue, including neuronal tissue, from excessive damage in a variety of experimental situations (Serhan *et al.*, 2002). The production of resolvins is favoured by the higher EPA and DHA status brought about by increased oral intake of these fatty acids.

Receptor-mediated effects

Quite recently, Oh *et al.* (2010) reported that a membrane G-protein coupled receptor called GPR120, which is able to bind long-chain fatty acids, is highly expressed on adipocytes and on inflammatory macrophages. A chemical agonist of GPR120 called GW9508 inhibited inflammatory responsiveness of macrophages, suggesting that GPR120 is involved in anti-inflammatory signalling. EPA and DHA promoted GPR120-mediated gene activation in cultured macrophages, and the anti-inflammatory effects of DHA did not occur in GPR120 knockdown cells. Thus, EPA and DHA might act on inflammatory cells via GPR-120 to reduce inflammatory responses. Oh *et al.* (2010) also demonstrated that DHA-induced translocation of the glucose transporter GLUT4 to the surface of cultured adipocytes was abolished by GPR120 knockout, suggesting that GPR120 mediates some of the favourable metabolic actions of DHA. These observations suggest effects of omega-3 fatty acids that do not involve either their incorporation into cell membrane phospholipids or a modification of lipid mediator production.

1.3.2 Increased intake of marine omega-3 fatty acids is beneficial to health

Through the mechanisms of action outlined above and the resulting modifications of cell and tissue function, marine omega-3 fatty acids exert physiological actions (Ruxton *et al.*, 2005; Calder and Yaqoob, 2009). These are summarized in Table 1.3, where they are linked to certain health or clinical benefits. A number of risk factors for cardiovascular disease are modified in a beneficial way by increased intake of marine omega-3 fatty acids: these include blood pressure (Geleijnse *et al.*, 2002), platelet reactivity and thrombosis (BNF, 1992), plasma triglyceride concentrations (Harris, 1996), vascular function (Nestel *et al.*, 2002), heart rate variability (von Schacky, 2008) and inflammation (Calder, 2006). As a result, increased marine omega-3 fatty acid intake or status has been associated with a reduced risk of cardiovascular morbidity and mortality in epidemiological studies (Calder, 2004; Harris *et al.*, 2008; Saravanan *et al.*, 2010; de Caterina, 2011; Mozaffarian and Wu, 2011). This most likely comes about because the more favourable risk factor profile would act to slow or limit atherosclerosis, the buildup of fatty material within the vascular wall. However, marine omega-3 fatty acids have been demonstrated to reduce mortality even in persons with advanced cardiovascular disease (Anonymous, 1999; Bucher *et al.*, 2002; Marchioli *et al.*, 2002; Studer *et al.*, 2005; Yokoyama *et al.*, 2007). Their action cannot relate to limiting atherosclerosis because the persons studied already have atherosclerosis. Instead, marine omega-3 fatty acids must have some action on the heart or within the vascular wall that reduces the likelihood of having a cardiovascular event (e.g. heart attack or stroke) or of such an event being fatal. The favoured mechanism here is a reduction in cardiac arrhythmias for which there is substantial evidence from cell culture and animal studies (Leaf *et al.*, 2003; Reiffel and McDonald, 2006), but less strong evidence from human studies (Reiffel and McDonald, 2006; von Schacky, 2008; Brouwer *et al.*, 2009). A second mechanism involved could be a reduction in inflammation within the vascular wall which would make it less likely that atherosclerotic plaques would rupture (Thies *et al.*, 2003; Cawood *et al.*, 2010; Calder, 2012b).

A number of non-cardiovascular actions of marine omega-3 fatty acids have also been documented in humans (Table 1.3), suggesting that increased intake of these fatty acids could be of benefit in protecting against or

Table 1.3 Summary of the physiological roles and potential clinical benefits of marine omega-3 fatty acids

Physiological role of marine omega-3 fatty acids	Potential clinical benefit	Target
Regulation of blood pressure	Decreased blood pressure	Hypertension; CVD*
Regulation of platelet function	Decreased likelihood of thrombosis	Thrombosis; CVD
Regulation of blood coagulation	Decreased likelihood of thrombosis	Thrombosis; CVD
Regulation of plasma triglyceride concentrations	Decreased plasma triglyceride concentrations	Hypertriglyceridaemia; CVD
Regulation of vascular function	Improved vascular reactivity	CVD
Regulation of cardiac rhythm	Decreased arrhythmias	CVD
Regulation of heart rate	Increased heart rate variability	CVD
Regulation of inflammation	Decreased inflammation	Inflammatory diseases (arthritis, inflammatory bowel diseases, psoriasis, lupus, asthma, cystic fibrosis, dermatitis, neurodegeneration, . . .); CVD
Regulation of immune function	Improved immune function	Compromised immunity
Regulation of fatty acid and triglyceride metabolism	Decreased triglyceride synthesis and storage	Weight gain; weight loss; obesity
Regulation of bone turnover	Maintained bone mass	Osteoporosis
Regulation of insulin sensitivity	Improved insulin sensitivity	Type-2 diabetes
Regulation of tumour cell growth	Decreased tumour cell growth and survival	Some cancers
Regulation of visual signalling (via rhodopsin)	Optimised visual signaling	Poor infant visual development (especially pre-term)
Structural component of brain and central nervous system	Optimised brain development – cognitive and learning processes	Poor infant and childhood cognitive processes and learning

*CVD cardiovascular disease.
Source: Reproduced with permission from Calder and Yaqoob, 2009.

treating many conditions. For example, they have been used successfully in rheumatoid arthritis (Calder, 2008b) and, in some studies, in inflammatory bowel diseases (Calder, 2008c), and may be useful in other inflammatory conditions (Calder, 2006). Beneficial effects of DHA within neural tissue may relate to important structural and functional roles. Thus, DHA has an essential structural role in the eye and brain, and its supply early in life when these tissues are developing is known to be of vital importance in terms of optimising visual and neurological development (SanGiovanni *et al.*, 2000a, b). Therefore, assuring an adequate supply of marine omega-3 fatty acids, especially DHA, in women during pregnancy and lactation, and in infants once breast feeding ceases, is really important.

Other studies have highlighted the potential for marine omega-3 fatty acids to contribute to enhanced mental development (Helland *et al.*, 2003) and improved childhood learning and behaviour (Richardson, 2004) and to reduce the burden of psychiatric illnesses in adults (Freeman *et al.*, 2006), although these remain controversial areas of possible action which require more robust scientific support. There may also be a role for marine omega-3 PUFA, DHA in particular, in preventing neurodegenerative disease of ageing (Solfrizzi *et al.*, 2010), and the production of protectins, especially neuroprotectin D1 (also called protectin D1), appears to be crucial for this effect (Lukiw *et al.*, 2005). The effects of marine omega-3 PUFA on health outcomes are likely to be dose-dependent, but clear dose–response data have not been identified in most cases, although Mozaffarian and Rimm (2006) have proposed dose–response profiles for several cardiovascular risk factors.

1.3.3 Recommendations for the intake of marine omega-3 fatty acids

The clear demonstration of physiological actions of marine omega-3 fatty acids that result in reduced risk of disease and in improved health outcomes, along with an increased understanding of the molecular and cellular mechanisms underlying those actions, indicates a strong need to set recommendations for the intake of these important fatty acids. However, the exact requirement for marine omega-3 fatty acids in order to maintain health is not known and this has impeded the setting of clear recommendations to achieve public health. Furthermore, there has been a lack of clarity about the extent to which EPA and DHA can be synthesised in humans so long as there is sufficient intake of the precursor α-linolenic acid. Nevertheless, the recognition of the benefits of marine omega-3 fatty acids has resulted in some recommendations to increase the intake of fish and, more specifically, of EPA+DHA by various government, non-government and professional bodies.

In the UK the recommendation is for an intake of at least two fish meals per week including at least one of oily fish (Scientific Advisory Committee on Nutrition and Committee on Toxicity, 2004). This was translated into an EPA+DHA recommendation of at least 450 mg/day (Scientific Advisory Committee on Nutrition and Committee on Toxicity, 2004). The International Society for the Study of Fatty Acids and Lipids suggested a target intake of 650 mg EPA+DHA per day (Simopolous *et al.*, 1999), later modified to a minimum intake of 500 mg/day (International Society for the Study of Fatty Acids and Lipids, 2004). In France an official recommendation for a target intake of 400–500 mg/day EPA+DHA with at least 100–120 mg DHA was made (French Agency for Food Environmental and Occupational Health Safety, 2003). The target intake for Australia and New Zealand is 430–610 mg/day (NHMRC, 2006).

Recently, the Food and Agriculture Organisation of the United Nations (FAO) and the European Food Safety Authority (EFSA) have made recommendations. The FAO recommended a minimum intake of 250 mg EPA+DHA per day for adult males and for non-pregnant/non-lactating adult females (FAO, 2010). For pregnant or lactating females the minimum intake was recommended to be 300 mg EPA+DHA per day of which at least 200 mg should be DHA (FAO, 2010). They also made recommendations for DHA intake for infants aged up to 2 years. For children, the recommendations for EPA+DHA in mg/day were 100–150 for those aged 2–4 years, 150–200 for those aged 4–6 years and 200–250 for those aged 6–10 years (FAO, 2010). The EFSA recommended an intake of 250 mg/day of EPA+DHA as being adequate, with an additional 100–200 mg/day of DHA being needed in pregnancy (EFSA, 2010). For infants and children aged 6 months to 2 years the EFSA recommended 100 mg DHA per day, while for children aged 2–18 years the EFSA commented that advice should be consistent with that for adults. An international consensus group recommended an intake of DHA of at least 200 mg/day for pregnant women (Koletzko *et al.*, 2007).

Recommendations have also been made for persons who have survived a heart attack or who have high blood triglyceride concentrations. For the secondary prevention of myocardial infarction, 1 g per day of EPA+DHA is recommended by the American Heart Association (Kris-Etherton *et al.*, 2002), the European Society for Cardiology and European Atherosclerosis Society (Van de Werf *et al.*, 2008) and a network of British Societies (JBS2, 2005). This recommendation is based upon the dose used in the GISSI-Prevenzione trial which demonstrated a reduction in risk of mortality, cardiovascular mortality and sudden death when ethyl esters of marine omega-3 fatty acids were used (Anonymous, 1999). For triglyceride lowering, a marine omega-3 fatty acid dose of 2–4 g/day is recommended (Kris-Etherton *et al.*, 2002).

In those individuals not regularly consuming oily fish, the intake of these fatty acids is likely to be <0.2 g/day and perhaps even much lower than this (Meyer *et al.*, 2003). Strategies to increase intake of marine omega-3 PUFA include eating oily fish, consuming fish oil capsules or liquid and eating foods specifically enriched in these fatty acids.

1.4 Health effects of α-linolenic acid

The foregoing discussion has centred upon the marine omega-3 PUFA for which there is much evidence for human health benefit and an increasing understanding of the multiple mechanisms involved, and for which a number of recommendations for increased intake have been made. The major plant omega-3 PUFA, α-linolenic acid, is an essential fatty acid and may have human health benefits either in its own right or by acting as a precursor for synthesis of the longer chain more unsaturated derivatives using the pathway shown in Fig. 1.2. These possibilities have been reviewed in some detail (Arterburn *et al.*, 2006; Burdge and Calder, 2006). Studies in humans using acute ingestion of stable isotopically-labelled α-linolenic acid have demonstrated some conversion to EPA and to DPA, but much more limited conversion to DHA, although this may be greater in young adult women than in men (Burdge *et al.*, 2002; Burdge and Wootton, 2002), possibly because of upregulation of the Δ^6 desaturase by female sex hormones. Little is known about the extent of α-linolenic acid conversion to EPA and DHA in infancy and childhood, in the elderly or during pregnancy and lactation, times when synthesis of marine omega-3 fatty acids might be important or desirable. A number of studies have examined the effect of chronic (i.e. weeks to months) consumption of increased amounts of α-linolenic acid. These studies confirm that increasing α-linolenic acid intake increases the EPA (and DPA) content of plasma lipids, platelets, leukocytes and erythrocytes, but that DHA content does not increase (Arterburn *et al.*, 2006; Burdge and Calder, 2006); these findings are in agreement with the stable isotope studies. Such studies with α-linolenic acid have demonstrated some effects on cardiovascular risk factors and on inflammatory markers but, where these are reported, they are typically weaker than the effects achieved from increasing consumption of EPA+DHA, and may be due to the increased appearance of EPA (Caughey *et al.*, 1996; Zhao *et al.*, 2004).

1.5 Future trends

Research in the area of omega-3 fatty acids will undoubtedly continue for the foreseeable future. There are likely to be many more studies with marine omega-3 fatty acids focusing on risk factor profiles and on clinical outcomes, especially in the areas of childhood cognition, mental performance and behaviour; age-related cognitive decline and dementia; and cancer. These studies will aim to identify clinically relevant effects and dose–response relationships (or at least effective doses) with an aim to support existing or new dietary recommendations or to develop new therapeutic strategies. Although DHA has vital and unique roles in the brain and eye, in other areas affected by marine omega-3 fatty acids it remains unclear whether EPA or DHA is the more effective (Mori and Woodman, 2006). It seems likely that these two metabolically related fatty acids will have overlapping but different functionalities (Mori and Woodman, 2006), and this prospect will be further explored in future research. Future research will also aim to further elucidate mechanisms of action; the recent discovery of a role for GPR120 in mediating the effects of DHA (Oh *et al.*, 2010) indicates that there is still much to be discovered about how EPA and DHA act to beneficially alter cell function. Linked to this, the biological activities of novel chemical mediators produced from EPA and DHA is likely to be an area of intense research activity.

Away from the marine omega-3 fatty acids, there is likely to be enhanced examination of the ability of plant-derived omega-3 fatty acids such as stearidonic acid (18:4 ω-3) to mimic the functional effects of EPA and DHA (Deckelbaum *et al.*, 2012). Further to this, studies will need to better identify the ability of plant omega-3 fatty acids to be converted to EPA and DHA in different sub-groups of the population including pregnant and lactating women, infants, children, girls of child-bearing age, the elderly and those with particular diseases. This will give much improved insight into the extent to which different sub-groups of the population can meet their demand for marine omega-3 fatty acids from endogenous biosynthesis and the extent to which these fatty acids need to be supplied preformed.

Finally, given that the only really naturally rich food source of EPA and DHA is seafood and that only a minority of people regularly eat seafood, especially oily fish, there is likely to be a significant focus on developing foods enriched or fortified with EPA and DHA. The level of enrichment that can be achieved may be limited either by metabolic processes in farm animals (in the case where farm animal feeding is used to enrich foods like eggs, meat and milk in EPA and DHA) or by food technology, processing and storage considerations. If food enrichment or fortification is to be used with the aim of delivering more EPA and DHA to consumers, the type of food used as a vehicle for delivery must be carefully considered as it does not make sense to deliver healthy marine omega-3 fatty acids within a matrix of less healthy components (Calder and Deckelbaum, 2008).

1.6 Conclusion

Current intakes of EPA and DHA are low in many, perhaps most, individuals living in Western countries. A good natural source of these fatty acids is seafood, especially oily fish. Fish oil capsules contain these fatty acids too, with a standard 1 g capsule providing about 0.3 g of EPA+DHA; more concentrated forms are also available in capsules. EPA and DHA are readily incorporated into transport (blood lipids), functional (cell and tissue) and storage (adipose) pools in humans. This incorporation is dose-dependent and follows a kinetic pattern that is characteristic for each pool. Incorporation is most rapid into blood lipids, followed by platelets and white cells, followed by erythrocytes. At sufficient levels of incorporation into cells, EPA and DHA influence the physical nature of cell membranes and membrane protein-mediated responses, lipid mediator generation, cell signalling and gene expression in many different cell types. Through these mechanisms, EPA and DHA influence cell and tissue physiology and the way cells and tissues respond to external signals. In most cases, the effects seen are compatible with improvements in disease biomarker profiles or in health-related outcomes. An important aspect of this is the requirement for marine omega-3 fatty acids, especially DHA, in early growth and development of the brain and visual system, meaning that adequate provision to the foetus and to the newborn infant is essential.

As a result of their effects on cell and tissue physiology, EPA and DHA play a role in achieving optimal health and in protection against disease. Marine omega-3 fatty acids not only protect against cardiovascular morbidity but also against mortality. In some situations, for example rheumatoid arthritis, they may be beneficial as therapeutic agents, although a high intake is required. On the basis of the recognised health improvements brought about by these fatty acids, recommendations have been made to increase their intake. This can be achieved through increased consumption of oily fish or fish oil capsules. The plant omega-3 fatty acid, α-linolenic acid, can be converted to EPA but in humans conversion to DHA appears to be poor. Effects of α-linolenic acid on human health-related outcomes appear to be due to conversion to the EPA.

1.7 Sources of further information and advice

Journals

Key research and state of the art review articles are published in many scientific journals, several of which are devoted specifically to lipids and fatty acids. These include *Progress in Lipid Research*, *Current Opinion in Lipidology*, the 'Lipid metabolism and therapy' section of *Current Opinion in Clinical Nutrition and Metabolic Care*, *Biochimica et Biophysica Acta–Molecular and Cell Biology of Lipids*, *Journal of Lipid Research*, *Prostaglandins Leukotrienes and Essential Fatty Acids*, *Lipids*, and *Lipids in Health and Disease*.

Books

- GURR MI, HARWOOD JL, FRAYN KN (2002) *Lipid Biochemistry* (5th edn). Oxford: Blackwell.
- NETTLETON JA (1995) *Omega-3 Fatty Acids and Health*. New York: Chapman & Hall.
- WATSON RA (ed.) (2009) *Fatty Acids in Health Promotion and Disease Causation*. Urbana, IL: AOCS Press.

Reports

- BNF (1999) *Briefing Paper: n-3 Fatty Acids and Health*. London: British Nutrition Foundation.
- FAO (2010) *Fats and Fatty Acids in Human Nutrition: Report of an Expert Consultation*. Rome: Food and Agricultural Organisation of the United Nations.

Websites

- American Oil Chemists' Society (www.aocs.org).
- Global Organization for EPA and DHA Omega-3 (www.goedomega3.com).
- International Society for the Study of Fatty Acids and Lipids (www.issfal.org).

1.8 References

ANONYMOUS (1999) Dietary supplementation with n-3 polyunsaturated fatty acids and vitamin E after myocardial infarction: results of the GISSI-Prevenzione trial. *Lancet* 354: 447–55.

ARTERBURN LM, HALL EB and OKEN H (2006) Distribution, interconversion, and dose response of n-3 fatty acids in humans. *Am J Clin Nutr* 83: 1467S–76S.

ARTERBURN LM, OKEN HA, BAILEY HALL E, HAMERSLEY J, KURATKO CN and HOFFMAN JP (2008) Algal-oil capsules and cooked salmon: nutritionally equivalent sources of docosahexaenoic acid. *J Am Diet Assoc* 108: 1204–9.

BLONK MC, BILO HJ, POPP-SNIJDERS C, MULDER C and DONKER AJ (1990) Dose–response effects of fish oil supplementation in healthy volunteers. *Am J Clin Nutr* 52: 120–27.

BNF (1992) *Unsaturated Fatty Acids: Nutritional and Physiological Significance*. London: Chapman & Hall.

BNF (1999) *Briefing Paper: N-3 Fatty Acids and Health*. London: British Nutrition Foundation.

BROUWER IA, RAITT MH, DULLEMEIJER C, KRAEMER DF, ZOCK PL, MORRIS C, KATAN MB, CONNOR WE, CAMM JA, SCHOUTEN EG and MCANULTY J (2009) Effect of fish oil on ventricular tachyarrhythmia in three studies in patients with implantable cardioverter defibrillators. *Eur Heart J* 30: 820–26.

BUCHER HC, HENGSTLER P, SCHINDLER C and MEIER G (2002) N-3 polyunsaturated fatty acids in coronary heart disease: a meta-analysis of randomized controlled trials. *Am J Med* 112: 298–304.

BURDGE GC and CALDER PC (2006) Dietary α-linolenic acid and health-related outcomes: a metabolic perspective. *Nutr Res Rev* 19: 26–52.

BURDGE GC and WOOTTON SA (2002) Conversion of α-linolenic acid to eicosapentaenoic, docosapentaenoic and docosahexaenoic acids in young women. *Brit J Nutr* 88: 411–20.

BURDGE GC, JONES AE and WOOTTON SA (2002) Eicosapentaenoic and docosapentaenoic acids are the principal products of α-linolenic acid metabolism in young men. *Brit J Nutr* 88: 355–63.

CALDER PC (2004) N-3 fatty acids and cardiovascular disease: evidence explained and mechanisms explored. *Clin Sci* 107: 1–11.

CALDER PC (2006) N-3 polyunsaturated fatty acids, inflammation, and inflammatory diseases. *Am J Clin Nutr* 83: 1505S–19S.

CALDER PC (2008a) The relationship between the fatty acid composition of immune cells and their function. *Prostaglandins Leukot Essent Fatty Acids* 79: 101–8.

CALDER PC (2008b) PUFA, inflammatory processes and rheumatoid arthritis. *Proc Nutr Soc* 67: 409–18.

CALDER PC (2008c) Polyunsaturated fatty acids, inflammatory processes and inflammatory bowel diseases. *Mol Nutr Food Res* 52: 885–97.

CALDER PC (2012a) Mechanisms of action of (n-3) fatty acids. *J Nutr* 142: 592S–9S.

CALDER PC (2012b) The role of marine omega-3 (n-3) fatty acids in inflammatory processes, atherosclerosis and plaque stability. *Mol Nutr Food Res* 56: 1073–80.

CALDER PC and DECKELBAUM RJ (2008) Omega-3 fatty acids: time to get the messages right! *Curr Opin Clin Nutr Metab Care* 11: 91–3.

CALDER PC and YAQOOB P (2009) Understanding omega-3 polyunsaturated fatty acids. *Postgrad Med* 121: 148–57.

CAUGHEY GE, MANTZIORIS E, GIBSON RA, CLELAND LG and JAMES J (1996) The effect on human tumor necrosis factor α and interleukin 1β production of diets enriched in n-3 fatty acids from vegetable oil or fish oil. *Am J Clin Nutr* 63: 116–22.

CAWOOD AL, DING R, NAPPER FL, YOUNG RH, WILLIAMS JA, WARD MJ, GUDMUNDSEN O, VIGE R, PAYNE SP, YE S, SHEARMAN CP, GALLAGHER PJ, GRIMBLE RF and CALDER PC (2010) Eicosapentaenoic acid (EPA) from highly concentrated n-3 fatty acid ethyl esters is incorporated into advanced atherosclerotic plaques and higher plaque EPA is associated with decreased plaque inflammation and increased stability. *Atherosclerosis* 212: 252–9.

CLARKE SD (2004) The multi-dimensional regulation of gene expression by fatty acids: polyunsaturated fats as nutrient sensors. *Curr Opin Lipidol* 15:13–18.

DE CATERINA R (2011) n-3 Fatty acids in cardiovascular disease. *N Engl J Med* 364: 2439–50.

DECKELBAUM RJ, WORGALL TS and SEO T (2006) N-3 fatty acids and gene expression. *Am J Clin Nutr* 83:1520S–5S.

DECKELBAUM RJ, CALDER PC, HARRIS WS, AKOH CC, MAKI KC, WHELAN J, BANZ WJ and KENNEDY E (2012) Conclusions and recommendations from the symposium, Heart Healthy Omega-3s for Food: Stearidonic Acid (SDA) as a Sustainable Choice. *J Nutr* 142: 641S–3S.

EFSA (2010) Scientific opinion on dietary reference values for fats, including saturated fatty acids, polyunsaturated fatty acids, monounsaturated fatty acids, *trans* fatty acids, and cholesterol. *EFSA J* 8: 1461, available at: http://www.efsa.europa.eu/fr/scdocs/doc/1461.pdf [accessed February 2013].

FABER J, BERKHOUT M, VOS AP, SIJBEN JW, CALDER PC, GARSSEN J and VAN HELVOORT A (2011) Supplementation with a fish oil-enriched, high-protein medical food leads to rapid incorporation of EPA into white blood cells and modulates immune responses within one week in healthy men and women. *J Nutr* 141: 964–70.

FAO (2010) *Fat and fatty acids in human nutrition: Report of an expert consultation*. Rome: Food and Agriculture Organisation of the United Nations.

FREEMAN MP, HIBBELN JR, WISNER KL, DAVIS JM, MISCHOULON D, PEET M, KECK JR PE, MARANGELL LB, RICHARDSON AJ, LAKE J and STOLL AL (2006) Omega-3 fatty acids: evidence basis for treatment and future research in psychiatry. *J Clin Psychiatry* 67: 1954–67.

French Agency for Food Environmental and Occupational Health Safety (2003) *The Omega 3 Fatty Acids and the Cardiovascular System: nutritional benefits and claims*. Maisons-Alfort: AFSSA, available at: http://www.afssa.fr/Documents/NUT-Ra-omega3EN.pdf [accessed January 2013].

GELEIJNSE JM, GILTAY EJ, GROBBEE DE, DONDERS ART and KOK FJ (2002) Blood pressure response to fish oil supplementation: meta-regression analysis of randomized trials. *J Hypertens* 20: 1493–9.

GURR MI, HARWOOD JL and FRAYN KN (2002) *Lipid Biochemistry* (5th edn). Oxford: Blackwell.

HARRIS WS (1996) N-3 fatty acids and lipoproteins: comparison of results from human and animal studies. *Lipids* 31: 243–52.

HARRIS WS, WINDSOR SL and DUJOVNE CA (1991) Effects of four doses of n-3 fatty acids given to hyperlipidemic patients for six months. *J Am Coll Nutr* 10: 220–27.

HARRIS WS, MILLER M, TIGHE AP, DAVIDSON MH and SCHAEFER EI (2008) Omega-3 fatty acids and coronary heart disease risk: Clinical and mechanistic perspectives. *Atherosclerosis* 197: 12–24.

HEALY DA, WALLACE FA, MILES EA, CALDER PC and NEWSHOLME P (2000) The effect of low to moderate amounts of dietary fish oil on neutrophil lipid composition and function. *Lipids* 35: 763–8.

HELLAND IB, SMITH L, SAAREM K, SAUGSTAD OD and DREVON CA (2003) Maternal supplementation with very-long-chain n-3 fatty acids during pregnancy and lactation augments children's IQ at 4 years of age. *Pediatrics* 111: e39–44.

International Society for the Study of Fatty Acids and Lipids (2004) *Recommendations for the intake of polyunsaturated fatty acids in healthy adults*, ISSFAL Policy Statement No. 3, June, available at: http://www.issfal.org/news-links/resources/publications/PUFAIntakeReccomdFinalReport.pdf [accessed February 2013].

JBS2 (2005) Joint British Societies' Guidelines on prevention of cardiovascular disease in clinical practice. British Cardiac Society. British Hypertension Society. Diabetes UK. HEART UK. Primary Care Cardiovascular Society. Stroke Association. *Heart* 91 (Suppl. 5): v1–v52.

JUMP DB (2002) Dietary polyunsaturated fatty acids and regulation of gene transcription. *Curr Opin Lipidol* 13: 155–64.

JUMP DB (2008) N-3 polyunsaturated fatty acid regulation of heparic gene transcription. *Curr Opin Lipidol* 19: 242–7.

KATAN MB, DESLYPERE JP, VAN BIRGELEN APJM, PENDERS M and ZEGWAARS M (1997) Kinetics of the incorporation of dietary fatty acids into serum cholesteryl esters, erythrocyte membranes and adipose tissue: an 18 month controlled study. *J Lipid Res* 38: 2012–22.

KOLETZKO B, CETIN I, BRENNA JT, Perinatal Lipid Intake Working Group; Child Health Foundation, Diabetic Pregnancy Study Group, European Association of Perinatal Medicine, European Association of Perinatal Medicine, European Society for Clinical Nutrition and Metabolism, European Society for Paediatric Gastroenterology, Hepatology and Nutrition – Committee on Nutrition, International Federation of Placenta Associations and International Society for the Study of Fatty Acids and Lipids (2007) Dietary fat intakes for pregnant and lactating women. *Brit J Nutr* 98: 873–7.

KRIS-ETHERTON PM, HARRIS WS, APPEL LJ and AMERICAN HEART ASSOCIATION NUTRITION COMMITTEE (2002) Fish consumption, fish oil, omega-3 fatty acids, and cardiovascular disease. *Circulation* 106: 2747–57.

LAPILLONNE A, CLARKE SD and HEIRD WC (2004) Polyunsaturated fatty acids and gene expression. *Curr Opin Clin Nutr Metab Care* 7: 151–6.

LEAF A, KANG JX, XIAO YF and BILLMAN GE (2003) Clinical prevention of sudden cardiac death by n-3 polyunsaturated fatty acids and mechanisms of prevention of arrhythmias by n-3 fish oils. *Circulation* 107: 2646–52.

LUKIW WJ, CUI JG, MARCHESELLI VL, BODKER M, BOTKJAER A, GOTLINGER K, SERHAN CN and BAZAN NG (2005) A role for docosahexaenoic acid-derived neuroprotectin D1 in neural cell survival and Alzheimer disease. *J Clin Invest* 115: 2774–83.

MARCHIOLI R, BARZI F, BOMBA E, CHIEFFO C, DI GREGORIO D, DI MASCIO R, FRANZOSI MG, GERACI E, LEVANTESI G, MAGGIONI AP, MANTINI L, MARFISI RM, MASTROGIUSEPPE G, MININNI N, NICOLOSI GI, SANTINI M, SCHWEIGER C, TAVAZZI L, TOGNONI G, TUCCI C and VALAGUSSA F (2002) Early protection against sudden death by n-3 polyunsaturated fatty acids after myocardial infarction – Time-course analysis of the results of the Gruppo Italiano per lo Studio della Sopravvivenza nell'Infarto Miocardico (GISSI)-Prevenzione. *Circulation* 105: 1897–903.

MARSEN TA, POLLOK M, OETTE K and BALDAMUS CA (1992) Pharmacokinetics of omega-3 fatty acids during ingestion of fish oil preparations. *Prostaglandins Leukot Essent Fatty Acids* 46: 191–6.

MEYER BJ, MANN NJ, LEWIS JL, MILLIGAN GC, SINCLAIR AJ and HOWE PR (2003) Dietary intakes and food sources of omega-6 and omega-3 polyunsaturated fatty acids. *Lipids* 38: 391–8.

MILES EA and CALDER PC (1998) Modulation of immune function by dietary fatty acids. *Proc Nutr Soc* 57: 277–92.

MORI TA and WOODMAN RJ (2006) The independent effects of eicosapentaenoic acid and docosahexaenoic acid on cardiovascular risk factors in humans. *Curr Opin Clin Nutr Metab Care* 9: 95–104.

MOZAFFARIAN D and RIMM EB (2006) Fish intake, contaminants, and human health: evaluating the risks and the benefits. *J Am Med Assoc* 296: 1885–99.

MOZAFFARIAN D and WU JHY (2011) Omega-3 fatty acids and cardiovascular disease. *J Am Coll Cardiol* 58: 2047–67.

NESTEL P, SHIGE H, POMEROY S, CEHUN M, ABBEY M and RAEDERSTORFF D (2002) The n-3 fatty acids eicosapentaenoic acid and docosahexaenoic acid increase systemic arterial compliance in humans. *Am J Clin Nutr* 76: 326–30.

NHMRC (2006) *Nutrient reference values for Australia and New Zealand including recommended dietary intakes*. Canberra: National Health and Medical Research Council. Available at: http://www.nhmrc.gov.au/publications/synopses/n35syn.htm [accessed January 2013].

NICOLAOU A and KAFATOS G (2004) *Bioactive Lipids*. Bridgwater: The Oily Press.

OH DY, TALUKDAR S, BAE EJ, IMAMURA T, MORINAGA H, FAN W, LI P, LU WJ, WATKINS SM and OLEFSKY JM (2010) GPR120 is an omega-3 fatty acid receptor mediating potent anti-inflammatory and insulin-sensitizing effects. *Cell* 142: 687–98.

POPP-SNIJDERS C, SCHOUTEN JA, VAN BLITTERSWIJK WJ and VAN DER VEEN EA (1986) Changes in membrane lipid composition of human erythrocytes after dietary supplementation of (n-3) fatty acids: maintenance of membrane fluidity. *Biochim Biophys Acta* 854: 31–7.

REES D, MILES EA, BANERJEE T, WELLS SJ, ROYNETTE CE, WAHLE KWJW and CALDER PC (2006) Dose-related effects of eicosapentaenoic acid on innate immune function in healthy humans: a comparison of young and older men. *Am J Clin Nutr* 83: 331–42.

REIFFEL J and MCDONALD A (2006) Antiarrhythmic effects of omega-3 fatty acids. *Am J Cardiol* 98: 50i–60i.

RICHARDSON AJ (2004) Clinical trials of fatty acid treatment in ADHD, dyslexia, dyspraxia and the autistic spectrum. *Prostaglandins Leukot Essent Fatty Acids* 70: 383–90.

RINGBOM T, HUSS U, STENHOLM A, FLOCK S, SKATTEBØL L, PERERA P and BOHLIN L (2001) Cox-2 inhibitory effects of naturally occurring and modified fatty acids. *J Nat Prod* 64: 745–9.

RUXTON CHS, CALDER PC, REED SC and SIMPSON MJA (2005) The impact of long-chain n-3 polyunsaturated fatty acids on human health. *Nutr Res Rev* 18: 113–29.

SANDERS TAB and ROSHANAI F (1983) The influence of different types of ω3 polyunsaturated fatty acids on blood lipids and platelet function in healthy volunteers. *Clin Sci* 64: 91–9.

SANGIOVANNI JP, PARRA-CABRERA S, COLDITZ GA, BERKEY CS and DWYER JT (2000a) Meta-analysis of dietary essential fatty acids and long-chain polyunsaturated fatty acids as they relate to visual resolution acuity in healthy preterm infants. *Pediatrics* 105: 1292–8.

SANGIOVANNI JP, BERKEY CS, DWYER JT and COLDITZ GA (2000b) Dietary essential fatty acids, long-chain polyunsaturated fatty acids, and visual resolution acuity in healthy fullterm infants: a systematic review. *Early Hum Dev* 57: 165–88.

SARAVANAN P, DAVIDSON NC, SCHMIDT EB and CALDER PC (2010) Cardiovascular effects of marine omega-3 fatty acids. *Lancet* 376: 540–50.

SCHUCHARDT JP, SCHNEIDER I, MEYER H, NEUBRONNER J, VON SCHACKY C and HAHN A (2011) Incorporation of EPA and DHA into plasma phospholipids in response to different omega-3 fatty acid formulations – a comparative bioavailability study of fish oil vs. krill oil. *Lipids Health Dis* 10: 145.

SCIENTIFIC ADVISORY COMMITTEE ON NUTRITION AND COMMITTEE ON TOXICITY (2004) *Advice on Fish Consumption: Benefits and Risks*. London: TSO.

SERHAN CN, CLISH CB, BRANNON J, COLGAN SP, GRONERT K and CHIANG N (2000a) Anti-inflammatory lipid signals generated from dietary n-3 fatty acids via cyclooxygenase-2 and transcellular processing: a novel mechanism for NSAID and n-3 PUFA therapeutic actions. *J Physiol Pharmacol* 4: 643–54.

SERHAN CN, CLISH CB, BRANNON J, COLGAN SP, CHIANG N and GRONERT K (2000b) Novel functional sets of lipid-derived mediators with antinflammatory actions generated from omega-3 fatty acids via cyclooxygenase 2-nonsteroidal antiinflammatory drugs and transcellular processing. *J Exp Med* 192: 1197–204.

SERHAN CN, HONG S, GRONERT K, COLGAN SP, DEVCHAND PR, MIRICK G and MOUSSIGNAC R-L (2002) Resolvins: a family of bioactive products of omega-3 fatty acid transformation circuits initiated by aspirin treatment that counter pro-inflammation signals. *J Exp Med* 196: 1025–37.

SIMOPOLOUS AP, LEAF A and SALEM N (1999) Essentiality and recommended dietary intakes for omega-6 and omega-3 fatty acids. *Ann Nutr Metab* 43: 127–30.

SOLFRIZZI V, FRISARDI V, CAPURSO C, D'INTRONO A, COLACICCO AM, VENDEMIALE G, CAPURSO A and PANZA F (2010) Dietary fatty acids in dementia and predementia syndromes: Epidemiological evidence and possible underlying mechanisms. *Ageing Res Rev* 9:184–99.

STUDER M, BRIEL M, LEIMENSTOLL B, GLASS TR and BUCHER HC (2005) Effect of different antilipidemic agents and diets on mortality: a systematic review. *Arch Intern Med* 165: 725–30.

THIES F, GARRY JMC, YAQOOB P, RERKASEM K, WILLIAMS J, SHEARMAN CP, GALLAGHER PJ, CALDER PC and GRIMBLE RF (2003) Association of n-3 polyunsaturated fatty acids with stability of atherosclerotic plaques: a randomised controlled trial. *Lancet* 361: 477–85.

VAN DE WERF F, BAX J, BETRIU A, BLOMSTOM-LUNDQVIST C, CREA F, FALK V, FILIPPATOS G, FOX K, HUBER K, KASTRATI A, ROSENGREN A, STEG PS, TUBARO M, VERHEUGT F, WEDINGER F and WEIS M (2008) Management of acute myocardial infarction in patients presenting with persistent ST-segment elevation. *Eur Heart J* 29: 2909–45.

VISIOLI F, RISÉ P, BARASSI MC, MARANGONI F and GALLI C (2003) Dietary intake of fish vs. formulations leads to higher plasma concentrations of n-3 fatty acids. *Lipids* 38: 415–18.

VON SCHACKY C (2008) Omega-3 fatty acids: antiarrhythmic, proarrhythmic or both? *Curr Opin Clin Nutr Metab Care* 11: 94–9.

VON SCHACKY C, FISCHER S and WEBER PC (1985) Long term effects of dietary marine ω-3 fatty acids upon plasma and cellular lipids, platelet function, and eicosanoid formation in humans. *J Clin Invest* 76: 1626–31.

YAQOOB P (2009) The nutritional significance of lipid rafts. *Annu Rev Nutr* 29: 257–82.

YAQOOB P, PALA HS, CORTINA-BORJA M, NEWSHOLME EA and CALDER PC (2000) Encapsulated fish oil enriched in α-tocopherol alters plasma phospholipid and mononuclear cell fatty acid compositions but not mononuclear cell functions. *Eur J Clin* Invest 30: 260–74.

YOKOYAMA M, ORIGASA H, MATSUZAKI M, MATSUZAWA Y, SAITO Y, ISHIKAWA Y, OIKAWA S, SASAKI J, HISHIDA H, ITAKURA H, KITA T, KITABATAKE A, NAKAYA N, SAKATA T, SHIMADA K and SHIRATO K. JAPAN EPA LIPID INTERVENTION STUDY (JELIS) INVESTIGATORS (2007) Effects of eicosapentaenoic acid on major coronary events in hypercholesterolaemic patients (JELIS): a randomised open-label, blinded endpoint analysis. *Lancet* 369: 1090–98.

ZHAO G, ETHERTON TD, MARTIN KR, WEST SG, GILLIES PJ and KRIS-ETHERTON PM (2004) Dietary alpha-linolenic acid reduces inflammatory and lipid cardiovascular risk factors in hypercholesterolemic men and women. *J Nutr* 134: 2991–7.

1.9 Appendix: abbreviations

CVD	cardiovascular disease
DHA	docosahexaenoic acid
DPA	docosapentaenoic acid
EPA	eicosapentaenoic acid
PUFA	polyunsaturated fatty acid

2

Sources of omega-3 fatty acids

A. P. Bimbo, Consultant, USA

DOI: 10.1533/9780857098863.1.27

Abstract: This chapter discusses the concerns that have been raised about how sources of marine oils will be able to keep up with the growing demand for these products in the omega-3 market. Traditional and other sources such as krill, microalgae, transgenic plants and other sources of fish oil are discussed. The chapter contains many tables using 10-year average catch data to demonstrate other sources of marine oils aside from the traditional anchovy/sardine sources with conservative estimates for production of these other oils. The chapter also compiles fatty acid profile data on these other sources from historic as well as current information.

Key words: krill oil, microalgae oils, fish oils, cod liver oil, transgenic plants, omega-3 fatty acids.

2.1 Introduction

In a recent online web article Daniels (2011) reported that the market for omega-3 food, beverage and supplements in the USA is worth over US$5 billion with a saturation point nowhere in sight. He mentioned that the total omega-3 market was recently valued at almost US$8 billion (€5.57 billion). A 2011 Packaged Facts report (Packaged Facts, 2011) mentions that the global market for EPA/DHA omega-3 products is projected to jump from $25.4 billion in 2011 to $34.7 billion in 2016.

The supply of eicosapentaenoic acid (EPA) and docosahexaenoic acid (DHA) is dominated by the fish oil players according to the Global Organization for EPA and DHA (GOED) omega-3. Fish oils represented about 80 % of the 2011 global market for omega-3 for human consumption according to GOED (2012), with 75 % of this used in dietary supplements.

So, while the demand for omega-3 products continues to increase, with no end to this growth in sight, environmentalists are predicting the demise of the global capture fisheries and especially the small forage fish that are expected to support this growing market. Objections to the catching of the fish come in spite of the fact that many commercial fisheries have undergone major changes, including the imposition of quotas, and many of them are now certified by third-party independent groups whose purpose is to ensure that the catch is sustainable and traceable. This certification process was demanded by the same groups who now attack these endeavors and actually criticize the certification groups for becoming too 'commercial'.

There are also the dire predictions that the end of the wild fisheries as we know them will take place around the year 2050, unless.... The 'unless', seems to periodically change as the industry is required to meet new quotas, reduction in fishing areas, sustainability certification, onboard and satellite monitoring and other regulations. One report (Pikitch *et al.*, 2012) recommended a reduction of 40–60 % in the landings of fish used for oil production in order to protect the species. Lawler (2011) went a little further recently and mentioned that perhaps the best way to protect the marine environment from over-exploitation would be to simply stop eating fish.

In addition to the attacks on the fishing industry, there have also been some suggestions that the available fish oil sources for the omega-3 market will be 'used up' in a relatively short period of time because of the 'rapid' growth in the market. Therefore, the omega-3 industry is concerned about whether there will be any fish and/or any other sources of raw material and the availability of suitable fish oils for this market. This chapter will attempt to bring this situation into perspective.

2.2 Background

When you look at the UN's Food and Agriculture Organization (FAO) statistics specifically for total fish landings, you find that the growth has been about 9.6 % per year between 1950 and 2010, the latest year for the data. Total fish landings are composed of wild capture and farmed fish. When you separate the two components you find that the capture fisheries have remained relatively static over the period 1985–2010, growing around 0.31 % per year (averaging about 76.7 mmt) while the farmed fish component grew about 25 % per year over the same period. If you extrapolate the data, it shows that the two lines will cross around the year 2050; however, this can be manipulated by how many years are included in the dataset. In 2010 aquaculture and wild caught fish represented 34 % and 66 %, respectively, of the world's fish production. Figure 2.1 shows the historical growth of wild-caught and farm-raised fish over the period 1990–2010 projected out to 2055.

While aquaculture is a major consumer of fish oil and competes with the omega-3 supply chain for this product, it can also be a source of raw material for the omega-3 market when the by-products or cuttings are converted to fishmeal and oil. In fact, both farmed and wild salmon oil are presently used in some omega-3 products and others may follow in the future.

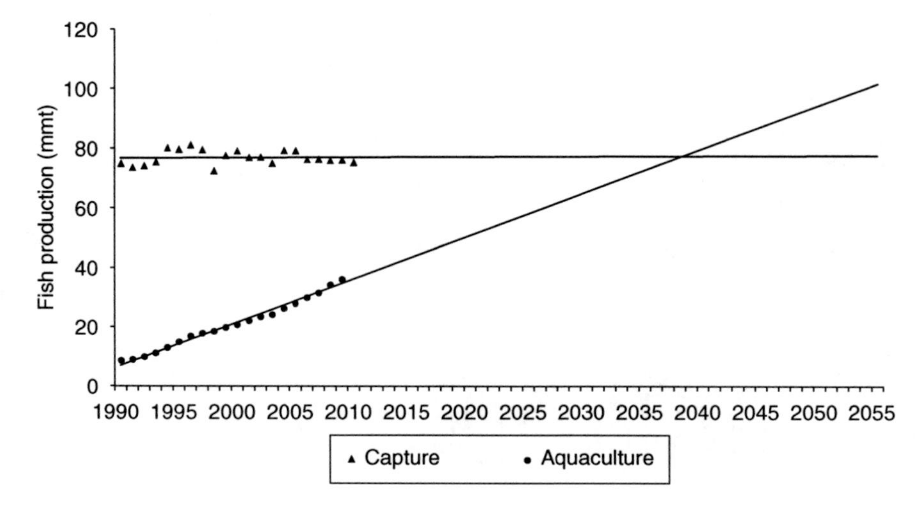

Fig. 2.1 Global fisheries capture and aquaculture production since 1990, projected to 2055. (Source: FAO, 2012)

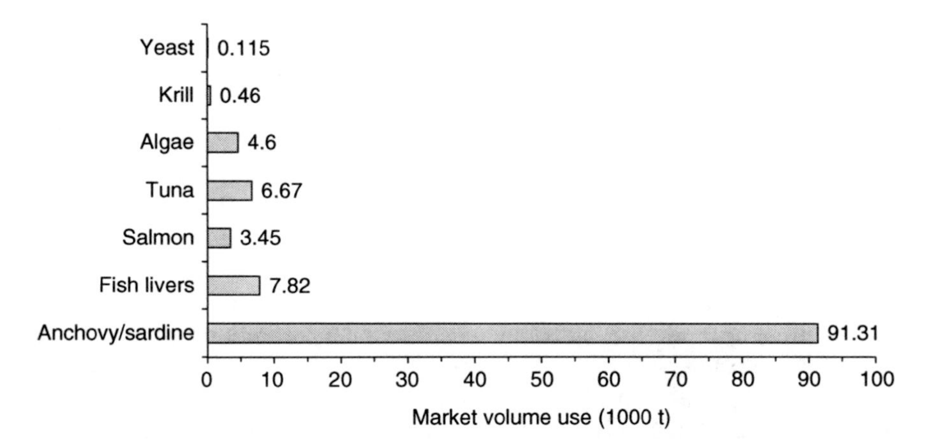

Fig. 2.2 Anchovy and sardines dominate the raw materials for the omega-3 market. (Source: Bimbo 2012a. Used with permission from GOED Exchange)

According to a recent presentation (GOED, 2012), anchovy and sardine oil account for about 80 % of the omega-3 finished product market with fish liver oils, salmon, tuna, algae or single-cell oils, krill, yeast and possibly plant oils accounting for the other 20 %. This can be seen in Fig. 2.2.

When you calculate the amount of crude fish oil that will be needed to produce the current weighted finished product mix (80 % triglyceride oils, 2.27 % low concentrates, 5.18 % middle concentrates and 2.55 % high concentrates) you find that at the current mix there is a 47 % loss of by-product. This can be seen in Fig. 2.3 where the data has been projected to the year 2025.

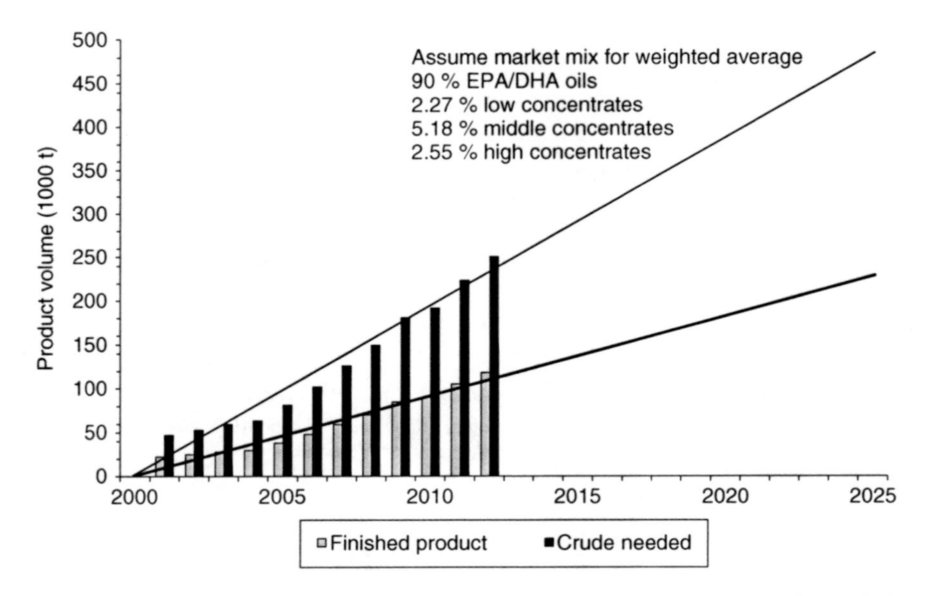

Fig. 2.3 Estimated sales of omega products all categories and crude fish oil needed. (Source: Bimbo 2012. Used with permission from GOED Exchange)

The difference between the crude oil input and the finished product output represents by-product material consisting of saturated and mono and di-unsaturated fatty acids. Depending on the starting oil, this by-product mix could contain large amounts of C16:1, C18:1, C18:2, C20:1 and C22:1 fatty acids. As a matter of information, C18:1 is currently being marketed as an omega-9 and C16:1 as an omega-7 fatty acid.

The price of crude fish oil is influenced by many situations, among them El Niño atmospheric occurrences, low fish oil yields, reduced fish catch (from lower quotas, fishing moratoriums and fishermen strikes), environmental disasters (tsunamis, hurricanes, volcanic eruptions and oil spill disasters) and commodity price fluctuations (from droughts, heavy rains or green energy mandates).

The historical fluctuations in price and fish oil production in Chile and Peru are shown in Fig. 2.4. El Niño events represented by arrows clearly show reductions in fish catch and the corresponding increase in crude fish oil prices. The period 2001 forward includes two El Niños, tsunamis, earthquakes in Chile, Peru and Japan, volcanic eruptions, a major oil spill in the US Gulf of Mexico and green energy mandates in the USA and elsewhere that have impacted the global commodity markets. There were predictions of another El Niño event in 2012–2013 but so far it has not developed into a strong event. However, in anticipation of the possible effect of the El Niño on the anchovy resource, the Peruvian government has severely limited the catch quotas for the late 2012–early 2013 fishing season.

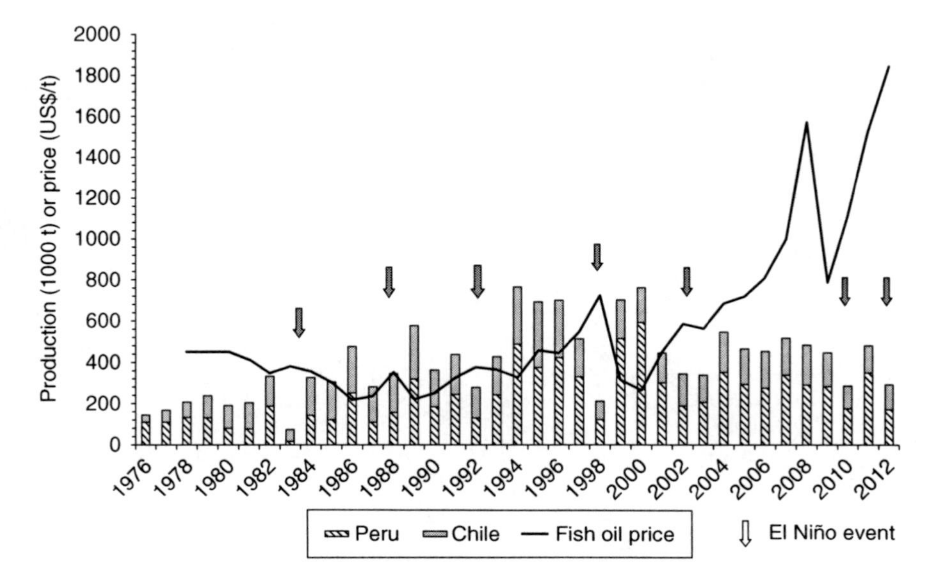

Fig. 2.4 Crude fish oil price and Peru and Chile fish oil production of anchovy, sardine and horse mackerel oil through 2012, estimated. (Source: Oil World, 2012. Used with permission from ISTA Mielke GmbH – Oil World, Global Research and Analysis)

The omega-3 market supply chain is also evolving. At one time there were clear demarcation lines between the crude oil producers, the semi-refiners, the full refiners and the nutraceutical oil companies such that the flow of product was relatively easy to manage and trace. Today there has been consolidation at all levels of the supply chain with some companies vertically integrating and others expanding via acquisitions and mergers. Companies at the lower end of the chain are installing refineries and concentration capabilities which allow them to participate in the 'value-added' revenue in the market. In some cases, crude virgin salmon oil is being successfully marketed directly to the consumer or through supplement companies, avoiding all the intermediaries in the supply chain. Consolidation among the companies at the upper end of the supply chain is also occurring and probably will continue in the future. This new supply chain can be seen in Fig. 2.5.

As the supply chain evolves and companies at the base begin to expand upwards, it will force the companies above them to also move upwards towards the more concentrated products. As more and more concentrated products are produced, the by-products (saturates and mono and di-unsaturates) will increase in volume. The economics of the entire process will depend upon what companies do with these by-products. One possibility is to convert these by-products to biodiesel products. Since the by-products are already in ethyl ester form, using them in biodiesel should be a relatively easy conversion if the product can meet the ASTM D6751–12 specifications

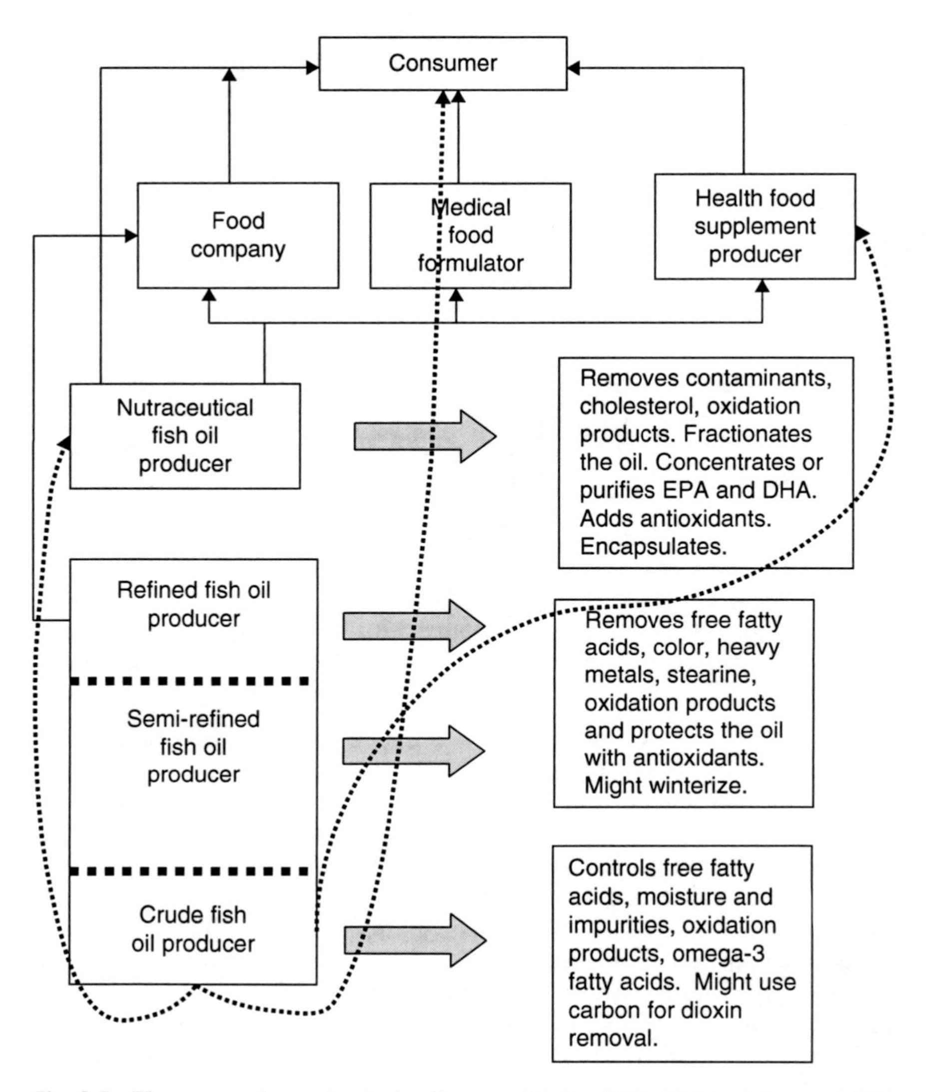

Fig. 2.5 The omega-3 supply chain. (Source: Bimbo 2012. Used with permission from GOED Exchange)

(ASTM, 2010). A comparison of the price of feed-grade menhaden oil and the USA average selling price of B100 biodiesel is shown in Fig. 2.6. Other possibilities for these by-products would be in the oleochemical field. Bimbo and Crowther (1992) and Bimbo (1996) have already reviewed some of these 'industrial applications' for marine oils and derivatives. A recent report by Transparency Market Research (2012) mentioned that the global oleochemical market was more than 13 million tons in 2010 and is expected to reach 15 million tons by 2018. Figure 2.7 shows the yield of finished

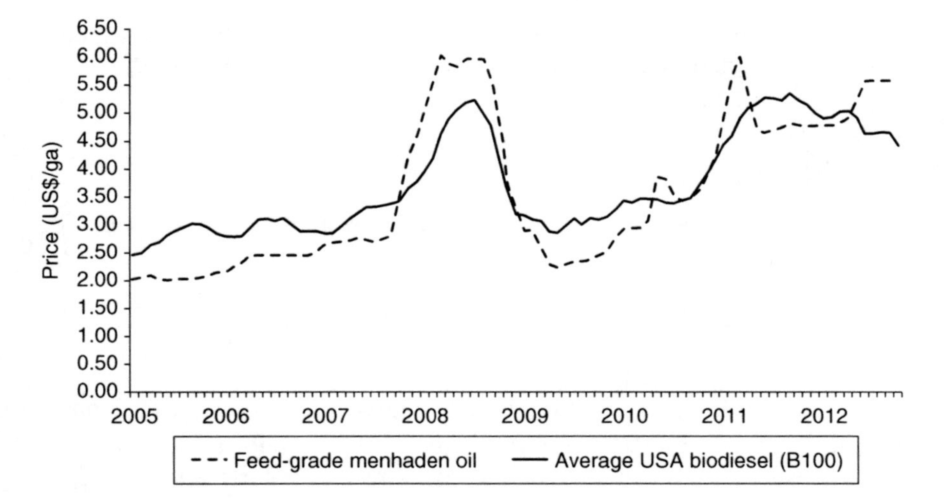

Fig. 2.6 Comparison of prices of feed grade menhaden fish oil and USA average B100 biodiesel through November 30, 2012. (Source: The Jacobsen Feed Bulletin, 2012. Used with permission from the Jacobsen Publishing Company)

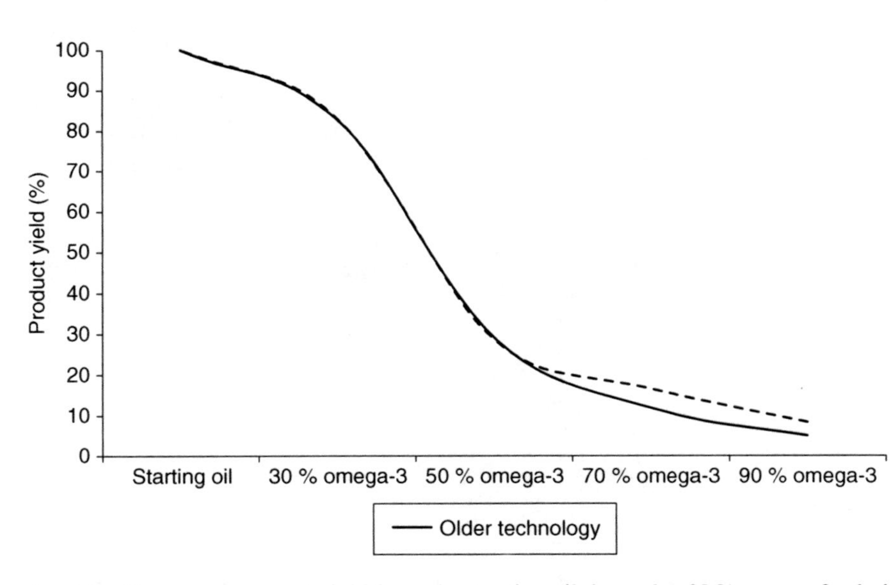

Fig. 2.7 Estimated percent yield from the starting oil through a 90 % omega-3 ethyl ester. (Sources: Breivik 1992, GOED 2012. Used with permission from GOED Exchange)

product as you move from the starting 30 % omega-3 oils to the very highly concentrated pharmaceutical grade products on the market today.

2.3 Marine oils in perspective

A number of entities or countries are the major producers of fish oils. For this chapter I have removed Denmark and Sweden from the EU 27 group and included them in the Scandinavia group. Marine oil production over the period 2002–2011 is shown in Table 2.1. The 'Others' category of countries account for about 87 000 tons of fish oil production. These can be seen in Table 2.2.

Fish oil production has been relatively stable over the period 2002–2011, averaging about 1 mmt. There were major El Niño events in 1998 and 2010 and a predicted event in 2012 which have affected and can affect the production in Peru and Chile dramatically. Any effect on production has a corresponding effect on the price of the fish oil.

In the context of this chapter, marine oils refer to fish body oils, fish liver oils, crustacean, mammal and cephalopod oils. According to FAO statistics, through the year 2010 (most current data available), fish body oils are the predominant product in this category, representing almost all of the production with small amounts of mammal and squid oil (FAO, 2012). This data can be seen in Fig. 2.8.

Unfortunately FAO does not collect detailed information about the composition of the global market for marine oil production so we find the fish body oils not easily identified (nei) as the predominant category. This

Table 2.1 Global fish oil production in major countries, 10-year average

	Volume (1000 t)	Proportion of global production (%)
EU 25*	48.32	4.76
Scandinavia	207.58	20.44
Peru	274.25	27.00
Chile	161.74	15.93
USA	76.68	7.55
Japan	112.49	11.08
Morocco	30.31	2.98
Canada	5.15	0.51
Mexico	18.65	1.84
Panama	8.81	0.87
Ecuador	5.78	0.57
South Africa	5.55	0.55
Others	86.86	5.93
Totals	1042.17	

Source: Oil World, 2012. Used with permission from ISTA Mielke GmbH – Oil World, Global Research and Analysis.
*Denmark and Sweden were removed from EU27 and included in Scandinavia.

Table 2.2 Fish oil production in other countries, 10-year average

	Volume (1000 t)	Proportion of global production (%)
Russia	3.78	0.37
Angola	3.67	0.36
Argentina	4.78	0.47
Brazil	3.36	0.33
China	14.90	1.47
India	5.04	0.50
Indonesia	5.65	0.56
Thailand	7.98	0.79
South Korea	3.44	0.34
Turkey	15.34	1.52
Vietnam	18.92	1.86
Total of other countries	86.86	

Source: Oil World, 2012. Used with permission from ISTA Mielke GmbH – Oil World, Global Research and Analysis.

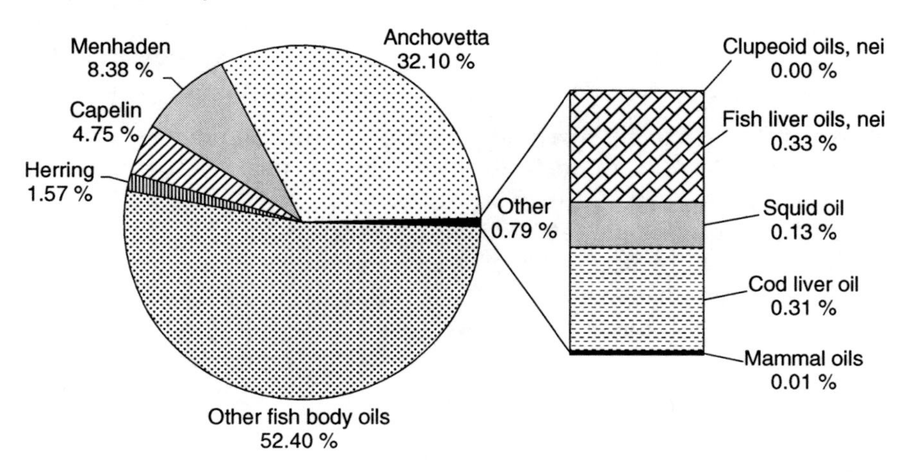

Fig. 2.8 Composition of global marine oil production. 10-year average production 1.07 mmt. (Source: FAO, 2012)

nei category would include pollock, salmon, tuna, hoki, sand eel, mixed white fish, catfish, dogfish, sprat, horse mackerel, sardines/pilchards and mackerel among others. Presumably, individually measured, the volume of these oils would be low or the suppliers of the information just do not feel that this information is important. Since FAO does report volumes as low as 29 mt, one would suspect that the reporting countries just do not want to or are unable to provide the required data or there is a confidential commercial reason for the lack of data. So the question becomes, besides the easily accessible oils – anchovy, menhaden, capelin, and the liver oils – what other oils might be available for the omega-3 market and where can they be found?

2.3.1 Raw material sources

The raw material utilized for the production of the various marine oils comes essentially from two sources – the targeted pelagic fisheries (including herrings, sardines and anchovies, and a miscellaneous pelagic fish group) and by-products from the edible fisheries, for example the tuna and bonito group. The other species used for the production of marine oils include krill, squid and, to a lesser extent, marine mammals. While the raw material landed for direct production of marine oil and fishmeal is 100 % utilized, the raw material destined for the edible market essentially yields 50 % edible meat and 50 % by-product composed of 15 % heads, 14 % frames, 4 % skin and 17 % viscera (including the livers). Generally, these by-products are utilized for the production of marine oils and fishmeal, but there are many locations around the world where this material is simply discarded into the sea or landfill. In some cases, the fish are processed aboard the fishing vessel and it is simply easier to discard the by-product into the sea than to preserve, store and transport it to a land-based facility. Space on fishing vessels is at a premium and generally only valuable fish or possibly livers are preserved for transport to the shore-based facility.

According to the FAO (1986), the main sources of raw material for marine oil production normally come from three areas:

- Industrial fish caught specifically for fishmeal and oil production which represents 15–20 % of the landings or approximately 16–21 mmt of fish using the FAO 2000–2010 average data.
- By-catch or incidental catch from other fisheries. There have been estimates that the by-catch from edible fish operations is about 7 mmt and almost 2 mmt that comes from the shrimp fishery. It has been reported that the EU fish quota regulations cause 1 mmt of fish to be discarded each year.
- By-products (cuttings or trimmings) from the edible fisheries that represent about 50 % of the fish destined for food use. This represents a potential of about 42–44 mmt of waste using the 2000–2010 FAO average fish landing data. Only a portion of that potential resource is currently utilized.

In terms of the omega-3 market there is a fourth category which includes krill (crustacean) and squid (mollusk), the genetically modified oilseeds, marine algae, yeasts and fungi (the single-cell oils).

2.3.2 Production

The crude marine oils are mostly produced by the wet reduction process which essentially separates the liquids from the solids, then separates the water from the oil and finally dries the protein cake to produce fishmeal. There are many variations on the process but the wet rendering process is the primary process used. Chapter 3 describes the process in more detail.

Other processing methods might employ solvent extraction, and enzymatic digestion to release the lipids. However, no matter what the process is called, it will involve removal of the water followed by separation and recovery of the lipids.

Some oils contain relatively large amounts of phospholipids, which are generally lipid soluble except in the presence of water, which causes them to hydrate and precipitate out of the oil. Krill, some fish heads and some farmed fish (catfish), for example, do not process successfully when the wet reduction process is used because the phospholipid fraction causes emulsions which are difficult to handle in the process. These oils can be processed by dry rendering (similar to how poultry is processed) or by producing a very high fat protein meal and then solvent extracting the neutral lipid and/or the phospholipid from the dried protein.

2.3.3 Markets

Marine oils are used in a diverse group of markets including industrial or technical, animal feed, pet food, aquaculture, food and of course the omega-3 market. The marine oil market has been evolving over the last 20 years. This can be seen in Fig. 2.9. For many years the primary market for marine oils was in the hydrogenated form for margarine, shortening and baking fats. This market eventually dissolved as the issue of *trans* fatty acids developed. There was a switch over to aquaculture as the primary market but, as fish oil prices rose, the aquaculture industry began looking for less expensive substitutes. In recent years, the omega-3 market has begun to develop rapidly and there have been concerns about the sources of these oils. The omega-3 market, which includes foods, supplements, infant formula and

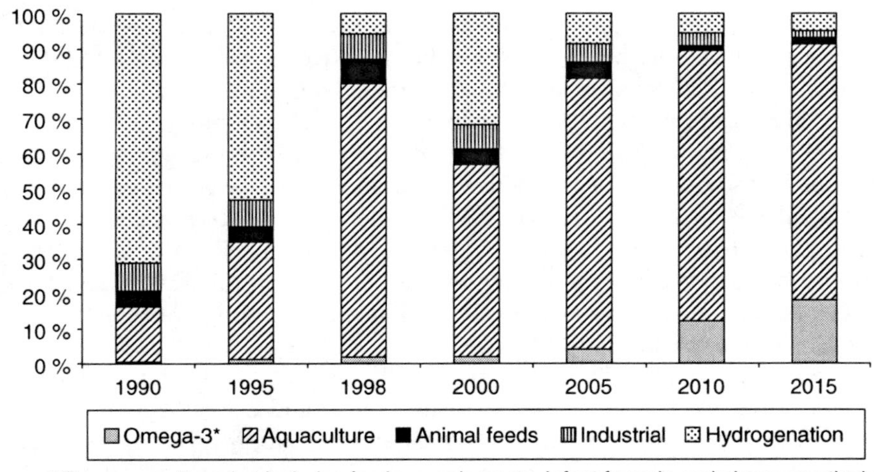

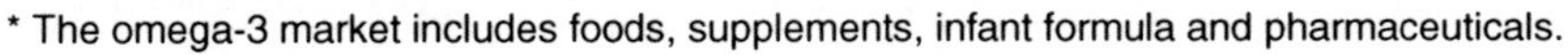

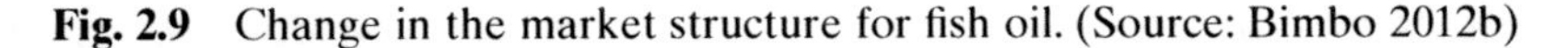

Fig. 2.9 Change in the market structure for fish oil. (Source: Bimbo 2012b)

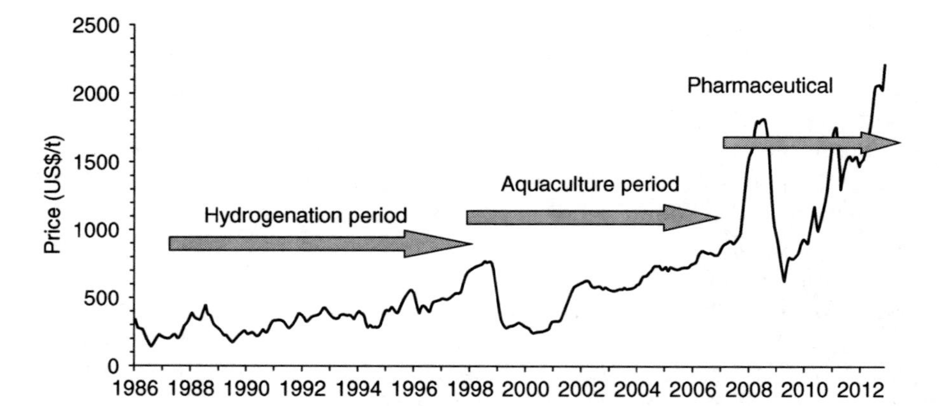

Fig. 2.10 Historic prices of crude fish oil (CIF) NW Europe, any origin through Nov. 22.2012. (Source: Oil World, 2012. Used with permission from ISTA Mielke GmbH - Oil World, Global Research and Analysis)

pharmaceuticals, requires special oils with high levels of the long-chain omega-3 fatty acids EPA and DHA, low levels of contaminants and low levels of oxidation. The omega-3 market is generally more capable of paying higher prices for the most desirable oils than the other users and this has helped to keep the price of marine oils high. The historical price (CIF: cost, insurance and freight) evolution of generic fish oil delivered into northwest Europe can be seen in Fig. 2.10. While still a relatively small segment of the overall marine oil market, concerns have already been raised about the stability of the raw material supply for the omega-3 market, since it seems to be concentrated in the Peruvian anchovy fishery.

The omega-3 market seems to feel that the most desirable fish oils, the anchovy and sardine, might reach their maximum availability in the next several years. At that point, it will be necessary to find other oil sources for this market. This has also caused some companies to take positions in the raw material supplier companies through joint ventures and investments in order to secure their supply of raw material. The fish oil producing companies have also been in an acquisition mode to secure a larger percentage of the available quota of fish resulting in further consolidation of the fishery. And, the fish oil producers are beginning to move their products up the supply chain to capture more added value for their products. While all this is happening, there has also been consolidation among the companies further up the market supply chain.

According to GOED (2012), the production of omega-3 products is projected to reach somewhere between 190 000 and 225 000 t by the year 2020. The data in Fig. 2.3, which used a weighted average requirement for crude fish oil, based on the current mix of 90 % triglyceride oils and 10 % concentrates, suggests that by 2025 the demand for crude fish oil could reach 450 000 t or more if the amount of concentrate production increases.

There are several prescription-grade fish oil products in the pipeline moving towards US FDA approval (in fact, Amarin's AMR101 product, now called Vascepa®, received US FDA approval on July 26, 2012) (Amarin, 2012) and if these products gain market acceptance (they are >90 % omega-3) that will put a strain on the source of acceptable oils or perhaps force the utilization other marine oil sources.

The production of Peruvian anchovy oil has ranged from a low of 175 000 to a high of 350 000 mt over the same 10-year period with a five-year average of 295 000 mt. At some point, it is possible that all the Peruvian anchovy oil will be diverted into the omega-3 market. However, that much demand will increase the price and, as has happened before, the buyers will begin looking for substitutes. There are other oils suitable for this market, but they are not the 'low hanging fruit' or easily accessible oils. It will take some effort to get these oils into this market and, if there is genuine concern about the supply, then now is the time to start 'cultivating' these alternative sources.

2.4 Current and alternative marine oils

The remainder of this chapter will deal with some of these alternative sources of omega-3 oils. Some of these oils might be considered targets of last resort because of the high levels of saturates and mono-unsaturates. However, there are a number of other oils that could be considered 'borderline'. In other words, they have a sufficient amount of omega-3 to support the market, but the cost to extract or concentrate these fatty acids will be somewhat higher than the costs for the Peruvian anchovy, and there are other oils (for example tuna) that are simply being burned as fuel oil. The use of these marginal oils will depend on finding markets for the higher levels of by-product fatty acids. If a market can be developed for the saturates and monounsaturates, separately from the omega-3 market, then the economics of producing the omega-3 concentrates from these oils will be more competitive.

In all cases described, there is a need to establish a 'what if' scenario so that all the calculations are on the same level. For this chapter, I have used the following conservative assumptions:

- Edible fish yield 46 % by-product which contains 2 % recoverable oil.
- Fish destined for the reduction industry are 100 % usable and contain 5 % recoverable oil.
- Fish livers represent 13 % of the fish and contain 50 % oil.
- Fish heads represent 15 % of the fish and contain 10 % oil.
- Krill is converted to krill meal and is 100 % usable. It contains 5 % lipid but only 2 % is recovered.
- Squid yields 25 % by-product which contains 2 % recoverable oil.

2.5 Krill and single-cell marine oils

2.5.1 Krill

Krill is considered the largest biomass in the world (estimated to be about 500 mmt) and has been utilized in Japan for centuries. FAO did not start keeping statistics on krill until the early 1970s when there was a global initiative to find unexploited marine sources of protein. Because of the size of the biomass, krill was considered one of the sources with great possibilities. Landings increased rapidly during the mid-1970s until mid-1980s with research conducted on the protein fraction in the USSR and eastern European countries on food and animal feed products. Unfortunately the products ran into regulatory problems because of high fluoride in the krill meat and shell and the US FDA requirement that krill products be treated as food additives instead of foods. The catch dropped off in the mid-1980s until the fluoride issue was resolved and then quickly increased. The collapse of the Soviet Union in the 1990s essentially ended the exploitation of krill since the main participants in the fishery were the Soviet Union and the eastern European countries and Japan. In recent times the catch has been gradually increasing but has not reached those previous levels. The potential exists, and the use of krill oil in the omega-3 market is expected to further exploit the large biomass. The Antarctic krill total acceptable catch (TAC) is about 6 mmt with a precautionary trigger limit of about 1 mmt. The five-year average catch has been about 142 000 t and, while the 2011–2012 season forecast was for 401 000 t, the preliminary catch only reached 156 000 t. The historical growth in the catch of Antarctic krill is shown in Fig. 2.11.

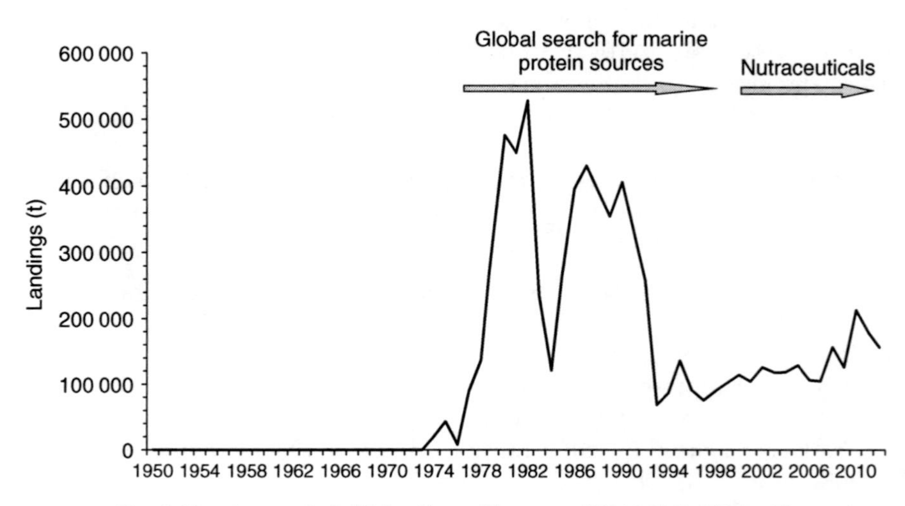

Fig. 2.11 Antarctic krill landings. (Sources: CCAMLR 2012a, b)

Table 2.3 Antarctic krill catch, 5-year average

Species	Country and % of krill catch	Total landings listed countries (mmt)	100 % by-product (mmt)	2 % oil yield (t)
Antarctic krill, 5 year average landings[1]	Japan (19 %), South Korea (26 %), Norway (36 %), Poland (5 %), Russian Federation (4 %), Ukraine (8 %), China (1 %), India (2 %)	0.142	0.142	2840
Antarctic krill, 2012 preliminary landings[2]		0.156	0.156	3120
Antarctic krill precautionary limit 2012[2]		1.0	1.0	20000

Sources: [1]CCAMLR, 2012a; [2]CCAMLR, 2012b.

Today, the targeting of krill for their oil has increased dramatically because of the interest in krill phospholipids. Much of this increase has been due to the increased Norwegian catch. The 10-year average catch shows Norway accounting for 27 % while the five-year average catch has Norway at 36 % with Japan and South Korea as the other major players in the fishery. This can be seen in Table 2.3.

According to GOED (2012), 999 t of krill oil were shipped in 2009. Neptune Bioresources, Aker Biomarine, Enzymotec and Rimfrost/Olympic Seafood are all expanding production capacity. There are several possible oil products that can be produced from krill, and the fatty acid profile of these products is shown in Table 2.4.

2.5.2 Single-cell oils

There have been many reports in the literature describing the potential for single-cell oils as a possible substitute for crude petroleum. Weyer *et al.* (2010) reported that while the literature has been promoting microbial oil production as 38000 gallons/acre/year (134.5 t per acre per year the theoretical value), a more realistic range covering different latitudes was in the 4350–5700 gallons/acre/year (15–20 t per acre per year) range. A benchmark 5000 t per year would require 250–323 acres if production was in open ponds. Vegetable oils, on the other hand, have been promoted (depending on the crop) as being able to supply 48 (soybean)–635 (palm) gallons per acre per year or 0.17–2.22 t per acre per year (Christi, 2007). Of course,

Table 2.4 Omega-3 fatty acid content of krill oil products

Species	% Total fatty acids								
	Saturates	Monoenes	C18:3 n-3	C18:4 n-3	C20:5 n-3	C22:5 n-3	C22:6 n-3	EPA+DHA	Total omega-3
Whole krill oil[1]	24	19	1		15	1	6	21	24
Whole krill oil[2]	35	28		4	17	1	10	27	31
Whole krill lipid[3]	37	30	1	3	15	1	8	23	28
Phospholipid fraction[3]	18	20			23	1	33	56	58
Triglyceride fraction[3]	46	38	1	3	4		1	5	10

Sources: [1]Aker Biomarine Antarctic AS, 2010; [2]Neptune Technologies & Bioresources, 2008; [3]Sclabos *et al.*, 2011.

normal soybean oil and palm oil would not provide any long-chain omega-3 fatty acids.

During the development stage to produce biofuels from single-cell oils, it became apparent that some of these oils could possibly fit into the overall development of the omega-3 market. Many companies have spent a great deal of time and effort collecting samples of micro-organisms that have the potential to produce oils in high volume, with lipid contents reaching 50–60 %. The lipid composition of these organisms can be manipulated by the growing conditions and composition of the nutrients fed to them. Several organisms are already being used in the omega-3 industry and they, have been successful in this market, although primarily in niche markets. However, we are now witnessing the crossover from the biofuels industry to the omega-3 industry by a number of companies. In order to compete in the bio-energy market you must have large volumes of product produced at a relatively low price (the commodity market). Target prices of US$2/gallon (US$0.565/kg) are difficult to achieve without government subsidies. When you look at the omega-3 market, crude fish oils are selling for US$1.50–2.00/kg and higher, and products in the omega-3 market for US$5–15/kg. So the omega-3 market is attractive because the potential selling price will be much higher than the biofuel market and it is not necessary to produce commodity volumes of the lipid.

For the photobioreactor (PBR), we should assume the following conditions:

- Production 2000 h/year.
- Turnaround 72 h = 28 batches per year.
- 50 % lipid in the biomass.
- 200 g/l dry biomass (1.7 lb/gal).
- 100 g/l oil (0.85 lb/gal).

We can compare the approximate production of oil from PBR to that from open ponds (OP). This can be seen in Table 2.5.

Table 2.5 Comparison of photobioreactors and open ponds for the production of single-cell oils

	Photobioreactor (PBR)		Open ponds (OP)	
Volume	100 m^3 = 100000 l		14 acres	
2012 cost, US$	17.52/gal	5.02/kg oil	9.28/gal	2.66/kg oil
Future target cost, US$	>10.00/gal	>2.86/kg oil	5.45/gal	1.56/kg oil
Production	280 t of oil per year		280 t of oil per year	

Sources: Haq, 2012; Rapier, 2012.

There are many potential organisms that can be used for the production of single-cell oils and the companies involved in this developing industry have culture libraries of these organisms capable of producing a variety of oils with different fatty acid profiles. Table 2.6 compares the fatty acid composition of several single-cell organisms being used for the production of these oils.

2.6 Wild fish and other marine oils

Fish oils are still the main source of omega-3 fatty acids. The following species-specific catch tables are based on the UN's FAO statistical database (FAO, 2012). This data is usually about two years behind since it takes that long to accumulate and process the data from all the participating countries. For this chapter we have used a 10-year average figure for the landings (2001–2010). The FAO data, while country specific for landings, is not necessarily country specific for fish oil production. The fish body oil nei represents 52 % of the fish oil production and includes some major sources of omega-3 oils. This makes it difficult to break out the fish oil production by species. On the other hand, statistical publications are very specific about volumes of fish oil production by country but do not identify the species and, for some countries, there are multiple species being landed and processed and possibly naturally blended.

So the data in the following tables are estimates of what the oil production might be, based on the assumption that, except for the known species used specifically for fishmeal and oil production, the fish are used for edible purposes and the calculations for by-product and fish oil are done according to the outline previously mentioned in this chapter. The purpose of the following detailed tables is to demonstrate that there are other sources of potential omega-3 oils, should the traditional sources become less available. However, these other sources might require further work to develop the resource and market.

2.6.1 Anchovy

When we look at the global catch of anchovy which fall into the *Engraulidae* family we find that Peru, Chile, Ecuador and Panama account for about 73 % of the 11.16 mmt landed, which means that other countries who land anchovy represent 27 % of those landings or 3.11 mmt. The 27 % is represented by over 60 countries but seven of them account for 20 %. If we assume that these countries use their anchovy for fishmeal and oil purposes, then using the previously designated 'what if' data we find that there is a potential 156 000 mt source of 'other' anchovy oil. Table 2.7 shows these other sources. Data from the literature show that all of these other anchovy species could be suitable substitutes for or additions to the current Peruvian anchovy fish oil. This can be seen in Table 2.8.

Table 2.6 Omega-3 fatty acid content of potential single-cell oil sources

Species	% Total fatty acids								
	Saturates	Mono-unsaturates	C18:3 n-3	C18:4 n-3	C20:5 n-3	C22:5 n-6	C22:6 n-3	EPA+DHA	Total omega-3
Ulkenia[1]	39					11	46	46	47
Schizochytrium[2]	35	3		1	3	14	35	38	39
Nannochloropsis[4]	28	31			35			35	35
Nannochloropsis oceanica[4]	30	29			19			19	19
Schizochytrium[3]	37	2			3	14	38	41	42
Porphyridium cruentum[7]	45	4			20			20	21
Chlorella minutissima [5]	30	26			34			34	34
Thraustochytrid[6]	37	3			2	16	37	39	41
Porphyridium aerugineum[7]	39	4			24			24	25
Isochrysis galbana[8]	20	16	4	13	1	1	16	17	33
Pavlova[8]	21	16	2	4	18		13	31	37
Phaeodactylum tricornutum[8]	28	29		3	28			28	32
Rhodomonas baltica[8]	17	4	12	5	4	2		4	22
Nannochloropsis oceanica[8]	37	23	1		23			23	24
Schizochytrium[9]	42	5			1	8	40	41	42
Crypthecodinium cohnii[10]	38	17					42	42	42
Schizochytrium[10]	32	1			3	16	40	43	44
Yarrowia lipolytica[11]	6	7	4		36			36	43
Chlorella protothecoides[12]	15	68	1						1
Marine *Chlorella*[13]	23	27	1		37			37	39

Sources: [1]Lonza, 2010; [2]Martek, 2003; [3]Doughman *et al.*, 2007; [4]Bae and Hur, 2011; [5]Seto *et al.*, 1984; [6]Miller *et al.*, 2008; [7]Klyacbko-Gurvlch *et al.*, 1994; [8]Patil *et al.*, 2007; [9]Ocean Nutrition Canada, 2011; [10]Ryan *et al.*, 2009; [11]DuPont, 2010; [12]Solazyme, 2010; [13]Makuta and Fujita, 1986.

Table 2.7 Anchovy, *Engraulidae* family, 10-year average landings

Species	Country and % of *Engraulidae* catch	Total landings listed countries (mmt)	By-product (mmt)*	5 % oil yield (t)*
Peruvian anchovy (73 %)*	Chile (11 %), Peru (61 %), Ecuador + Panama (1 %)	8.05	8.05	402 500
Japanese anchovy (14 %)	China (8 %), Japan (4 %), South Korea (2 %)	1.48	1.48	74 000
European anchovy (5 %)	Turkey (3 %)	0.60	0.60	30 000
Stolephorus anchovies nei (2 %)	Indonesia (2 %)	0.20	0.20	10 000
Southern African anchovy (2 %)	South Africa (2 %)	0.23	0.23	11 500
Other anchovy (5 %)		0.60	0.60	30 000
Total		11.16		558 000

*Assuming 100 % converted to fishmeal and fish oil and 5 % oil yield.
Source: FAO, 2012.

Table 2.8 Omega-3 fatty acid content of oils and lipids from anchovy

Species	% Total fatty acids								
	Saturates	Mono-unsaturates	C18:3 n-3	C18:4 n-3	C20:5 n-3	C22:5 n-3	C22:6 n-3	EPA+DHA	Total omega-3
Peruvian anchovy[1]	31	25	1	2	22	2	9	31	36
European anchovy[2]	31	19	2		8		19	27	29
European anchovy[3]	34	20	2		11		16	28	29
European anchovy[4]	31	33	2	1	7	1	12	19	23
Brazil enchova[5]	33	37	3		4	2	13	17	23
Northern anchovy[6]	41	20	1		16	3	16	32	35
Peruvian anchovy[7]	31	24	1	3	17	2	9	26	34
European anchovy[8]	36	29	1	1	10	1	16	26	30

Sources: [1]Bimbo, 1998; [2]Kose, personal communication, 2011; [3]Tufan *et al.*, 2011; [4]Ustiin *et al.*, 1996; [5]Visentainer *et al.*, 2007; [6]Litz, 2008; [7]Ackman, 2005; [8]Oksuz and Ozyılmaz, 2010.

2.6.2 Sardine/pilchard and other clupeoids

Sardines and pilchards fall into the *Clupeidae* family. This includes sardines, pilchards, menhaden, herring, shad, sprat and other *Clupeidae* fish. Sardines and pilchards are landed by 11 countries and they represent 30 % of the landings. Atlantic and Gulf menhaden represent 7 % of the *Clupeidae* fish and are caught primarily in the USA, although other menhaden landings have been reported in Argentina and Brazil. Menhaden, sprat and thread herring are caught for fishmeal and oil production while the other *Clupeidae* fish may be used for food products. Using the previous described 'what if' calculations we have a potential 175 100 t of fish oil. However, at the present time, herring, sprat and shad might not be suitable because of the low omega-3 content of the oil. This reduces the total sardine/pilchard oil potential to 129 900 t. These calculations are shown in Table 2.9.

Herring, sprat and shad combined represent 24 % of the *Clupeidae* landings, but the oils are relatively low in omega-3. Atlantic menhaden is a better source of omega-3 than Gulf menhaden; however, Gulf menhaden should not be discounted. India, Indonesia, Malaysia and the Philippines account for almost 10 % of the *Clupeidae* landings and could offer about 17 000 t of oil. The sardinella group in this region is rich in EPA and DHA; however, the Indian oil sardine and fringescale sardinella seem to be richer sources than the Bali sardine. It is already well known that the Chilean sardine, South African/Namibian pilchard, Pacific sardine and the Japanese sardine are rich sources of omega-3. Thread herring and Pacific sardine from Mexico might also be an interesting possibility for omega-3 production. At one time, Pacific sardine oil routinely contained an 18:12 EPA–DHA composition. The fatty acid profiles of these oils are shown in Table 2.10.

2.6.3 Mackerels

Mackerel fall into the *scombridae* family and include chub, Atlantic, Indian and Spanish mackerels. Chub mackerel is the primary species representing about 43 % of the landings. Chub mackerel are caught by 10 countries with Chile, China, South Korea and Japan accounting for 74 % of the total landings. Atlantic mackerel account for 17 % of the mackerel landings with Norway, Ireland and the UK accounting for about 59 % of the landings. Indian mackerels account for about 13 % of the mackerel landings with Malaysia, India, the Philippines and Thailand accounting for about 77 % of the landings. This can be seen in Table 2.11. Indian and Chub mackerels seem to offer the best possibilities as new sources of omega-3 oils. This can be seen in Table 2.12.

2.6.4 Squid

Squid are mollusks and about 3.5 mmt are landed annually by about 93 countries. China, South Korea, Taiwan, Peru, Japan, Argentina, Thailand

Table 2.9 Sardine/pilchards and other members of the *Clupeidae* family, 10-year average landings

Species	Country and % of *Clupeidae* catch	Total landings listed countries (mmt)	By-product (mmt)	2 % oil yield (t)
Herring	Canada (2 %), Denmark (1 %), Iceland (3 %), Russian Federation (2 %), Sweden (1 %), USA (1 %), Netherlands (1 %), Norway (8 %), UK (1 %), Germany (1 %), Finland (1 %), Faeroe Islands (1 %), Chile (5 %)	2.64	1.21	24 200
Sardine/pilchard	China (2 %), India (3 %), Mexico (5 %), Morocco (7 %), South Africa (2 %), USA (1 %), Portugal (1 %)	2.64	1	20 000
Sardinellas	Indonesia (3 %), Thailand (3 %), Philippines (3 %), Nigeria (1 %), Netherlands (1 %), Venezuela + Bolivia (1 %), Senegal (1 %)	1.98	0.91	18 200
Gulf menhaden	USA (5 %)	0.48	0.48	76 800
Atlantic menhaden	USA (2 %)	0.21	0.21	10 500
Sprat	Denmark (2 %), Sweden (1 %), Poland (1 %)	0.79	0.79	15 800
Shad/alewife	Bangladesh (3 %)	0.56	0.26	5200
Thread herring	Brazil (3 %), Cuba (1 %), Ecuador (7 %), Mexico (70 %), Panama (16 %), USA (1 %), Venezuela and Bolivia (3 %)	0.22	0.22	4400
Total		9.52		175 100

Source: FAO, 2012.

Table 2.10 Omega-3 fatty acid content of oils and lipids from sardines/pilchards and other members of the *Clupeidae* family

Species	% Total fatty acids								
	Saturates	Mono-unsaturates	C18:3 n-3	C18:4 n-3	C20:5 n-3	C22:5 n-3	C22:6 n-3	EPA+DHA	Total omega-3
Chilean sardine[1]	32	23	2	3	11	2	17	28	35
Indian oil sardine[2,4,5]	39	22	2	2	15	2	14	29	36
Bali sardinella[3]	47	29			3		14	17	
Fringescale sardinella[4]	36	11			12		33	45	
Brazil sardine[6]	40	20	2		9	1	23	32	35
Chilean sardine[7]	38	25	3		19	3	3	22	29
Sprat[8]	26	47	2		6	1	9	15	18
Japanese sardine[9]	33	28	1	4	12	2	12	24	31
Atlantic herring[9]	28	49	1	4	6	1	6	12	19
Thread herring[10]	42	20	1	1	6	2	19	25	29
Spanish sardine[10]	38	17	1	1	6	1	27	33	36
Pacific sardine[11]	41	21	1		19	4	10	29	34
South African pilchard[12]	30	24	1	2	19	2	6	25	34
Portuguese sardine [12]	31	28	1	3	11	1	13	24	32
North Sea herring [12]	21	54	2	3	7	1	7	14	21
Japanese sardine[12]	31	28	1	2	17	2	10	27	33
Pacific herring[13]	29	47		1	8	1	10	18	20
Pacific herring[13]	26	48		1	9	1	9	18	21
Japanese sardine[14]	33	29		2	17		7	24	
Japanese sardine[15]	25	29	1	3	13	2	7	20	27
Black Sea sprat[16]	31	32	1				17	17	19
Black Sea shad[16]	31	35					21	21	22
Atlantic menhaden[17]	32	22	1	3	13	2	10	23	32
Gulf menhaden[17]	31	25	1	2	13	2	7	20	27
Gulf of California sardine[18]	32	24		2	20		12	32	35

Sources: [1]Ganga *et al.*, 1998; [2]Chakraborty *et al.*, 2010; [3]Khoddami *et al.*, 2009; [4]Som, 2010; [5]Liyanage *et al.*, 1989; [6]Visentainer *et al.*, 2007; [7]Cornejo, personal communication, 2012; [8]Bimbo, 1998; [9]Ando *et al.*, 1992; [10]Hale, 1984; [11]Litz, 2008; [12]Ackman, 2005; [13]Huynh *et al.*, 2007; [14]Hayashi and Kishimura, 1993; [15]Toru Takagi, personal communication, 1993; [16]Stancheva *et al.*, 2012; [17]Bimbo, 1989; [18]Gámez-Mezaa *et al.*, 1999.

Table 2.11 Mackerel, *Scombridae* family, 10-year average landings

Species	Country and % of *Scombridae* catch	Total landings listed countries (mmt)	By-product (mmt)	2 % oil yield (t)
Atlantic mackerel 17 %	Denmark (1 %), Germany (1 %), Ireland (2 %), Netherlands (1 %), Norway (4 %), Russian Federation (1 %), Spain (1 %), UK (4 %), Canada (1 %), Faeroe Islands (1 %), Iceland (1 %), USA (1 %)	0.69	0.32	6400
Chub mackerel 43 %	Chile (7 %), China (10 %), Ecuador (1 %), Japan (11 %), South Korea (4 %), Morocco (2 %), Peru (2 %), Russian Federation (1 %), Taiwan (1 %)	1.80	0.83	16 600
Indian mackerels 13 %	Malaysia (3 %), India (2 %), Indonesia (1 %), Pakistan (1 %), Philippines (2 %), Thailand (3 %)	0.53	0.24	4800
Other mackerel 27 %	Other countries	1.15	0.48	9600
Total		4.17	1.65	33 000

Source: FAO, 2012.

Table 2.12 Omega-3 fatty acid content of oils and lipids from various mackerel

Species	% Total fatty acids								
	Saturates	Mono-unsaturates	C18:3 n-3	C18:4 n-3	C20:5 n-3	C22:5 n-3	C22:6 n-3	EPA+DHA	Total omega-3
Indian mackerel[1]	39	25	1	2	11	2	14	25	29
Indian mackerel[2]	33	18	2	2	9	1	19	28	35
Spanish mackerel[2]	47	26	1	1	5	1	14	27	22
Spotted mackerel[3]	36	22		1	6	2	18	24	27
Atlantic mackerel[4]	30	30	2		8	1	12	20	22
Chub mackerel[5]	35	23	1	1	5	3	21	26	30
Mackerel[6]	24	47	1	4	7	1	8	15	14

Sources: [1]Nisa and Asadullah, 2011; [2]Liyanage *et al.*, 1989; [3]Osako *et al.*, 2006; [4]Khiari, 2010; [5]Hale and Brown, 1983; [6]Bimbo, 1998.

and Chile account for about 68 % of the landings. Squid has less waste than other species; assuming 25 % by-product and a 2 % oil yield would yield about 18 000 t of potential squid oil. According to the FAO database, the five-year average production of squid oil is about 600 t with most of it produced in South Korea and Japan. According to Uddin *et al.* (2010), on a dry basis squid viscera can be as high as 40 % lipid. The potential yields and catch data are shown in Table 2.13. Squid oil is a rich source of omega-3 fatty acids with very high levels of DHA. This seems to range across most of the squid species as can be seen in Table 2.14.

2.6.5 Jack and horse mackerels

Chilean jack mackerel (jurel), also called horse mackerel, is the primary species in the *Carangidae* group and represents about 52 % of the total landings. There is very little information on the other species, but it is assumed that if the fish are being used for food then the by-products either are or could be converted into fishmeal and oil, especially in the countries where the fishmeal and oil industry is well established (Chile, Japan, Peru, Ecuador, Ireland, Namibia and South Africa). Catch data, locations and potential yields are shown in Table 2.15.

Except for Chilean jack mackerel, there is very little information on the fatty acid composition of the fat in horse mackerel. Perhaps the by-products are processed with other species and a mixed fish oil is produced. One paper from authors in Spain and Norway reported that wild Mediterranean horse mackerel tend to congregate around fish cages feeding on juvenile fish and perhaps fish pellets from the cages (Fernandez-Jover *et al.*, 2007). The authors sampled the wild fish from areas around the cages and control areas with no fish cages and reported the differences in fatty acid composition. Chilean jack mackerel oil composition, on the other hand, is well documented and is known to be higher in DHA than in EPA. The available fatty acid data on horse mackerel is shown in Table 2.16.

2.6.6 Sand eels

Sand eels, members of the *Ammodytidae* family, are caught primarily by Denmark with smaller catches by Norway and Sweden. In Denmark, they are also called tobis and, at certain times of the year, the oil is very red in colour. Sand eel catch data is shown in Table 2.17. In 2012, the sand eel quota was reduced to 0.18 mmt which would reduce the oil yield to 9 000 mt in Table 2.17. The fatty acid composition of sand eel is borderline and could be used as a source of omega-3 fatty acids. This is shown in Table 2.18.

2.6.7 Atlantic and Pacific cod

Cod is a member of the *Gadidae* family. The Atlantic cod is a food fish and its liver oil is the primary source of cod liver oil. The livers represent

Table 2.13 Squid, 10-year average landings

Species	Country and % of squid catch	Total landings listed countries (mmt)	25 % By-product (mmt)	2 % Oil yield (t)
Argentine shortfin squid	Argentina (5 %), China (3 %), Japan (1 %), South Korea (3 %), Taiwan (4 %)	0.59	0.15	3000
Cephalopods nei	China (1 %), India (2 %), Vietnam (6 %)	0.34	0.09	1800
Common squids nei	Indonesia (1 %), Philippines (2 %), Thailand (2 %)	0.22	0.06	1200
Bobtail squids nei	China (5 %), Thailand (1 %)	0.36	0.09	1800
Japanese flying squid	Japan (7 %), South Korea (6 %)	0.45	0.11	2200
Jumbo flying squid	Chile (3 %), China (2 %), Japan (1 %), Mexico (2 %), Peru (8 %), Taiwan (1 %)	0.64	0.16	3200
Various squids nei	Japan (1 %), USA (2 %), Falkland Islands (1 %), Russian Federation (2 %), China (10 %), South Korea (1 %), Malaysia (2 %)	0.58	0.15	3000
Others		0.30	0.08	1600
Total		3.48		17800

Source: FAO, 2012.

Table 2.14 Omega-3 fatty acid content of oils and lipids from various squid

Species	% Total fatty acids								
	Saturates	Mono-unsaturates	C18:3 n-3	C18:4 n-3	C20:5 n-3	C22:5 n-3	C22:6 n-3	EPA+DHA	Total omega-3
Squid[1]	31	28	1	4	12	1	19	31	37
Indian squid[5]	41	14	2		8		12	20	27
Squid[2]	25	23		1	2		31	33	36
Squid[3]	36	8			10	1	43	53	54
Arrow squid[8]	31	20			14	1	38	52	52
Flying squid[4]	26	8			18		44	62	
Magister armhook squid medium[6]	22	35	1	1	13		20	33	37
North Pacific bobtail squid[6]	23	29			19	1	20	39	41
Squid[7]	28	34		1	14		13	27	
Broad squid[8]	35	14			14	1	34	48	49

Sources: [1]Adlercreutz and Lyberg, 2008; [2]Sigurgisladottir and Palmadottir, 1993; [3]Soltan and Gibson, 2008; [4]Dunne *et al.*, 2010; [5]Chedoloh *et al.*, 2011; [6]Iverson *et al.*, 2002; [7]Hayashi and Kishimura, 1993; [8]Vlieg and Body, 1988.

Table 2.15 Jack and horse mackerel, 10-year average landings

Species	Country and % of total jack and horse mackerel catch	Total landings listed countries (mmt)	46 % by-product (mmt)	2 % oil yield (t)
Chilean jack mackerel*	Chile (35 %), China (3 %), Ecuador (1 %), Peru (6 %) Vanuatu (2 %), Faeroe Islands (1 %), Germany (1 %), Lithuania (1 %), Netherlands (1 %), Poland (1 %)	1.85	1.85	37 800
Japanese jack mackerels	China (2 %), Japan (6 %), South Korea (1 %)	0.31	0.14	2800
Atlantic horse mackerel	Iceland (1 %), Ireland (1 %), Netherlands (2 %), Norway (1 %)	0.25	0.12	2400
Cape horse mackerel	Namibia (8 %), South Africa (1 %)	0.34	0.16	3200
Jack and horse mackerel nei	Angola (1 %), India (1 %), Lithuania (1 %), Mauritania (1 %), New Zealand (1 %), Russian Federation (2 %), Spain (1 %), Thailand (1 %), Cyprus (1 %), Latvia (1 %)	0.46	0.21	4200
Carangids nei	India (1 %), Malaysia (1 %), Philippines (2 %), Thailand (1 %)	0.23	0.11	2200
Others		0.11	0.05	1000
Total		3.55		52 800

*The 2012 quota for Chilean jack mackerel was reduced to 0.30 mmt plus an additional 0.12 mmt within Peru's 200 mile exclusion zone. That quota would reduce the Chilean jack mackerel catch to 0.42 mmt and result in an oil yield of 8400 t, reducing the total oil available to 24 000 t.
Source: FAO, 2012.

Table 2.16 Omega-3 fatty acid content of oil and lipids from various jack and horse mackerel

Species	% Total fatty acids								
	Saturates	Monounsaturates	C18:3 n-3	C18:4 n-3	C20:5 n-3	C22:5 n-3	C22:6 n-3	EPA+DHA	Total omega-3
Chilean jack mackerel[3]	33	30	1	1	11	3	18	29	34
Jack mackerel[1]	26				9	3	19	28	
Jack mackerel[2]	26	33			11	2	12	23	25
Jack mackerel[4]	31	27	1	2	13	2	15	28	33
Mediterranean horse mackerel[5]	36	16			6	1	35	41	44
Black Sea horse mackerel[6]	38	23					18	18	20
Black Sea horse mackerel[7]	38	38	1		4	1	15	19	21

Sources: [1]O'Connor *et al.*, 2007; [2]Nichols, 2007; [3]Cornejo, personal communication, 2012; [4]Bimbo, 1998; [5]Fernandez-Jover *et al.*, 2007; [6]Stancheva *et al.*, 2012; [7]Huang *et al.*, 2012.

Table 2.17 Sand eel, *Ammodytes* family, 10-year average landings

Species	Country and % of total sand eel catch	Total landings listed countries (mmt)	100 % by-product (mmt)	5 % oil yield (t)
Sand eels	Denmark (50 %), Norway (10 %), Sweden (4 %), Faeroe Islands (1 %), Germany (1 %)	0.48	0.48	24000
Pacific sand lance	China (23 %, Japan (9 %), South Korea (1 %)	0.24	0.24	12000
Total		0.72		36000

Source: FAO, 2012.

Table 2.18 Omega-3 fatty acid content of sand eel oil and lipids

Species	% Total fatty acids								
	Saturates	Mono-unsaturates	C18:3 n-3	C18:4 n-3	C20:5 n-3	C22:5 n-3	C22:6 n-3	EPA+DHA	Total omega-3
Sand eel[1]	23	42	1	5	11	1	11	22	29
Sand eel[2]	24	37	1	6	13	1	12	25	32
Pacific sand eel total lipid[3]	29	24	1	3	13	1	19	32	44

Sources: [1]Bimbo, 1998; [2]Jakobsen, 2001; [3]Iverson *et al.*, 2002.

about 13 % of the fish weight and contain about 50 % oil. There is a general shortage of cod liver oil that is partially satisfied by other fish liver oils not easily identified (nei) by FAO. The Pacific cod is the third largest fishery in Alaska, is regulated by quota, MSC certified and the oil could supplement Atlantic cod liver oil. Catch data for cod is shown in Table 2.19. The fatty acid profiles for Atlantic and Pacific cod liver oil are similar. This is shown in Table 2.20.

2.6.8 Wild Pacific salmon

On average, almost 1 mmt of wild Pacific salmon (five species) are landed each year. The USA (Alaska), Japan and the Russian Federation account for 97 % of these landings. Most of the oil in the wild Pacific salmon is in the heads which represent about 15 % of the fish weight. The average fat content in the heads is 10 %. For this chapter we assumed that 6 % is recoverable. The catch and potential yields for wild Pacific salmon are shown in Table 2.21. Wild Pacific salmon have a moderate amount of omega-3 fatty acids in the oil. However, the fishery is MSC certified and the oil is in demand, especially in the 'virgin' or natural form (unrefined). The fatty acid profiles of wild Pacific salmon oil are shown in Table 2.22.

2.6.9 Walleye (Alaska) pollock

Alaska pollock is a member of the *Gadidae* family and represents a sizeable resource of fish. Pollock is about 32 % of the US total landings and 58 % of the Alaska landings. Alaska pollock livers represent about 10 % of the weight of the fish and contain, on average, about 50 % lipid. The US fishery is MSC certified and the Russian fishery is under evaluation at this time. Table 2.23 outlines the catch and potential yield of fish oil from the Alaska pollock. Pollock oil can be used as a liver oil or a fish oil. The fatty acid profile is borderline in the omega-3 area, but there are Alaska pollock omega-3 products on the market today. Table 2.24 presents some fatty acid data on Alaska pollock oil.

2.6.10 Norway pout and blue whiting

The Norway Pout fishery is relatively small and confined principally to Norway and Denmark. The by-products are probably blended into other fishery by-products and not available as a separate product. Blue whiting is a large fishery primarily confined to the EU and northern European countries with a smaller catch controlled by 25 other countries. Table 2.25 reports the landings and potential yield of fish oil from these fisheries. Blue whiting fish oil is a potential source of omega-3 fatty acids and Table 2.26 presents some fatty acid profile data on blue whiting, southern blue whiting and Norway pout.

Table 2.19 Cod, *Gadidae* family, 10-year average landings

Species	Country and % of cod catch	Total landings listed countries (mmt)	13 % liver waste (mmt)	50 % oil yield (t)
Atlantic cod	Canada (2 %), Denmark (3 %), Faeroe Islands (3 %), France (1 %), Germany (1 %), Greenland (1 %), Iceland (16 %), Latvia 1 %, Norway (18 %), Poland (1 %), Russian Federation (16 %), Spain (1 %), Sweden (1 %), UK (2 %), USA (1 %)	0.87	0.11	55 000
Pacific cod*	Japan (3 %), Russian Federation (5 %), USA (19 %), South Korea (1 %)	0.35	0.05	25 000
Other cod		0.03	0.00	1950
Total		1.25		81 950

*The Gulf of Alaska Pacific cod quota was 59 563 t in 2010 (giving a potential 3872 t of oil).
Source: FAO, 2012.

Table 2.20 Omega-3 fatty acid content of cod liver oils

Species	% Total fatty acids								
	Saturates	Mono-unsaturates	C18:3 n-3	C18:4 n-3	C20:5 n-3	C22:5 n-3	C22:6 n-3	EPA+DHA	Total omega-3
Atlantic cod[1]	23	22	1	1	15	1	28	43	46
Cod liver, Atlantic[2]	18	43	3	3	11	1	13	24	31
Cod liver, Pacific	9	54	1	1	10	3	13	20	30
Pacific cod[3]	22	28			11		27	38	42
Cod liver oil Spain[4]	21	43	1	2	9	1	11	20	25
Cod liver oil Sweden[5]	21	44	2	3	10	1	15	25	27
Cod liver oil Poland[5]	19	52		2	9	1	12	21	23
Cod liver oil Poland[5]	23	44	1	2	10	3	13	23	26
Cod liver oil Iceland[5]	18	53	1	2	10	1	13	23	24

Sources: [1]Sigurgisladottir and Palmadottir, 1993; [2]Bimbo, personal data, 2011; [3]Iverson *et al.*, 2002; [4]Guil-Guerrero and Belarbi, 2001; [5]Kolanowski, 2010.

Table 2.21 Wild Pacific salmon, *Salmonidae* family, 10-year average landings

Species	Country and % of wild Pacific salmon catch	Total landings listed countries (mmt)	27 % by-product (mmt)	6 % oil yield (t)
Pacific salmon, five species	Canada (2 %), Japan (37 %), Russian Federation (25 %), USA (29 %)	0.89	0.24	14400
		OR		
Pacific salmon heads only, 15 % of the fish weight		0.89	0.13	7800

Source: FAO, 2012.

Table 2.22 Omega-3 fatty acid content of wild Pacific salmon oil

Species	% Total fatty acids								
	Saturates	Mono-unsaturates	C18:3 n-3	C18:4 n-3	C20:5 n-3	C22:5 n-3	C22:6 n-3	EPA+DHA	Total omega-3
Wild Pacific salmon[1]	21	32	1	2	9	3	11	20	27
Wild Pacific salmon[2]	18	34	1	1	8	2	8	16	22

Sources: [1]Lane, personal communication, 2012; [2]Oliveira *et al.*, 2010.

Table 2.23 Alaska pollock and saithe *Gadidae* family, 10-year average landings

Species	Country and % of Alaska pollock and saithe catch	Total landings listed countries (mmt)	66 % by-product (mmt)	5 % oil yield (t)
Alaska pollock	Japan (7 %), North Korea (2 %), South Korea (1 %), Russian Federation (35 %), USA (40 %)	2.85	1.88	94 000
Saithe	Faeroe Islands (2 %), France (1 %), Iceland (2 %), Norway (7 %)	0.41	0.27	13 500
		OR		
Pollock livers*		3.3	0.36	90 000

*Pollock livers represent about 11 % of the fish weight and contain 50 % lipid. The assumption used here is that 25 % of the lipid could be recovered. The Bering Sea/Aleutian Island quota for the USA was 1.2 mmt in 2012.
Source: FAO, 2012.

Table 2.24 Omega-3 fatty acid content of pollock oil and lipids

Species	% Total fatty acids								
	Saturates	Mono-unsaturates	C18:3 n-3	C18:4 n-3	C20:5 n-3	C22:5 n-3	C22:6 n-3	EPA+DHA	Total omega-3
Alaska pollock oil[1]	33	43	1		14	1	6	20	22
Alaska pollock liver oil[2]	15	50		1	9	1	4	13	15
Alaska pollock oil[2]	15	52		1	9	1	4	13	16
Alaska pollock oil[3]	21	43		2	9	1	6	15	18

Sources: [1]Cowger, personal communication, 2009; [2]Oliveira, 2010; [3]Bimbo, 1998.

Table 2.25 Norway pout, blue whiting and southern blue whiting, *Gadidae* family, 10-year average landings

Species	Country and % of Norway pout, blue whiting or southern blue whiting catch	Total landings listed countries (mmt)	100 % by-product (mmt)	2 % oil yield (t)
Norway pout	Denmark (66 %), Norway (31 %), Faeroe Islands (2 %)	0.07	0.07	1400
Blue whiting	Denmark (3 %), Faeroe Islands (14 %), France (1 %), Germany (1 %), Iceland (17 %), Ireland (2 %), Netherlands (4 %) Norway (35 %), Russian Federation (16 %) Spain (2 %), Sweden (1 %), UK (3 %)	1.7	1.70	34 000
Southern blue whiting	Argentina (26 %), Chile (22 %), Japan (21 %), New Zealand (22 %), Spain (3 %), Ukraine (3 %)	0.14	0.14	2800
Total		1.91		38 200

Source: FAO, 2012.

Table 2.26 Omega-3 fatty acid content of Norway pout, blue whiting and southern blue whiting oils and lipids

Species	% Total fatty acids								
	Saturates	Mono-unsaturates	C18:3 n-3	C18:4 n-3	C20:5 n-3	C22:5 n-3	C22:6 n-3	EPA+DHA	Total omega-3
Norway pout[1]	22	22	1	1	14	1	33	47	50
Norway pout[2]	20	44	1	3	9	1	14	23	28
Norway pout[3]	20	42	1	3	9	1	14	23	27
Blue whiting[3]	26	9			21		29	50	
Southern blue whiting[4]	24	18			8	1	40	48	50
Blue whiting[3]	20	49	1	3	7	1	8	15	19

Sources: [1]Sigurgisladottir and Palmadottir, 1993; [2]Bimbo, 1998; [3]Dunne *et al.*, 2010; [4]Vlieg and Body, 1988.

2.6.11 Blue grenadier (hoki)

The New Zealand hoki fishery is relatively small, is MSC certified and operates under a quota system. Hoki livers represent 10 % of the weight of the fish and contain up to 50 % lipid. The lipid can be very high in DHA. Table 2.27 reports the landings and potential yield of fish oil from the New Zealand hoki and Argentine hake fisheries. Table 2.28 shows the fatty acid profile of the lipid from the New Zealand hoki and Argentine hake.

2.6.12 Capelin

Capelin belong to the *Osmeridae* family which includes smelts. Capelin represent about 98 % of the landings in this family and seven countries account for most of this. Table 2.29 reports the capelin landings and potential oil yield from these fish. Capelin represents a sizeable amount of the global fish oil production. The capelin fish oil, however, is relatively low in omega-3 fatty acids. This is reported in Table 2.30.

2.6.13 Tuna and bonito

Tuna and bonito like mackerel are members of the *Scombridae* family. Tuna and bonito present a special case since they represent a number of different species. Tuna are migratory fish and are caught in all the major oceans by well over 150 countries. Some species are considered endangered, but the small tuna are considered sustainable. Table 2.31 reports the tuna and bonito landings. Skipjack and yellow fin make up about 68 % of the global landings. Tuna oil is rich in DHA, which distinguishes it from other marine oils and makes it much more attractive for the infant formula market. Table 2.32 reports the fatty acid profiles of a number of different tuna and bonito species.

2.7 Species farmed for marine oils

Farmed fish represented 32 % of the total fish landings in 2010, up from 20 % in 1999. China is the major aquaculture producer, representing about 56 % of the production followed by India and Vietnam. Figure 2.12 compares the major aquaculture-producing countries over the period 2001–2010.

2.7.1 Farmed salmon and trout

Atlantic salmon and rainbow trout represent about 6 % of the farmed fish produced globally. There is also a small amount of Pacific coho salmon

Table 2.27 New Zealand hoki and Argentine hake, *Merluccidae* family, 10-year average landings

Species	Country and % of hoki or hake catch	Total landings listed countries (mmt)	46 % by-product (mmt)	2 % oil yield (t)
Hoki (blue grenadier)	Australia (3 %), Japan (6 %), South Korea (4 %), New Zealand (81 %), Ukraine (4 %)	0.18	0.08	1600
Argentina hake	Argentina (85 %), Brazil (1 %), Falkland Islands (1 %), Spain (4 %), Uruguay (9 %)	0.07	0.03	600
Total		0.25		2200

Note: The 2011–2012 TAC for New Zealand hoki was set at 0.13 mmt which would yield about 1200 t of fish oil. The Argentine hoki fishery landed 70000 t of fish in 2011.
Source: FAO, 2012.

Table 2.28 Omega-3 fatty acid content of New Zealand hoki, Argentine hake and other hake oils or lipids

Species	% Total fatty acids								
	Saturates	Mono-unsaturates	C18:3 n-3	C18:4 n-3	C20:5 n-3	C22:5 n-3	C22:6 n-3	EPA+DHA	Total omega-3
Blue grenadier (hoki)[1]	31	18			7	2	38	45	48
Blue grenadier (hoki)[4]	30	28			5	2	31	36	38
Argentine hake[2]	22	40		4	7		14	21	29
North Sea whiting[3]	24	26	1	1	9		30	39	41
NZ hake[5]	35	51			2	1	7	9	10
Pacific hake[6]	13	20		1	6		4	10	11

Sources: [1]Nichols *et al.*, 1998; [2]Mendez, 1997; [3]Sigurgisladottir and Palmadottir, 1993; [4]Soltan and Gibson, 2008; [5] Vlieg and Body, 1988; [6] Oliveira, 2010.

Table 2.29 Capelin, *Osmeridae* family, 10-year average landings

Species	Country and % of capelin catch	Total landings listed countries (mmt)	100 % by-product (mmt)	5 % oil yield (t)
Capelin	Canada (3 %), Denmark (2 %), Faeroe Islands (4 %), Greenland (2 %), Iceland (56 %), Norway (24 %), Russian Federation (9 %)	0.89	0.89	44 500
Total		0.89		44 500

Source: FAO, 2012.

Table 2.30 Omega-3 fatty acid content of capelin oil and lipids

Species	% Total fatty acids								
	Saturates	Mono-unsaturates	C18:3 n-3	C18:4 n-3	C20:5 n-3	C22:5 n-3	C22:6 n-3	EPA+DHA	Total omega-3
Capelin oil[1]	19	57	1	1	9	1	6	15	17
Capelin total lipid[2]	25	29		1	13	2	25	38	42
Capelin[3]	18	56	1	3	8		6	14	16

Sources: [1]Jakobsen, 2001; [2]Iverson *et al.*, 2002; [3]Bimbo, 1998.

Table 2.31 Tuna and bonito, *Scombridae* family, 10-year average landings

Species	Country and % of tuna or bonito catch	Total landings listed countries (mmt)	46 % by-product (mmt)	2 % oil yield (t)
Skipjack	China (1 %), Ecuador (2 %), France (1 %), Ghana (1 %), Indonesia (5 %), Iran (1 %), Japan (6 %), South Korea (3 %), Maldives (2 %), Marshall Islands (1 %), Papua New Guinea (3 %), Philippines (3 %), Seychelles (1 %), Spain (3 %), Sri Lanka (1 %), Taiwan (3 %), USA (2 %), Vanuatu (1 %)	2.35	1.08	21 600
Albacore	Japan (1 %)	0.26	0.12	2400
Yellow fin	Ecuador (1 %), France (1 %), Indonesia (2 %), Iran (1 %), Japan (1 %), South Korea (1 %), Mexico (2 %), Papua New Guinea (1 %), Philippines (2 %), Spain (1 %), Sri Lanka (1 %), Taiwan (1 %), Venezuela and Bolivia (1 %)	1.26	0.58	11 600
Bigeye	Taiwan (1 %)	0.45	0.21	4200
Longtail	Indonesia (2 %), Iran (1 %), Thailand (1 %)	0.25	0.12	2400
Kawakawa	Indonesia (3 %), Philippines (1 %),	0.31	0.14	2800
Frigate and bullet	Indonesia (2 %)	0.35	0.16	3200
Other tuna and bonito	Other countries (3 %)	0.14	0.06	1200
Total		5.37		49 400

Source: FAO, 2012.

Table 2.32 Omega-3 fatty acid content of tuna and bonito oils and lipids

Species	% Total fatty acids								
	Saturates	Mono-unsaturates	C18:3 n-3	C18:4 n-3	C20:5 n-3	C22:5 n-3	C22:6 n-3	EPA+DHA	Total omega-3
Yellow fin tuna[1]	35	19	1	3	7	2	21	28	33
Tuna Japan[2]	27	22	1	1	6	1	29	35	38
Tuna[3]	31	28	1	2	10	2	20	30	36
Kawakawa[4]	51	22			2		15	17	
Tuna[5]	29	23	1	1	7	1	26	33	38
Tuna[6]	31	32	1	1	6	1	20	26	32
Tuna[7]	26	22	1	1	12	2	28	40	42
Albacore tuna[8]	32	29			6	1	26	32	33
Skipjack tuna[8]	33	32			8	2	20	28	30
Slender tuna[8]	31	38			8	2	14	22	24
Southern blue fin tuna[8]	33	43			3	1	13	16	17
Tuna[9]	33	28	1	1	6	2	22	28	32

Sources: [1]Liyanage *et al*., 1989; [2]Kolanowski, 2010; [3]Puleva Biotech, 2006; [4]Khoddami *et al.*, 2012; [5]Clover Corporation Ltd, 2001; [6]Ross Products Div. Abbott Laboratories, 2001; [7]Nichols, 2007; [8]Vlieg and Body, 1988; [9]Bimbo, 1998.

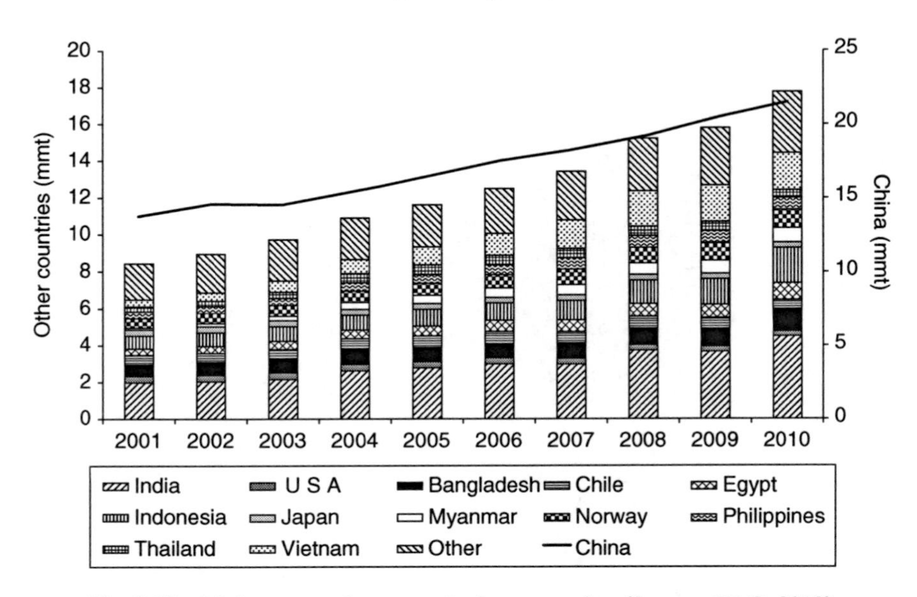

Fig. 2.12 Major aquaculture-producing countries. (Source: FAO, 2012)

produced in Chile. There is a potential (based on the 10-year average production) for about 19000 t of fish oil if all the by-products are recovered and processed. It is difficult to say how much salmon oil is actually produced globally since there are no individual statistics reported and no way to reliably estimate the oil yields. They are probably reported as fish oils not easily identified (nei). Table 2.33 reports the production of farmed salmon and trout and the potential fish oil that can be produced from the by-product.

Farmed salmon can be a relatively rich source of omega-3 fatty acids, but the level of these omega-3s will depend on what the fish are fed. One good measure of this is to look for the level of linoleic acid C18:2n-6 in the oil. Normal wild fish will have levels in the area of 1 %. Farmed fish can be as high as 9–10 % linoleic acid which would indicate that vegetable oil has been fed to the fish. As the price of fishmeal and fish oil increases, there is an incentive within the aquaculture industry to seek substitutes.

Fishmeal is a concentrated source of many nutrients including amino acids, macro and micro minerals, and lipids primarily in the omega-3 form. While herbivores can thrive on vegetable diets, the carnivorous fish have a nutritional requirement for amino acids and omega-3 fatty acids found in fish. The aquaculture industry has succeeded in replacing a large amount of the fishmeal and fish oil in the farmed fish diets, but at the expense of increasing the omega-6 content and reducing the omega-3 content of the fish flesh. The marker for the omega-6 in the farmed fish is linoleic acid and

Table 2.33 Farmed salmonids, 10-year average production

Species	Country and % of farmed salmonid production	Total landings listed countries (mmt)	46 % by-product (mmt)	2 % oil yield (t)
Atlantic salmon	Australia (1 %), Canada (5 %), Chile (15 %), Faeroe Islands (2 %), Norway (30 %), UK (7 %)	1.25	0.58	11 600
Pacific salmon (Coho)	Chile (5 %)	0.15	0.07	1400
Rainbow trout	Chile (7 %), Denmark (2 %), France (2 %), Germany (1 %), Iran (2 %), Italy (2 %), Norway (3 %), Spain (1 %), Turkey (2.58 %), USA (1.14 %)	0.61	0.28	5600
Others		0.03	0.01	0.00
Total		2.04		18 600

Source: FAO, 2012.

the higher the linoleic acid in the fish lipid, the more vegetable oil has been fed. For example, canola oil can have 15–30 %, soybean oil 48–59 %, sunflowerseed oil 48–74 % and safflowerseed oil 69–83 % linoleic acid. Fish oils, on the other hand, contain about 1–2 % linoleic acid. When these vegetable oils are substituted for fish oil in the diets of salmonids and other carnivorous fish, the fish fat incorporates the fatty acids from the diet into the fish lipids, hence the higher linoleic acid in the fat of the farmed salmonids. Table 2.34 reports the fatty acid profiles of some farmed salmon and trout. Where possible, some wild Atlantic salmon lipid composition is also included.

2.7.2 Farmed river eels

Eels are farmed in China, Japan and Taiwan among other countries. As with other farmed species, the level of omega-3 will depend on what they are fed. Table 2.35 reports the production and potential fish oil that might be produced from farmed eels. Table 2.36 reports the fatty acid composition of a number of eel species. The European eel seems to be a potential source of oil with a high omega-3 fatty acid composition.

2.7.3 Farmed catfish

Catfish are not generally considered a good source of omega-3 fatty acids since their feed is somewhat similar to poultry feed and the fat reflects the vegetable oil fatty acid profiles. Almost 2 mmt of catfish (10-year average) are produced each year globally. In 2010, 3.2 mmt were produced so catfish could be a major raw material if the omega-3 content were higher. Table 2.37 reports the various species of catfish produced and potential fish oil that might be available. Table 2.38 shows that it is possible to produce a high omega-3 catfish oil, as shown in the Japanese data.

2.7.4 Farmed fish (China)

China is the dominant player in the aquaculture sector, producing about 56 % of the farmed fish or about 17 mmt of fish (10-year average) (FAO, 2012). Various carp are the major species farmed, and they collectively represent about 79 % of the Chinese production. It is difficult to determine if any of the farmed fish generate usable waste on a scale that could supply the production of fishmeal and oil. However, collectively there could be 6 mmt of waste available and at a 2 % oil yield that would produce about 122 000 t of fish oil. Judging by the volume of tilapia fillets imported by the USA, there is the possibility that sufficient waste is generated in China. Common, grass, silver, bighead and crucian carp account for 73 % of the carp production in China. Table 2.39 reports the production and potential fish oil that could be produced from the by-products of carp in China.

Table 2.34 Omega-3 fatty acid content of various farmed salmonid oils and lipids

Species	% Total fatty acids								
	Saturates	Mono-unsaturates	C18:2 n-6	C18:3 n-3	C20:5 n-3	C22:5 n-3	C22:6 n-3	EPA+DHA	Total omega-3
Farmed salmon, Chile[1]	26	34	3	1	10	5	14	24	32
Farmed Atlantic salmon[2]	24	31	7		7	4	16	23	27
Farmed salmon Turkey[3]	28	35	11	1	3	2	17	20	24
Farmed salmon[4]				1	9	2	11	18	24
Atlantic salmon, Tasmania[5]	30	332	2		8	3	20	28	32
Rainbow trout, farmed USA[6]	28	28	12	1	5		12	17	19
Coho salmon, farmed USA	22	35	4	1	5		10	15	17
Rainbow trout and lake trout[7]			9	1	4		13	17	20
Wild Atlantic salmon[7]			3	1	5		7	12	17
Wild Atlantic salmon[8]	25	43	1	1	6	2	11	17	21
Farmed Atlantic salmon[8]	20	42	9	3	5	3	8	13	24
Farmed New Zealand King salmon[9]	17	21	4		4	1	6	10	12

Sources: [1]Pesquera Pacific Star, personal communication, 2005; [2]Nichols, 2007; [3]Ustiin *et al.*, 1996; [4]Bimbo, 2007; [5]Ho and Paul, 2009; [6]Nettleton, 2000; [7]van Vliet and Katan, 1990; [8]Tammeras, 2011; [9]Pauga, 2009.

Table 2.35 Farmed river eels, *Anguillidae* family, 10-year average production

Species	Country and % of farmed river eel catch	Total landings listed countries (mmt)	46 % by-product (mmt)	2 % oil yield (t)
All eel species	China (71 %), Denmark (1 %), Indonesia (1 %), Japan 9 %, South Korea (2 %), Netherlands (2 %), Taiwan (12 %), Italy (1 %), Malaysia (1 %)	0.24	0.11	2200
Total		0.24		2200

Source: FAO, 2012.

Table 2.36 Omega-3 fatty acid content of farmed eel oils and lipids

Species	% Total fatty acids								
	Saturates	Mono-unsaturates	C18:2 n-6	C18:3 n-3	C20:5 n-3	C22:5 n-3	C22:6 n-3	EPA+DHA	Total omega-3
European eel[1]	25	28	1		6		25	31	33
Shortfin eel[2]	30	35	4	3	4	3	6	10	18
European eel[3]			5	1	3		6	9	12

Sources: [1]Kissil *et al.*, 1987; [2]Hirt-Chabbert and Andrés, 2011; [3]van Vliet and Katan, 1990.

Table 2.37 Farmed catfish, 10-year average production

Species	Country and % of farmed catfish production	Total landings listed countries (mmt)	46 % by-products (mmt)	2 % oil yield (t)
Amur catfish	China (14 %)	0.28	0.13	2600
Hybrid catfish	Thailand (6 %)	0.12	0.06	1200
Channel catfish	China (8 %), USA (13 %)	0.42	0.19	3800
North African catfish	Nigeria (2 %), Uganda (1 %)	0.07	0.03	600
Pangas catfish	Cambodia (1 %), Indonesia (3 %), Myanmar (1 %), Vietnam (28 %)	0.64	0.29	5800
Striped catfish	Bangladesh (5 %), Thailand (1 %)	0.12	0.06	1200
Torpedo-shaped catfish	Indonesia (5 %), Malaysia (1 %), Nigeria (1 %), Vietnam (1 %)	0.16	0.07 0.07	1400 1400
Yellow catfish	China (5 %)	0.11	0.05	1000
Total		1.92		17600

Source: FAO, 2012.

Table 2.38 Omega-3 fatty acid content of farmed catfish oil and lipids

Species	% Total fatty acids								
	Saturates	Mono-unsaturates	C18:2 n-6	C18:3 n-3	C20:5 n-3	C22:5 n-3	C22:6 n-3	EPA+DHA	Total omega-3
Catfish, Japan[1]	29	16	4	1	3	3	21	24	28
Catfish Japan[1]	25	39	9	1	4	1	14	18	20
Catfish, USA[1]	29	43	13	1	1	1	4	5	6
Catfish, Thailand[1]	37	41	11				2	2	3
Tra catfish[2]	43	35	8	1		1	5	5	7
Channel catfish, farmed USA[3]	22	51	13	1	1		2	3	4
Farmed catfish oil USA[4]	24	58	14	1			1	1	2

Sources: [1]Shirai, 2011; [2]Ho and Paul, 2009; [3]Nettleton, 2000; [4]Bimbo personal information, 1994.

Table 2.39 Chinese farmed carp, *Cyprinidae* family, 10-year average production

Species	% of total Chinese farmed fish	Total landings (mmt)	46 % by-product (mmt)	2 % oil yield (t)
Bighead carp	11	1.97	0.91	18200
Black carp	2	0.29	0.13	2600
Common carp	13	2.18	1.00	20000
Crucian carp	10	1.78	0.82	16400
Grass carp	20	3.44	1.58	31600
Silver carp	19	3.13	1.44	28800
Wuchang bream	3	0.53	0.24	4800
Total		13.32	6.12	122400

Source: FAO, 2012.

As with catfish, one would not expect carp to be a rich source of omega-3 fatty acids and, for the most part, the data supports that except for bighead and silver carp. A recent paper published by Li *et al.* (2011) indicated that these carp raised in China had high levels of omega-3 fatty acids in the lipid. These two species should be of interest. The data is reported in Table 2.40.

China's production of farmed marine species (carp would be considered a freshwater species) has also been increasing over the last 10 years and, in 2010, the 800000 t represented about 5 % of the Chinese farmed fish production. The marine fish are represented by a number of species, including some not easily identified (nei) as shown in Fig. 2.13. Collectively, these fish could yield about 6000 t of fish oil which might have a relatively high omega-3 component since the marine fish require a diet which contains these fatty acids. This data is reported in Table 2.41.

2.8 Sustainability and certifications

In recent years, raw material sustainability has become a big issue in the overall seafood industry and this includes the sourcing for marine oil production. Various entities have been involved in certification programmes based on the UN's FAO Code of Conduct for Responsible Fisheries (FAO, 2011). The code is voluntary and was developed in 1995 as a set of principles for all countries, fishing entities, governmental or non-governmental organizations, and all persons concerned with the conservation of fishery resources and management of fisheries to help guide the management and development of fisheries. Generally, most certification programmes involve third

Table 2.40 Omega-3 fatty acid content of Chinese farmed carp lipids

Species	% Total fatty acids								
	Saturates	Mono-unsaturates	C18:2 n-6	C18:3 n-3	C20:5 n-3	C22:5 n-3	C22:6 n-3	EPA+DHA	Total omega-3
Crucian carp	23	35	17	3	2	1	7	9	12
Bighead carp	26	23	5	5	14	2	13	27	35
Grass carp	23	37	16	8	1	1	3	4	14
Common carp	36	42	6	3	1	1	2	3	6
Black carp	23	36	18	9	1	1		1	12
Silver carp	27	19	2	4	14	3	16	30	36

Source: Li *et al.*, 2011.

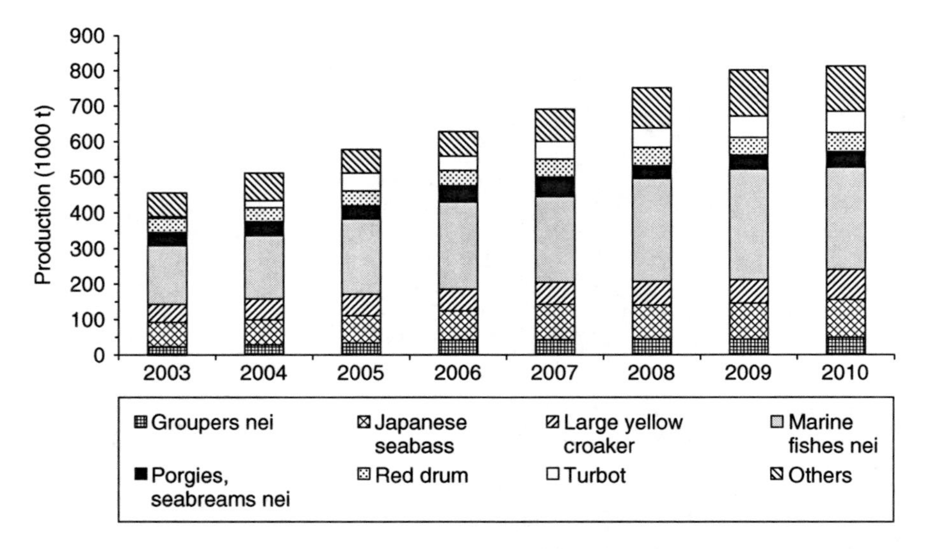

Fig. 2.13 Chinese marine fish aquaculture production. (Source: FAO, 2012)

Table 2.41 Chinese marine fish aquaculture production, 5-year and 10-year averages

Species	Production (mmt)	46 % by-product (mmt)	2 % oil yield (t)
Marine fish, 10-year average	0.59	0.27	5400
Marine fish, 5-year average	0.74	0.34	6800

Source: FAO, 2012.

parties in the assessment of the raw material source. Adherence to the Code implies that the fish are caught and processed in a sustainable manner and that the impact on the environment is minimal.

Under the Code's heading 8.4 Fishing Operations, sub-paragraph 8.4.5:

> States with relevant groups from industry, should encourage the development and implementation of technologies and operational methods that reduce discards. The use of fishing gear and practices that lead to the discarding of catch should be discouraged and the use of fishing gear and practices that increase survival rates of escaping fish should be promoted.

Under the heading 11.1 Responsible Fish Utilization, sub-paragraph 11.1.8:

> States should encourage those involved in fish processing, distribution and marketing to: a) reduce post-harvest losses and waste; b) improve the use of by-catch to the extent that this is consistent with responsible fisheries management practices; and c) use the resources, especially water and energy, in particular wood, in an environmentally sound manner.

In other words, there should be minimal waste and the discards utilization should be improved. On the other hand, the FAO document entitled *Guidelines for the Ecolabelling of Fish and Fishery Products from Marine Capture Fisheries* (FAO, 2009) only mentions discards twice and does not mention by-product or waste utilization at all. The FAO Guidelines for ecolabelling, like the FAO Code, are voluntary and used by certification groups to set principles for a credible fishery certification and ecolabelling scheme. The key points of these guidelines are that ecolabelling programmes have:

- objective, third-party fishery assessment using scientific evidence;
- transparent processes with built-in stakeholder consultation and objection procedures;
- standards based on the three factors – sustainability of target species, ecosystems and management practices (MSC, 2012a).

In the opinion of this writer, discarding 40–60 % of the catch as waste is not a very sustainable use of fisheries resources. While a considerable amount of by-product is currently utilized for fishmeal and oil production, silage, hydrolyzates and other products, and will probably be used more in the future, there are some certified fisheries that may discard the by-catch and by-products at sea. Perhaps utilization of the by-product and discards should play a more prominent part in the overall certification process as an incentive for these fisheries to make better use of their raw materials.

Two of the major groups involved in the certification of the raw material are the Marine Stewardship Council (MSC) and the Friend of the Sea (FOS). Both groups utilize third party inspectors for the fishery assessment and certification process and also certify products. The three main principles of MSC's fishery standard are: (i) sustainable fish stocks, (ii) minimizing environmental impact and (iii) effective management. These main principles are supported by 31 more detailed criteria (MSC, 2012b). MSC's Chain of Custody certification ensures that any seafood product with the MSC ecolabel is traceable back to an MSC certified sustainable fishery. FOS certifies products which originate from certified fisheries. Their criteria for sustainable fisheries require:

- target stock not over-exploited;
- fishery to generate a maximum 8 % discards;
- no by-catch of endangered species;
- no impact on the seabed;
- compliance with regulations; for total acceptable catch (TAC), illegal, unreported and unregulated (IUU) catch, flag of convenience (FOC), etc.
- social accountability;
- gradual reduction of carbon footprint (FOS, 2012a).

Table 2.42 Friend of the Sea (FOS) approved fisheries

Species	Catch method	Location
Anchovies	Purse seine	Croatia; Morocco; Peru Austral Group; Argentina Centauro S.A. fleet
Cod and blue cod	Longline	Iceland; New Zealand Leigh Fishery
Mackerel	Purse seine	Morocco; Peru Austral Group
Menhaden	Purse seine	USA (Atlantic and Gulf of Mexico)
Salmon	Longline, troll, purse seine	New Zealand Lee Fishery; Canada; USA-Alaska SPC fleet; Alaska interocean fleet
Sardines	Purse seine	Morocco
Squid	Line and handline	Chile Seatec fleet; Vietnam
Tuna	Longline, pole and line, troll, handline, purse seine	Brazil; Ecuador; Ireland BIM Fleet; Maldives; Oman; New Zealand Leigh Fishery; Philippines Frabelle Fleet; Philippines; Senegal Asociacion Atuneros Caneros Dakar; South Africa AKA Global Fish fleet; Spain Pevaeche fleet; Sri Lanka

Source: FOS, 2012a.

Some of the species used for the production of fishmeal and oil have been certified by these organizations and any overlap between them is minimal. As of the end of September 2012, over 30 fisheries have received FOS certification. Some of these can be seen in Table 2.42 (FOS, 2012b). Among the highlights are the anchovy fisheries of Peru, and Argentina, the US menhaden fishery, the sardine fisheries of Morocco and Portugal and the wild salmon fisheries of Canada, New Zealand and USA-Alaska. The FOS certified fish oil and omega-3 products can be seen in Table 2.43 (FOS, 2012c).

The MSC program includes about 286 fisheries, either certified or in assessment through the end of September 2012. A partial list of the certified fisheries can be seen in Table 2.44 (MSC, 2012c). Among the highlights are the Alaska wild salmon fishery, the US Alaska pollock fishery, the US Alaska Pacific cod fishery, the Mexican Gulf of California sardine fishery and the New Zealand hoki fishery. A partial list of the MSC fisheries in assessment can be seen in Table 2.45 (MSC, 2012c). A list of MSC labeled fish oil or omega-3 products can be seen in Table 2.46 (MSC, 2012d). Because certification is an ongoing process any list is going to change so the reader is advised to go to the links in the appropriate references to get an updated list of fisheries and/or products that have been certified.

Table 2.43 Friend of the Sea (FOS) certified fish oil, krill and omega-3 products

Country	Omega-3	Fish oil	Krill oil and krill products
Australia		Health World Ltd	
Canada			Neptune Technologies and Bioresources
Colombia	Naturmega SA		
Denmark	Biosym		
Finland	Suomen Bioteeki Oy		
France	Winterisation Europe	Winterisation Europe; Polaris	Natesis
Germany	Goerlich Pharma International GmbH	Dr. Loges + Co. GmbH	
Morocco		Sovapec – Maromega	
Norway	Pharma Marine AS Calamarine; Epax AS; VitOmega; Amundsen Omega3 AS; Norway Omega AS	Pharma Marine; Epax AS; GC Rieber Oils AS; Napro Pharma- BASF; Hofseth Biocare (farmed fish oil)	Olympic Seafood
Peru		Anchoveta, Austral; Anchoveta Copeinca	
Sweden	Cardinova AB; VitoPharma; Eskimo 3	Cardinova AB	
Switzerland			Oleosea SA
UK	Healthspan Ltd (Vitempo)		
USA	Omega Protein; Nordic Naturals	Omega Protein; Nordic Naturals; Nexgen Pharma	
Vietnam		New Life Health Products Joint Stock Company	

Source: FOS, 2012c.

Table 2.44 Marine Stewardship Council (MSC) partial list of certified fisheries

Species	Fishery name
Krill	Aker Biomarine Antarctic krill
Salmon	Alaska salmon; Iturup Island pink and chum salmon; British Columbia pink salmon; British Columbia sockeye salmon; Northeast Sakhalin Island trap net pink salmon; Annette Islands Reserve salmon; Ozernaya River sockeye salmon
Anchovy	Argentina anchovy
Herring	Astrid Fiske North Sea herring; Danish Pelagic Producers Organization Atlanto Scandian herring; Danish Pelagic Producers Organization North Sea herring; Faroese Pelagic Organization Atlanto-Scandian herring; Norway North Sea and Skagerrak herring; Norway spring spawning herring; Pelagic Freezer Trawler Association North Sea herring; Pelagic Freezer-Trawler Association Atlanto-Scandian herring pelagic trawl; SPPO North Sea herring; SPSG Ltd Atlanto Scandian herring; SPSG Ltd North Sea herring; SPSG West of Scotland herring pelagic trawl; CSHMAC Celtic Sea herring; Hastings Fleet pelagic herring
Tuna	Canadian Highly Migratory Species Foundation (CHMSF) British Columbia albacore tuna North Pacific; PNA Western and Central Pacific skipjack tuna; Tosakatsuo Suisan pole and line skipjack tuna; Mexico Baja California pole and line yellowfin and skipjack tuna; New Zealand albacore tuna troll; American Albacore Fishing Association – Pacific north and south; American Western Fish Boat Owners Association (WFOA) Albacore tuna North Pacific
Sardine/pilchard	Cornwall sardine, UK; Gulf of California, Mexico – sardine; South Brittany sardine purse seine; Portugal sardine purse seine
Mackerel	Danish Pelagic Producers Organization North East Atlantic mackerel; Irish Pelagic Sustainability Association (IPSA) western mackerel; Irish Pelagic Sustainability Group (IPSG) western mackerel pelagic trawl; North East Atlantic mackerel pelagic trawl, purse-seine and handline; Pelagic Freezer-Trawler Association North East Atlantic mackerel pelagic trawl; SPPO North East Atlantic mackerel; Scottish Pelagic Sustainability Group Ltd western component of north east Atlantic mackerel
Alaska pollock	Gulf of Alaska pollock; Bering Sea and Aleutian Islands pollock

Table 2.44 *Continued*

Species	Fishery name
Cod	DFPO Denmark Eastern Baltic cod; IGP Icelandic cod; Fiskbranschens Sweden Eastern Baltic cod; Atlantic cod and haddock longline, handline and Danish seine; Faroe Island North East Arctic cod; Germany Eastern Baltic cod; Küstenfischer Nord eG Heiligenhafen Germany Eastern Baltic cod; Norway North East Arctic cod; Comapêche and Euronor cod and haddock; Barents Sea cod and haddock; Pescafria-Pesquera Rodrigez Barents Sea cod; UK Fisheries Ltd/DFFU/Doggerbank Northeast Arctic cod, haddock and saithe; Bering Sea and Aleutian Islands Pacific cod; Gulf of Alaska Pacific cod
Hoki	New Zealand hoki; Argentina hoki
Dogfish	British Columbia spiny dogfish; US Atlantic spiny dogfish
Hake	South Africa hake trawl

Source: MSC, 2012c.

Table 2.45 Marine Stewardship Council (MSC) partial list of fisheries in assessment

Species	Fishery name
Salmon	British Columbia chum; Hokkaido Fall chum salmon Set Net; Sakhalin Island Aniva Bay trap net pink salmon
Pollock	Russia Bering Sea pollock; Russia Navarinsky pollock; Russia Sea of Okhotsk pollock
Thread Herring	Gulf of California, Mexico thread herring
Tuna	Fiji albacore tuna longline; Maldives pole & line and handline tuna; Maldives pole & line skipjack tuna; Southeast US North Atlantic big eye tuna and yellowfin tuna
Hake	Chile hake trawl; New Zealand EEZ hake trawl fishery; Cornish hake gill net; Grupo Regal Spain hake longline; DFPO Denmark North Sea, Skagerrak & Kattegat hake
Sprat	SPPO North Sea and Baltic herring and sprats; CSHMAC Celtic Sea sprat trawl
Herring	NAFO Division 4R Atlantic herring purse seine; Samherji Norwegian & Icelandic herring trawl and seine; SPPO North Sea and Baltic herring and sprats; Western Baltic spring spawning herring;
Sardine/pilchard	CSHMAC Celtic Sea sardine trawl

Source: MSC, 2012c.

Table 2.46 Marine Stewardship Council (MSC) partial list of labelled fish oil, krill and omega-3 products

Brand	Product	Distribution countries
54 degrees North	Alaska Pollock Omega-3 with Vitamin D	USA
Barlean's Organic Oils	Ideal Omega 3 orange flavored	USA
Barlean's Organic Oils	Wild & Whole Krill Oil	USA
Blackmores	Optimal Health Eco Krill and Eco Krill Super Strength	Australia, New Zealand
Cleanmarine	Krill Oil	Ireland, UK
CVS pharmacy	100 % Pure Omega-3 Krill Oil	USA
CVS pharmacy	Extra Strength Omega-3 Krill Oil	USA
Dr. Mercola	Virgin Salmon Oil Dietary Supplement	Australia, Canada, USA
Dr. Ron's	Ultra Pure 100 % Pure Natural Astaxanthin in Wild Alaskan Sockeye Salmon Oil	Canada, USA
Dr. Ron's	Ultra-Pure 100 % Pure Wild Antarctic Krill Oil	USA
Gold Seal	Wild salmon oil	USA
Healthspan	Krill Oil	UK
meijer	Omega-3 Super Krill Oil	USA
Nutrilys	Del Mar Wild Antarctic Krill Oil	USA
Nutrilys	Del Mar Wild Alaskan Sockeye Salmon Oil, also with Vitamin D3, also with Astaxanthin	USA
Nutrilys	Neuromer Huille de Saumon Sauvage Sockeye d'Alaska	France
Nycomed	NEW-TON Omega 3 PLUS	Belgium, Luxembourg
Schiff	MegaRed Omega-3 Krill Oil and Extra Strength Krill Oil	USA
Schiff	MegaRed Joint Care Krill Oil	USA
Spring Valley	100 % Pure Omega-3 Krill Oil	USA
up&up	100 % pure omega-3 krill oil	USA
Vital Choice	Wild Antarctic Krill Oil	USA
Vital Choice	Wild Alaskan Sockeye Salmon Oil; also with Vitamin D3	Canada, USA
Vital Choice	Wild Alaska Salmon Oil with Rhodiola; also with Curcumin	USA
Vital Choice	Vital Red Astaxanthin in Wild Alaskan Sockeye Salmon	Canada, USA

Table 2.46 *Continued*

Brand	Product	Distribution countries
Vitempo	ECO Krill Oil	France
Walgreens	Extra Strength Omega-3 Krill Oil	USA
Walgreens	100 % Pure Omega-3 Krill Oil	USA
Wildcatch	Sockeye salmon oil supplements	USA

Source: MSC, 2012d.

2.9 Plant sources

For as long as I can remember there has always been a level of competition between fish oils and vegetable oils. In the industrial market, fish oil was able to compete because it was always the least expensive oil on the commodity market and industrial processes were designed to make fish oil 'similar' to vegetable oils so that they could be utilized as drying oils in paints and other coatings. Making them similar always involved reduction or 'neutralization' of the long-chain polyunsaturates, which were too reactive for most industrial processes. Therefore industry employed polymerization (heat bodying under inert gas) or oxidation (blowing with air) or a combination of both processes to achieve this reduction in reactivity. In paints, for example, the high polyunsaturated fatty acids in fish oil caused white paint to yellow after a short period of time making fish oil inferior to vegetable oils. In animal feeds (except farmed fish), high levels of the polyunsaturated fatty acids made chickens, eggs and pork taste fishy.

With the advent of omega-3 fatty acids, we finally achieved the factor that exploited the difference between fish oils and vegetable oils, in effect displacing the 'same' characteristics with the 'unique' characteristics, namely the omega-3 fatty acids. Around the same time, the vegetable oil companies were working on methods to eliminate the traces of the shorter chain omega-3 fatty acid C18:3 n-3, α-linolenic acid (ALA), in soybean oil which were causing shelf-life problems in cooking oils, margarines and shortening.

As the omega-3 market developed, along with concerns about supply, research to genetically modify vegetable oil sources to enhance the omega-3 and even force the plant to produce the longer chain omega-3 fatty acids began to develop. Long-range concerns within the fishing industry centred on production because there was a limited amount of fish and fish oil available and the vegetable oil producers could simply plant more acres to increase production. We now seem to be in the early stages of realizing those concerns.

The primary omega-3 fatty acid in the plant kingdom is ALA C18:3 n-3 which, in humans, is not efficiently converted to the longer chain omega-3 fatty acids. In addition to the marine oils, krill and single-cell oils as sources of these long-chain omega-3 fatty acids, there have been and continue to be developments in the genetic modification of oilseed crops so that they produce some level of the long-chain omega-3 fatty acids in the lipid. The long chain omega-3 fatty acids would be specifically the C20:5 n-3 (EPA) and C22:6 n-3 (DHA) fatty acids although, so far, some plants have been modified to produce C18:4 n-3, stearidonic acid (SDA). SDA is metabolically formed by the desaturation of ALA. Because SDA bypasses the rate-limiting step in the conversion of ALA to the omega-3 fatty acids EPA and DHA, it forms more EPA and possibly DHA in the body when consumed. Both ALA and SDA are converted to EPA; what differs is their conversion efficiency. ALA is inefficiently converted to EPA – it is either converted to energy or to SDA as part of its normal conversion to EPA. ALA intake enriches red blood cell EPA levels from 0.2 to 7 %. In contrast, SDA enriches red blood cell EPA levels from 16.7 % to as much as 26 %. James *et al.* (2003) concluded that SDA was metabolized to tissue EPA three to five times more efficiently than ALA in humans. There are some plants that are naturally high in linolenic acid and some contain SDA and γ-linolenic acid (GLA). These are shown in Table 2.47.

Watkins in 2009 interviewed several companies for *Inform* magazine. The purpose of the interview was to determine the current status of genetic modification of oilseeds and the timetable for bringing these products to commercialization. Although some companies declined to comment, those who did and who were working in the omega-3 area reported timeframes of about five to seven years or roughly 2014–2016 for commercialization. Oils not generally related to the omega-3 area had shorter timeframes for commercialization. In 2008, Johnson reported that Dow Agrisciences and Martek (now DSM) were working jointly on a project to produce DHA in the canola seed oil. This information is shown in Table 2.48.

The Arcadia product SONOVA™ 400, a high GLA product, was approved by the US FDA for use in dietary supplements in December 2009 and commercially marketed in mid-2010. The DuPont and Monsanto high SDA soybean oil is now ready for commercial release. In fact, USDA (2012) published in the July 13, 2012 *US Federal Register*:

> We are advising the public of our determination that a soybean line developed by the Monsanto Co., designated as event MON 87769, which has been genetically engineered to produce stearidonic acid, an omega-3 fatty acid not found in conventional soybean, is no longer considered a regulated article under our regulations governing the introduction of certain genetically engineered organisms.

There are a number of experimental transgenic lines, either developing or already developed, which contain the long-chain omega-3 fatty acids. The

Table 2.47 Omega-3 fatty acid content of some plant sources

Species	% Total fatty acids					
	Saturates	Mono-unsaturates	C18:2 n-6	C18:3 n-3	C18:3 n-6	C18:4 n-3
Soybean oil[2]	14	23	55	8		
Canola oil[1]	6	62	22	10		
Flaxseed oil[2]	9	15	15	61		
Echium oil[3]	11	19	19	29	10	12
Corn gromwell[5]	8	9	13	43	6	20
Hemp seed oil[2]	7	9	56	22	4	2
Blackcurrent seed oil[2]	8	11	48	13	17	3
Evening primrose oil[2]	7	8	76		9	
Borage oil[2]	17	17	42		24	
Echium oil[4]	11	18	15	29	12	13
Chia [6]	11	8	19	57		
Chia [7]	11	8	19	61		
SDA omega 3 soybean oil[8]	17	17	23	11	7	23

Sources: [1]ISEO, 2006; [2]Callaway, 2004; [3]Croda, 2006; [4]King and Sons Ltd, 2000; [5]Bentley personal communication, 2012; [6]Coates, 2013; [7]NSRI, 2012; [8]Monsanto, 2009.

progression from stems to leaves to seeds seems to take the most time for development. Some of these transgenic lines and the fatty acid compositions of their seeds is shown in Table 2.49. A very recent publication (Petrie *et al.*, 2012) from CSIRO Australia now reports:

> In conclusion, the production of high levels of DHA has been a major goal of the metabolic engineering community. This study resulted in the accumulation of up to 15 % DHA in a land plant seed oil, a level that exceeds the 12 % level generally found in commodity bulk fish oil. A high n3/n6 ratio was also observed. We look forward to the application of this technology in crop species: 1 hectare of a Brassica napus crop containing 12 % DHA in seed oil would produce as much DHA as approximately 10 000 fish. (This is a simplified calculation based on 10 000 kg fish = 1 000 kg oil = 120 kg DHA. Assumptions are that average fish = 1 kg, fish oil yield is 10 % by mass, average DHA is 12 %. For smaller size and less oily fish, the number of equivalent fish increases and for larger fish, the number of fish would decrease. Similarly, 1 ha *B. napus* = 2.5 T seed = 1 000 kg oil = 120 kg DHA. Assumptions are that *B. napus* seed contains 40 % oil by weight, 12 % DHA). (Copyright: © 2012 Petrie *et al.*)

Table 2.48 Projects and timetable in the development of transgenic plants with long chain omega-3 fatty acids in the seeds

Company/Institution	Plant(s)	Product 1	Product 2	Product 3	Timetable
BASF Germany[1]	Canola oil (*Brassica napus*)	Omega-6 fatty acid arachidonic acid (ARA) for infant food formulas	Omega-3 fatty EPA for food, feed and dietary supplement applications	Mixture of EPA and DHA for food, feed and dietary supplement applications	Commercial levels of ARA and EPA have been obtained in canola oil. Commencement of commercial production is envisaged sometime within the next five to seven years.
CSIRO, Australia[1,2]	Canola (*Brassica napus*) and cottonseed (*Gossypium hirsutum*)		Produce oil containing EPA and DHA	Produce oil containing EPA and DHA	The technology has progressed beyond proof-of concept stage. Commercial production of omega-3 LC-PUFA canola and/or cottonseed is targeted to begin in 2015.
National Research Council of Canada[1]	Ethiopian mustard (*Brassica carinata*)	The proportion of nervonic acid (24:1 Δ^{15}) has been raised from 2 % in (non-transformed wild type) to 45 % in the transgenic			Stable fourth-generation transgenic lines were tested under confined field trials in 2007 and 2008. Limited scale-up will follow in 2010.
Agriculture and Agri-Food Canada[2]	Flax (*Linum usitatissimum*)	Increased the oil content up to 50 % and linolenic acid up to 59–60 %			Seed of these improved varieties already is available and is being marketed as Prairie Thunder, Shape flax, and FP2214. Oil is expected to be available for use by the food industry in two or three years.

Arcadia Biosciences, USA[3, 6, 7]	Safflower (*Carthamus tinctorius*)	High-GLA (>40 %)		In the process of completing pre-commercialization activities. Seed is currently available for planting for a Phase I rollout. The product SONOVA™ 400 was subsequently approved by the USFDA for use in dietary supplements in December 2009 and commercially marketed in mid-2010.
Monsanto Co., USA in collaboration with Solae LLC[3]	Soybeans	Stearidonic acid (C18:4) levels increased from 0 to 20 %.		Seed and oil will be available in three to five years. The USDA subsequently approved the transgenic seed line in July 2012. The USFDA affirmed the GRAS status of the SDA soybean oil in 2009.
Dow Agrisciences/ Martek[4]	Canola	High DHA		Unavailable
DuPont[5]	Soybean		High EPA and DHA	High EPA oil phase 1 2014

Sources: [1]Watkins, 2009a; [2]Watkins, 2009b; [3]Watkins, 2009c; [4]Johnson, 2008; [5]Broglie, 2006; [6]Watkins, 2010; [7]Bioriginal, 2009.

Table 2.49 The omega-3 and omega-6 fatty acid content of seed oil in some transgenic plant lines in development

% Total fatty acids							
C18:2 n-6	C18:3 n-3	C18:3 n-6	C18:4 n-3	C20:4 n-6	C20:5 n-3	C22:5 n-3	C22:6 n-3
Seeds from transgenic brassica lines[1]							
7	11	20	6	5	1		
17	11	13	3	1	3		
29	14	1	1	3	2		
10	8	18	4	2	4		
27	13	2	1	6	4		
Cultivated tobacco, flax, brassica, other oilseeds[2,5]							
		29		2			
		17	11	1	1		
		12	1	2	20	1	
		27	2	2	20	1	
			12				
		27	5	6	20	4	
4	30		6		2	2	15
Wild tobacco[3]							
13	40	2	2			2	3
14	56		1		1		
13	45	2	1			2	3
Oilseeds including model plants[4]							
			10				
					5		1
			1	2	26		
				22			
				7	15		2

Sources: [1]Ruiz-Lopez *et al.*, 2012a; [2]Ruiz-Lopez *et al.*, 2012b; [3]Petrie *et al.*, 2010; [4]Nichols *et al.*, 2010; [5]Petrie *et al.*, 2012.

The data from this study appears in Table 2.49 and seems to be ahead of the timetable reported for CSIRO in Table 2.48.

2.10 Conclusion and future trends

The entire omega-3 market supply chain is in a state of transition with mergers, acquisitions and joint ventures taking place at all levels of the market. The clear lines in the supply chain are being blurred by these actions and this is forcing some of the more sophisticated companies to move up the supply chain towards the more 'value-added' concentrate products. As you move up this chain of supply, the level of by-product increases to the point where there will be an effect on the supply of raw materials. The availability of fish oil is limited and perhaps 60–65 % of the volume of fish oil available is suitable or borderline suitable for this market.

Should the EU and others enforce regulations regarding discards or the full utilization of the landed fish, this might improve the sourcing of raw materials coming from fish since it will require utilization of the by-products. While krill is a major biomass that is not even remotely fished to its quota limits, there would probably be an environmental uproar if the catch did approach these limits.

That leaves single-cell oils and transgenic plants. Single-cell oils are being produced today in large volumes for the biofuel industry. One company, Solazyme, has a joint venture with Bunge in Brazil to produce 130 million gallons of product by 2014. If they can do that, they certainly can produce an oil for the omega-3 market in smaller but still reasonable volumes from appropriate organisms. Other companies are also moving ahead with the production of single-cell oils so these would probably begin to fill some needs in the short to medium term, two to five years. In the medium to longer term, two to seven years, we should begin to see oils coming from transgenic plants with EPA and/or DHA in the lipid. Monsanto and DuPont's high SDA oil is poised to enter the market within the next year or so, but there is still no indication that the market will accept such an oil since it will have the GMO label on it. CSIRO in Australia recently reported that they have achieved levels of DHA that exceed the 12 % level generally found in bulk fish oil. The development should be applicable in oilseed crops since 1 ha of the plant containing 12 % DHA in the seed oil would produce as much DHA as approximately 10 000 fish.

All of these current and potential future products will generate large volumes of by-product. The single-cell oil production results in two products, the single-cell oil and the spent biomass. Each of these fractions is about 50 % of the production. The spent biomass is targeting the fishmeal replacement market. However, fishmeal is a complete ingredient, balanced in protein, lipid and minerals. Most replacements require fortification to compete with fishmeal so the issue will become an economic one. Can these replacements compete with fishmeal on price and nutrient content after they are fortified and, if so, are the feeding results comparable? The protein meal from the transgenic process must be utilized in order to make the operation economically feasible. The same is true for the single-cell oil process; the spent biomass and/or the biomass with the oil in it must be able to compete on price and functionality in order for the overall process to be economically feasible.

As new fish by-products become available it is going to be necessary to screen them for omega-3 content. In preparing this chapter, it is quite clear that most of the data available is a total lipid extract of either the edible portion of the fish or the whole fish ground up since these raw materials are not currently being used to manufacture fish oil. A total lipid analysis does not necessarily indicate what a fish oil produced from those fish would look like since the mechanical processing would eliminate any phospholipid from the oil unless it is solvent extracted. It is therefore recommended that analyses be run on the oil 'cooked' and squeezed out of the fish or fish by-product. This cooking could be something as simple as placing the fish or by-product in a bag and inserting the bag into boiling water until the lipid is released as oil An analysis of this oil would probably be quite different from the total lipid extract of the fish and would be more valuable in determining whether the oil would be suitable for the omega-3 market. In reviewing the literature for this chapter, I came across a number of Master and Doctoral dissertations in which the total lipid extract was used to characterize the omega-3 content of the lipid. It would be valuable to the omega-3 market to see some dissertations where the lipid was mechanically expressed from the fish or fish by-product as a better reflection of what a fish oil would look like.

2.11 References

ACKMAN RG (2005) 'Fish oils', in SHAHIDI, F. (ed.), *Bailey's Industrial Oil and Fat Products* (6th edn), Hoboken, NJ: Wiley Interscience, 279–317.

ADLERCREUTZ P and LYBERG A-M (2008) *A polyunsaturated fatty acid (PUFA) enriched marine oil comprising eicosapentaenoic acid (EPA) and docosahexaenoic acid (DHA), and a process of production thereof.* WO 2008/133573 Al.

AKER BIOMARINE ANTARCTIC AS (2010) GRAS notification – high phospholipid krill oil, GRN000371, available at: http://www.accessdata.fda.gov/scripts/fcn/gras_notices/GRN000371.pdf [accessed January 2013].

AMARIN CORPORATION (2012) 'Amarin announces FDA approval of Vascepa(TM) (icosapent ethyl) capsules for the reduction of triglyceride levels in adult patients with severe hypertriglyceridemia', press release, 26 July, available at: http://files.shareholder.com/downloads/AMRN/2266558371x0x586350/7f7dbe6f-10f4-477a-98a2-1439493b53b5/AMRN_News_2012_7_26_General_Releases.pdf [accessed February 2013].

ANDO Y, NISHIMURA K, AOYANAGI M and TAKAGI T (1992) 'Stereospecific analysis of fish oil triacyl-*sn*-glycerols', *JAOCS* 69, 417–424.

ASTM (2010) *ASTM D6751-12 Standard Specification for Biodiesel Fuel Blend Stock (B100) for Middle Distillate Fuels.* West Conshohocken, PA: ASTM International.

BAE JH and HUR SB (2011) 'Selection of suitable species of *Chlorella*, *Nannochloris*, and *Nannochloropsis* in high- and low-temperature seasons for mass culture of the rotifer *Brachionus plicatilis*', *Fish Aquat Sci* 14, 323–332, available at: http://www.e-fas.org/Upload/files/E-FAS/13_%EB%B0%B0%EC%A7%84%ED%9D%AC_2011_61_2011_12_26.pdf [accessed January 2013].

BIMBO AP (1989) 'Fish oils: past and present food uses', *JAOCS* 66, 1717–1726.

BIMBO AP (1996) 'Uses for refined fish oils in the industrial market', *Proceedings of the International Fishmeal and Oil Manufacturers Association (IFOMA), Workshop on future opportunities for fish oil*, Cape Town, 22 November, 64–86.

BIMBO AP (1998) 'Guidelines for characterizing food-grade fish oil', *INFORM* 9, 473–483.

BIMBO AP (2007) 'Processing of marine oils', in BREIVIK H (ed.), *Long-chain Omega-3 Specialty Oils.* Bridgwater: The Oily Press, 77–109.

BIMBO AP (2012a) 'Raw material sources for omega 3 fatty acids', presented at the 2012 GOED Exchange, Boston, June 6–8, available from: http://www.goedexchange.com/ [accessed 7 August 2012 – requires a login].
BIMBO AP (2012b) 'Fish meal and oil', in GRANATA LA, FLICK GJ JR, MARTIN RE (eds), *The Seafood Industry; Species, Products, Processing and Safety (2nd edn)*. Chichester: Wiley-Blackwell, 348–373.
BIMBO AP and CROWTHER JB (1992) 'Marine oils: fishing for industrial uses'. *Inform* 3, 988–1001.
BIORIGINAL (2009) 'SONOVA™ 400 High GLA Safflower Oil Receives FDA Acceptance As New Dietary Ingredient', joint press release, Bioriginal Food and Science Corp. and Arcadia Biosciences Inc. Press release, 14 December, available at: http://www.bioriginal.com/news/press_details.php?newsID=73 [accessed January 2013].
BREIVIK H (1992) Concentrates: A Scandinavian viewpoint. Paper presented at the AOCS Short Course, *Modern Applications of Marine Oils*, Toronto, 7–8 May. Urbana, Ill, AOCS.
BROGLIE R (2006) Translating discovery research into commercial products, in *NABC Report 18: Agricultural Biotechnology: Economic Growth Through New Products, Partnerships and Workforce Development*. Ithaca, NY: National Agricultural Biotechnology Council, 193–198, available at: http://nabc.cals.cornell.edu/pubs/pubs_reports.cfm#nabc18 [accessed January 2013].
CALLAWAY JC (2004) 'Hempseed as a nutritional resource: an overview', *Euphytica* 140, 65–72, available at: http://www.finola.com/Hempseed%20Nutrition.pdf [accessed January 2013].
CHAKRABORTY K, VIJAYAGOPAL P, CHAKRABORTY RD and VIJAYAN KK (2010) 'Preparation of eicosapentaenoic acid concentrates from sardine oil by *Bacillus circulans* lipase'. *Food Chem* 120, 433–442.
CHEDOLOH R, KARRILA TT and PAKDEECHANUAN P (2011) Fatty acid composition of important aquatic animals in Southern Thailand. *Int Food Res J* 18: 783–790.
CHRISTI Y (2007) 'Biodiesel from microalgae'. *Biotechnol Adv* 25, 294–306.
CLOVER CORPORATION LTD (2001) GRAS notification – Hi DHA tuna oil, GRN 0097, available at: http://www.accessdata.fda.gov/scripts/fcn/gras_notices/203487a.pdf [accessed January 2013].
COATES W (2013) *Composition of flax and chia seed*, available at: http://azchia.com/flax_us_chia/ [accessed February 2013].
CRODA (2006) Application for the approval of refined echium oil (stearidonic acid-rich oil from *Echium plantagineum*). Goole: Croda Chemicals Europe Ltd, available at: http://www.food.gov.uk/multimedia/pdfs/refiinedechiumapplication.pdf [accessed January 2013].
CCAMLR (2012a) Preliminary report of the Thirty-first Meeting of the Scientific Committee. Hobart: Scientific Committee for the Conservation of Antarctic Marine Living Resources, Hobart, 22–26 October, available at: http://www.ccamlr.org/en/sc-camlr-xxxi [accessed January 2013].
CCAMLR (2012b) *CCAMLR Statistical Bulletin* 24 (2002–2011). Hobart: Commission for the Conservation of Antarctic Marine Living Resources, available at: http://www.ccamlr.org/en/document/publications/ccamlr-statistical-bulletin-vol-24–2002%E2%80%932011 [accessed January 2013].
DANIELS S (2011) *All-conquering omega-3 set for further growth*. NutraIngredients.com special edition: omega-3, available at: http://www.nutraingredients.com/Consumer-Trends/All-conquering-omega-3-market-set-for-further-growth [accessed January 2013].
DOUGHMAN SD, KRUPANIDHI S and SANJEEVI CB (2007) 'Omega-3 fatty acids for nutrition and medicine: considering microalgae oil as a vegetarian source of EPA and DHA', *Curr Diabetes Rev* 3, 198–203.

DUNNE PG, CRONIN DA, MARTINE H, BRENNAN T and GORMLEY R (2010) 'Determination of the total lipid and the long chain omega-3 polyunsaturated fatty acids, EPA and DHA, in deep-sea fish and shark species from the north-east Atlantic', *J FisheriesSciences.com* 4, 269–281.

DUPONT (2010) GRAS notice – EPA rich triglyceride oil, GRN 0355, available at: http://www.accessdata.fda.gov/scripts/fcn/gras_notices/GRN000355.pdf [accessed January 2013].

FAO (1986) *The production of Fish Meal and Oil*, FAO Fisheries Technical Paper 142 Rev 1. Rome: Food and Agriculture Organization of the United Nations.

FAO (2009) *Guidelines for the ecolabelling of fish and fishery products from marine capture fisheries* revision 1. Rome: Food and Agriculture Organization of the United Nations, available at: http://www.fao.org/docrep/012/i1119t/i1119t.pdf [accessed January 2013].

FAO (2011) *Code of conduct for responsible fisheries*. Rome: Food and Agriculture Organization of the United Nations, available at: http://www.fao.org/docrep/013/i1900e/i1900e.pdf [accessed January 2013].

FAO (2012) FishStatJ – software for fishery statistical time service. Release: 2.0.0 a tool for fishery statistics analysis. Rome: Food and Agriculture Organization of the United Nations, available at: http://www.fao.org/fishery/statistics/software/fishstatj/en [accessed January 2013].

FERNANDEZ-JOVER D, JIMENEZ JA, SANCHEZ-JEREZ P, BAYLE-SEMPERE J, CASALDUERO FG, LOPEZ J and DEMPSTER T (2007) 'Changes in body condition and fatty acid composition of wild Mediterranean horse mackerel (*Trachurus mediterraneus*, Steindachner, 1868) associated to sea cage fish farms. *Mar Environ Res* 63, 1–18.

FOS (2012a) Fisheries – Introduction. Milan: Friend of the Sea, available at: http://www.friendofthesea.org/fisheries.asp [accessed 25 October 2012].

FOS (2012b) Friend of the Sea Approved Fisheries and Fleets. Milan, available at: http://www.friendofthesea.org/fisheries.asp?ID=7 [accessed 25 October 2012]

FOS (2012c) Certified Products. Milan: Friend of the Sea, available at: http://www.friendofthesea.org/certified-products.asp [accessed 25 October 2012].

GÁMEZ-MEZAA N, HIGUERA-CIAPARAB I, CALDERON DE LA BARCAB AM, VÁZQUEZ-MORENOB L, NORIEGA-RODRÍGUEZA J and ANGULO-GUERREROC O (1999) 'Seasonal variation in the fatty acid composition and quality of sardine oil from *Sardinops sagax caeruleus* of the Gulf of California', *Lipids* 34, 639–642.

GANGA A, NIETO S, SANHUEZ J, ROMO C, SPEISKY H and VALENZUELA A (1998) 'Concentration and stabilization of n-3 polyunsaturated fatty acids from sardine oil', *JAOCS* 75, 733–736.

GOED (2012) 'Global supply and demand trends in omega-3 fish oils', *IFFO Market Forum*, Miami, FL, 17 April, available at: http://portal.sliderocket.com/GOED-omega3/IFFO-Miami-Meeting-2012 [accessed January 2013].

GUIL-GUERRERO JL and BELARBI E (2001) 'Purification process for cod liver oil polyunsaturated fatty acids', *JAOCS* 78, 477–484, available at: http://lib3.dss.go.th/fulltext/Journal/J.AOCS/J.AOCS/2001/no.5/2001v78n5p477–484.pdf [accessed January 2013].

HALE MB (1984) 'Proximate chemical composition and fatty acids of three small coastal pelagic species'. *Mar Fisheries Rev* 46, 19–21.

HALE MB and BROWN T (1983) 'Fatty acids and lipid classes of three underutilized species and changes due to canning'. *Mar Fisheries Rev* 45, 4–6.

HAQ Z (2012) Biofuels Design Cases, DOE Office of Biomass Program, available at: http://www.usbiomassboard.gov/pdfs/tac_design_case_haq.pdf [accessed January 2013].

HAYASHI K and KISHIMURA H (1993) 'Separation of eicosapentaenoic acid-enriched triglycerides by column chromatography on silicic acid'. *Bull Fac Fish Hokkaido*

Univ, 44, 24–31, available at: http://eprints2008.lib.hokudai.ac.jp/dspace/bitstream/2115/24106/1/44(1)_P24–31.pdf [accessed January 2013].

HIRT-CHABBERT JA (2011) *Adding value to New Zealand eels by aquaculture*. PhD thesis, Auckland University of Technology, New Zealand, available at: http://aut.researchgateway.ac.nz/bitstream/handle/10292/1387/Hirt-ChabbertJ.pdf?sequence=3 [accessed January 2013].

HO BT and PAUL DR (2009) 'Fatty acid profile of Tra catfish (*Pangasius hypophthalmus*) compared to Atlantic Salmon (*Salmo solar*) and Asian Seabass (*Lates calcarifer*)', *Int Food Res J* 16, 501–506, available at: http://www.ifrj.upm.edu.my/16 %20(4)%202009/06 %20IFRJ-2008–153 %20Vietnam-%20Australia%20 2nd %20proof.pdf [accessed January 2013].

HUANG L-T C, BULBUL U, WEN P-C, GLEW RH and AYAZ FA (2012) 'Fatty acid composition of 12 fish species from the Black Sea', *J Food Sci* 77, 512–518.

HUYNH MD, KITTS DD, HU C and TRITES AW (2007) 'Comparison of fatty acid profiles of spawning and non-spawning Pacific herring, *Clupea harengus pallasi*', *Comp Biochem Physiol*, Part B 146 504–511.

ISEO (2006) *Food Fats and Oils* (9th edn). Washington DC: Institute of Shortening and Edible Oils, available at: http://www.cocoscience.com/pdf/food_fats_n_oils_compositions_of_various.pdf [accessed January 2013].

IVERSON SJ, FROST KJ and LANG SLC (2002) 'Fat content and fatty acid composition of forage fish and invertebrates in Prince William Sound, Alaska: factors contributing to among and within species variability', *Mar Ecol Prog Ser* 241, 161–181, available at: http://fatlab.biology.dal.ca/docs/data/2002/Iverson%20etal%20 MEPS2002 %20copy.pdf [accessed January 2013].

JACOBSON FEED BULLETIN (2012) Subscription database available at: https://www.thejacobsen.com/ [accessed January 2013].

JAKOBSEN JV (2001) *Fish trial with crude and carbon filtered fish oils from Denmark and Iceland*, Research Report 2001–2, Nor Aqua Innovation AS, available at: http://www.iffo.net/downloads/Research%20reports/IFOMA%201978–2001/2001/Fish%20trials%20with%20crude%20and%20carbon%20filtered%20 fish%20oils%202001–2.pdf [accessed January 2013].

JAMES MJ, URSIN VM and CLELAND LG (2003) 'Metabolism of stearidonic acid in human subjects: comparison with the metabolism of other n-3 fatty acids'. *Am J Clin Nutr* 77, 1140–1145.

JOHNSON A (2008) 'Biotech canola could offer even healthier oil', *Farm and Ranch Guide*, June 19, available at: http://www.theprairiestar.com/news/agri-tech/biotech-canola-could-offer-even-healthier-oil/article_ea2a618b-9de6-5f61-9208-bffa267c81b9.html [accessed February 2013].

KHIARI Z (2010) Functional and bioactive components from mackerel (*Scomber scombrus*) and blue whiting (*Micromesistius poutassou*) processing waste. PhD thesis, Dublin Institute of Technology, Ireland.

KHODDAMI A, ARIFFIN AA, BAKAR J, RAVICHANDRAN S and GHAZALI HM (2009) 'Fatty acid profile of the oil extracted from fish waste (head, intestine and liver) (*Sardinella lemuru*)', *World Appl Sci J* 7, 127–131.

KHODDAMI A, ARIFFIN AA, BAKAR J and GHAZALI HM (2012) 'Quality and fatty acid profile of the oil extracted from fish waste (head, intestine and liver) (*Euthynnus affinis*)', *Afr J Biotechnol*, 11, 1683–1689, available at: http://www.academicjournals.org/ajb/PDF/pdf2012/24Jan/Khoddami%20et%20al.pdf [accessed January 2013].

KING JK and SONS LTD (2000) Submission to the UK Food Standards Agency for the approval of echium oil as a novel food, available at: http://www.food.gov.uk/multimedia/pdfs/echiumapp.pdf [accessed January 2013].

KISSIL GW, YOCINGSOM A and COWEY CB (1987) 'Capacity of the European eel (*Anguilla anguilla*) to elongate and desaturate dietary linoleic acid', *J Nutr* 117, 1379–1384.

KLYACBKO-GURVLCH GL, DOUCHA J, KOPEZKIL J, RYABYKH IE and SEMENEOKO VE (1994) 'Comparative investigation of fatty acid composition in lipids of various strains of *Porphyridium cruentum* and *Porphyridium aerugineum*', *Russ J Plant Physiol* 41, 281–289.

KOLANOWSKI W (2010) 'Omega-3 lc PUFA contents and oxidative stability of encapsulated fish oil dietary supplements', *Int J Food Prop* 13, 498–511.

LAWLER S (2011) 'Tuna or not tuna? The real cost of taking a fish out of water', available at: http://theconversation.edu.au/tuna-or-not-tuna-the-real-cost-of-taking-a-fish-out-of-water-2825 [accessed January 2013].

LI G, SINCLAIR AJ and DUO LI J (2011) 'Comparison of lipid content and fatty acid composition in the edible meat of wild and cultured freshwater and marine fish and shrimps from China', *J Agric Food Chem* 59, 1871–1881.

LITZ MNC (2008) Ecology of the northern subpopulation of Northern Anchovy (*Engraulis mordax*) in the California Current Large Marine Ecosystem. MSc thesis, Oregon State University, USA.

LIYANAGE DW, WIJESUNDERA DRC and WIKRAMANAYAKE TW (1989) 'Some nutritionally important fatty acids in seven varieties of fish eaten in Sri Lanka' , *Ceylon J Med Sci* 32, 23–32.

LONZA (2010) GRAS notification – Ulkenia DHA oil derived from *Ulkenia* sp, GRN 000319, available at: http://www.accessdata.fda.gov/scripts/fcn/gras_notices/GRN000319.pdf [accessed January 2013].

MAKUTA M and FUJITA T (1986) 'Effects of EPA and use in health foods', *Japan Food Sci* 25, 29–35.

MARTEK (2003) GRAS notification–DHA algal oil derived from *Schizochytrium* sp., GRN 00137, available at: http://www.accessdata.fda.gov/scripts/fcn/gras_notices/706545A.PDF [accessed January 2013].

MÉNDEZ E (1997) 'Seasonal changes in the lipid classes and fatty acid compositions of hake (*Merluccius hubbsi*) liver oil', *JAOCS* 74, 1173–1175.

MILLER MR, NICHOLS PD and CARTER CG (2008) 'N-3 oil sources for use in aquaculture – alternatives to the unsustainable harvest of wild fish, *Nutr Res Rev* 21, 85–96.

MONSANTO (2009) GRAS notice – stearidonic (SDA) omega-3 soybean oil, GRN 00283 available at: http://www.accessdata.fda.gov/scripts/fcn/gras_notices/grn000283.pdf [accessed January 2013].

MSC (2012a) How we meet best practice. London: Marine Stewardship Council, available at: http://www.msc.org/about-us/credibility/how-we-meet-best-practice [accessed 23 October 2012].

MSC (2012b) MSC environmental standard for sustainable fishing. London: Marine Stewardship Council, available at: http://www.msc.org/about-us/standards/standards/msc-environmental-standard [accessed 25 October 2012].

MSC (2012c) Track a fishery. London: Marine Stewardship Council, available at: http://www.msc.org/track-a-fishery [accessed 23 October 2012].

MSC (2012d) Sustainable seafood product finder. London: Marine Stewardship Council, available at: http://www.msc.org/where-to-buy/product-finder [accessed 23 October 2012].

NEPTUNE TECHNOLOGIES & BIORESOURCES (2008) GRAS notification – high phospholipid krill oil, GRN 000242, available at: http://www.accessdata.fda.gov/scripts/fcn/gras_notices/grn000242.pdf, [accessed 19 July 2012].

NETTLETON JA (2000) Fatty acids in cultivated and wild fish, in IIFET (International Institute of Fisheries Economics & Trade), *Microbehavior and macroresults: proceedings of the tenth biennial conference of the International Institute of Fisheries Economics and Trade presentations*, Corvallis, OR, 10–14 July, available at: http://oregonstate.edu/dept/iifet/2000/papers/nettleton2.pdf [accessed January 2013].

NICHOLS PD (2007) 'Fish oil sources', in BREIVIK H (ed.), *Long Chain Omega-3 Specialty Oils*. Bridgwater: The Oily Press, 23–42.

NICHOLS PD, VIRTUE P, MOONEY BD, ELLIOTT NG and YEARSLEY GK (1998) *Seafood the good food: the oil content and composition of Australian commercial fishes, shellfishes and crustaceans*. Deakin: Fisheries Research and Development Corporation.

NICHOLS PD, PETRIE J and SINGH S (2010) 'Long-chain omega-3 oils – an update on sustainable sources', *Nutrients* 2, 572–585, available at: www.mdpi.com/2072-6643/2/6/572/pdf [accessed January 2013].

NISA K and ASADULLAH K (2011) 'Seasonal variation in chemical composition of the Indian mackerel (*Rastrelliger kanagurta*) from Karachi coast', *Iran J Fish Sci* 10, 67–74.

NSRI (2012) 'Chia seed – *Salvia hispanica* l. technical sheet'. Winter Park, FL: Nutritional Science Research Institute, available at: http://www.nsrinews.com/abstracts/Chia_Technical_Sheet.pdf [accessed January 2013].

OCEAN NUTRITION CANADA (2011) DHA-rich algal oil from *Schizochytrium* sp. ONC T18, A submission to the UK Food Standards Agency requesting consideration of substantial equivalence to DHA-rich algal oil from *Schizochytrium* sp. authorized in accordance with Regulation (EC) No. 258/97, submitted 10th October. Dartmouth, available at: http://www.food.gov.uk/multimedia/pdfs/dharich [accessed January 2013].

OIL WORLD (2012) 'Global analysis of all major oilseeds, oils and oilmeals supply, demand and price outlook', Thomas Mielke ed., ISTAMielke GmbH, Hamburg.

OLIVEIRA ACM (2010) *Purification of pollock oil using short path distillation*. Fairbanks, AK: Pollock Conservation Cooperative Research Center, available at: http://www.sfos.uaf.edu/pcc/projects/08/oliveira/Purification_of_pollock_oil_FINAL_report_Oliveira_2010.pdf [accessed January 2013].

OLIVEIRA ACM, LAPIS TJ, POPP T, HIMELBLOOM B, SMILEY S, BECHTEL PJ and CRAPO CC (2010) 'The chemical composition and oxidative stability of Alaska commercial salmon oils', in BECHTEL PJ and SMILEY S (eds), *A Sustainable Future: Fish Processing Byproducts*. Fairbanks, AK: Alaska Sea Grant College Program, Univ of Alaska, 241–257.

OKSUZ A and OZYILMAZ A (2010) 'Changes in fatty acid compositions of Black Sea anchovy (*Engraulis encrasicolus* L. 1758) during catching season', *Turk J Fish Aquat Sci* 10, 381–385.

OSAKO K, SAITO H, HOSSAIN MA, KUWAHARA K and OKAMOTO A (2006) 'Docosahexaenoic acid levels in the lipids of spotted mackerel *Scomber australasicus*', *Lipids* 41, 713–720.

PACKAGED FACTS (2011) 'Omega-3: Global Product Trends and Opportunities' available from: http://www.packagedfacts.com/Omega-Global-Product-6385341/ [accessed January 2013].

PATIL V, KALLQVIST T, OLSEN E, VOGT G and GISLERØD HR (2007) 'Fatty acid composition of 12 microalgae for possible use in aquaculture feed', *Aquacult Int* 15, 1–9, available at: http://moritz.botany.ut.ee/~olli/b/Patil07.pdf [accessed January 2012].

PAUGA M (2009) The effects of consuming farmed salmon compared to salmon oil capsules on long chain omega 3 fatty acids and selenium status in humans. MSc thesis, Massey University, New Zealand.

PETRIE JR, SHRESTHA P, LIU Q, MANSOUR MP, WOO CC, ZHOU X-R, NICHOLS PD, GREEN AG and SINGH SP (2010) 'Rapid expression of transgenes driven by seed-specific constructs in leaf tissue: DHA production', *Plant Methods* 6, 8 pages, available at: http://www.plantmethods.com/content/pdf/1746-4811-6-8.pdf [accessed January 2013].

PETRIE JR, SHRESTHA P, ZHOU X-R, MANSOUR MP, LIU Q, BELIDE S, NICHOLS PD and SINGH SP (2012) 'Metabolic engineering plant seeds with fish oil-like levels of DHA', *PLoS ONE* 7(11), 7 pages, available at: http://www.plosone.org/article/info%3Adoi%2F10.1371%2Fjournal.pone.0049165 [accessed January 2013].

PIKITCH E, BOERSMA PD, BOYD IL, CONOVER DO, CURY P, ESSINGTON T, HEPPELL SS, HOUDE ED, MANGEL M, PAULY D, PLAGÁNYI É, SAINSBURY K and STENECK RS (2012) *Little fish, big impact: managing a crucial link in ocean food webs*. Washington, DC: Lenfest Ocean Program, available at: http://www.lenfestocean.org/foragefishreport [accessed January 2013].

PULEVA BIOTECH (2006) GRAS notification – Eupoly-EPA and Eupoly-DHA derived from fish oils, GRN 00193, available at: http://www.accessdata.fda.gov/scripts/fcn/gras_notices/grn000193.pdf [accessed January 2013].

RAPIER R (2012) *Current and Projected Costs for Biofuels From Algae and Pyrolysis Energy Tribune*, 9 May, available at: http://www.energytribune.com/articles.cfm/10570/Current-and-Projected-Costs-for-Biofuels-from-Algae-and-Pyrolysis [accessed January 2013].

ROSS LABORATORIES DIVISION ABBOTT LABORATORIES (2001) GRAS notification – GRAS determination for docosahexaenoic acid rich oil derived from tuna and arachidonic acid rich oil derived from *Mortierella alpina*, GRN 0094, available at: http://www.accessdata.fda.gov/scripts/fcn/gras_notices/grn000094A.pdf [accessed January 2013].

RUIZ-LOPEZ N, HASLAM RP, VENEGAS-CALERÓN M, LI T, BAUER J, NAPIER JA and SAYANOVA O (2012a) Enhancing the accumulation of omega-3 long chain polyunsaturated fatty acids in transgenic *Arabidopsis thaliana* via iterative metabolic engineering and genetic crossing, *Transgenic Res* 21, 1233–1243.

RUIZ-LOPEZ N, SAYANOV O, NAPIER JA and HASLAM RP (2012b) 'Metabolic engineering of the omega-3 long chain polyunsaturated fatty acid biosynthetic pathway into transgenic plants *J Exp Bot* 63, 2397–2410.

RYAN AS, KESKE MA, HOFFMAN JP and NELSON EB (2009) 'Clinical overview of algal-docosahexaenoic acid: effects on triglyceride levels and other cardiovascular risk factors', *Am J Therap* 16, 183–192, available at: http://www.algen-dha.com/pdf/DHA_studie_trygliceride.pdf. [accessed January 2013].

SCLABOS KATEVAS D, TORO GUERRA RR and CHIONG LAY MM (2011) *Solvent-free process for obtaining phospholipids and neutral enriched krill oils*, United States Patent Application US 20110224450 Al, available from: http://patft.uspto.gov/netahtml/PTO/search-bool.html [accessed February 2013].

SETO A, WANG HL and HESSELTINE CW (1984) 'Culture conditions affect eicosapentaenoic acid content of chlorella minutissima', *JAOCS* 61, 892–894.

SHIRAI N (2011) 'Fish sources of various lipids including n-3 polyunsaturated fatty acids and their dietary effects', in HERNANDEZ EM, HOSOKAWA M (eds), *Omega-3 Oils Applications in Functional Foods*. Urbana, IL: AOCS Press, 61–71.

SIGURGISLADOTTIR S and PALMADOTTIR H (1993) 'Fatty acid composition of thirty-five Icelandic fish species. *JAOCS* 70, 1081–1087.

SOLAZYME (2010) GRAS Application 0331 GRAS Notice for an ingredient algal oil (*Chlorella*), available at: http://www.accessdata.fda.gov/scripts/fcn/gras_notices/GRN000331.pdf [accessed January 2013].

SOLTAN S and GIBSON RA (2008) 'Levels of omega 3 fatty acids in Australian seafood', *Asia Pac J Clin Nutr* 17, 385–390.

SOM CRS (2010) Bioactivity Profile of Polyunsaturated Fattyacid extracts from *Sardinella longiceps* and *Sardinella fimbriata* – A Comparative Study. PhD thesis, Cochin University of Science and Technology, India.

STANCHEVA M, GALUNSKA B, DOBREVA AD and MERDZHANOVA A (2012) 'Retinol, alpha-tocopherol and fatty acid content in Bulgarian Black Sea fish species', *Grasas y Aceites* 63, 152–157, available at: http://www.google.com/url?sa=t&rct=j&q=&esr

c=s&frm=1&source=web&cd=6&ved=0CF4QFjAF&url=http%3A%2F%2Fgrasasyaceites.revistas.csic.es%2Findex.php%2Fgrasasyaceites%2Farticle%2Fdownload%2F1367 %2F1364&ei=8je1T5vSMcOJ6AG9s4z3Dw&usg=AFQjCNHhRT4IAlzLqyKtHmMfVjBEbOE3tA&sig2=w5NEtv67FOxeJEVwEhPKaA [accessed January 2013].

TØMMERÅS S (2011) Fat, fatty acids and fat soluble nutrients in fillet of farmed and wild Atlantic salmon (*Salmo salar* L.). Masters Degree, University of Tromso UIT, available at: http://munin.uit.no/bitstream/handle/10037/3475/thesis.pdf?sequence=2 [accessed January 2013].

TRANSPARENCY MARKET RESEARCH (2012) *Global Oleochemicals Market (Glycerine, Fatty Acids, Fatty Alcohols), Downstream Application Potential, 2010–2018*. Albany, NY, available at: http://www.transparencymarketresearch.com/global-oleochemicals-market.html [accessed January 2012].

TUFAN B, KORAL S and KOSE S (2011) 'Changes during fishing season in the fat content and fatty acid profile of edible muscle, liver and gonads of anchovy (*Engraulis encrasicolus*) caught in the Turkish Black Sea', *Int J Food Sci Technol* 46, 800–810.

UDDIN MDS, AHN H-M, KISHIMURA H and CHUN B-S (2010) 'Production of valued materials from squid viscera by subcritical water hydrolysis' *J Environ Biol* 31(5), 675–679, available at: http://www.jeb.co.in/journal_issues/201009_sep10/paper_21.pdf [accessed January 2013].

USDA (2012) 'Monsanto Co.; Determination of nonregulated status of soybean genetically engineered to produce stearidonic acid', Submission for OMB Review: Comment Request, *Federal Register* 77(135), 41350.

USTIIN G, AKOVA A and DANDIK L (1996) 'Oil content and fatty acid composition of commercially important Turkish fish species, *JAOCS* 73, 389–391.

VAN VLIET T and KATAN MB (1990) 'Lower ratio of n-3 to n-6 fatty acids in cultured than in wild fish', *Am J Clin Nutr* 51, 1–2, available at: http://edepot.wur.nl/49245 [accessed January 2013].

VISENTAINER JV, NOFFS MD, CARVALHO PO, DE ALMEIDA VV, DE OLIVEIRA CC and DE SOUZAO NE (2007) 'Lipid content and fatty acid composition of 15 marine fish species from the southeast coast of Brazil', *JAOCS* 84, 543–547.

VLIEG P and BODY DR (1988) 'Lipid contents and fatty acid composition of some New Zealand freshwater finfish and marine finfish, shellfish, and roes'. *N Z J Mar Freshwater Res* 22, 151–162.

WATKINS C (2009a) 'Oilseeds of the Future: Part 1', *Inform* 20, 276–279, available at: http://www.aocs.org/Membership/FreeCover.cfm?itemnumber=1086 [accessed January 2013].

WATKINS C (2009b) 'Oilseeds of the Future: Part 2', *Inform* 20, 342–344, available at: http://www.aocs.org/Membership/FreeCover.cfm?itemnumber=1096 [accessed January 2013].

WATKINS C (2009c) 'Oilseeds of the Future: Part 3', *Inform* 20, 408–410, available at: http://www.aocs.org/Membership/FreeCover.cfm?itemnumber=1097 [accessed January 2013].

WATKINS C (2010) 'First high-GLA safflower oil on market', *Inform* 21, 338–339, available at: http://www.aocs.org/Membership/FreeCover.cfm?itemnumber=3541 [accessed January 2013].

WEYER KM, BUSH DR, DARZINS AL and WILLSON BD (2010) 'Theoretical maximum algal oil production', *Bioenerg Res* 3, 204–213.

Part II

Stabilisation of fish oil and foods enriched with omega-3 fatty acids

3

Impact of extraction, refining and concentration stages on the stability of fish oil

Å. Oterhals and G. Vogt, Nofima, Norway

DOI: 10.1533/9780857098863.2.111

Abstract: Crude fish oil is produced by processing whole fish from capture fisheries or by-products of the fish filleting industry. Before the oil can be used in food applications, oxidation products, pigments and off-flavour compounds must be removed. This type of refining is known to have a negative impact on the oxidative stability of the fish oil, due to the removal of natural antioxidants in the crude oil during the refining process. The majority of research has been carried out on the effect of removing α-tocopherols and phospholipids, but other natural antioxidants and synergists should also be taken into account. Improvements in the quality of the crude oil and minimal use of refining methods can contribute to an initially reduced oxidation level, the retention of natural antioxidants and an increase in the oxidative stability of the final food-grade fish oil.

Key words: fish oil extraction, quality, refining process, oxidative stability, endogenous antioxidants, omega-3 fatty acids.

3.1 Introduction

Crude fish oil can be produced by processing either whole fish from capture fisheries or by-products of the fish filleting industry. The high content of polyunsaturated fatty acids (PUFA) in fish oils makes them susceptible to oxidative processes, resulting in hydroperoxides. When hydroperoxides decompose, secondary oxidation products are created, such as aldehydes, ketones and acids, which have a fishy, rancid flavour and are consequently not suitable for foods. High oxidation levels might also lead to the loss of PUFA, and are linked to possible negative health effects (EFSA, 2010; VKM, 2011). The oxidation of fish oil takes place wherever oxygen is present or there is a risk of exposure, including during raw material storage and handling and in all processing steps in crude fish oil production, such as oil storage and transportation, refining and concentration operations and formulation and storage of the final product.

Refining of fish and other edible oils is known to have a negative impact on their oxidative stability (Ferrari *et al.*, 1996; Wanasundara *et al.*, 1998; Cmolik *et al.*, 2008; Oterhals and Berntssen, 2010), due to the removal of intrinsic antioxidants from the crude oil during the various refining operations. To slow down and limit the level of oxidation during crude oil extraction and refining, care should be taken to avoid exposure to oxygen and to retain any endogenous antioxidants in the fish raw material, so that these are carried over to the extracted fish oil. In combination with added antioxidants, this will contribute to an improvement of the oxidation level and stability of the final refined consumer product.

3.1.1 Raw material and fish oil quality regulations

The European Community has implemented hygiene, quality and process requirements for the raw materials used in fish oil intended for human consumption. The raw material has to meet certain criteria (Commission Regulation (EC) 853/2004) including:

(i) Sourced from approved establishments (including vessels).
(ii) Derived from fishery products that are fit for human consumption.
(iii) Transported and stored in hygienic conditions.
(iv) Chilled as soon as possible.

The food business operator may refrain from chilling the fishery products when whole fishery products are used directly in the preparation of fish oil for human consumption and the raw material is processed within 36 h of loading, provided that the freshness criteria are met and the total volatile basic nitrogen (TVB-N) value of the unprocessed fishery products does not exceed the following limits (Commission Regulation (EC) 1022/2008):

- 25 mg N/100 g of flesh for *Sebastes* spp., *Helicolenus dactylopterus*, *Sebastichthys capensis*.
- 30 mg N/100 g of flesh for species belonging to the *Pleuronectidae* family except *Hippoglossus* spp.
- 35 mg N/100 g of flesh for *Salma salar* and species belonging to the *Merlucciidae* and *Gadidae* family.
- 60 mg N/100 g of whole fishery products used directly for the preparation of fish oil for human consumption. Member States may set limits at a higher level for certain species pending the establishment of specific Community legislation.

No regulations or legislation regarding quality (freshness) requirements for fish used for the production of fishmeal and fish oil exist outside the European Union (EFSA, 2010). Moreover, the TVB-N criterion of a maximum of 60 mg N/100 g for whole fish is not based on scientific evidence; it is actually a spoilage criterion used for the assessment of ice-stored gutted fish and fish fillets that is also implemented in the feed industry as a criterion for high quality fishmeal and fish oil, e.g. Norse-LT 94 and NorSalmOil, which have a maximum of 50 and 90 mg TVB-N/100 g, respectively (http://www.norsildmel.no/).

Increased attention has also been given to the content of persistent organic pollutants (POPs) in food as a result of several severe contamination episodes (SCF, 2000). POPs were defined by the Stockholm Convention in 2001 (UNEP, 2001) on the basis of their persistency, bioaccumulation factor, potential for long-range environmental transport and adverse effect on human health or the environment. If the crude oil contains POPs above the maximum permitted levels (MPLs), the refining process must include a decontamination step. Current EU legislations for food-grade fish oil include MPLs for polychlorinated dibenzo-*p*-dioxins (PCDDs), polychlorinated dibenzofurans (PCDFs) and polychlorinated biphenyls (PCBs) (Commission Regulation (EU) No 1259/2011), as well as polycyclic aromatic hydrocarbons (PAHs) (Commission Regulation (EC) No 1881/2006).

3.1.2 Crude and refined oil quality standards

The quality of crude fish oil varies depending on the type and quality of the fish raw material, the processing conditions and the crude oil storage conditions. A general outline of the quality parameters used in the industry is given in Table 3.1; however, this is based on figures gathered by the International Fishmeal and Fish Oil Organization (IFFO) in the 1980s and does not incorporate current quality and process requirements for raw materials used in fish oil intended for human consumption. No official information is available regarding the variation in crude oil quality currently experienced by the refining industry. The introduction of maximum TVB-N levels (Commission Regulation (EC) 1022/2008) can be expected to have a

Table 3.1 Crude fish oil quality guidelines

Moisture	<0.5 %
Free fatty acids	2–5 %
Peroxide value (PV)	3–20 meq/kg
Anisidine value (AV)	4–60
TOTOX (2 × PV + AV)	10–60
Color	Up to Gardner 14
Iron	0.5–7.0 ppm
Copper	<0.3 ppm
Phosphorous	5–100 ppm

Source: Young, 1986a.

Table 3.2 Specifications given in selected fish oil monographs

Test	GOED* EPA and DHA oils	Eur. Ph. 1192 Cod-liver oil (type A)	Eur. Ph. 1912 Fish oil, rich in omega-3 acids (type 1)
Acid value	3 mg/g KOH	2 mg/g KOH	0.5 mg/g KOH
Peroxide value (PV)	5 meq/kg	10 meq/kg	10 meq/kg
Anisidine value (AV)	20	30	30
TOTOX (2 × PV + AV)	26	–	–
Oligomers	–	–	1.5 %
Unsaponifiable matter	–	1.5 %	1.5 %
PCDD/Fs	2 pg/g WHO-TEQ	–	–
Dioxin-like PCBs	3 pg/g WHO-TEQ	–	–
PCDD/Fs + dioxin-like PCBs	4 pg/g WHO-TEQ	–	–
PCBs†	0.09 mg/kg	–	–
Lead (Pb)	0.1 mg/kg	–	–
Cadmium (Cd)	0.1 mg/kg	–	–
Mercury (Hg)	0.1 mg/kg	–	–
Inorganic arsenic (As)	0.1 mg/kg	–	–

*Not applicable for cod liver oil. Omega-3 may be in the form of triglycerides or ethyl esters.
†Sum of IUPAC congeners 28, 52, 101, 118, 153, 180.

significant effect on the free fatty acid (FFA) level but less impact on other specifications such as the peroxide value, anisidine value and moisture content.

A Voluntary Monograph quality standard for fully refined eicosapentaenoic (EPA) and docosahexaenoic (DHA) oils has been developed by the industry through the Global Organization of EPA and DHA Omega-3 (GOED; http://www.goedomega3.com/). The standard (GOED, 2012; Table 3.2) is somewhat more strict than current official regulations with regard to maximum levels of PCDD/F and PCB, and also states that the colour of the product should be from pale, light-yellow to orange and the odour bland to mild fish-like. Several pharmaceutical monographs have also been developed to cover different products on the market (VKM, 2011): the specifications given in two of these are listed in Table 3.2. Although intended for medicinal products, these standards are also increasingly being used as a reference point for the purchase and sale of marine oils for food applications. Work on a new Codex Alimentarius Edible Fish Oil Standard was initiated in 2011, including fatty acid specifications for named oils; the standard is expected to be finalized in 2015.

Food-grade fish oil should have a low oxidation level and be light coloured with a bland to mild fish-like flavour (Bimbo, 1998). To obtain oil that meets these requirements, several purification steps are necessary in order to remove FFAs, pigments, off-flavours, POPs and other impurities while preserving the omega-3 fatty acid content.

3.2 Methods for the extraction, refining and concentration of fish oil

3.2.1 The fishmeal and oil process

Fish oil and fishmeal are produced using an integrated manufacturing process relying on a wet rendering method. The raw material is heat coagulated; mechanical dewatering and separation is then carried out to extract the oil phase, followed by thermal dewatering steps to concentrate the solubles and obtain dried fishmeal (FAO, 1986; Søbstad, 1992; Schmidtsdorff, 1995). The industrial-scale unit operations are fairly standardized worldwide, although some differences can be observed in the technology used and process layout adopted, depending on the type of raw material used and the target product quality (Bimbo, 2011). Enzyme-assisted extraction technology enables the use of gentler process conditions combined with the production of protein hydrolysate. Organic solvent extraction technology is only used in marine phospholipid production and will not be covered here.

A general outline of the unit operations used in the conventional manufacturing process for fishmeal and oil is given in Fig. 3.1. After heat treatment to 90–95 °C in a continuous screw cooker, the fish raw material is run over a strainer to remove the free water and oil phase before entering the screw press. The material entering the mechanical press is transported

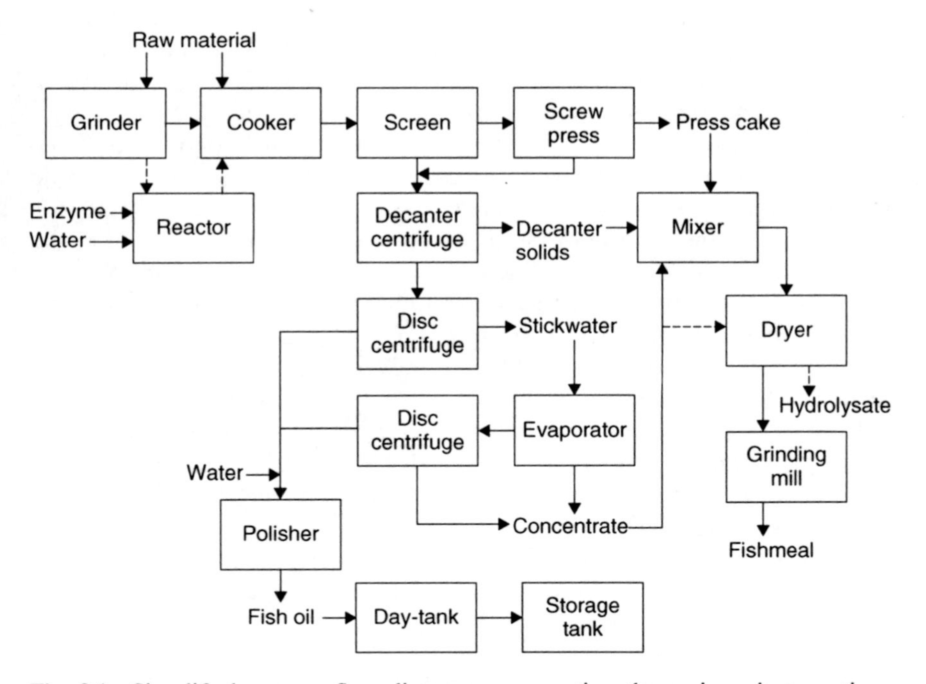

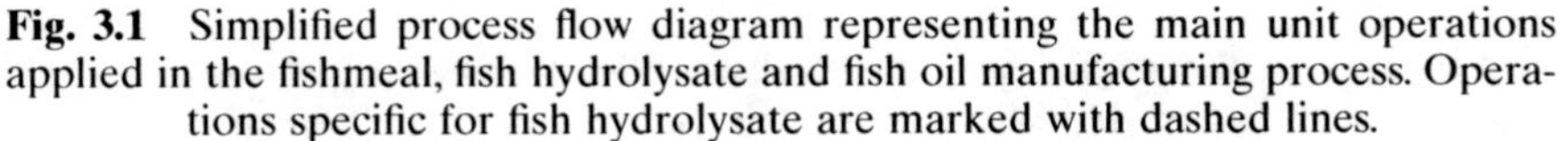

Fig. 3.1 Simplified process flow diagram representing the main unit operations applied in the fishmeal, fish hydrolysate and fish oil manufacturing process. Operations specific for fish hydrolysate are marked with dashed lines.

by counter-rotating screws of reducing height. The compression ratio, normally 1:3.5–4 in a fish press, causes fish oil and water to be squeezed out of the coagulated material and through the sieve plates. The water and oil, together with solubles and fine particles, are collected in the bottom of the press and mixed with the oil/water phase removed by the strainer. The combined liquid streams are heated to above 90 °C and run over a decanter centrifuge to remove suspended fine solids before oil separation by a disc centrifuge.

In the Condec process the screw cooker is exchanged with a scraped heat exchanger, thus reducing the heating time from 15–20 min to less than 2 min (Søbstad, 1992). In addition, the screw press is replaced with a decanter centrifuge. The screw press–decanter centrifuge–disc centrifuge system may also optionally be replaced with a three-phase decanter centrifuge, which significantly reduces the residence time at high temperature for the oil phase.

In the production of fish protein hydrolysate, the raw material is heated up to 50–60 °C in a batch or continuous reactor with the addition of a protease. After a defined residence time, the hydrolysate is heated up to above 90 °C to inactivate the enzyme, before the oil and solids are separated by a strainer and/or a decanter centrifuge. The separated liquid phase (stickwater) is concentrated in an evaporator. The stickwater concentrate might optionally be separated a second time to further reduce the fat content. To produce fishmeal, the presscake and decanter solids are mixed with concentrate and dried to a final moisture content of 6–10 %. Fish protein hydrolysate is formulated either as a concentrate or spray-dried powder.

The separated oil is polished by mixing with hot water followed by separation over a disc centrifuge, and is then pumped to a day-tank to settle residual impurities (i.e. water, protein, particles, etc.). The settled sludge is removed from the bottom of the day-tank before the oil is pumped to the final storage tank. Normally no active cooling of the oil is carried out, and the slow cooling process secures a favourable reduced viscosity during this settling operation. Any residual impurities will continue to settle in the storage tank and should be routinely removed from the bottom. On shipment, the oil is heated to 25–30 °C using hot water or steam coils at the bottom of the storage tank, thus ensuring the melting of any solid fraction (stearin), product homogeneity and reduced viscosity before the oil is pumped to a transport container or bulk ship carrier. The same temperature conditions are used when the oil is discharged. A detailed description of the practice for the storage and transport of edible oils and fats in bulk is given in the FAO/WHO code of practice (Codex Alimentarius, 2011).

3.2.2 Factors influencing crude oil quality

The quality of the crude fish oil obtained is principally dependent on the raw material type and quality and the processing conditions used. Increased

TVB-N in the raw material is linked to an increase in the FFA level of the extracted oil due to bacterial and endogenous lipase and phospholipase activity (de Koning 1995; Aidos *et al.*, 2003; Wu and Bechtel, 2009). The activity of spoilage bacteria is also linked to the development of biogenic amines used as quality criteria in fishmeal (Opstvedt *et al.*, 2000; Aidos *et al.*, 2003). If FFA levels are high, the sensory properties of the crude oil are affected: train oil and acidic attributes develop, and the oil takes on a darker colour (Oterhals, unpublished results).

The oxidation parameters that are usually measured, however, are less influenced by the TVB-N level. Studies by Aidos *et al.* (2003) and Wu and Bechtel (2009) found that the peroxide value and conjugated diene content were not correlated to storage time and temperature and either remained at the initial level or decreased. With regard to secondary oxidation products, the anisidine value remained relatively unchanged in crude oil extracted from ageing herring by-products (Aidos *et al.*, 2003), while the level of thiobarbituric acid reactive substances (TBARS) decreased in oil from ageing pollock by-products (Wu and Bechtel, 2009). These observations may be explained by the breakdown of hydroperoxides during the elevated temperature conditions used in the crude oil extraction process and their reaction with amino acids, which leads to the formation of hydrophilic tertiary products that are then found in the water phase.

There have been few studies carried out on the impact of different processing conditions on oil quality parameters. Aidos *et al.* (2003) reported that a coagulation temperature of between 90 and 100 °C had no effect during the processing of herring by-products. However, the FFA content, oxidation level and oxidative stability were all positively influenced by increasing the pump speed (i.e. by a reduced residence time in the scraped heat exchanger) and negatively influenced by increased decanter speed. Skåra *et al.* (2004) found that the processing method did not affect oxidation level or stability in a study comparing the use of a three-phase decanter versus a two-stage separation process (i.e. two-phase decanter followed by a disc centrifuge) for salmon by-product processing. Processing of the liquid phase involves several transfer steps, including residence time in intermediate buffer tanks, between separation stages. In the conventional manufacturing process for fishmeal and oil, it is not standard industry practice to use nitrogen cover in the buffer tanks to minimize oxygen exposure. However, the high temperature conditions (90–95 °C) used in the separation process ensure a moisture saturated atmosphere above the liquid with a low oxygen partial pressure. This might also explain the lack of effect reported by Skåra *et al.* (2004).

To minimize the activity of endogenous lipase and protease, the raw material should be heated up to above the inactivation temperature as quickly as possible: this can be achieved by pumping hot press- or decanter liquid back to the cooker. The added hot liquid facilitates a rapid temperature increase as well as improving heat transfer in the cooker. In some plants a waste heat exchanger is used to preheat the raw material, using the vapour phase from the indirect fishmeal steam driers. Although this type of heat integration can contribute to a reduction in the overall energy consumption, the added low-temperature residence time might also lead to increased enzymatic breakdown of the raw material with a resulting negative impact on oil quality, i.e. an increased FFA level, which is also reported in oil separated from silage (Reece, 1980). Oil with a low FFA level can be obtained using active enzymatic hydrolysis of the by-products: for example, Gbogouri *et al.* (2006) obtained oil with an acid value <0.7 mg KOH/g from salmon heads.

After separation of the oil, the water is removed and the oil is therefore no longer protected from oxygen exposure. Some producers use inert gas cover to minimize oxidation of the oil at this stage. During bulk ship transportation, the oil is exposed to oxygen during transfer operations and in the onboard storage tanks. In a study conducted by the Norwegian fish oil industry, a 500 t parcel of capelin oil was tracked throughout transportation (Oterhals, unpublished results). No increase in the oxidation level measured by the peroxide value and the anisidine value could be observed between the oil sample taken from the storage tank before shipment and the average sample taken during offloading of the boat. Capelin oil contains relatively low levels of EPA and DHA and is known to have a high oxidative stability compared to other fish oils. It may therefore not be possible to generalize these findings to other types of fish oil; instead, targeted studies should be carried out for different types of fish oil and different transportation systems.

3.2.3 Fish oil refining, decontamination and concentration

Fish oil refining and concentration operations have been extensively reviewed by others (Bimbo, 2007; Breivik, 2007; Hamm, 2009) and only a short overview will be provided here. The principal objective of the refining process is to remove colour bodies, trace metals, phospholipids, oxidation products and organic pollutants, and to obtain light-coloured oil with a bland flavour and low oxidation level (Table 3.2): this is achieved through chemical and physical refining operations (Fig. 3.2).

Degumming of the oil is facilitated by the addition of small amounts of phosphoric or citric acid to the oil at 90–100 °C in order to hydrate the phospholipids, with the subsequent addition of water followed by separation. The process also contributes to the reduction of the metal content and removal of proteinaceous matter from the oil. Enzymatic degumming has been developed as a gentler alternative; however, the phospholipase step requires a long residence time and the process is unable to catalyse the hydrolysis of non-hydratable phosphatides under industrial conditions (Dijkstra, 2010).

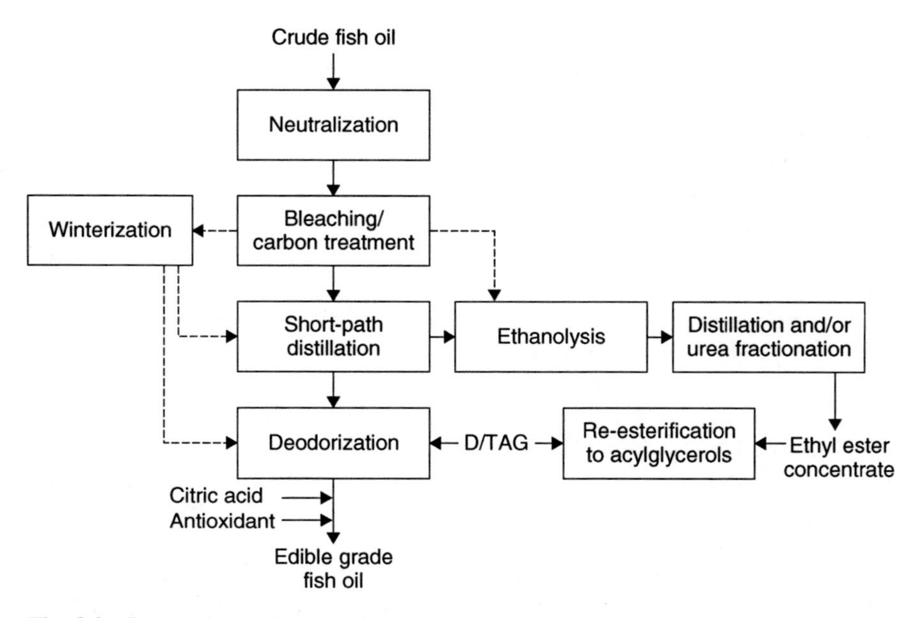

Fig. 3.2 Processing steps used in the production of edible grade fish oil and ethyl ester concentrate. Dotted lines indicate optional processing routes.

The use of degumming is not always necessary for a high quality crude fish oil, since the required refining effects can be achieved in the subsequent alkali and bleaching stages. Alkali-refining or neutralization is used to reduce the FFA level to below 0.1 %, which is achieved through the addition of aqueous alkali followed by separation of the soap-containing aqueous phase. The process is followed by a hot water washing stage to remove any traces of remaining soap. An additional effect on residual soap content can also be achieved by the acidification of the water with citric or phosphoric acid. The alkali-refining process also facilitates the removal of phospholipids, proteinaceous and insoluble matter, and metals. Before the bleaching stage, the oil is vacuum dried to remove water. It is then treated with acid-activated bleaching earth (0.5–2 %) at 80–100 °C under continuous mixing and reduced pressure (<50 mbar). The vacuum is broken with nitrogen before filtration to remove the bleaching earth and adsorbed compounds, i.e. pigments, phospholipids, soap, oxidation products and trace metals.

The activated carbon treatment used to remove POPs can either be combined with the bleaching process or performed as a separate stage under similar process conditions. Activated carbon has been shown to be highly effective for the removal of PCDD/Fs but less effective for the removal of PCBs, particularly mono-*ortho* PCBs (Oterhals *et al.*, 2007). It has long been used for the removal of PAHs in edible oils (Leon-Camacho *et al.*, 2003) and is also able to remove pesticides to some extent (Ortiz *et al.*, 2011). Fish oil contains variable amounts of high melting triglycerides (stearin) that can be removed by a chilling operation (winterization) followed by filtration of the crystallized lipids. The separated stearin fraction shows only a minor reduction in the omega-3 content and could be used as hardstock in soft spread formulations (Bimbo, 2007). The winterization step can optionally be skipped to preserve the natural composition of the fish oil. As an alternative to activated carbon, short-path distillation can be used to remove POPs. The optimal operation conditions have been found to be a temperature of around 200 °C with the addition of a working fluid (Oterhals *et al.*, 2010).

In the deodorization step, volatile compounds in the fish oil are removed by the injection of steam at 180 °C and <3 mbar. A higher temperature improves the stripping efficiency, but has the potential disadvantage of thermally-induced formation of polymers, cyclic fatty acid monomers (CFAM) and *trans* isomers (Fournier *et al.*, 2006). In addition to the removal of off-flavour compounds, the deodorization stage also facilitates the thermal breakdown of residual hydroperoxides and the removal of organochlorine pesticides and PCBs (Hilbert *et al.*, 1998). During cool-down, citric acid is usually added to the deodorized fish oil as a chelating agent and antioxidant. The final fish oil product should have a peroxide value below 0.1 meq kg^{-1} immediately after the deodorization process.

Concentrated omega-3 fatty acids are preferentially used in nutraceutical and pharmaceutical products but might find some application in functional foods if the lipid content is a restricting factor. Among the many techniques developed (Breivik, 2007; Rubio-Rodriguez *et al.*, 2010), urea fractionation and short-path distillation are the most commonly used in the industry. Short-path distillated oil should preferably be used as the starting material to ensure the absence of POPs and cholesterol. In both cases, the triacylglycerols are converted to ethyl esters (ethanolysis) before the fractionation process (Fig. 3.2).

The production of ethyl esters is performed by a chemical (NaOH and KOH and their alkoxides) or enzymatic (lipase) catalysed reaction whereby the fish oil is hydrolysed to FFAs and further esterified with ethanol. The resulting ethyl esters allow for the fractional distillation of the long-chain fatty acids at lower temperatures and separation by urea complexation. When they come into contact with urea in ethanol, most straight-chain fatty acids form complexes with crystallized urea as the mixture cools. The selectivity is dependent on several factors (Breivik, 2007) but, in general, it is the saturated fatty acids that are most easily trapped into the channel of the urea complex, followed by monounsaturated fatty acids. The crystals can then be removed by filtration leaving a concentrate of omega-3 PUFA. Concentration by short-path distillation is carried out in two steps. In the first step, the light fraction (short-chain fatty acids) is removed as a distillate. The residue is distilled a second time and the bulk oil collected as distillate (omega-3 concentrate) while the heavy residue products are discarded. Rossi *et al.* (2011) studied the optimal temperature conditions for squid oil and found that these were 120 °C for stage one and 140 °C for stage two. The obtained omega-3 ethyl ester concentrate can be converted back to a mixed di/triacylglycerol (D/TAG) by lipase-catalysed re-esterification with glycerol (Fig. 3.2) or inter-esterification (Xu *et al.*, 2007).

3.3 Impact of extraction, refining and concentration stages on oil stability

Fish contains several endogenous anti- and pro-oxidants. The endogenous protection mechanisms against oxidation are based on several types of systems, including enzymes, molecular antioxidants and a combination of these (Kitts 1997; Undeland *et al.*, 1998; Maestre *et al.*, 2011; VKM, 2011). Under physiological conditions, continuous production of reactive oxygen species occurs. The major role of the protection mechanisms is to control and remove these reactive oxygen species and to regulate the oxidative stress.

Important enzymatic systems include glutathione peroxidase (GPS), superoxide dismutase (SOD), which catalyses the dismutation of superoxides into hydrogen peroxide, and catalase, which decomposes hydrogen peroxide. Molecular antioxidants include ascorbic acid, α-tocopherol, ubiquinone (Q10) and carotenoids. Ascorbic acid can function as a chelator and oxygen scavenger, but also as a superoxide scavenger. Tocopherol acts as a peroxyl radical scavenger, and ubiquinone may have a similar effect. Among the carotenoids, it has been suggested that astaxanthine (as found in salmonidae) reacts with peroxyl radicals. The antioxidant action of phospholipids appears contradictory: it may be that they function as metal chelators, along with other components such as polyamines, amino acids and peptides.

The enzyme-mediated antioxidant systems decline *post mortem* and are totally inactivated during heat treatment of the raw material prior to fat separation. Ascorbic acid is partially lost during the early *post mortem* stages (Undeland *et al.*, 1998). Any water-soluble anti- and pro-oxidants preferentially partition into the water phase during the process and end up in the concentrate or fishmeal product. As yet, there are no quantitative studies examining the effect of raw material quality and process conditions on the carryover of endogenous anti- and pro-oxidative compounds from fish to extracted fish oil. Compounds reported in crude fish oil that may affect oxidative stability include α-tocopherol, retinol, carotenoids, polyamines, phospholipids, peptides and trace metals.

The edible fish oil refining process is designed to remove FFAs, phospholipids, trace metals, colour bodies, hydroperoxides, oxidation products, POPs and off-flavour compounds. The processing steps applied (Fig. 3.2) are based on chemical reactions and liquid–liquid extraction, adsorption and volatilization technology. Pro-oxidative compounds are removed during these processing steps: this should generally improve the oxidative stability of the refined product. However, published studies on marine and vegetable oil refining have in fact revealed the opposite effect, with more refining steps leading to reduced stability (Ferrari *et al.*, 1996; Wanasundara *et al.*, 1998; Cmolik *et al.*, 2008; Oterhals and Berntssen, 2010). On the whole, the crude oil has been found to be most stable and its alkali-refined and bleached counterpart least stable. The deodorization of fish oil has a small positive effect (Wanasundara *et al.*, 1998) and molecular distillation can provide either a positive or negative effect depending on the processing conditions used (Oterhals and Berntssen, 2010).

Similar negative processing effects have been documented in vegetable oil refining, although some differences in the order of oxidative stability have been reported. Jung *et al.* (1989) studied the effects of soybean oil refining and found that the oxidative stability of the oil decreased as follows: crude > deodorized > degummed > alkali-refined > bleached. Yoon and Kim (1994) studied rice bran oil, reporting the following order of oxidative stability: crude ≥ degummed > bleached ≈ deodorized > alkali-refined oil. Finally, Gordon and Rahman (1991) studied coconut oil, with the following oxidative stability hierarchy: degummed > bleached > crude >> deodorized. The findings are attributed to the co-removal of natural antioxidants (tocopherol and phospholipids) and pro-oxidants (trace metals) or to the decomposition of hydroperoxides in the oil during the refining steps. Ideally, refining protocols should be developed that maximize the retention of the natural antioxidants. This is, however, often not compatible with the target chemical and sensory product specifications.

The degumming step is designed to remove phospholipids in the crude oil. Several studies have reported that phospholipids have a positive effect on oxidative stability in fish lipid systems (Saito and Ishihara, 1997); this effect is primarily attributed to the side-chain moieties that contain amine and hydroxyl groups or to decomposition products such as choline and ethanolamine. Phosphatidic acid derivatives did not show any antioxidative effect. The reported phosphorous level in crude fish oil is 5–100 ppm (Young, 1986b), and is heavily dependent on the water washing or polishing regime used. The phosphorous level corresponds roughly to 159–3170 ppm acetone insolubles (List *et al.*, 1978). Phospholipids have an amphiphilic nature and are further reduced during the alkali-refining step; their polar nature also results in effective adsorption to bleaching clay and silica. The removal of phospholipids, or a low initial level of phospholipids in the crude oil, is needed to minimize emulsion loss during the alkali-refining step and to optimize the performance of the bleaching clay.

Among the natural antioxidants, tocopherols have been given the most attention in edible oil and food systems, and a synergistic effect with phospholipids has been reported (Bandarra *et al.*, 1999). Young (1986b) reported levels of between 25 and 60 ppm in various fish oils, while Scott and Latshaw (1991) reported 117 ppm in menhaden oil. The variability might be due to different levels of fat at the time of processing. Only α-tocopherol is found in fish oil, at levels that are generally much lower than the levels of tocopherols and tocotrienols found in vegetable oils (Ferrari *et al.*, 1996; Gunstone and Harwood, 2007). Increased POP levels have been observed in the extracted crude oil with reduced fat levels from pelagic fish species (Mundell *et al.*, 2003), and a similar effect might also be expected for other lipid-soluble compounds.

The reduction of tocopherols during vegetable oil refining has been studied by several authors. High retention of tocopherols has been observed throughout the degumming, alkali-refining, bleaching and winterization steps in commercial vegetable oil refining (Ferrari *et al.*, 1996). However, a major reduction (14–57 %) in the total tocopherols was observed after the deodorization step (Ferrari *et al.*, 1996). The effect is strongly linked to the deodorization temperature used (Cmolik *et al.*, 2008), with 100 % retention estimated if the temperature is kept below 209 °C. Optimization studies by De Greyt *et al.* (1999) have revealed that tocopherol removal is mainly affected by the amount of sparging steam, pressure and temperature. Comparative results have been observed in experimental marine oil refining with a 23–26 % reduction of α-tocopherol after 4 h of deodorization at 100 °C (Wanasundara *et al.*, 1998). Scott and Latshaw (1991) used similar deodorization conditions and observed a 20 % reduction of α-tocopherol in menhaden oil. They also observed a significant reduction (27 %) after the bleaching step, while Oterhals and Berntssen (2010) observed a small increase (4 %) of the α-tocopherol level in herring oil after the alkali-refining and bleaching step. This was attributed to the partitioning of non-polar compounds in the lipid phase during the alkali-refining step with a consistent increase proportional to the amount of FFAs removed as water-soluble sodium salts (Oterhals *et al.*, 2007). After short-path distillation, the retention of α-tocopherol varied between 36 and 100 % and was influenced by evaporator temperature, feed rate and amount of distillate. Activated carbon adsorption is widely used in the industry to reduce the level of PCDD/F–PCB–TEQ (sum of dioxins, furans and dioxin-like PCBs toxic equivalent), and has been shown to have no effect on the oxidation level (Maes *et al.*, 2005; Oterhals *et al.*, 2007) or oxidative stability of the fish oil (Maes *et al.*, 2005).

Generally, the loss of oxidative stability in refined marine oils compared to crude marine oils has been explained by the removal of α-tocopherols and phospholipid synergists. However, the full retention of α-tocopherol after alkali-refining and bleaching in studies by Oterhals and Berntssen (2010) indicates that such mechanisms are less likely to fully explain the observed reduction (24 %) in oxidative stability. Other compounds found in marine oils, such as retinol (Tesoriere *et al.*, 1996), carotenoids (Shimidzu *et al.*, 1996), peptides and peptide–lipid oxidation products (Hidalgo and Zamora, 2006), polyamines (Løvaas, 1991) and phenolic compounds (Lin and Hwang, 2002) should be considered as possible contributing factors.

Carotenoids and retinol might be found in high levels in fish oil, and it is generally accepted that an increasing number of conjugated double bonds is associated with a greater quenching activity against singlet oxygen ($^1O_2$) (Shimidzu *et al.*, 1996). Both compounds are, however, quantitatively removed by bleaching clay (Scott and Latshaw, 1991). Peptides are removed by both alkali-refining and bleaching operations. Peptide–lipid oxidation products are more lipophilic and we are not aware of any studies examining the retention of such compounds during refining operations. Polyamines like spermine, spermidine and putrescine are fully protonated at neutral pH but probably exist as neutral compounds in an oil phase. They are soluble in water, and loss during the alkali-refining and bleaching stages might be expected based on their chemical properties. Lin and Hwang (2002) reported no loss of phenolics after alkali-refining, bleaching and deodorization but 28 % reduction after short-path distillation.

The level of natural antioxidants in crude fish oils is very low compared to that of the added antioxidants in stabilized oils for human consumption. The quantitative effects of these compounds during and after the refining operations are not fully understood, and further studies are required to explore the nature and potential of natural antioxidants in marine oils. Improved carryover of these compounds during refining operations might significantly contribute to the stability of the oil and could also have synergistic effects with other antioxidants added to the final product.

3.4 Conclusion and future trends

In any refining operation, a high-quality crude product is desirable in order to obtain a final product with the highest possible quality. Processing conditions, along with the type and quality of the raw material, are known to have a direct impact on crude fish oil quality parameters, including the level of FFAs, α-tocopherol and oxidation products. The introduction of food hygiene and TVB-N criteria (maximum TVB-N of 60 mg/100 g) for fish raw materials destined for use in producing fish oil for human consumption will contribute to improvements in the general quality of crude fish oil. However, further studies are required to assess the potential improvements in crude fish oil quality with even lower spoilage levels. An increasing demand for high-quality fish oil for human consumption will drive the implementation of food hygiene improvements at processing plants, the extensive use of cooling using ice or refrigerated water, and faster processing of the fish after it is caught.

The utilization of fresh by-products from the fish farming industry has opened up new possibilities for the production of high-quality and extra low oxidized fish oil. The processing plant could be situated adjacent to the fish filleting line, allowing direct processing of the fresh by-products. The quality that can be obtained in this way has been demonstrated by Skåra *et al.* (2004) based on Atlantic salmon by-products (head, frame bones and skin) stored at 4 °C for 24 h and processed in a small-scale production plant consisting of a mincer, scraped-surface heat exchanger (90–95 °C), decanter centrifuge and oil polisher. At optimum testing conditions, they obtained salmon oil with an anisidine and peroxide value of <1 meq/kg and an FFA level of <0.2 %.

There has also been increased focus on the combined production of marine protein hydrolysates owing to their bioactive properties and many potential application areas (Kim and Wijesekara, 2010). In a protein hydrolysis study carried out by Gbogouri *et al.* (2006) based on frozen Atlantic salmon heads, a fish oil peroxide value of 1.5 meq/kg and acid value of 0.7 mg/g KOH was obtained. The heads were crushed after thawing at 4 °C, mixed with water and hydrolysed for 2 h at 50–55 °C under nitrogen before heating to 95 °C and oil separation.

The possible separation of oil from cod liver below the protein denaturation temperature has been demonstrated by Jansson and Elvevoll (2010). High-quality cod liver oil was obtained using an extraction temperature of 27 °C (FFA level 0.9 %, peroxide value 1.0 meq kg^{-1} and anisidine value 0.6). Cod liver oil extracted at low temperature (40 °C) compared with conventional high-temperature conditions (90 °C) also resulted in improved sensory properties and oxidative stability after refining and deodorization (Jansson *et al.*, 1994). To avoid emulsion problems pelagic fish raw material must be gently heated to around the protein denaturation temperature of 50–60 °C (Lohne, 1976).

Rubio-Rodriguez *et al.* (2012) studied the use of supercritical carbon dioxide fluid extraction under mild conditions (25 MPa, 313 K) as a possible alternative to wet rendering and enzymatic extraction; this method may offer a lower oxidation level and a reduction in FFA content. However, a major economical drawback is the need to dry the raw material before supercritical fluid extraction.

These low-temperature and/or enzyme-assisted extraction technologies, combined with the use of high-quality material, will in the future contribute to improvements in crude oil quality and a reduction in the need for extensive refining of the oil to obtain a bland flavour. The combination of gentle extraction and minimum refining methods will also contribute to the preservation of natural antioxidants and to improvements in the oxidative stability of food-grade fish oil. The use of added antioxidants during the extraction process and nitrogen blanketing of the separated crude oil could also have a positive impact.

3.5 Sources of further information and advice

- ACKMAN, R.G. (2005) Fish oils, in SHAHIDI, F. (ed.), *Bailey's Industrial Oil and Fat Products* (6th edn). Hoboken, NJ: Wiley. Volume 3, 279–317.

- BIMBO, A.P. (2011) *The Production and Processing of Marine Oils*. The AOCS Lipid Library, available at: *http://lipidlibrary.aocs.org/processing/marine/index.htm* [accessed January 2013].
- BREIVIK, H. (2007) *Long-Chain Omega-3 Specialty Oils*. Bridgwater: The Oily Press.
- FAO (1986) The Production of Fish Meal and Oil, FAO Fisheries Technical Paper 142. Rome: Food and Agriculture Organization of the United Nations, available at: http://www.fao.org/docrep/003/X6899E/X6899E00.HTM [accessed January 2013].
- ROSSELL, B. (2009) *Fish Oils*. Leatherhead: Leatherhead Publishing; Chichester: Wiley-Blackwell.
- RUITER, A. (1995) *Fish and Fishery Products. Composition, Nutritive Properties and Stability*. Oxford: CAB International.
- SHAHIDI, F. (2005) *Bailey's Industrial Oil and Fat* (6th edn), volume 5: Edible Oil and Fat Products: Processing Technologies. Hoboken, NJ: Wiley.

3.6 References

AIDOS, I., VAN DER PADT, A., BOOM, R. M. and LUTEN, J. B. (2003) 'Quality of crude fish oil extracted from herring byproducts of varying states of freshness', *J Food Sci* 68, 458–465.

BANDARRA, N. M., CAMPOS, R. M., BATISTA, I., NUNES, M. L. and EMPIS, J. M. (1999) 'Antioxidant synergy of alpha-tocopherol and phospholipids', *J Am Oil Chem Soc* 76, 905–913.

BIMBO, A. P. (1998) 'Guidelines for characterizing food-grade fish oil', *INFORM* 9, 473–483.

BIMBO, A. P. (2007) 'Processing of marine oils', in BREIVIK, H. (ed.), *Long-Chain Omega-3 Specialty Oils*. Bridgwater: The Oily Press, 77–109.

BIMBO, A. P. (2011) *Edible Oil Processing. The Production and Processing of Marine Oils*. The AOCS Lipid Library, available at: http://lipidlibrary.aocs.org/processing/marine/index.htm [accessed January 2013].

BREIVIK, H. (2007) 'Concentrates', in BREIVIK, H. (ed.), *Long-Chain Omega-3 Specialty Oils*. Bridgwater: The Oily Press, 111–140.

CMOLIK, J., POKORNY, J., REBLOVA, Z. and SVOBODA, Z. (2008) 'Tocopherol retention in physically refined rapeseed oil as a function of deodorization temperature', *Eur J Lipid Sci Technol* 110, 754–759.

Codex Alimentarius (2011) *Recommended International Code of Practice for the Storage and Transport of Edible Fats and Oils in Bulk*, CAC/RCP 36 – 1987 (Rev.1-1999, Rev.2-2001, Rev.3-2005, Rev.4-2011). Rome: FAO, available at: http://www.codexalimentarius.net/download/standards/101/CXP_036e.pdf [accessed January 2013].

Commission Regulation (EC) 853/2004. Regulation of the European Parliament and the Council laying down specific hygiene rules on the hygiene of food stuffs, *OJ* L139, 55.

Commission Regulation (EC) 1881/2006 of 19 December 2006 setting maximum levels for certain contaminants in foodstuffs, *OJ* L364, 5–24.

Commission Regulation (EC) 1022/2008 of 17 October 2008 amending Regulation (EC) No 2074/2005 as regards the total volatile basic nitrogen (TVB-N) limits, *OJ* L277, 18–20.

Commission Regulation (EU) 1259/2011 of 2 December 2011 amending Regulation (EC) No 1881/2006 as regards maximum levels for dioxins, dioxin-like PCBs and non dioxin-like PCBs in foodstuffs, *OJ* L320, 18–23.

DIJKSTRA, A. J. (2010) 'Enzymatic degumming', *Eur J Lipid Sci Technol* 112, 1178–1189.

DE GREYT, W. F., KELLENS, M. J. and HUYGHEBAERT, A. D. (1999) 'Effect of physical refining on selected minor components in vegetable oils', *Lipid/Fett* 11, 428–432.

DE KONING, A. J. (1995) 'The free fatty acid content of fish oil, part IV. Rates of free fatty acid formation from phospholipids and neutral lipids in anchovy (*Engraulis capensis*) stored at various temperatures', *Lipid/Fett* 97, 341–346.

EFSA (2010) 'Scientific opinion on fish oil for human consumption. food hygiene, including rancidity', *EFSA J* 8(10), 1874, available at: http://www.efsa.europa.eu/en/efsajournal/doc/1874.pdf [accessed February 2013].

EUR. PH. (2011) *European Pharmacopoeia* (7th edn). Strasbourg: Council of Europe, European Directorate for the Quality of Medicine.

FAO (1986) *The Production of Fish Meal and Oil*, FAO Fisheries Technical Paper 142. Rome: Food and Agriculture Organization of the United Nations, available at: http://www.fao.org/docrep/003/X6899E/X6899E00.HTM [accessed January 2013].

FERRARI, R. A., SCHULTE, E., ESTEVES, W., BRUHL, L. and MUKHERJEE, K. D. (1996) 'Minor constituents of vegetable oils during industrial processing', *J Am Oil Chem Soc* 73, 587–592.

FOURNIER, V., DESTAILLATS, F., JUANEDA, P., DIONISI, F., LAMBELET, P., SEBEDIO, J. L. and BERDEAUX, O. (2006) 'Thermal degradation of long-chain polyunsaturated fatty acids during deodorization of fish oil', *Eur J Lipid Sci Technol* 108, 33–42.

GBOGOURI, G. A., LINDER, M., FANNI, J. and PARMENTIER, M. (2006) 'Analysis of lipids extracted from salmon (*Salmo salar*) heads by commercial proteolytic enzymes', *Eur J Lipid Sci Technol* 108, 766–775.

GOED (2012) *GOED Voluntary Monograph (v. 4). Omega-3 EPA, Omega-3 DHA, Omega-3 EPA & DHA*. Salt Lake City, UT: Global Organization for EPA and DHA Omega-3, available at: http://www.goedomega3.com/images/stories/files/goedmonograph.pdf [accessed February 2013].

GORDON, M. H. and RAHMAN, I. A. (1991) 'Effect of processing on the composition and oxidative stability of coconut oil', *J Am Oil Chem Soc* 68, 574–576.

GUNSTONE, F. D. and HARWOOD, J. L. (2007) 'Occurrence and characterization of oils and fats', in GUNSTONE, F. D., HARWOOD, J. L. and DJIKSTRA, A. J. (eds), *The Lipid Handbook*. Boca Raton, FL: CRC Press, Taylor & Francis Group, 37–141.

HAMM, W. (2009) 'Processing of fish oil', in ROSSELL, B. (ed.), *Fish Oils*. Leatherhead: Leatherhead Publishing; Chichester: Wiley-Blackwell, 81–98.

HIDALGO, F. J. and ZAMORA, R. (2006) 'Peptides and proteins in edible oils: Stability, allergenicity, and new processing trends', *Trends Food Sci Technol* 17, 56–63.

HILBERT, G., LILLEMARK, L., BALCHEN, S. and HØJSKOV, C. S. (1998) 'Reduction of organochlorine contaminants from fish oil during refining', *Chemosphere* 37, 1241–1252.

JANSSON, S. and ELVEVOLL, E. (2000) *Process for separating lipids and proteins from biological material*, WO Patent 00/23545.

JANSSON, S., STRØM. T., OLSEN, R. L. and ELVEVOLL, E. O. (1994) 'Quality of cod liver oils extracted at low and high temperature', abstract, LIPIDFORUM conference, *Lipids from the sea for food and health foods – Practical aspects*, Sandefjord, Norway, 10–11 March.

JUNG, M. Y., YOON, S. H. and MIN, D. B. (1989) 'Effects of processing steps on the contents of minor compounds and oxidation of soybean oil', *J Am Oil Chem Soc* 66, 118–120.

KIM, S. K. and WIJESEKARA, I. (2010) 'Development and biological activities of marine-derived bioactive peptides: a review', *J Funct Foods* 2, 1–9.

KITTS, D. (1997) 'An evaluation of the multiple effects of the antioxidant vitamins', *Trends Food Sci Technol* 8, 198–203.

LIST, G. R., HEAKIN, A. J., EVANS, C. D., BLACK, L. T. and MOUNTS, T. L. (1978) 'Factor for converting elemental phosphorus to acetone insolubles in crude soybean oil', *J Am Oil Chem Soc* 55, 521–522.

LEON-CAMACHO, M., VIERA-ALCAIDE, I. and RUIZ-MENDEZ, M. W. (2003) 'Elimination of polycyclic aromatic hydrocarbons by bleaching of olive pomace oil', *Eur J Lipid Sci Technol* 105, 9–16.

LIN, C. C. and HWANG, L. S. A. (2002) 'Comparison of the effects of various purification treatments on the oxidative stability of squid visceral oil', *J Am Oil Chem Soc* 79, 489–494.

LOHNE, P. (1976) 'Fettfraskilling – ny kunnskap kan åpne for flere prosessmuligheter', *Meldinger fra SSF* No 3, 9–14.

LØVAAS, E. (1991) 'Antioxidative effects of polyamines', *J Am Oil Chem Soc* 68, 353–358.

MAES, J., DE MEULENAER, B., VAN HEERSWYNGHELS. P., DE GREYT, W., EPPE, G., DE PAUW, E. and HUYGHEBAERT, A. (2005) 'Removal of dioxins and PCB from fish oil by activated carbon and its influence on the nutritional quality of the oil', *J Am Oil Chem Soc* 82, 593–597.

MAESTRE, R., PAZOS, M. and MEDINA, I. (2011) 'Role of the raw composition of pelagic fish muscle on the development of lipid oxidation and rancidity during storage', *J Agric Food Chem* 59, 6284–6291.

MUNDELL, D., MAGNUSSEN, M. P., MAGNUSSON, J. R. and VANG, G. (2003) *Dioxin and PCBs in Four Commercially Important Pelagic Fish Stocks in the North East Atlantic*, available at: http://www.hfs.fo/pls/portal/docs/PAGE/HFS/WWW_HFS_FO/UMSITING/KUNNANDITILFAR/KUNNANDITILFARRITG/DIOXIN AND PCB IN PELAGIC FISH.PDF [accessed January 2013].

OPSTVEDT, J., MUNDHEIM, H., NYGÅRD, E., AASE, H. and PIKE, I. H. (2000) 'Reduced growth and feed consumption of Atlantic salmon (*Salmo salar* L.) fed fish meal made from stale fish is not due to increased contents of biogenic amines', *Aquaculture* 188, 323–327.

ORTIZ, X., CARABELLIDO, L., MARTI, M., MARTI, R., TOMAS, X. and DIAZ-FERRERO, J. (2011) 'Elimination of persistent organic pollutants from fish oil with solid adsorbents', *Chemosphere* 82, 1301–1307.

OTERHALS, Å. and BERNTSSEN, M. H. G. (2010) 'Effects of refining and removal of persistent organic pollutants by short-path distillation on nutritional quality and oxidative stability of fish oil', *J Agric Food Chem* 58, 12250–12259.

OTERHALS, Å., SOLVANG, M., NORTVEDT, R. and BERNTSSEN, M. H. G. (2007) 'Optimization of activated carbon-based decontamination of fish oil by response surface methodology', *Eur J Lipid Sci Technol* 109, 691–705.

OTERHALS, Å., KVAMME, B. and BERNTSSEN, M. H. G. (2010) 'Modeling of a short-path distillation process to remove persistent organic pollutants in fish oil based on process parameters and quantitative structure properties relationships', *Chemosphere* 80, 83–92.

REECE, P. (1980) 'Control and reduction of free fatty acid concentration in oil recovered from fish silage prepared from sprat', *J Sci Food Agric* 31, 147–155.

ROSSI, P. C., PRAMPARO, M. DEL C., GAICH, M. C., GROSSO, N. R. and NEPOTE, V. (2011) 'Optimization of molecular distillation to concentrate ethyl esters of eicosapentaenoic (20:5 omega-3) and docosahexaenoic acids (22:6 omega-3) using simplified phenomenological modeling', *J Sci Food Agric* 91, 1452–1458.

RUBIO-RODRIGUEZ, N., BELTRAN, S., JAIME, I., DE DIEGO, S. M., SANZ, M. T. and CARBALLIDO, J. R. (2010) 'Production of omega-3 polyunsaturated fatty acid concentrates: a review', *Innov Food Sci Emerg Technol* 11, 1–12.

RUBIO-RODRIGUEZ, N., DE DIEGO, S. M., BELTRAN, S., JAIME, I., TERESA SANZ, M. and ROVIRA, J. (2012) 'Supercritical fluid extraction of fish oil from fish by-products: a comparison with other extraction methods', *J Food Eng* 109, 238–248.

SCF (2000) *Opinion of the SCF on the Risk Assessment of Dioxins and Dioxin-like PCBs in Food. Adopted on 22 November 2000*. Brussels: European Commission Health & Consumer Protection Directorate-General.

SCOTT, K. C. and LATSHAW, J. D. (1991) 'Effects of commercial processing on the fat-soluble vitamin content of menhaden fish oil', *J Am Oil Chem Soc* 68, 234–236.

SHIMIDZU, N., GOTO, M. and MIKI, W. (1996) 'Carotenoids as singlet oxygen quenchers in marine organisms', *Fisheries Sci* 62, 134–137.

SCHMIDTSDORFF, W. (1995) 'Fish meal and fish oil – Not only by-products', *in*: RUITER, A. *Fish and Fishery Products. Composition, Nutritive Properties and Stability*. Oxford: CAB International, 347–376.

SKÅRA, T., SIVERTSVIK, M. and BIRKELAND, S. (2004) 'Production of salmon oil from filleting byproducts – effects of storage conditions on lipid oxidation and content of omega-3 polyunsaturated fatty acids', *J Food Sci* 69, E417–E421.

SØBSTAD, G. E. (1992) 'Marine oil separation, purification technology', *INFORM* 3, 827–830.

SAITO, H. and ISHIHARA, K. (1997) 'Antioxidant activity and active sites of phospholipids as antioxidants', *J Am Oil Chem Soc* 74, 1531–1536.

TESORIERE, L., BONGIORNO, A., PINTAUDI, A. M., DANNA, R., DARPA, D. and LIVREA, M. A. (1996) 'Synergistic interactions between vitamin A and vitamin E against lipid peroxidation in phosphatidylcholine liposomes' *Arch Biochem Biophys* 326, 57–63.

UNDELAND, I., EKSTRAND, B. and LINGNERT, H. (1998) 'Lipid oxidation in herring (*Clupea harengus*) light muscle, dark muscle, and skin, stored separately or as intact fillets', *J Am Oil Chem Soc* 75, 581–590.

UNEP (2001) *Stockholm Convention on Persistent Organic Pollutants*. Geneva: United Nations Environmental Program. Available at: http://chm.pops.int/ [accessed January 2012].

VKM (2011) *Description of the processes in the value chain and risk assessment of decomposition substances and oxidation products in fish oils*. Opinion of Steering Committee of the Norwegian Scientific Committee for Food Safety, Oslo, available at: http://english.vkm.no/dav/0fd42c8b08.pdf [accessed January 2013].

WANASUNDARA, U. N., SHAHIDI, F. and AMAROWICZ, R. (1998) 'Effect of processing on constituents and oxidative stability of marine oils', *J Food Lipids* 5, 29–41.

WU, T. H. and BECHTEL, P. J. (2009) 'Quality of crude oil extracted from aging walleye Pollock (*Theragra chalcogramma*) byproducts', *J Am Oil Chem Soc* 86, 903–908.

XU, X., H-KITTIKUN, A. and ZHANG, H. (2007) 'Enzymatic processing of omega-3 specialty oils', in Breivik, H. (ed.), *Long-Chain Omega-3 Specialty Oils*. Bridgwater: The Oily Press, 141–164.

YOON, S. H. and KIM, S. K. (1994) 'Oxidative stability of high fatty-acid rice bran oil at different stages of refining', *J Am Oil Chem Soc* 71, 227–229.

YOUNG, F. V. K. (1986a) *The Refining and Hydrogenation of Fish Oil*, IAFMM Fish Oil Bulletin No. 17. St Albans: International Association of Fish Meal Manufacturers.

YOUNG, F. V. K. (1986b) *The chemical and physical properties of crude fish oils for refiners and hydrogenators*, IAFMM Fish Oil Bulletin No. 18. St Albans: International Association of Fish Meal Manufacturers.

4

Stabilization of omega-3 oils and enriched foods using antioxidants

C. Jacobsen, A.-D. M. Sørensen and N. S. Nielsen, Technical University of Denmark, Denmark

DOI: 10.1533/9780857098863.2.130

Abstract: Foods enriched with omega-3 polyunsaturated fatty acids (PUFA) are highly susceptible to lipid oxidation due to their high degree of unsaturation. Addition of antioxidants is therefore often necessary in order to prevent oxidation. However, antioxidant efficacy is not easy to predict in complex food systems as it is influenced by many different factors. This chapter will briefly discuss the major factors influencing antioxidant efficacy in heterophasic food systems enriched with omega-3 fatty acids. Moreover, the efficacy of different antioxidants in a range of different omega-3 enriched foods will be reviewed.

Key words: tocopherol, EDTA, phenolic antioxidants, ascorbic acid, neat oils, emulsified foods.

4.1 Introduction

Omega-3 polyunsaturated fatty acids (PUFA) are highly susceptible to lipid oxidation due to their high degree of unsaturation. Lipid oxidation will give rise to formation of undesirable fishy off-flavours and unhealthy compounds such as free radicals and reactive aldehydes. In severe cases, lipid oxidation may also reduce the level of omega-3 PUFA and thereby the nutritional value of these lipids. Lipid oxidation therefore poses a major challenge to food producers when they want to use omega-3 PUFA in food applications. A prerequisite for successful development of foods with a high omega-3 PUFA content is therefore that lipid oxidation is prevented or at least delayed as long as possible. Unfortunately, the lipid oxidation and antioxidant mechanisms in multiphase food systems are very complex and many factors can influence the rate and extent of lipid oxidation, as well as the efficacy of different antioxidants in such systems. Oxidation mechanisms in multiphase systems are dealt with in Chapter 12. This chapter will briefly introduce the basic lipid oxidation and antioxidant reactions and will review the most important factors affecting antioxidant effects. Subsequently, the current knowledge on the efficacy of different antioxidants in omega-3 PUFA enriched food systems will be discussed. Most attention will be devoted to omega-3 enriched food emulsions as the literature on other omega-3 enriched foods is scarce. However, antioxidant effects in muscle foods will also be touched upon.

4.2 Lipid oxidation and antioxidant reactions

The basic lipid oxidation processes consist of the following steps (Fig. 4.1). In the initiation step, the polyunsaturated lipid will, in the presence of coloured sensitizers and light, metal ions, haeme iron or heat, form free lipid radicals (L•). Subsequently, the very reactive free lipid radicals will react with oxygen whereby lipid peroxyl radicals (LOO•) are formed. The peroxyl radical will react with a new lipid molecule whereby the lipid hydroperoxides (peroxides, LOOH) are formed. The peroxides are also termed primary oxidation products and they are tasteless. However, peroxides may, in the presence of heat, haeme iron or metal ions, be decomposed into secondary volatile oxidation products (volatiles). Several food ingredients contain

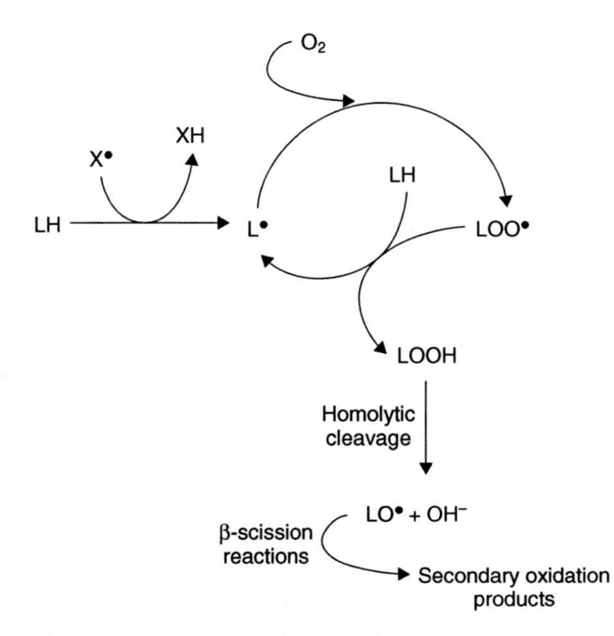

Fig. 4.1 Oxidation mechanism of polyunsaturated lipids. LH: unsaturated lipid; X•: radical initiator; L•: lipid alkyl radical; LO•: lipid alkoxyl radical; LOO•: lipid peroxyl radical; LOOH: lipid hydroperoxide.

trace levels of metal ions. Therefore, metal-catalysed decomposition of peroxides is regarded as the most important driving force for lipid oxidation in many food systems. The decomposition of lipid hydroperoxides takes place via metal catalysed, homolytic (unimolecular) cleavage of the oxygen–oxygen bond in the peroxide (LOOH), generating a highly reactive alkoxyl lipid radical ($LO^•$) and a hydroxyl ion (OH^-). The alkoxyl lipid radicals may initiate new reactions, but usually degrade rapidly by carbon–carbon cleavage on either side of the radical to form different volatile decomposition products (off-flavours) (Frankel, 2005). Hence, the metal catalysed decomposition of lipid peroxides not only generates free radicals, which initiate further oxidation reactions, but also leads to the formation of secondary volatile oxidation compounds, which are responsible for the off-flavours formed owing to oxidation. The off-flavours formed from omega-3 PUFA oxidation are particularly unpleasant and the sensory threshold for many of these oxidation products is low (Frankel, 2005).

Antioxidants are compounds that are able to retard or inhibit lipid oxidation. Antioxidants are classified as primary or secondary antioxidants based on their mechanism of action. However, some antioxidants have more than one mechanism of action and are referred to as multiple-function antioxidants. Primary antioxidants, also referred to as chain-breaking antioxidants, are characterized by their ability to react directly with free radicals and convert them to more stable, non-radical products. In the initiation and propagation steps, antioxidants react with lipid, alkoxyl and peroxyl radicals. In particular, the formation of stable lipid alcohols and the trapping of alkoxyl radicals with antioxidants are important reactions. These reactions inhibit further decomposition into aldehydes and other volatile oxidation products and the antioxidant radicals ($A^•$) formed are less reactive than lipid, alkoxyl and peroxyl radicals. In addition, antioxidant radicals can terminate autoxidation by reacting directly with the various lipid radicals. Phenolic compounds with one or more hydroxyl groups are often effective chain-breaking antioxidants because they can donate H-atoms to the free radicals and because they produce stable and relatively unreactive phenoxyl radicals after the donation of the H-atom. In the phenoxyl radical, the unpaired electron is delocalized around the aromatic structure and is therefore stabilized by high resonance energy. Examples of synthetic phenolic compounds are butylated hydroxytoluene (BHT), butylated hydroxyanisole (BHA), propyl gallate and tertiary butyl hydroquinone (TBHQ). Examples of natural phenolic compounds are tocopherol, caffeic acid and coumaric acid.

Phenolic antioxidants can also show pro-oxidant activity. This may be because the phenoxyl radical is less resonance stabilized whereby it can have a tendency to act as a chain carrier. This means that the phenoxyl radical reacts with lipids which donate a hydrogen atom to the phenoxyl radical whereby the lipid is turned into a lipid radical ($L^•$) and the phenoxyl radical reverts to a phenolic antioxidant (A). Owing to their ability to donate electrons, phenolic compounds can also act as pro-oxidants by reducing the less reactive Fe^{3+} to Fe^{2+} as will be further discussed later.

Secondary antioxidants can inhibit lipid oxidation by several different mechanisms, including chelation of transition metals, oxygen scavenging, synergism between antioxidants and singlet oxygen quenching. Metal chelators are the most important secondary antioxidants. They exert their function by inactivating the metals, which will prevent the metal ions from decomposing lipid hydroperoxides to reactive radicals. Examples of metal chelators are EDTA (ethylenediaminetetra-acetic acid, synthetic compound), polyphosphates, phytate and lactoferrin.

4.2.1 Factors affecting antioxidant efficacy

Irrespective of the complexity of the food system, the efficacy of antioxidants is highly influenced by their actual concentration. At high concentrations, some antioxidants such as tocopherol may have the opposite effect and become pro-oxidants. Furthermore, added antioxidants may act synergistically with endogenous antioxidants to obtain improved antioxidative effects. However, pro-oxidant effects of endogenous and added antioxidants may also occur if the total concentration becomes too high.

As far as the antioxidant efficacy in foods is concerned, the complexity of the food systems has to be taken into consideration. Thus, most foods comprise different phases and constituents, for example, air, water, lipid and solid particles. Oil-in-water (o/w) emulsions, such as milk, mayonnaise and salad dressing, and water-in-oil (w/o) emulsions, such as margarine and butter, are widely consumed groups of such complex food systems. In both types of emulsions (o/w and w/o), the oil and the aqueous phases are separated by an interface made up by emulsifiers, which are compounds with both lipophilic and hydrophilic properties. In solid foods, such as energy bars, the physical structure may be even more complex and is not well described in the literature. The heterophasic nature makes the mechanisms of lipid oxidation in most foods more complex than those in neat oil systems, and oxidation reactions can be affected by a number of different factors as described in Chapter 12. Likewise, antioxidant efficacy can be affected by a number of factors, which will be summarized in the following.

In emulsions, the antioxidant will partition into the oil phase, into the water phase or at the interface and this will influence its efficacy. The relationship between antioxidant partitioning and antioxidant efficacy is also called 'the polar paradox' (Porter, 1993; Frankel *et al.*, 1994; Huang *et al.*, 1996). According to the polar paradox, polar antioxidants such as ascorbic acid are more active in non-polar media like neat oils than they are in their more non-polar counterparts (e.g. ascorbyl palmitate), whereas non-polar antioxidants are more active in more polar systems like emulsions. For several years, attempts have been made to use the polar paradox theory to predict antioxidant effects in emulsified systems. However, in several cases the experimental data did not agree with the predictions made from this theory. Recent research on lipophilization of polar antioxidants has led to the so-called cut-off theory, which encompasses and expands the polar paradox theory (Laguerre *et al.*, 2009, 2010). In brief, this theory states that the efficacy of polar antioxidants such as ascorbic acid in emulsions can be increased by lipophilizing the antioxidants up to a certain length of the alkyl group esterified to the polar antioxidant. Beyond the optimal chain length of the alkyl group, the efficacy of the lipophilized antioxidant will decrease. The cut-off theory has been confirmed in simple o/w emulsions with antioxidants such as rosmarinic acid (Laguerre *et al.*, 2010), chlorogenic acid (Laguerre *et al.*, 2009) and dihydrocaffeic acid (DHCA) (Sørensen *et al.*, 2012b). In contrast, a recent study performed with rutin and lipophilized rutin (rutin laurate (C12) and rutin palmitate (C16)) as antioxidants in o/w emulsions, performed by Lue (2009) did not, however, support the cut-off effect, because the esters were consistently less effective when compared with rutin. However, only two different chain lengths were evaluated, so the cut-off effect could occur before C12 in this system with this antioxidant. So far, only one study has been performed to evaluate the effect of lipophilized antioxidants in complex food emulsion, namely fish oil enriched milk (Sørensen *et al.*, 2012a), as will be discussed in Section 4.4.1.

The increasing activity of antioxidants with increasing chain length up to the optimum chain length has been explained by the improved ability of the antioxidant to localize at the oil–water interface where oxidation takes place. The decreasing efficacy of antioxidants lipophilized with alkyl chains longer than the optimum chain length has been explained by the possible ability of the lipophilized compound to form micelles in the aqueous phase. Such micellization would mean that less antioxidant is present at the oil–water interface and therefore the antioxidant effect is lower (Laguerre *et al.*, 2009).

Recent data have also suggested that other factors, such as the interactions between the antioxidants, iron and the emulsifier, and the pH of the emulsion, will influence the antioxidant efficacy and, in some food emulsions, this may be at least as important as the partitioning of the antioxidants (Sørensen *et al.*, 2008). The examples below, from studies on antioxidant effects in neat fish oil as well as complex food systems, illustrate that with our current knowledge it is very difficult to predict antioxidant efficacy in omega-3 enriched foods.

4.3 Antioxidant protection of oils and oil-based products

4.3.1 Neat fish oils

The industry often uses antioxidants such as tocopherols, citric acid or its esters, ascorbyl palmitate or propyl gallate to protect fish oil against oxidation. Recently, there has also been an increasing interest in using natural antioxidants such as rosemary extracts.

Kulås and Ackman (2001) studied the effect of α-tocopherol (50–2000 mg/kg), γ-tocopherol (100–2000 mg/kg) and δ-tocopherol (100–2000 mg/kg) on the formation and decomposition of hydroperoxides in purified fish oil stored at 30 °C in the dark. Fish oil was purified by multi-layer column chromatography using hexane as a solvent. Due to the removal of natural antioxidants, purified fish oil oxidized very rapidly with no apparent induction period. The relative ability of the tocopherols to retard the formation of hydroperoxides decreased in the order α-tocopherol > γ-tocopherol > δ-tocopherol at a low level of addition (100 mg/kg), but a reverse order of activity was found when the tocopherol concentration was 1000 mg/kg. Based on measurements of lipid hydroperoxide formation, it was found that inversion of activity occurred for α-tocopherol at 100 mg/kg and for γ-tocopherol at 500 mg/kg, whereas the antioxidant activity of δ-tocopherol increased with level of addition up to 1500–2000 mg/kg. None of the tocopherols displayed any pro-oxidant activity.

Later Kulås *et al.* (2002) studied how α-, γ- and δ-tocopherol (100 or 1000 mg/kg) influenced the distribution of volatile secondary oxidation products in fish oil. They particularly focused on oxidation products expected to be important for adverse flavour formation. The tocopherol type and concentration affected not only the overall formation of volatile secondary oxidation products but also the composition of this group of oxidation products. Interestingly, although α-tocopherol was an active inhibitor of overall volatile formation, it appeared to direct the formation of the more flavour-potent aldehydes, such as heptadienal, when used in a high concentration.

The antioxidant properties of naturally-occurring flavonols, namely quercetin and quercetin glycosides, have been compared with those of a common food antioxidant, BHT, in fish oil by Huber *et al.* (2009). They found that glycosylation enhanced the antioxidant activity of quercetin and that quercetin-3-O-glucoside exhibited a better antioxidant activity than BHT in bulk fish oil. Recently, Martín *et al.* (2012) investigated the ability of supercritical extracts of rosemary, α-tocopherol or a mixture of the two to inhibit lipid oxidation in 'ultra high' omega-3 concentrates from fish oil as triacylglycerols (TAG) or ethyl esters (EE). Accelerated oxidation conditions at temperatures ranging from 50–70 °C using the Rancimat showed that both rosemary extracts and α-tocopherol in concentrations of 500 mg/kg reduced lipid oxidation, when added individually. They also found that the two antioxidants acted synergistically when used together in a ratio of 1:1. A storage experiment at room temperature in the dark confirmed that a mixture (1:1) of the two antioxidants in a total concentration of 500 mg/kg significantly reduced oxidation in both types of concentrates as measured by peroxide values (PV) and anisidine values (AV) (Fig. 4.2).

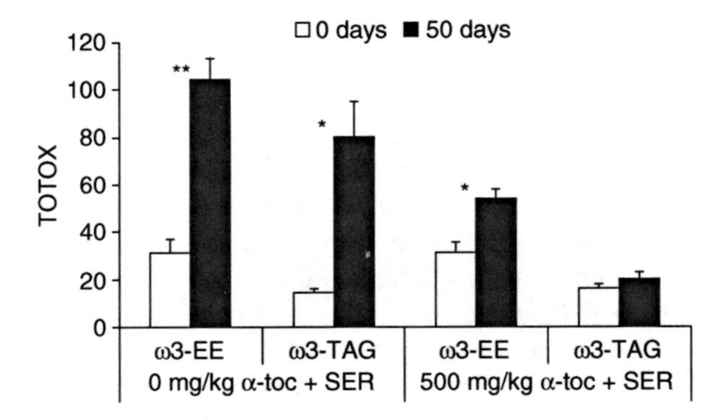

Fig. 4.2 TOTOX value (2 × peroxide value + anisidine value) of ultra-high omega-3 concentrates as ethyl esters (EE) or triacylglycerides (TAG) in absence (0 mg/kg) and presence (500 mg/kg) of the binary mixture of the antioxidants α-tocopherol (α-toc) plus rosemary extract (SER) after 50 days of storage at room temperature in the dark. Data are presented as mean values (n = 4) ± standard deviation. Values within the same antioxidant treatment and type of sample (EE or TAG) are significantly different if $p \leq 0.05$ (*), $p \leq 0.01$ (**). Reprinted from *Food Research International* 45, 336–341. Martín, D., Terrón, A., Fornari, T., Reglero, G., Torres, C. F., Oxidative stabilization of ultra-high omega-3 concentrates as ethyl esters or triacylglycerols, Copyright (2012), with permission from Elsevier.

4.3.2 Omega-3 enriched mayonnaise

Mayonnaise is an o/w emulsion with a high oil content (70–80 %) and a low pH (~4). The oxidative stability of mayonnaise prepared with fish oil (70 %) and without antioxidants is very poor, with a shelf-life of only one day at room temperature (Jafar *et al.*, 1994). Several studies on the efficacy of different antioxidants in mayonnaise have been carried out in products in which 20 % of the rapeseed oil was substituted with fish oil, as will be summarized in the following. The total lipid content in this mayonnaise was 80 %.

Despite the fact that a large number of antioxidants have been evaluated in fish oil enriched mayonnaise, only the metal chelator EDTA was found to be an efficient antioxidant in this food system (Jacobsen *et al.*, 2001a). This was explained by the finding that the low pH together with iron present in egg yolk, which is used as the emulsifier in mayonnaise, are responsible for the fast lipid oxidation rate in fish oil enriched mayonnaise (Jacobsen *et al.*, 2001b). Hence, a strong metal chelator is required to prevent lipid oxidation in fish oil enriched mayonnaise. Other metal chelators were also evaluated in fish oil enriched mayonnaise, namely lactoferrin and phytic acid, but either of these metal chelators efficiently prevented lipid oxidation and thereby off-flavour formation in this food system (Nielsen *et al.*, 2004). The antioxidative effect of lactoferrin seemed to be concentration dependent, since it had a slight antioxidative activity at low concentrations and showed pro-oxidant activity at high concentrations. The different antioxidative efficacies of EDTA, lactoferrin and phytic acid were suggested to be due to the different binding constants of the metal chelators to Fe^{2+} or that EDTA might be less sensitive to pH values around 4 than the other metal chelators (Nielsen *et al.*, 2004; Jacobsen *et al.*, 2008). Interestingly, EDTA was shown to work efficiently even at very low concentrations (6 mg/kg). The good antioxidative effect of EDTA is in accordance with a previous study by Jafar *et al.* (1994), who found that the shelf-life of mayonnaise based on only fish oil could be increased by 48 days by addition of citric acid or sodium citrate and propyl gallate in the oil phase and EDTA and ascorbic acid in the aqueous phase. However, they did not evaluate the effect of adding only EDTA.

Ascorbic acid and ascorbyl palmitate were shown to act as strong pro-oxidants, which gave rise to formation of fishy off-flavours immediately after addition to the mayonnaise. Furthermore, the pro-oxidative effect of ascorbic acid increased with increasing concentrations (40 to 800 mg/kg) (Jacobsen *et al.*, 1999a). Additional experiments on the oxidative stability of fish oil enriched mayonnaise with ascorbic acid added indicated that ascorbic acid induced iron release from the oil–water interface into the aqueous phase and that this effect of ascorbic acid was strongest at low pH (3.8–4.2) (Jacobsen *et al.*, 2001b). It was proposed by the authors that iron release from the interface was a result of broken ion bridges between iron and egg yolk proteins, whereby iron ions become accessible as initiators for the lipid oxidation. Moreover, in the presence of ascorbic acid or ascorbyl palmitate, lipid oxidation was further increased due to its ability to reduce Fe^{3+} to Fe^{2+} ions that rapidly catalyse lipid oxidation (Jacobsen *et al.*, 1999a, 2001b). Furthermore, a combination of ascorbic acid, lecithin and tocopherol (A/L/T) as antioxidants in the mayonnaise did not protect the fish oil against oxidation, but instead promoted oxidation. This finding was probably due to the properties described above for ascorbic acid alone in fish oil enriched mayonnaise (Jacobsen *et al.*, 2001b).

Both propyl gallate (40 mg/kg) and gallic acid (200 mg/kg) acted as pro-oxidants in mayonnaise (Jacobsen *et al.*, 1999b, 2001a). The pro-oxidative effects of propyl gallate and gallic acid were suggested to be due to their ability to reduce metal ions to their more active form, for example, the reduction of Fe^{3+} to Fe^{2+}.

Mixtures of tocopherols were found to have a concentration-dependent effect in fish oil enriched mayonnaise. Moreover, their effect also depended on whether a water- or oil-soluble tocopherol mixture was used (Jacobsen *et al.*, 2000). With an oil-soluble tocopherol mixture, sensory analysis and determination of volatile oxidation products showed weak antioxidative effects at lower tocopherol concentrations ($\leq$ 32 mg/kg) with the highest protection at 16 mg/kg. In contrast, pro-oxidative effects were observed at higher concentrations. Addition of a tocopherol mixture as a water-soluble preparation in mayonnaise generally exerted pro-oxidative effects on fishy flavour. These observations suggest that tocopherol does not have an unequivocal effect on fishy odour and flavour in mayonnaise. The poor effect of tocopherol observed in mayonnaise may be a result of the high levels of tocopherols already present in the oils used in the mayonnaise (rapeseed oil 64 % and fish oil 16 %). Since tocopherol has only been evaluated as mixtures in mayonnaise, it cannot be ruled out that better effects may be exerted by γ-tocopherol alone, as this antioxidant was observed to have antioxidative effects in salad dressing, as will be described below. However, rapeseed oil has a very high level of γ-tocopherol, so the question is whether additional γ-tocopherol will have any effect in mayonnaise. Moreover Jacobsen *et al.* (2001b) suggested that the crucial step in the formation of fishy odour and flavour in mayonnaise is the metal-catalysed breakdown of peroxides from omega-3 PUFA located in the aqueous phase or at the o/w interface. If this is the case, tocopherol can only to a limited extent reduce off-flavour formation by inhibiting deterioration of omega-3 PUFA inside the oil droplets because the reactions between the omega-3 PUFA and the radicals formed from the decomposed peroxides will take place at the o/w interface.

4.3.3 Mayonnaise-based salads

Sørensen *et al.* (2009) reported that addition of 1 % of oregano, thyme or rosemary to fish oil enriched tuna salads slowed down the formation of volatiles during storage, indicating that addition of spices could increase the oxidative stability compared to the standard tuna salad with fish oil. On the basis of the volatiles data, it could be concluded that oregano had the strongest antioxidative effect, followed by rosemary and thyme. However, the dry spices lead to undesirable flavors from the spices in the traditional tuna salads and further studies are therefore needed to evaluate whether extracts from such spices could be used as antioxidants.

4.3.4 Dressing

Only one antioxidant study on fish oil enriched dressing has been reported in the literature (Let *et al.*, 2007a). In this study, the salad dressing was prepared with 25 % fat of which 40 % was fish oil. Whey protein was used as emulsifier and a mixture of guar gum, xanthan gum and acetylated distarch adipate were added as stabilizers. The antioxidative effects of γ-tocopherol, ascorbyl palmitate and EDTA were tested either alone or in combination. Similar to the findings for mayonnaise, EDTA was a very efficient antioxidant, which inhibited oxidation by approximately 80 % at both concentrations evaluated (10 and 50 mg/kg). Moreover, the lipophilic γ-tocopherol was found to exert an intermediate antioxidative effect (ca 40 % inhibition) on peroxide formation irrespective of the amount added (Let *et al.*, 2007a). However, for the volatiles a concentration-dependent effect was observed. The highest protection (66 % inhibition) was obtained with the lowest concentration (22 mg/kg). A concentration-dependent effect was also observed for ascorbyl palmitate. At low concentrations (5 mg/kg), ascorbyl palmitate slightly reduced oxidation, whereas it acted as a pro-oxidant at high concentrations (30 mg/kg). Interestingly, the efficacy of EDTA could be further improved when used in combination with ascorbyl palmitate and tocopherol (Let *et al.*, 2007a). The strong effects of the metal chelator EDTA and the poor effects of tocopherol and ascorbyl palmitate when added alone suggest that metal catalysed oxidation is also very important in salad dressing. The metal content has been suggested to be relatively low in salad dressing (Jacobsen *et al.*, 2008), and these authors therefore found it surprising that metal catalysed oxidation is so prominent in a whey protein emulsified salad dressing. Jacobsen *et al.* (2008) suggested that a low pH in combination with even small levels of protein-bound metal ions can intensify metal catalysed oxidation in food emulsions and that this could explain the important role of metal ions in this food system, in which pH is around 4.

4.3.5 Margarine

Traditional margarine has a high fat content (~82 %) and is a w/o emulsion. Margarine is a solid–liquid emulsion and therefore the diffusion rate of different components in this system, such as antioxidants and pro-oxidants, may be lower compared to a liquid–liquid emulsion such as milk.

There is only one antioxidant study on margarine available in the literature. This study was performed by Young (1990) who produced fish oil enriched margarine in which 20 % of the soybean oil was substituted with fish oil. Two different antioxidant mixtures – 150 mg/kg Grindox® 117 (ascorbyl palmitate, propyl gallate and citric acid) and 200 mg/kg Grindox® 109 (BHA, BHT, propyl gallate and citric acid) – were evaluated in margarine with and without fish oil enrichment. No significant difference between the two antioxidant mixtures was found. However, preliminary sensory tests indicated a better flavour stability when Grindox® 109 (BHA, BHT) was added to margarine, whereas chemical measurements indicated that Grindox® 177 (ascorbyl palmitate) had a stronger antioxidative effect (Young, 1990). The oxidative stability could be further improved by addition of EDTA (150 mg/kg).

4.4 Antioxidant protection of other food products

4.4.1 Milk

Several studies on the effect of adding various antioxidants to milk enriched with fish oil have been reported by our laboratory. In these studies, milk contained 1.5 % fat of which either 0.5 % (absolute value) or all the oil was fish oil. From these studies it is evident that fish oil enriched milk will oxidize rapidly if precautions to avoid oxidation are not taken. Let *et al.* (2004) demonstrated that the most oxidatively stable omega-3 enriched milk was obtained by the addition of rapeseed oil together with fish oil (1:1). Apart from the diluting effect of adding rapeseed oil to the fish oil, it was suggested that the rapeseed oil also provided an 'antioxidative' effect due to its high content of γ-tocopherol. Moreover, γ-tocopherol was also found to be a good antioxidant when added directly to milk enriched with fish oil (no rapeseed oil) in a concentration of 1.7 mg/kg (Let *et al.*, 2005). When added in lower (0.8 mg/kg) or higher (3.3 mg/kg) concentrations, it had only weak antioxidant effects. Importantly, addition of a combination of α- and γ-tocopherol to omega-3 enriched milk was found to have pro-oxidative effects. In contrast, pure α-tocopherol in a concentration of 1.1 mg/kg had weak antioxidative effects. Pro-oxidative effects of the combination of α- and γ-tocopherol was suggested to be due to a too high concentration of α-tocopherol in the fish oil enriched milk, resulting from the fact that the fish oil itself used for the milk systems contained high concentrations of α-tocopherol. Other studies have also shown that α-tocopherol can have pro-oxidative effects in high concentrations (Huang *et al.*, 1994; Kulås and Ackman, 2001).

Apart from addition of rapeseed oil to protect the fish oil enriched milk against oxidation, the most efficient antioxidant was found to be ascorbyl palmitate, which exerted a strong antioxidative effect at an addition level of only 1.5 mg/kg in milk with 1.5 % fat (Let *et al.*, 2005). Interestingly, in strawberry flavoured milk drink, which contained 5 % fat of which 2.5 % was enzyme-modified fish oil, ambiguous results were obtained (Jacobsen *et al.*, 2008). Thus, ascorbyl palmitate was found to be able to reduce the formation of lipid hydroperoxides and certain volatiles such as heptadienal when added in high concentrations (15 and 30 mg/kg). In contrast, ascorbyl palmitate promoted the formation of hexenal and nonadienal as well as fishy off-flavours when added in concentrations of 7.5 mg/kg and above, but reduced the formation of these two volatiles when added at a lower concentration of 3.75 mg/kg (Jacobsen *et al.*, 2008).

The much stronger antioxidative effect of ascorbyl palmitate in milk with 1.5 % fat compared to its effect in the milk drink with 5 % fat was suggested to be due to the different ascorbyl palmitate concentrations applied; it was speculated that ascorbyl palmitate may have a stronger antioxidative effect in milk drink if lower concentrations than 3.75 mg/kg are applied, and this needs further investigation (Jacobsen *et al.*, 2008). It was also speculated that the different compositions of the two milk systems might have influenced the efficacy of ascorbyl palmitate. Milk with 1.5 % fat did not contain any additives, whereas the milk drink contained mono- and diglycerides, carageenan and guar gum, which may interact at the o/w interface. Such interactions may have reduced the ability of ascorbyl palmitate to regenerate tocopherol (Jacobsen *et al.*, 2008).

The effect of EDTA was also investigated in the milk system. Interestingly, when a low fish oil concentration (0.5 % fish oil) or when a very high quality fish oil (PV < 0.2 meq/kg) was used for supplementation with 1.5 % fish oil, EDTA only slightly reduced oxidation. In contrast, EDTA seemed to efficiently inhibit lipid oxidation when a high concentration of fish oil of a lower quality (PV 1.5 meq/kg) was used (Let *et al.*, 2005). The reason for the better effects of EDTA in milk emulsions containing fish oil of a lower quality was most likely that oxidation was much more pronounced in this emulsion and therefore the effect of EDTA was easier to detect. This finding was supported by another study on milk drink containing 5 % fat, of which 0.5 % (absolute value) was enzyme-modified fish oil. In this system, EDTA effectively reduced off-flavour formation (Timm-Heinrich *et al.*, 2004).

Recently, Boroski *et al.* (2012) evaluated the antioxidative effect of oregano extract and oregano essential oil in a dairy beverage formulation consisting of skim milk powder and water supplemented with $FeSO_4$ and linseed oil (2 g/100 g). They did not evaluate the effect of substituting linseed oil with fish oil, but the results are included in this chapter as similar effects of the antioxidants may be expected in fish oil enriched milk. Borski *et al.* (2012) found that both oregano extract and oregano essential oil could reduce formation of conjugated dienes, hexanal and propanal and depletion of oxygen caused by heat- or light-induced oxidation. The oregano extract was more efficient than oregano essential oil in doing so. The effects of the antioxidants on sensory properties were, however, not evaluated.

Other natural extracts, namely, rosemary and green tea extracts, have been evaluated in fish oil enriched milk (1.5 % fat) in our laboratory (Sørensen, 2010). Both types of extracts efficiently reduced formation of lipid hydroperoxides and volatile oxidation products. Unfortunately, addition of the antioxidant extracts also resulted in undesirable off-flavours of rosemary and green tea and they can therefore not be used as antioxidants in this food system (Sørensen, 2010).

As previously mentioned, lipophilized antioxidants have been evaluated in fish oil enriched milk (Sørensen *et al.*, 2012a). This study evaluated the antioxidative effect of dihydrocaffeic acid, rutin, two dihydrocaffeates (octyl and oleyl dihydrocaffeate) and two rutin esters (rutin laurate and rutin palimitate) (Fig. 4.3). For both types of compounds, the medium-chain ester was a better antioxidant than the long-chain ester and the phenol. Moreover, the results of dihydrocaffeates as antioxidants in fish oil enriched milk confirmed the findings from an earlier study in o/w emulsion (Sørensen *et al.*, 2012b). However, for the milk system, the difference in efficacy between octyl and oleyl dihydrocaffeate seemed to be smaller than in the simple o/w emulsions. Nevertheless, the results of dihydrocaffeates and rutin ester in fish oil enriched milk seemed to support the previously mentioned cut-off effect despite the few alkyl chain lengths evaluated for each phenolipid.

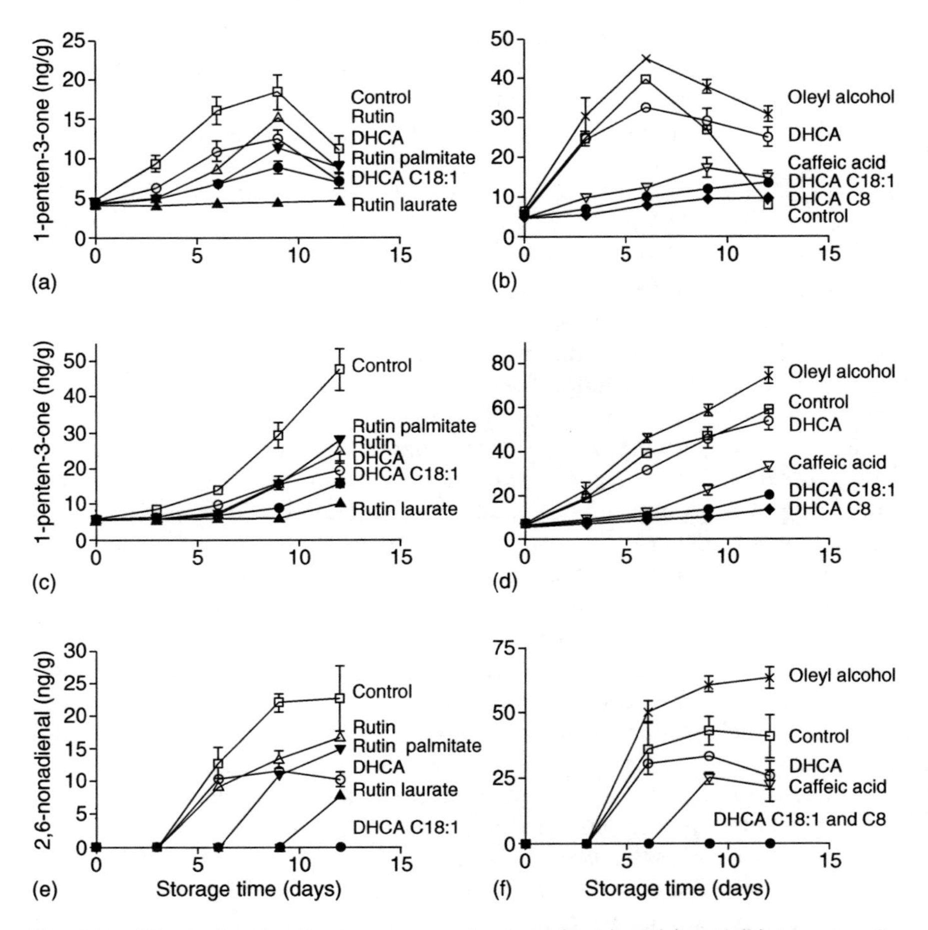

Fig. 4.3 Effect of antioxidants on concentrations (ng/g) of (a) and (b) 1-penten-3-one, (c) and (d) 1-penten-3-ol, (e) and (f) 2,6-nonadienal in milk. Bars indicate standard deviation of three measurements. DHCA: dihydrocaffeic acid; DHCA C8: octyl dihydrocaffeate; DHCA C18:1: oleyl dihydrocaffeate. Reprinted from Sørensen, A.-D., M., Petersen, L.K., de Diego, S., Nielsen, N.S., Lue, B.-M., Yang, Z., Xu, X. and Jacobsen, C. The antioxidative effect of lipophilized rutin and dihydrocaffeic acid in fish-oil-enriched milk. *Eur. J. Lipid Sci Technol.* 114, 434–445. Copyright (2012) with permission from Wiley-VCH.

4.4.2 Yoghurt and drinking yoghurt

Several studies have shown that yoghurt and drinking yoghurt enriched with omega-3 fatty acids have good sensory stability (Kolanowski *et al.*, 1999; Jacobsen *et al.*, 2006; Nielsen *et al.*, 2007). On the basis of these findings, it can be concluded that yoghurt could be easier to enrich with omega-3 PUFA than milk. This is probably the reason why only one study has evaluated the effect of adding antioxidants to this food system (Nielsen *et al.*, 2007). In this study, it was found that addition of citric acid ester (50, 100 and 200 mg/kg) to the drinking yoghurt did not have any effect. In contrast, addition of EDTA (50 mg/kg) seemed to have a slight antioxidative effect in drinking yoghurt after addition of iron ions (50 mg/kg), even though the presence of this pro-oxidant did not result in significantly more oxidation (Nielsen *et al.*, 2007).

4.4.3 Fitness bars and bread

Studies on the effects of antioxidant in fish oil enriched solid matrices such as breads or bread-like products are very scarce and only two studies have investigated antioxidant effects in fish oil enriched energy bars (Nielsen and Jacobsen, 2009; Horn *et al.*, 2009). In the first study, the effect of EDTA on oxidation in fitness bars enriched with emulsified fish oil was investigated. Surprisingly, EDTA (100–2000 mg/kg) decreased the oxidative stability compared to energy bars without EDTA. The authors suggested that the EDTA:iron ratio was too low to obtain an antioxidative effect in this system. They based this hypothesis on the fact that the concentration of EDTA must be sufficient to chelate all the iron, otherwise preferential chelation of Fe^{3+} over Fe^{2+} takes place, leaving the more active oxidation catalyst Fe^{2+} free to work.

Horn *et al.* (2009) evaluated the effect of the hydrophilic antioxidant, caffeic acid, in energy bars at 3.75–15 mg/kg. Similar to EDTA, caffeic acid also decreased the oxidative stability. The authors ascribed the pro-oxidative effect of caffeic acid to its ability to reduce transition metal ions, which are more potent pro-oxidants than the unreduced form. The hydrophilic nature of caffeic acid was furthermore suggested to lead to a localization of caffeic acid that would favour reduction of metal ions over radical scavenging.

Two other antioxidants with different polarities/solubilities were tested in the same study, namely the amphiphilic ascorbyl palmitate and the lipophilic γ-tocopherol. Ascorbyl palmitate was added to energy bars in concentrations of 3.75–15 mg/kg and showed less pro-oxidative activity than caffeic acid, but still decreased oxidative stability, especially in the highest concentrations (Horn *et al.*, 2009). The authors suggested that the pro-oxidant activity of ascorbyl palmitate was caused by the same mechanism as that of caffeic acid, i.e. the ability of the 'antioxidant' to reduce transition metals to a more pro-oxidative form. As mentioned above, more or less similar results have been reported for fish oil enriched salad dressing. Thus, a high concentration of ascorbyl palmitate was found to be more pro-oxidative than a lower concentration in both systems (Let *et al.*, 2007b; Horn *et al.*, 2009). The concentration dependence of ascorbyl palmitate was suggested to exist because the antioxidative mechanism of ascorbyl palmitate is over-ridden by its ability to reduce transition metal ions when present in a high concentration (Horn *et al.*, 2009).

In contrast to the hydrophilic and amphiphilic antioxidants tested in energy bars, the lipophilic γ-tocopherol (5.5–55 mg/kg) had an antioxidative effect when added in concentrations above 22 mg/kg (Horn *et al.*, 2009). The authors suggested that the lipophilic nature of γ-tocopherol favoured an optimal localization of the antioxidant in order to carry out its antioxidative effect. However, in low concentrations, a pro-oxidative effect of γ-tocopherol was observed, which is contradictory to other studies on the effects of tocopherols, in which pro-oxidative effects were found for high concentrations of tocopherols (Huang *et al.*, 1994).

Taken together, the proposed ability of caffeic acid and ascorbyl palmitate to act as pro-oxidants because they reduced Fe^{3+} to Fe^{2+} could indicate that metal catalysed oxidation to some extent is an important factor in energy bars. However, the finding that EDTA was also found to be pro-oxidative may suggest that the metal catalysing mechanism may be different from that observed in systems such as mayonnaise and dressing (Jacobsen *et al.*, 2001a; Let *et al.*, 2007a). The observed strong antioxidative effect of γ-tocopherol suggests that free radical scavengers can reduce lipid oxidation in energy bars. This could indicate that initiation of lipid oxidation by already existing free radicals present in the ingredients used for energy bars may be an important factor. The control of lipid oxidation may therefore perhaps be further improved by adding a combination of antioxidants with both free radical scavenging and metal-chelating properties. This deserves further investigation.

Only one study on the effect of the addition of antioxidants to omega-3 enriched bread has been reported in the literature (de Conto *et al.*, 2012). In this study, bread was enriched with microencapsulated fish oil and the antioxidative effect of rosemary extract was investigated. Different concentrations of both microencapsulated fish oil (0.00–5.00 g/100 g) and rosemary extract (0.000–0.100 g/100 g) were applied using a central composite rotational design. Among the responses evaluated were sensory acceptance tests for appearance, aroma, flavour texture and overall acceptance. All samples enriched with omega-3 oils presented acceptable sensory scores and the addition of rosemary extract did not affect sensory characteristics.

4.4.4 Fish and meat products

Relatively few studies are available on the stabilization of omega-3 enriched fish and meat products by antioxidants. Park *et al.* (2004) evaluated the antioxidative effect of EDTA in cod surimi enriched with 1.5 % algal oil. The algal oil was added either as neat oil or as an o/w emulsion. Two different algal oils were evaluated – one without antioxidants added and one with a mix of lipid-soluble antioxidants (1000 mg/kg tocopherol mixture, 1000 mg/kg rosemary extract and 500 mg/kg ascorbyl palmitate). EDTA did not have any effect in cod surimi with neat oil containing lipid-soluble antioxidants when evaluated by determination of PV and thiobarbituric acid reactive substances (TBARS). In contrast, an antioxidative effect of EDTA was observed when the algal oil was added to the cod surimi as an emulsion with lipid-soluble antioxidants.

Pérez-Mateos *et al.* (2006) also studied the oxidative stability of fish oil enriched surimi in the presence of different antioxidants. In this study, surimi was made from pollock muscle to which menhaden oil or a fish oil concentrate was added, each in two concentrations (7.0 or 11.6 % for menhaden oil and 1.7 or 2.8 % for the fish oil concentrate). Menhaden oil contained a mixture of tocopherols plus TBHQ added by the fish oil manufacturer, whereas the fish oil concentrate only contained a mixture of tocopherols. Surimi enriched with menhaden oil received better sensory scores than surimi enriched with fish oil concentrate, mainly due to the fact that the latter had a fishy taste. Rosemary (750 mg/kg) or tea extracts (650 mg/kg) were able to partially mask this fishy taste, but both extracts seemed to have weak pro-oxidative effects in surimi with menhaden oil (Pérez-Mateos *et al.*, 2006).

Olsen *et al.* (2006) evaluated the antioxidative effect of addition of citric acid (3300 mg/kg) or EDTA (75 mg/kg) to salmon paté containing 14 % cod liver oil. The fish oil producer had added α-tocopherol (1075 mg/kg), lecithin (1050 mg/kg) and ascorbyl palmitate (375 mg/kg) to the cod liver oil which was used in this experiment. Analysis of secondary volatile oxidation products by gas chromatography – mass spectroscopy (GC–MS) as well as sensory analysis suggested that neither citric acid nor EDTA could prevent lipid oxidation in this food system. In fact, citric acid and EDTA even slightly promoted formation of volatile oxidation products. EDTA had a small positive impact on the sensory perception of the samples, whereas citric acid seemed to slightly increase scores for rancidity. The authors suggested that the poor effect of citric acid was partly due to the fact that addition of citric acid reduced pH, which in some cases has been shown to increase oxidation. Likewise, it was suggested that the increased formation of volatiles in samples with EDTA was due to a too low EDTA concentration.

The antioxidative effects of rosemary, mixed tocopherols, TBHQ or ascorbyl palmitate in extruded salmon jerky snacks have recently been evaluated (Kong *et al.*, 2011). In this product additional omega-3 oils was not added, but is included in this chapter as it is one of the rare studies on antioxidants in omega-3 rich snack products. Rosemary inhibited formation of lipid hydroperoxides better than the other antioxidants, but none of the antioxidants significantly inhibited malonaldehyde levels, which is a measure for secondary oxidation products. Rosemary also inhibited loss of pigments (astaxanthin) better than any of the other antioxidants.

The effects of adding antioxidant cocktails to different meat products enriched with algal oil were investigated by Lee *et al.* (2005, 2006). The results of these studies are further discussed in Chapter 10 on enrichment of meat products with omega-3.

4.5 Future trends

Traditionally, the industry has mainly used free radical chain-breaking synthetic antioxidants for the prevention of oxidation in foods. As mentioned above, this strategy seems to be less efficient in preventing lipid oxidation in many food systems enriched with omega-3 PUFA. With our increased understanding of the important role of trace metals, emulsifiers and processing conditions in lipid oxidation processes, more efforts will be dedicated to using this knowledge to develop alternative strategies to retard lipid oxidation in real foods with omega-3 PUFA oils. One such strategy may be an increased use of natural metal chelators, including plant extracts, with both radical scavenging and metal chelating properties.

4.6 Conclusion

As illustrated in this chapter, antioxidants can increase the oxidative stability of omega-3 enriched foods. However, it should be noted that in several cases antioxidants, such as propyl gallate, tocopherol and ascorbyl palmitate, which have traditionally been used by the food industry, are not very efficient in omega-3 PUFA containing foods. Moreover, the same antioxidant exerts completely different effects in different food systems. Therefore, a better quantitative understanding of the effects of antioxidants in real food systems is necessary. Research on lipophilized antioxidants is on-going in several research groups in the world and hopefully this research will help us to better understand the structure–activity relationship of antioxidants in complex food systems.

4.7 References

BOROSKI, M., GIROUX, H. J., SABIK, H., PETIT, H. V., VISENTAINER, J. V., MATUMOTO-PINTRO, P. T. and BRITTEN, M. (2012) 'Use of oregano extract and essential oil as antioxidants in functional dairy beverage formulations', *LWT–Food Science and Technology*, 47, 167–174.

DE CONTO, L. C., OLIVEIRA, R. S. P., MARTIN, L. G. P., CHANG, Y. K. and STED, C. J. (2012) 'Effects of the addition of microencapsulated omega-3 and rosemary extract on the technological and sensory quality of white pan bread', *LWT–Food Science and Technology*, 45, 103–109.

FRANKEL, E. N. (2005) *Lipid Oxidation*. Dundee: The Oily Press.

FRANKEL, E. N., HUANG, S.-W., KANNER, J. and GERMAN, B. (1994) 'Interfacial phenomena in the evaluation of antioxidants: Bulk oils vs emulsions', *J Agric Food Chem*, 42, 1054–1059.

HORN, A. F., NIELSEN, N. S. and JACOBSEN, C. (2009) 'Additions of caffeic acid, ascorbyl palmitate or γ-tocopherol to fish oil-enriched energy bars affect lipid oxidation differently', *Food Chem*, 112, 412–420.

HUANG, S.-W., FRANKEL, E. N. and GERMAN, J. B. (1994) 'Antioxidant activity of α- and γ-tocopherols in bulk oils and in oil-in water emulsions', *J Agric Food Chem*, 42, 2108–2114.

HUANG, S.-W., HOPIA, A., SCHWARZ, K., FRANKEL, E. N. and GERMAN, J. B. (1996) 'Antioxidant activity of α-tocopherol and trolox in different lipid substrates: Bulk oils vs oil-in-water emulsions', *J Agric Food Chem*, 44, 444–452.

HUBER, G. M., RUPASINGHE, H. P. V. and SHAHIDI, F. (2009) 'Inhibition of oxidation of omega-3 polyunsaturated fatty acids and fish oil by quercetin glycosides', *Food Chem*, 117, 290–295.

JACOBSEN, C., ADLER-NISSEN, J. and MEYER, A. S. (1999a) 'Effect of ascorbic acid on iron release from the emulsifier interface and on the oxidative flavor deterioration in fish oil enriched mayonnaise', *J Agric Food Chem*, 47, 4917–4926.

JACOBSEN, C., HARTVIGSEN, K., LUND, P., MEYER, A.S., ADLER-NISSEN, J., HOLSTBORG, J. and HØLMER, G. (1999b) 'Oxidation in fish oil enriched mayonnaise: 1. Assessment of propyl gallate as antioxidant by discriminant partial least squares regression analysis', *Z Lebensm Unters Forsch*, 210, 13–30.

JACOBSEN, C., HARTVIGSEN, K., LUND, P., ADLER-NISSEN, J., HØLMER, G. and MEYER, A. S. (2000) 'Oxidation in fish oil enriched mayonnaise: 2. Assessment of the efficacy of different tocopherol antioxidant systems by discriminant partial least squares regression analysis', *Eur Food Res Technol*, 210, 242–257.

JACOBSEN, C., HARTVIGSEN, K., THOMSEN, M. K., HANSEN, L. F., LUND, P., SKIBSTED, L. H., HØLMER, G., ADLER-NISSEN, J. and MEYER, A. S. (2001a) 'Lipid oxidation in fish oil enriched mayonnaise: Calcium disodium ethylenediaminetetraacetate, but not gallic acid, strongly inhibited oxidative deterioration', *J Agric Food Chem*, 49, 1009–1019.

JACOBSEN, C., TIMM, M. and MEYER, A. S. (2001b) 'Oxidation in fish oil enriched mayonnaise: Ascorbic acid and low pH increase oxidative deterioration', *J Agric Food Chem*, 49, 3947–3956.

JACOBSEN, C., LET, M. B., ANDERSEN, G. and MEYER, A. S. (2006) 'Oxidative stability of fish oil enriched yoghurts', in JACOBSEN, J., BAKAERT, C., SÆBØ, K., OEHLENSCHLÄGER, A. and LUTEN, J. (eds), *Seafood Research From Fish to Dish: Quality, Safety and Processing of Wild and Farmed Fish.* Wageningen: Wageningen Academic Publishers, pp. 71–86.

JACOBSEN, C., LET, M. B., NIELSEN, N. S. and MEYER, A. S. (2008) 'Antioxidant strategies for preventing oxidative flavour deterioration of foods enriched with n-3 polyunsaturated lipids: a comparative evaluation', *Trend Food SciTechnol*, 19, 76–93.

JAFAR, S. S., HULTIN, H. O., BIMBO, A. P., CROWTHER, J. B. and BARLOW, S. M. (1994) 'Stabilization by antioxidants of mayonnaise made from fish oil', *J Food Lipids*, 1, 295–311.

KOLANOWSKI, W., SWIDERSKI, F. and BERGER, S. (1999) 'Possibilities of fish oil application for food products enrichment with omega-3 PUFA', *Int J Food Sci Nutr*, 50, 39–49.

KONG, J. A., PERKINS, L. B., DOUGHERTY, M. P. and CAMIRE, M. E. (2011) 'Control of lipid oxidation in extruded salmon jerky snacks', *J Food Sci*, 76, C8–C13.

KULÅS, E. and ACKMAN, R. G. (2001) 'Different tocopherols and the relationship between two methods for determination of primary oxidation products in fish oil', *J Agric Food Chem*, 49, 1724–1729.

KULÅS, E., OLSEN, E. and ACKMAN, R. G. (2002) 'Effect of alpha-, gamma-, delta-tocopherol on the distribution of volatile secondary oxidation products in fish oil', *Eur J Lipid Sci Technol*, 104, 520–529.

LAGUERRE, M., GIRALDO, L. J. L., LECOMTE, J., FIGUEROA-ESPINOZA, M. C., BARÉA, B., WEISS, J., DECKER, E. A. and VILLENEUVE, P. (2009) 'Chain length affects antioxidant properties of chlorogenate esters in emulsion: the cutoff theory behind the polar paradox', *J Agric Food Chem*, 57 (23), 11335–11342.

LAGUERRE, M., GIRALDO, L. J. L., LECOMTE, J., FIGUEROA-ESPINOZA, M.-C., BARÉA, B., WEISS, J., DECKER, E. A. and VILLENEUVE, P. (2010) 'Relationship between hydrophobicity and antioxidant ability of 'phenolipids' in emulsion: a parabolic effect of the chain length of rosmarinate esters', *J Agric Food Chem*, 58, 2869–2876.

LEE, S., DECKER, E. A., FAUSTMAN, C. and MANCINI, R. A. (2005) 'The effects of antioxidant combinations on color and lipid oxidation in n-3 oil fortified ground beef patties', *Meat Sci*, 70, 683–689.

LEE, S., HERNANDEZ, P., DJORDJEVIC, D., FARAJI, H., HOLLENDER, R., FAUSTMAN, C. and DECKER, E. A. (2006) 'Effect of antioxidants and cooking on stability of n-3 fatty acids in fortified meat products', *J Food Sci*, 71, 233–238.

LET, M. B., JACOBSEN, C. and MEYER, A. S. (2004) 'Effects of fish oil type, lipid antioxidants and presence of rapeseed oil on oxidative flavour stability of fish oil enriched milk', *Eur J Lipid Sci Technol*, 106, 170–182.

LET, M. B., JACOBSEN, C., PHAM, K. A. and MEYER, A. S. (2005) 'Protection against oxidation of fish-oil-enriched milk emulsions through addition of rapeseed oil or antioxidants', *J Agric Food Chem*, 53, 5429–5437.

LET, M. B., JACOBSEN, C. and MEYER, A. S. (2007a) 'Ascorbyl palmitate, gamma-tocopherol, and EDTA affect lipid oxidation in fish oil enriched salad dressing differently', *J Agric Food Chem*, 55, 2369–2375.

LET, M. B., JACOBSEN, C. and MEYER, A. S. (2007b) 'Lipid oxidation in milk, yoghurt, and salad dressing enriched with neat fish oil or pre-emulsified fish oil', *J Agric Food Chem*, 55, 7802–7809.

LUE, B.-M. (2009) *Enzymatic lipophilization of bioactive compounds in ionic liquids*, PhD thesis, Aarhus University, Denmark.

MARTÍN, D., TERRÓN, A., FORNARI, T., REGLERO, G. and TORRES, C. F. (2012) 'Oxidative stabilization of ultra-high omega-3 concentrates as ethyl esters or triacylglycerols', *Food Res Int*, 45, 336–341.

NIELSEN, N. S. and JACOBSEN, C. (2009) 'Methods for reducing lipid oxidation in fish-oil-enriched energy bars', *Int J Food Sci Technol*, 44, 1536–1546.

NIELSEN, N. S., PETERSEN, A., MEYER, A. S., TIMM-HEINRICH, M. and JACOBSEN, C. (2004) 'Effects of lactoferrin, phytic acid, and EDTA on oxidation in two food emulsions enriched with long-chain polyunsaturated fatty acids', *J Agric Food Chem*, 52, 7690–7699.

NIELSEN, N. S., DEBNATH, D. and JACOBSEN, C. (2007) 'Oxidative stability of fish oil enriched drinking yoghurt', *Int Dairy J*, 17, 1478–1485.

OLSEN, E., VEBERG, A., VOGT, G., TOMIC, O., KIRKHUS, B., EKEBERG, D. and NILSSON, A. (2006) 'Analysis of early lipid oxidation in salmon pate with cod liver oil and antioxidants', *J Food Sci*, 71, S284–S292.

PARK, Y., KELLEHER, S. D., McCLEMENTS, D. J. and DECKER, E. A. (2004) 'Incorporation and stabilization of omega-3 fatty acids in surimi made from cod, *Gadus morhua*', *J Agric Food Chem*, 52, 597–601.

PÉREZ-MATEOS, M., LANIER, T. C. and BOYD, L. C. (2006) 'Effects of rosemary and green tea extracts on frozen surimi gels fortified with omega-3 fatty acids', *J Sci Food Agric*, 86, 558–567.

PORTER, W. L. (1993) 'Paradoxical behavior of antioxidants in food and biological systems', *Toxicol Ind Health*, 9, 93–122.

SØRENSEN, A.-D. M. (2010) *The influence of ingredients or lipophilized antioxidants on the oxidative stability of fish oil enriched food systems*, PhD thesis, National Food Institute, Technical University of Denmark. ISBN 978-87-92158-92-5

SØRENSEN, A.-D. M., HAAHR, A.-M., BECKER, E. M., SKIBSTED, L. H., BERGENSTÅHL, B., NILSSON, L. and JACOBSEN, C. (2008) 'Interactions between iron, phenolic compounds, emulsifiers, and pH in omega-3-enriched oil-in-water emulsions', *J Agric Food Chem*, 56, 1740–1750.

SØRENSEN, A.-D. M., NIELSEN, N. S. and JACOBSEN, C. (2009) 'Oxidative stability of fish oil enriched mayonnaise based salads', *Eur J Lipid Sci Technol*, 112, 476–487.

SØRENSEN, A.-D. M., PETERSEN, L. K., DE DIEGO, S., NIELSEN, N. S., LUE, B.-M., YANG, Z., XU, X. and JACOBSEN, C. (2012a) 'The antioxidative effect of lipophilized rutin and dihydrocaffeic acid in fish-oil-enriched milk', *Eur J Lipid Sci Technol*, 114, 434–445.

SØRENSEN, A.-D. M., NIELSEN, N. S., YANG, Z., XU, X. and JACOBSEN, C. (2012b) 'The effect of lipophilization of dihydrocaffeic acid on its antioxidative properties in fish-oil-enriched emulsion', *Eur J Lipid Sci Technol*, 114, 134–145.

TIMM-HEINRICH, M., XU, X., NIELSEN, N. S. and JACOBSEN, C. (2004) 'Oxidative stability of mayonnaise and milk drink produced with structured lipids based on fish oil and caprylic acid', *Eur Food Res Technol*, 219, 32–41.

YOUNG, F. V. K. (1990) 'Using unhydrogenated fish oil in margarine', *INFORM*, 1, 731–741.

5

Stabilization of omega-3 oils and enriched foods using emulsifiers

C. Genot, T.-H. Kabri and A. Meynier, INRA, France

DOI: 10.1533/9780857098863.2.150

Abstract: This chapter reviews the use of emulsifiers in delivery systems and foods enriched in omega-3 fatty acids. It begins by explaining the reasons why emulsifiers are required for formulation and stabilization of various multiphase systems, the focus being on oil-in-water emulsions, before going on to give an overview of the main classes of food-grade emulsifiers and their ability to stabilize emulsions and food formulations related to some of their molecular characteristics. The possible involvement of emulsifiers such as proteins and lecithins in delaying lipid oxidation is then presented, and the effects of emulsification and emulsifiers on flavour are also summarized. In conclusion, the potential for optimizing the bioavailability and the beneficial effects of polyunsaturated fatty acids through the control of lipid organization and the need for research in this area are underlined.

Key words: food-grade emulsifiers, lecithin, protein, oil/water interface, omega-3 PUFA oils, oxidation, formulated foods, omega-3 fatty acids.

5.1 Introduction

The market for foods enriched with oils containing polyunsaturated fatty acids (PUFA) from the n-3 series (omega-3 PUFA), has seen a dramatic expansion (see Chapter 2) in response to national and international nutritional recommendations regarding the dietary intake of lipids (AFSSA, 2010; EFSA, 2010a; Taneja and Singh, 2012). Indeed, numerous scientific papers have proven or reviewed the health benefits of these fatty acids (Yashodhara *et al.*, 2009), which are often provided in insufficient amounts by the diet (Astorg *et al.*, 2004; Bauch *et al.*, 2006; Sioen *et al.*, 2010; Meyer, 2011).

Once the legal specifications ensuring the safety of the ingredients have been met, the production and marketing of high-value omega-3 enriched products still needs to pass several additional barriers. Formulations containing omega-3 PUFA oils need to respond to technological and sensory criteria. Their appearance, texture and flavour (or taste) should be guaranteed to ensure their acceptability by the consumer. Ease of preparation and handling are also essential. In all cases, the final product or the intermediate delivery system should be stable during storage and keep its original properties during its entire shelf-life. However, the introduction of oils containing omega-3 fatty acids in a complex formulation poses problems related to their physical and chemical stabilities.

The chemical and physical stabilities of omega-3 formulations are interdependent phenomena characterized by complex multi-timescale kinetics. Physical instability of omega-3 PUFA formulations originates from the hydrophobic nature of the oils and their insolubility in water; it is driven by thermodynamic features and partially resolved through the use of emulsifiers (Friberg and Larsson, 1997; McClements, 2005). Chemical instability results from the high susceptibility of PUFA to become oxidized and to form various oxidative species in the presence of oxygen. It is dependent on many parameters, among them emulsified state and emulsifier characteristics (McClements and Decker, 2000; Genot *et al.*, 2003a, 2013; Frankel, 2005; Jacobsen *et al.*, 2008 and Waraho *et al.*, 2011). Thus emulsifiers play a part in both the physical and the chemical stabilization of the formulations. Finally, emulsifiers also contribute to the expression of the sensory properties (flavour and texture) of the final products.

The objective of this chapter is to provide an overview of the use of emulsifiers to stabilize omega-3 PUFA food formulations. We will show how emulsifiers can physically stabilize omega-3 PUFA oil formulations or foods, before presenting an overview of the range of emulsifiers that can be used for this purpose. Current knowledge of the influence of emulsifiers on lipid oxidation will also be summarized. In addition, as sensory aspects often determine consumer acceptability, the effect of emulsification and emulsifiers on the release of odorant compounds and on their sensory perception will be briefly covered. Examples of applications from the literature will be used to illustrate these different features.

5.2 Reasons for using emulsifiers

5.2.1 Characteristics of omega-3 polyunsaturated fatty acid (PUFA) oils

Omega-3 PUFA oils include oils from vegetal origin containing α-linolenic acid (LNA: C18:3 n-3) and oils mainly from marine origin characterized by their content in the long-chain PUFA (LC-PUFA) eicosapentaenoic acid (EPA: C20:5 n-3) and docosahexaenoic acid (DHA: C22:6 n-3) (see chapters 1 and 2). They also comprise chemically or enzymatically structured oils (Osborn and Akoh, 2002) and oils made of ethyl esters of the above LC-PUFA. With the exception of this last case, the fatty acids (FA) in the oils are esterified on the glycerol backbone of triacylglycerols (TAG) or possibly of diacylglycerols or phospholipids (PL). Due to their richness in PUFA, these oils have melting points well below zero degrees. They are liquid at ambient temperature. They are immiscible with water and have a low density of: 0.900–0.922 g.cm^{-3} (Bockish, 1998) or even lower (Sathivel *et al.*, 2003; Yin *et al.*, 2011). Thus, when mixed with an aqueous medium they tend naturally to separate and float over the aqueous medium. When omega-3 PUFA were introduced into a delivery system or a food product this natural destabilization must be counteracted. This is the primary reason for the use of emulsifiers in delivery systems and food formulations.

Edible oils also contain, in amounts depending on the extraction procedure and the refining degree, a lot of minor compounds such as lipophilic vitamins, phenolics and pigments, but also possibly free fatty acids, partial glycerides (mono- and diglycerides), polar lipids, traces of water, minerals, lipid oxidation products and odorant compounds. Many of these compounds are surface-active and chemically reactive. These compounds can actively contribute to the stabilization/destabilization of omega-3 PUFA delivery systems and enriched foods, but they can not generally ensure the long-term stability of the products in the current practice of food agrosystems. They could also contribute to the higher viscosity of the unrefined oils as compared to the refined ones (Sathivel *et al.*, 2003; Yin *et al.*, 2011).

5.2.2 Emulsions and other potential delivery systems: definitions

An *emulsion* is a basic structure for many products made in industries such as food processing, cosmetics and pharmaceuticals. The term 'emulsion' has been extended to all thermodynamically unstable multiphase systems comprising at least one hydrophilic phase (water) and a lipophilic phase (oil), the one being dispersed as droplets in the other. Emulsions are divided into oil-in-water (o/w) emulsions such as, for example, milk, mayonnaise, soups and sauces, and water-in-oil (w/o) emulsions, represented by butter, margarines and spreads (McClements, 2007; Kralova and Sjoblom, 2009). A schematic representation of o/w and w/o emulsions is provided in Fig. 5.1. In this chapter, we will focus on o/w emulsions as a basis for many delivery systems for incorporating omega-3 PUFA oil into food products and also look at microemulsions because these systems have great potential for future applications. The o/w emulsions are currently classified according to the size distribution of their oil droplets (McClements, 2012).

The term *emulsion*, or *macroemulsion*, refers to conventional emulsions for which the average droplet size is larger than the micrometre. Macroemulsions with droplet sizes >0.5 μm can be observed with an optical microscope. They are sensitive to the action of gravity following Stokes' law. Emulsions whose droplet size is centred around 100 nm or below (Salager *et al.*, 2001) are called *nanoemulsions*. These emulsions are transparent. Their preparation requires specific emulsification protocols involving

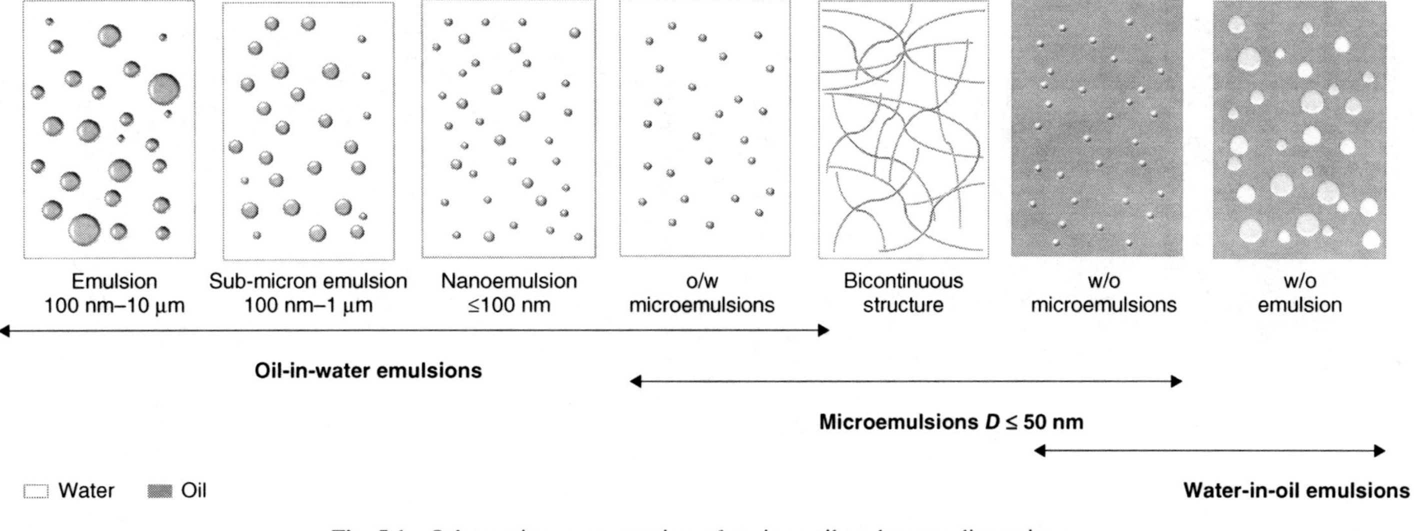

Fig. 5.1 Schematic representation of various oil and water dispersions.

high-energy (microfluidizer) or low-energy (phase-inversion) techniques. In between, *sub-micron emulsions* (200 nm < droplet size < 1 μm) present a milky appearance, as do macroemulsions. They are sometimes incorrectly named microemulsions. Nanoemulsions and sub-micron emulsions are thermodynamically unstable systems, but they are less sensitive to Stokes' law than conventional emulsions and kinetically less sensitive to other destabilization mechanisms. *Multilayer emulsions* are made of oil droplets successively coated by a charged emulsifier and a polymer with an opposite charge whereas *Pickering emulsions* are stabilized by solid particles. Finally, *multiple* o/w/o or w/o/w *emulsions* have been proposed to deliver active molecules with low solubility for specific applications.

Microemulsions are thermodynamically stable and isotropic mixtures of water, oil, surfactant and co-surfactant. They require low energy input, and they are characterized by internal structures of typical sizes (5–100 nm) well below the wavelengths of visible light, and are therefore transparent. Microemulsions are either organized as small size o/w or w/o emulsions, very similar to nanoemulsions, or as bicontinuous interpenetrated water and oil domains with alternate interfacial curvatures (Fig. 5.1). These structures, formed from the self-assembly of biomolecules, are the basis for the formation of oleogels. They could be promising tools for lipophilic compounds delivery, including omega-3 fatty acids (Marangoni and Garti, 2011).

5.2.3 Formation of emulsions – the emulsification process

The process that converts two separate immiscible liquids into an emulsion or that reduces the size of the droplets in a pre-existing emulsion is known as emulsification. This process requires an input of energy and the presence of emulsifier (Friberg and Larsson, 1997; McClements, 2005). The most common systems used in the manufacture of emulsions are rotor–stator, high-pressure, ultrasonic and membrane systems (Schultz *et al.*, 2004; McClements, 2005; Urban *et al.*, 2006; Jafari *et al.*, 2008).

High speed blenders are widely used in the food industry for the direct homogenization of oil and water phases. These blenders produce droplet sizes ranging from 2–10 μm. *Colloid mills* are based on the formation of a high-shear laminar flow between rotor and stator disks, which enables reduction of the droplet size of coarse or high-viscosity emulsions. The size of the oil droplets obtained with these blenders varies between 1 and 5 μm. Fine emulsions in the food industry are often prepared with *high-pressure valve homogenizers*. A coarse emulsion (primary emulsion) is forced from a pressure chamber through a valve by a high-pressure pump. A combination of intense shear, cavitational and turbulent flow conditions breaks the large droplets into smaller ones. Droplet size ranging from 0.1–2 μm are typically produced.

Ultrasonic homogenizers are well suited to producing small volumes of emulsions and are used in research laboratories when raw materials used to prepare emulsions are expensive. The main droplet disruption mechanism of these homogenizers is cavitation. The droplet sizes obtained can be very small (0.1 μm).

Membrane homogenizers are used to form emulsions by forcing one phase into the other through a solid membrane of controlled pore size. The major advantage of this technique is a very high energy yield because less energy is lost by viscous dissipation compared to the other techniques, but the technique cannot be used for preparing concentrated emulsions. Droplet size varies between 0.5 and 10 μm, depending on the size of the membrane pores and the oil and aqueous phase flows. Membrane emulsification has been proposed to prepare emulsions with well-defined droplet sizes and less broad droplet size distributions than the other techniques.

Additionally, low-energy techniques have been developed to produce nanoemulsions (Gutiérrez *et al.*, 2008; McClements, 2011). For instance, protein-stabilized nanoemulsions can be produced with a combined homogenization and amphiphilic solvent dissolution/evaporation approach (Lee and McClements, 2010), by the emulsion inversion point (EIP) method or by the phase inversion temperature (PIT) method (Sagalowicz and Leser, 2010). Microemulsions, in common with other self-assembly structures, require little energy for their formation, but they require a large amount of surfactants.

5.2.4 Destabilization of emulsions

The term 'emulsion stability' refers to the ability of an emulsion to resist changes in its physical properties over time (Friberg and Larsson, 1997; McClements, 2005). For oils having low water solubility, such as omega-3 oils, these changes are mainly due to three mechanisms of destabilization: creaming, coalescence and flocculation (Fig. 5.2). Emulsion stability, in static conditions (storage) and in dynamic conditions (handling and processing *post*-emulsification, for instance pumping, mixing, sterilization, freeze–thaw treatment, drying) is an important consideration even if the emulsion is only to be stored for a short period of time. Emulsion stability and the underlying mechanisms have been extensively described in many books and review papers (such as, for instance, those cited above). Therefore only the most important knowledge with regards to the contents of this chapter has been summarized below.

Flocculation is often the first stage of emulsion destabilization, because it facilitates creaming and coalescence. It occurs when two or more droplets come together to form an aggregate in which the droplets retain their individual integrity. Depending on the concentration of the lipid phase, the aggregates may either be separated by regions of the continuous phase or fill up the whole emulsion. Flocculation depends on the relative magnitude of electrostatic, steric, van der Waals, hydrophobic and depletion colloidal interactions, the first two being repulsive and the other three attractive.

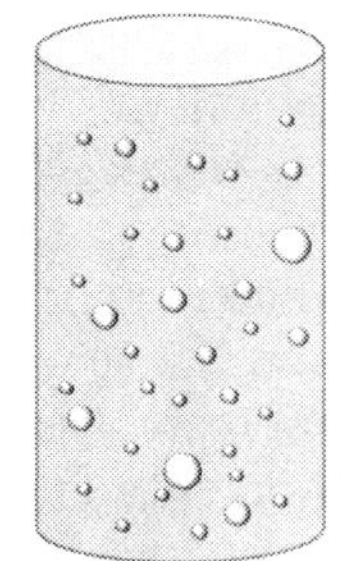

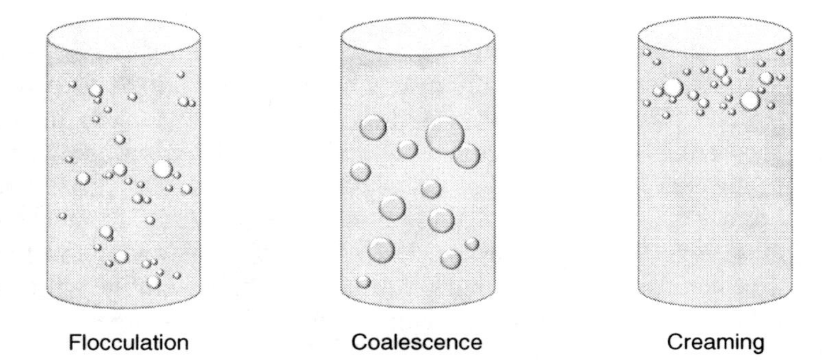

Fig. 5.2 Main mechanisms of emulsion destabilization.

When attractive forces prevail over repulsive ones, droplets remain in contact after collision. Aggregates, or flocs, are formed.

Coalescence is the process whereby two or more droplets merge to form a single larger droplet due to rupture of the interfacial film. Extensive droplet coalescence can eventually lead to the formation of a separate layer of oil on top of a sample, which is known as 'oiling off'. The probability of coalescence occurrence is proportional to the time when two droplets are close together. Coalescence is enhanced by high shear force and reduced viscosity of the continuous phase and depends on the properties of the interfacial film.

Creaming corresponds to the upward movement of droplets or droplet aggregates due to the fact that they have a lower density than the surrounding liquid, whereas sedimentation describes the downward movement of droplets when they have a higher density than the surrounding liquid. The velocity of creaming directly depends on the density difference between the dispersed and continuous phases, the square diameter of the droplets and the inverse viscosity of the continuous phase. Hydrocolloids, which increase the viscosity of the aqueous phase or which have gelling properties, are effective in preventing creaming. Nanoemulsions are very resistant to physical destabilization *via* creaming, flocculation or coalescence. Their very small oil droplets have low volume/surface ratio that enhances the relative part taken by the interfacial layer in the droplet's volume and mass fractions and in their overall properties. As this layer integrates water molecules interacting with the emulsifiers, especially in the case of polymeric emulsifiers, the density difference between water phase and oil droplets is reduced. This makes nanoemulsions relatively impervious to gravitational force. Moreover, the thickness of the interface compared to the size of the droplets favours steric stabilization (Sagalowicz and Leser, 2010).

5.2.5 The role of emulsifiers in the stabilization of emulsions

Mechanical energy alone is not sufficient to form a kinetically stable emulsion since two immiscible phases rapidly revert back after processing to their initial separate phases with oil at the top and water below; the presence of surface-active molecules is also required. This is why emulsions are produced by homogenizing oil and aqueous phases together in the presence of one or more emulsifiers (McClements, 2005).

Emulsifiers are surface-active agents that adsorb at the o/w interfaces created during the homogenization process (Fig. 5.3). They decrease the surface tension between the oil and the water phases (around 25 mN m^{-1} between pure triglycerides and water), the amount of energy needed for disrupting the droplets, namely the Laplace pressure, and the total free energy of the system. Indeed, the smaller the droplets, the more energy is

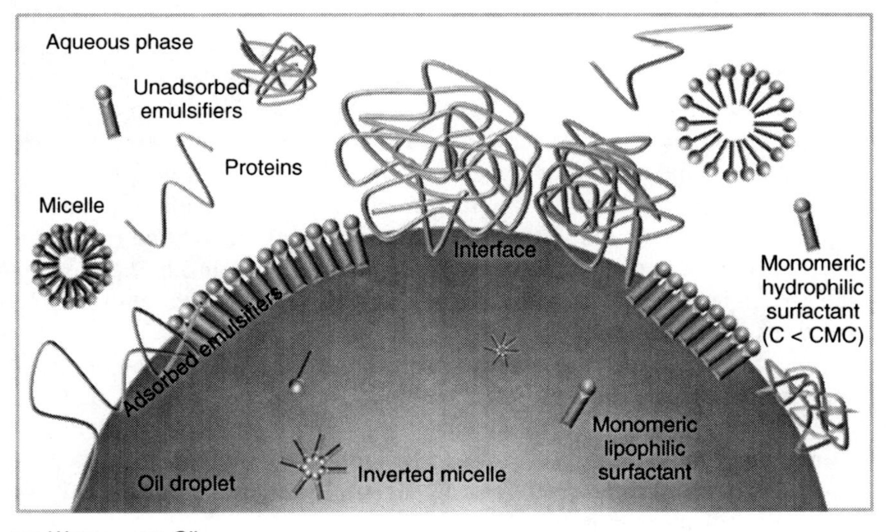

Fig. 5.3 Schematic representation of the partition of emulsifiers between interface, oil and water phase in an emulsion.

needed for breaking their surface. Emulsifiers facilitate the formation of emulsions by this means.

Emulsifiers also prevent the flocculation and coalescence of oil droplets by forming a protective layer generating steric or electrostatic repulsive interactions which slow down or prevent aggregation of the droplets. Flocculation can be inhibited by electrostatic repulsions taking place between charged interfaces owing to the charge carried by the adsorbed emulsifiers. However, in food systems, the best way to reduce the occurrence of flocculation phenomena is often to make use of steric interactions afforded by biopolymers. Indeed, when an emulsion is stabilized through electrostatic interactions, the system is pH- and ionic strength-sensitive, a screening or a decrease of the droplet charge provoking irreversible flocculation. In contrast, systems mainly stabilized by steric interactions are subject only to weak and easily reversible flocculation. They are also relatively insensitive to destabilization induced by freeze–thaw processes (McClements, 2005). From a practical point of view, steric repulsions require higher amounts of emulsifier (wt %) than electrostatic stabilization.

Coalescence is enhanced by an inelastic and uncharged film and by a slow migration of the emulsifier to the areas with low interface concentrations. In contrast, high concentrations of emulsifiers create a thick and elastic interfacial membrane, which hinders the droplets from merging together. Nevertheless, a large concentration of emulsifiers, which creates a low interfacial tension, could enhance the possibility of coalescence since the low tension, in addition to stabilizing the emulsion, also reduces the amount of energy needed for film rupture. Emulsifiers reduce creaming by controlling flocculation and coalescence, but also by favouring reduction of droplet size, thus limiting droplet velocity due to gravitational forces. Polymeric emulsifiers may also reduce creaming by limiting the difference in continuous- and dispersed-phase densities through the formation of a thick hydrated interface layer surrounding small sized droplets or by increasing the viscosity of the continuous phase.

The effectiveness and the ability of emulsifiers to produce emulsion droplets of small size and to prevent destabilization phenomena (aggregation, flocculation and/or coalescence) is highly variable and highly dependent on environmental conditions such as pH, temperature and storage conditions (Dickinson, 2009).

To summarize, in order to obtain a stable emulsion, different factors must be controlled among them:

- **the energy applied**: increasing the applied energy increases the chance of collisions and breakage of the droplets, allowing the emulsion to pass the emulsification zone more quickly;
- **the residence time of the emulsion droplets in the region of emulsification**: should be long enough to enable the adsorption of the emulsifier at the newly created interface;

- **the concentration of emulsifiers**: must be sufficient to cover the entire surface of the droplets and to reduce the surface tension. As a consequence, the total amount of emulsifier needed for emulsion stabilization increases dramatically when the targeted size of the oil droplet decreases;
- **the diffusion and adsorption rate of the emulsifiers**: the emulsifiers must move to the interface quickly enough to reduce interfacial tension and to stabilize the freshly formed droplets by forming a resistant layer;
- **the structure and physicochemical properties of the interfacial layer**: these comprise properties such as electric charge, thickness, surface coverage, surface tension, etc. which both the nature and the amounts of adsorbed emulsifiers depend (Fig. 5.3);
- **the interactions of the emulsifier with other ingredients**: the association between biopolymers and emulsifiers may lead to competition and flocculation of the droplets formed.

All these factors will also affect the oxidative stability of the emulsions as it will be summarized below.

The size distribution of emulsion droplets and the stability of the emulsion depend on the process of emulsification and on the nature and amount of emulsifiers. However, in many applications, emulsifiers are used in great excess, that is in quantities much higher than the quantities needed for coverage of the o/w interface. Industrial applications must also take into account cost, market availability, ease of use, compatibility with other ingredients and regulation (Guzey and McClements, 2007).

5.3 Emulsifiers for omega-3 polyunsaturated fatty acid (PUFA) delivery systems and emulsified foods

An emulsifier is defined as 'a single chemical or a mixture of components having a capacity for promoting emulsion formation and short-term stability by interfacial action' (Dickinson, 2003; Garti and Leser, 2001). Emulsifiers are amphiphilic molecules, i.e. they possess polar and non-polar regions that confer upon them the ability to adsorb at interfaces.

The most common emulsifiers used in the food industry are amphiphilic proteins, phospholipids and small-sized molecular surfactants (Charalambous and Doxastakis, 1989; McClements, 2005). They are of natural or synthetic origin and currently divided into two main groups (van Nieuwenhuyzen and Szuhaj, 1998; Kralova and Sjoblom, 2009):

- **low molecular weight emulsifiers** comprising lecithins (mainly composed of phospholipids), monoglycerides and their esters, diglycerides, sucroglycerides esters (sucrose esters), polysorbates (sorbitan esters) and glycolipids of microbial origin;
- **high molecular weight emulsifiers** comprising proteins and surface-active hydrocolloids.

Prior to homogenization, the emulsifier is usually dispersed in the phase in which it is the most soluble, so that water-soluble surfactants are dispersed in the aqueous phase and oil-soluble surfactants are dispersed in the lipid phase. Note that combinations of emulsifiers are generally present in real applications (Fig. 5.3).

5.3.1 Adsorption of emulsifiers at the oil-in-water (o/w) interface and stabilization of emulsions

The stabilization of an emulsion requires the presence of a surfactant or an amphiphilic polymer adsorbing at the o/w interface. The adsorption results in a reduction of the interfacial tension and in steric or electrostatic repulsions between droplets, reducing the occurrence of coalescence in the system. Various factors influence the stabilizing effect of emulsifiers. These include factors related to their intrinsic properties, such as their molecular size (low molecular weight emulsifiers diffuse more rapidly at the interface than biopolymers), their aptitude to decrease the interfacial tension (surface activity), the sizes of the hydrophobic and hydrophilic moieties in the molecules, their solubility in one or other of the emulsion phases or their charge (anionic or cationic, nonionic or zwitterionic nature).

In the case of a charged emulsifier, the distribution of the charges and the pK of the chemical groups involved should also be considered.

For polymeric emulsifiers such as proteins, their capacity to adsorb and to stabilize emulsions is determined by several additional parameters. The distribution of the hydrophilic and hydrophobic residues within the polymeric chain into separate hydrophilic and hydrophobic clusters or domains is more favourable to emulsion stabilization than a random distribution of the residues. The ability of the polymeric chain to change its conformation upon its adsorption at the interface (rigid or flexible polymer) is also an important factor.

Environmental conditions such as temperature or pH also influence the formation and stabilizing effect of the interface (Gupta and Muralidhara, 2001). The reasons are linked to their effect on characteristics of the emulsifiers such as the degree of hydration and size of their polar moieties, the liquid or solid state of the hydrophobic alkyl chains and the charge carried by the polar residues.

Stabilization of the emulsion droplets requires the rapid formation of a continuous monomolecular interfacial layer unless coalescence occurs during the emulsification process itself. Therefore, the emulsifier concentration in the total emulsion should be sufficient to provide enough molecules to cover the entire generated interface. A decrease in the surface load leads to an increase in interfacial tension and, ultimately, causes a destabilization of the system (Capek, 2004; McClements, 2005). In contrast, when emulsifier amounts exceed that which is needed only for interface coverage, unadsorbed emulsifiers will dissolve or form colloidal structures in the oil or in the aqueous phase depending on their solubility and how they were initially added to the system (Fig. 5.3). These unadsorbed fractions of emulsifiers can influence the physical and chemical stabilities of the delivery systems (Berton *et al.*, 2011a).

5.3.2 Low molecular weight emulsifiers

Molecular geometry of low molecular weight emulsifiers

One important feature to consider when looking at the ability of small-size amphiphilic molecules to stabilize o/w or w/o emulsions or other multiphase structures such as microemulsions and organogels is their molecular geometry and their packing at the interfaces (Friberg and Larsson, 1997; McClements, 2005; Marangoni and Garti, 2011). Small-size amphiphilic molecules are composed of a hydrophobic tail – one or more alkyl chains – that dives into the oil phase, and a hydrophilic head group oriented towards the aqueous phase (Fig. 5.3). When adsorbed at the interface, these molecules self-organize with more or less dense packing so that the lowest free energy of the monolayer can be obtained. The molecules tend to confer upon the interface an optimum curvature according to the respective sizes of the hydrophilic heads and the hydrophobic tails (Fig. 5.4).

The Israelachvili–Mitchel–Ninham packing parameter or shape factor (p) characterizes the geometric property of the amphiphiles (Israelachvili, 1992; Mouritsen, 2011).

$$p = v/La \quad [5.1]$$

where v and L are the molecular volume and length of the hydrophobic tail and a is the cross-sectional area of the hydrophilic head group. For instance, phosphatidylcholine (PC), composed of two fatty acid chains and a large headgroup, can be represented as large truncated cone, almost a cylinder. It exhibits a packing parameter close to 1 and is organized as lamellar mesophases in water. When adsorbed at the o/w interface, it tends to promote monolayers with zero or very limited curvature and therefore tends to hinder the formation of sub-micron or nanoscale oil droplets. To favour the formation of small oil droplets and the stabilization of o/w emulsions, PC can be used with cone-shaped molecules with $p < 1$, such as lysophospholipids (Hauser, 1987; Bueschelberger, 2004).

The packing of surfactant molecules is sensitive to the environmental conditions, such as temperature, pH and ionic strength, all of which influence the hydration of the polar head and/or the liquid–gel or solid state of the hydrocarbon chains. When mixtures of amphiphiles are used, as is most common in practice, mutual interactions or repulsion between molecules take place at the o/w interface. Thus, depending on the respective concentrations of the compounds, they organize either as ideal mixtures or patches (rafts) with complex structural and dynamic properties (Hennere *et al.*, 2009). This complex mesomorphism of the amphiphiles can be useful to design optimized delivery systems such as, for example, nanoemulsions and edible oleogels (Gutiérrez *et al.*, 2008; Marangoni and Garti, 2011).

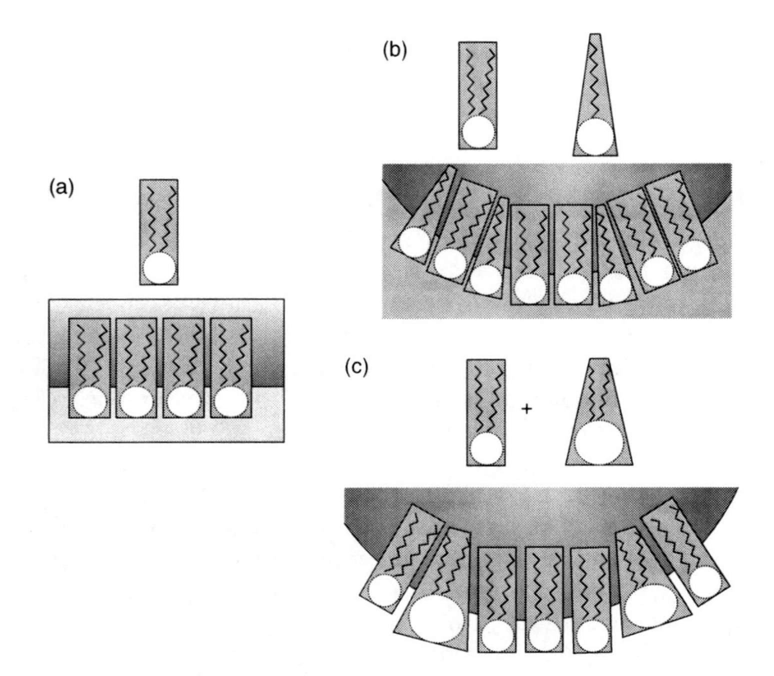

Fig. 5.4 Schematic representation of the effect of the molecular geometry of surfactant on o/w interface curvature and stabilization of oil droplets. The adsorption of surfactants with cylindrical geometry such as phospholipids with two acyl chains (for example phosphatidyl choline) leads to planar interfaces with low curvature (a) and formation of large oil droplets (> μm) with limited stability. Interface curvature and stabilization of oil droplets with small size (<< μm) can be achieved by mixing surfactants with cylindrical geometry with surfactants with truncated cone geometry such as monoacyl-phospholipids (b), for example lyso-phosphatidyl choline, or surfactants having a large polar head (c), such as tweens.

The hydrophilic–lipophilic balance (HLB)

The amphiphilic character of small-size emulsifiers can be characterized by the hydrophilic–lipophilic balance (HLB). The HLB concept, proposed by Griffin in 1949, is the best-known method to select a surfactant suitable for an application. This semiempirical method assigns the surfactant a HLB number according to its chemical structure. Several experimental and numeric methods have been developed over the years to determine HLB numbers (Friberg and Larsson, 1997; Stauffer, 2005). These methods, initially developed for nonionic surfactants, are mainly based on the respective sizes of the hydrophobic and hydrophilic moieties of the surfactant molecules. HLB numbers allow the ability of the surfactant to stabilise o/w or w/o emulsions to be predicted.

Surfactants with HLB values between 4 and 6 generally stabilize w/o emulsions whereas HLB values between 8 and 18 would stabilize o/w emulsions (Bos and van Vliet, 2001; Pichot *et al.*, 2010). Tabulated HLB numbers of many surfactants can be found in the literature. HLB numbers of surfactant mixtures can be calculated from their respective weight proportions.

Although very useful, the HLB method suffers from several shortcomings. The HLB number does not take into account parameters such as polar head hydration and hydrocarbon chain unsaturation. As a unique value is assigned for each surfactant, the effects of other components of the formulation are neglected. For instance, HLB number does not take into account the nature of the oil phase. This is why the concept of 'required HLB' or 'effective HLB value' has been introduced (Marszall and van Valkenburg, 1982). The required HLB is the HLB of the surfactant, or mixture of surfactants, which allows the most stable emulsion for a given system (processing conditions, oil phase, etc.) to be obtained. To estimate the required HLB, emulsions are prepared with the same aqueous and oily phases but different surfactants within range of HLB. The required HLB corresponds to the maximum stability of the emulsion (Salager *et al.*, 2001; McClements, 2005).

The characteristics of the aqueous phase are also ignored when using the HLB concept. For instance, interactions in the interfacial zone linked to the salinity of the aqueous phase or to the presence of alcohol are not taken into consideration. The effect of the temperature is also completely ignored. Therefore complementary methods such as determining the PIT can be used in addition to the HLB method to further optimize the formulation of the emulsions (Shinoda, 1967; Shinoda and Saito, 1969). Temperatures below the PIT favour the stability of o/w emulsions whereas w/o emulsions are obtained above this temperature. Ternary Winsor phase diagrams (Winsor, 1956) are also useful to determine the water/oil/surfactant ratios favouring one lipid/water organization or another or to determine the optimal amount of a co-surfactant needed to stabilize an emulsion. These methods are intended to optimize the stability of the emulsions and not the emulsification process.

Characteristics of o/w interfaces covered by low molecular weight emulsifiers

Due to their low molecular weight, surfactants are able to diffuse very rapidly to the o/w interfaces. This facilitates the stabilization of small oil droplets during emulsification by avoiding rapid coalescence of the droplets and the formation of sub-micron and nanoemulsions (McClements, 2011, 2012). They also present high surface activity and compete favourably with biopolymers at the interface (Nylander *et al.*, 1997). The surface load of the o/w interface covered by low molecular weight emulsifiers is usually in the range 1–2 mg m^{-2} (Genot *et al.*, 2013 and herein cited publications). Surfactant molecules are tightly packed at the interface, particularly polyoxyethylene sorbitan esters such as Tween® 20. In emulsions stabilized by these molecules, nearly 100 % of the droplet surface is actually covered. Surfactants form fluid interfaces with a substantial surface lateral diffusion coefficient. Surfactants are generally considered to be less efficient than proteins in avoiding interfacial film breaking and droplet coalescence. However, ionic surfactants induce electrostatic repulsions whereas nonionic surfactants such as polysorbates can exert steric repulsions because of their polyoxyethylene chains. Table 5.1 presents the main characteristics and recommended usages of various food-grade surfactants whose structures are presented in Figs. 5.5 and 5.6.

Lecithins

Lecithins are widely used in the food industry. They consist mainly of glycerophospholipids, PC being a main component of most lecithins together with other phospholipids such as phosphatidylethanolamine (PE) and phosphatidylinositol (PI) (Fig. 5.5). Technical lecithins also often contain appreciable quantities of lyso-phospholipids. Some lecithins may also contain sphingolipids and glycolipids, depending on their origin. Lecithins originate from various sources, but the main industrial sources are soya, rapeseed and sunflower seeds, and egg yolk. We could also mention milk lecithins and marine lecithins which could prove to have applications in the future due to their potential nutritional applications. Milk lecithins contain sphingomyelin while marine lecithins are characterized by their high LC omega-3 PUFA content (Kullenberg *et al.*, 2012). Both have been tested for their emulsifying properties in delivery emulsions and enriched foods (Horn *et al.*, 2011, 2012a; Lu *et al.*, 2012). Crude commercial lecithins usually contain around 35 % TAG. They can be fractionated and chemically or enzymatically modified. The HLB numbers of commercial lecithins are rarely higher than 9, commonly ranging between 2 and 7, but lecithins allow the formation of o/w emulsions, and occasionally w/o emulsions (Bueschelberger, 2004; Stauffer, 2005). However, emulsions stabilized only by lecithin are currently not very stable, with the exception of nanoemulsions.

Lecithins tend to form bilayers when dispersed in water, but their molecular organization depends on various parameters, such as their polar lipid composition, hydration, ionic strength, pH, temperature, presence of sterols, etc. (Akoh and Min, 2002; Bueschelberger, 2004; Kralova and Sjoblom, 2009). PC, which is amphoteric, is characterized by a relatively high HLB number and a geometry that is close to cylindrical. It organizes as lamellar structures in aqueous solution, forming uni- or multilamellar vesicles (liposomes) and monolayers at o/w interfaces. PE, also amphoteric, has an inverted cone-shaped geometry. It exhibits low HLB number and tends to form a hexagonal phase in water, and, when mixed with PC, it allows effective organization of the interface. The negative charge carried by PI contributes to electrostatic stabilization of the emulsions. Additionally, partial hydrolysis of lecithins is recognized to improve their emulsifying properties due to the steric hindrance (molecular geometry) of lysophospholipids ($p < 1$). Use of PC with aqueous soluble surfactants such as sugar esters or

Table 5.1 Classification and characteristics of low molecular weight surfactants used in food industry

Emulsifier	Abbreviation	EU number[1,2]	US FDA status[3,4]	Limit of use		HLB[3,4]	Solubility/ dispersibility	Emulsion type	Charge	Appearance[1]
				FAO/WHO expert committee[1,5]	European Union[2]					
Lecithin	–	E 322	184.1400 GRAS	Not limited	*Quantum satis*	<9	Soluble in oil Dispersible in water	w/o and o/w	Amphoteric to anionic	Brown highly viscous or semi-liquid or powder
Mono and diglycerides	–	E 471	184.1505 GRAS	Not limited	*Quantum satis*	3–6	Soluble in oil Dispersible in water	w/o	Nonionic	Pale straw to brown oily liquid to white or white slightly off-white waxy solid
Acid esters of mono- and diglycerides	ACETEM	E 472a	172.828	Not limited	*Quantum satis*	1.5	Soluble in oil	w/o	Anionic to nonionic	Colourless to ivory – oily to waxy depending on the fatty acids and the proportion of acetic acid
Lactic acid esters of mono- and diglycerides	LACTEM	E 472b	172.852	Not limited	*Quantum satis*	5–8	Soluble in oil Dispersible in hot water	o/w	Anionic to nonionic	Light yellow to amber – oily to waxy depending on fatty acids and lactic acid proportion
Citric acid esters of mono- and diglycerides	CITREM	E 472c	172.832	Not limited	*Quantum satis*	3–10*	Soluble in oil Dispersible in hot water	o/w	Anionic	White to ivory – oily to waxy depending on the fatty acids

(Continued)

Table 5.1 *Continued*

Emulsifier	Abbreviation	EU number[1,2]	US FDA status[3,4]	Limit of use		HLB[3,4]	Solubility/ dispersibility	Emulsion type	Charge	Appearance[1]
				FAO/WHO expert committee[1,5]	European Union[2]					
Diacetyltartaric acid esters of mono- and diglycerides	DATEM	E 472e	184.1101	0–50 mg/kg bw	*Quantum satis*	7–8	Soluble in methanol, ethanol and acetone Dispersible in water	o/w	Anionic to nonionic	Sticky viscous liquid – fat-like to waxy, flake or powder form
Sucrose esters of fatty acids	–	E 473	172.859	0–30 mg/kg bw	50 mg/kg (except beverages)	1–18	Soluble in water and ethanol	w/o and o/w	Nonionic	White to slightly greyish powder with saturated fatty acids Yellowish, pasty to waxy with unsaturated fatty acids
Sorbitan monostearate	SMS/Span 60	E 491	172.842	0–25 mg/kg bw	*Quantum satis*	4.7	Soluble above its melting point in oils Dispersible in hot water	w/o	Nonionic	Light cream to tan-coloured, hard waxy solid with a slight characteristic odour and bland taste

Sorbitan tristearate	STS/Span 65	E 492	GRAS	0–25 mg/kg bw	*Quantum satis*	2.1	Insoluble in cold water Dispersible in edible oils	w/o	Nonionic	Light cream to tan-coloured, hard waxy solid with a slight characteristic odour and bland taste
Sorbitan monolaurate	SML/Span20	E 493	–	0–25 mg/kg bw	*Quantum satis*	8.6	Soluble in water	o/w	Nonionic	Amber-coloured, oily liquid with a slight characteristic odour
Sorbitan mono-oleate	SMO/Span 80	E 494	–	0–25 mg/kg bw	*Quantum satis*	4.3	Soluble in water	w/o	Nonionic	Amber-coloured oily liquid with a slight characteristic odour
Polyoxyethylene sorbitan monolaurate	Polysorbate 20 Tween® 20	E 432	–	0–25 mg/kg bw	*Quantum satis*	16.7	Soluble in water, ethanol, methanol, ethyl acetate and dioxan	o/w	Nonionic	Lemon to amber-coloured, oily liquid at 25 °C, faint characteristic odour, warm somewhat bitter taste
Polyoxyethylene sorbitan mono-oleate	Polysorbate 80 Tween® 80	E 433	172.840	0–25 mg/kg bw	*Quantum satis*	15	Soluble in water, ethanol, methanol, ethyl acetate and toluene	o/w	Nonionic	Lemon to amber-coloured, oily liquid at 25 °C, faint characteristic odour, waxy somewhat bitter taste

(Continued)

Table 5.1 *Continued*

Emulsifier	Abbreviation	EU number[1,2]	US FDA status[3,4]	Limit of use		HLB[3,4]	Solubility/ dispersibility	Emulsion type	Charge	Appearance[1]
				FAO/WHO expert committee[1,5]	European Union[2]					
Polyoxyethylene sorbitan monostearate	Polysorbate 60 Tween® 60	E 435	172.836 GRAS	0–25 mg/kg bw	*Quantum satis*	14.9	Soluble in water, ethyl acetate and toluene	o/w	Nonionic	Lemon to amber-coloured oily liquid at 25 °C, faint characteristic odour and waxy, somewhat bitter taste
Polyoxyethylene sorbitan tristearate	Polysorbate 65 Tween® 65	E 436	172.838 GRAS	0–25 mg/kg bw	*Quantum satis*	10.5	Soluble in oil, petroleum ether, acetone, ether, dioxane, ethanol and methanol Dispersible in water	o/w	Nonionic	Lemon to amber-coloured oily liquid at 25 °C, faint characteristic odour and waxy, somewhat bitter taste
Polyglycerol esters of fatty acids	PGE	E 475	172.854	0–25 mg/kg bw	*Quantum satis*	6–11	Soluble in oil Dispersible in water	o/w	Nonionic	The product is a light yellow to amber-coloured, oily to hard waxy material of a consistency determined by the fatty acids.

GRAS = generally recognized as safe, bw = body weight, o/w = oil in water, w/o = water in oil.
*HLB of CITREM varies depending on the type and amount of fatty acids and citric acid, neutralization degree and pH; generally 9–11.
Sources: [1]http://www.emulsifiers.org/files/EFEMA_Index_of_Food_Emulsifiers.pdf; [2]http://eur-lex.europa.eu/LexUriServ/LexUriServ.do?uri=CELEX:32011R1130:EN:NOT; http://ec.europa.eu/food/food/chemicalsafety/additives/new_regul_en.htm; [3]McClements, 2005; [4]Whitehurst, 2004; [5]http://www.fao.org/food/food-safety-quality/scientific-advice/jecfa/jecfa-additives/en/.

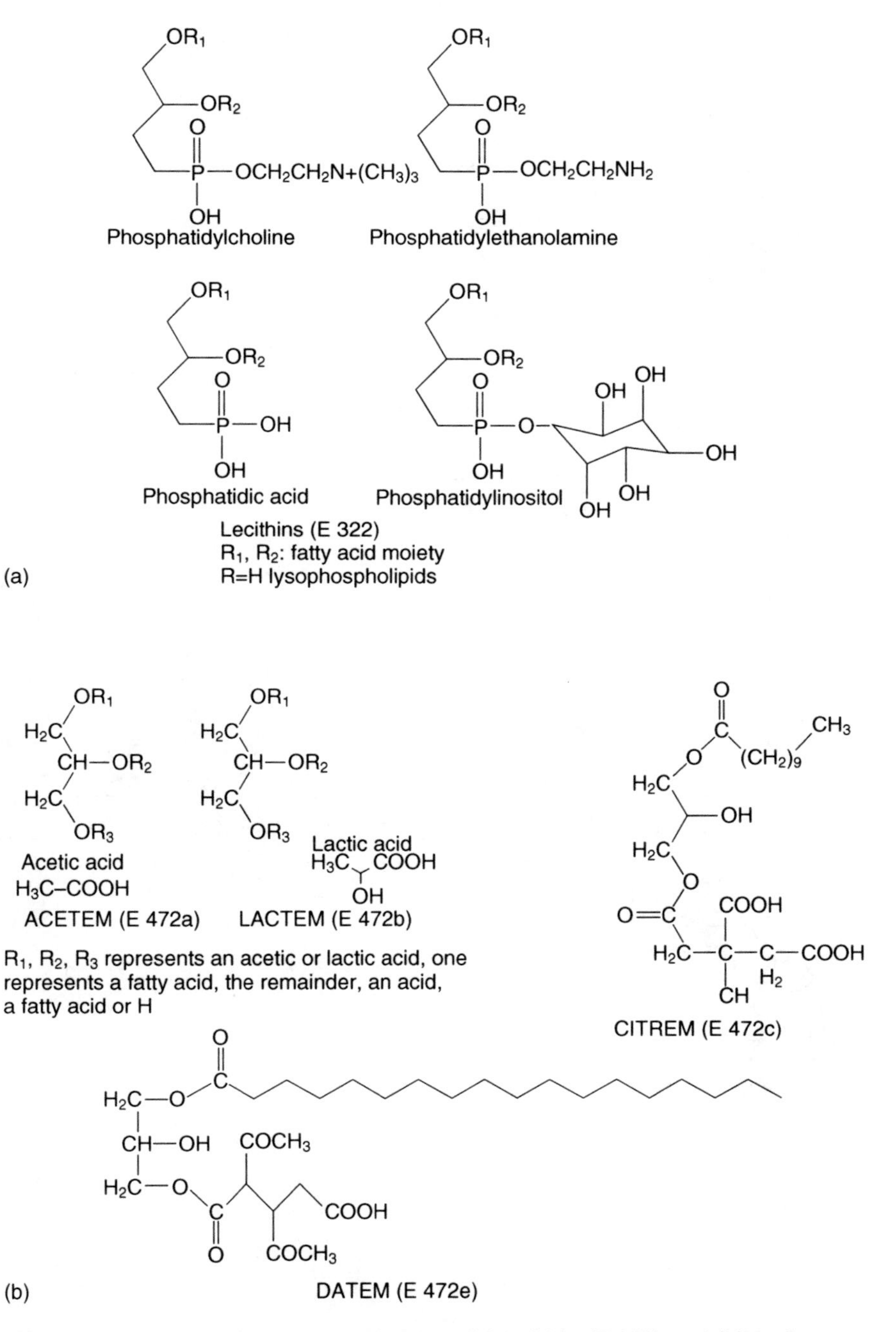

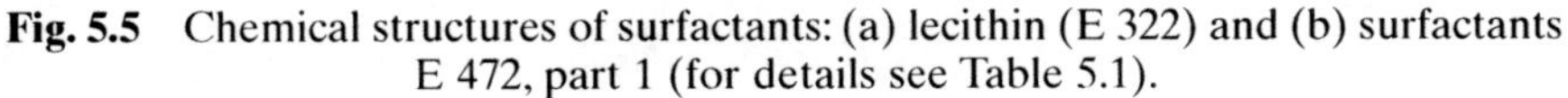

Fig. 5.5 Chemical structures of surfactants: (a) lecithin (E 322) and (b) surfactants E 472, part 1 (for details see Table 5.1).

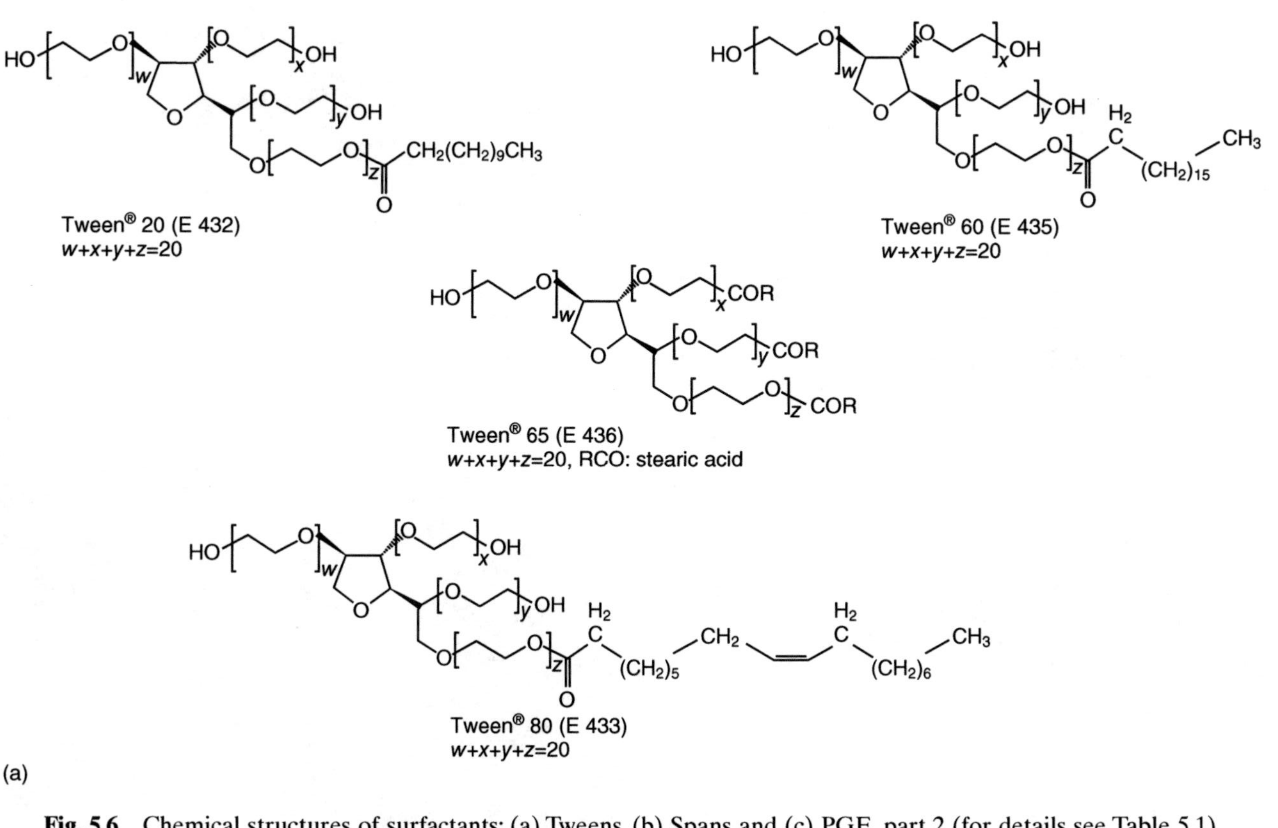

Fig. 5.6 Chemical structures of surfactants: (a) Tweens, (b) Spans and (c) PGE, part 2 (for details see Table 5.1).

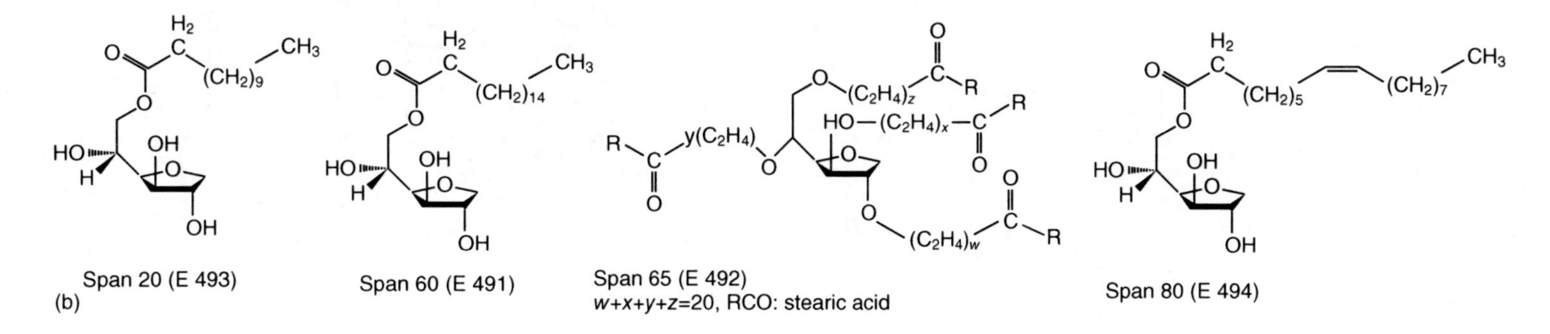

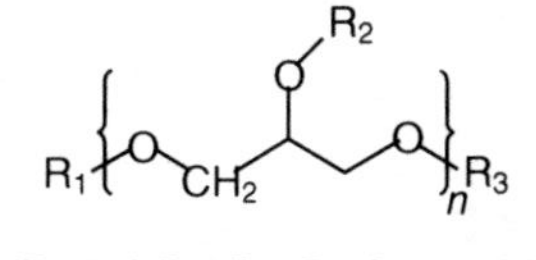

Fig. 5.6 *Continued*

polysorbates also facilitates the stabilization of sub-micron and nanoemulsions. Fatty acid chain length and unsaturation also influence emulsifying properties of lecithins. Synthetic PCs with shorter and saturated acyl hydrocarbon chains and PC mixtures having the lowest total number of carbon atoms were shown to favour the formation of small oil droplets, short-chain PCs being considered by the authors as the most potent emulsifiers (Nii and Ishii, 2004; Ishii and Nii, 2005).

Mono- and diglycerides

Mono- and diglycerides are produced by synthesis and considered to be GRAS (generally recognised as safe) ingredients and thus their use is not limited. Commercial mono- and diglycerides usually contain 45–55 % monoglycerides, 38–45 % diglycerides, 8–12 % triglycerides and 1–7 % free glycerol (Garti, 1999; Moonen and Bas, 2004; Stauffer, 2005). Hydrophobic in nature, these nonionic emulsifiers are not soluble in water but dissolve fully in oil. They are assigned a low HLB number (3–6) and stabilize w/o emulsions forming reversed micelles. They are also characterized by very complex phase-forming properties in the presence of water, oil and other co-solvents and by their ability to crystallize. These properties contribute to their functionality in various food formulations (for instance ice creams) and to their potential application in the design of oleogels (Larsson, 2004; Whitehurst, 2004; Marangoni and Garti, 2011).

Monoglycerides esters

Monoacylglycerols are also used as raw materials for making more lipophilic or more hydrophilic molecules for use in the cosmetic and food industries. Esters of monoglycerides with organic acids, such as acetic acid (acetic acid esters of monoglycerides – ACETEM), lactic acid (LACTEM), succinic acid, diacetyl tartaric acid (DATEM) and citric acid (CITREM) (Fig. 5.5), present very different polarities, surface activities and crystalline behaviours from those of the parent monoglycerides. These anionic molecules exhibit different abilities to emulsify and stabilize commercial formulations. DATEM, based on C16 and C18 chain length monoglycerides, are effective emulsifiers in liquid o/w emulsions because their interactions with the adsorbed proteins stabilize the interfacial film. CITREM are hydrophilic emulsifiers that contribute to the prevention of droplet coalescence in o/w emulsions.

Sucrose esters

Sugar esters represent a broad range of compounds made from a sugar and fatty acids. The sugar can be sucrose or one of the polyols, such as sorbitol or xylitol, but only sucrose esters of fatty acids and sucroglycerides are authorized by European regulation for use in a number of foods (EFSA, 2010b). Sucrose esters of fatty acids consist of a mixture of mono-, di- and tri-esters of sucrose with fatty acids. Commercial products are classified according to the mean number of esterified fatty acids on a sucrose molecule. They are nonionic and water-soluble surfactants whose phase behaviour is little influenced by temperature. Their lipophilic character increases with their degree of esterification and with the chain-length of the esterified fatty acid (carbon chain-lengths are 6–18). Sucrose esters covering a very wide range of HLB values (1–18) can be obtained with various potential applications.

Sucrose esters present low toxicity, are biodegradable and have been used for different therapeutic and cosmetic applications (Sadtler *et al.*, 2004). They have also been used to prepare micelles and microemulsions. They are reported to have good taste and aroma profiles and could be of interest as surfactants for the food, beverage and pharmaceutical industries (Nelen and Cooper, 2004; Szuts *et al.*, 2010).

Sorbitan esters, polysorbates and other esters of fatty acids

Sorbitan esters or Span© derive from the esterification of dehydrated sorbitol with fatty acids (Fig. 5.6). The esterification of the hydroxyl groups of sorbitol with fatty acids produces molecules varying in their degree of esterification and in their HLB. For example, sorbitan monolaurate and sorbitan monostearate exhibit HLB numbers of 8.6 and 4.7, respectively. They can be used to stabilize o/w and w/o emulsions respectively.

Sorbitan esters can react with ethylene oxide to give the polyoxyethylene derivatives, usually referred as *polysorbates* or Tweens®. Sorbitan monolaurate, monostearate, tristearate and mono-oleate form, respectively, polysorbate 20, polysorbate 60, polysorbate 65 and polysorbate 80. These non-ionic, water-soluble molecules exhibit a wide range of hydrophobicity, surface activity, HLB numbers and emulsifying properties. Polysorbate 20 and 60 with HLB numbers of 16.7 and 14.9, respectively, can stabilize o/w emulsions. Polysorbate 65 with an HLB of 10.5 is the most lipophilic; it exhibits low surface activity and emulsifying power (Cottrell and van Peij, 2004; Hasenhuettl, 2008).

Polysorbates, especially Tweens®, are widely used in model systems. They are food additives approved for use in food in the European Union with restricted usages (1000–5000 mg/kg depending on the food category). Their effective use in food applications is in fact limited as a result of consumer perception of synthetic molecules, environmental issues and cost. They also have been reported to affect taste and aroma. Other polyol esters of fatty acids, such as *polyglycerol esters* (PGE) and *propylene glycol monostearate* (PGMS) and the water-dispersible anionic sodium stearoyl lactylate (SSL), can also be used as food emulsifiers according to the food regulations.

Biosurfactants

Biosurfactants or bioemulsifiers are surface-active molecules synthesized by micro-organisms. They include glycolipids, such as sophorolipids and rhamnolipids. These molecules have the ability to provide low interfacial tension (Rosenberg and Ron, 1999).

Rhamnolipids from *Pseudomonas aeruginosa*, surfactin from *Bacillus subtilis*, emulsan from *Acinetobacter calcoaceticus* and sophorolipids from *Candida bombicola* are some examples of microbial-derived surfactants (Rosenberg and Ron, 1999; Nitschke and Costa, 2007). Because of their low toxicity, biodegradable nature, effectiveness at extreme temperatures, pH, salinity and biosynthesis (Garti, 1999; Rosenberg and Ron, 1999; Ron and Rosenberg, 2001; Nitschke and Costa, 2007), they could replace currently used chemical emulsifiers in some applications (Rosenberg and Ron, 1999), provided that each specific usage is allowed by the regulating authorities. Their use is also limited by the cost of production and insufficient experience in application.

5.3.3 High molecular weight emulsifiers

Proteins

Proteins are generally amphiphilic biopolymers that adsorb to the interfaces formed during emulsification with the hydrophilic groups in the aqueous phase and the lipophilic groups in the dispersed phase. This adsorption reduces the interfacial tension enough to ensure formation of stable oil droplets. Many proteins exhibit good ability to create and stabilize an emulsion. In addition to their functional properties, proteins have high nutritional value and are GRAS (Chen *et al.*, 2006). This is why they are widely used to stabilize food formulations.

Milk proteins, namely caseins and whey proteins, are used as emulsifiers in many emulsified food formulations. Egg proteins, meat and fish proteins and proteins isolated from legumes or cereals also exhibit good emulsifying properties (McClements, 2005). This function depends on characteristics of the biopolymers such as their molecular flexibility, molecular size, surface hydrophobicity, net charge and amino acid composition (Genot *et al.*, 2003b, 2013; Mootoosingh and Rousseau, 2006). Typical surface loads encountered for protein-stabilized interfaces range from 1.5–4.5 mg m^{-2} (Genot *et al.*, 2013 and herein cited references). Only the hydrophobic parts of the polypeptidic chain are actually in direct contact with the o/w interface, the other protein segments protruding into the aqueous phase (Fig. 5.3). Therefore the interface thickness of oil droplets covered by only one layer of protein varies from 1–15 nm, depending on the ability of the protein to modify its conformation and to spread at the interface. Due to the internal constraints and the arrangement of the polypeptidic chains onto the droplet surface, only 30–40 % of the interface is actually covered with proteins (Dickinson, 2009). Proteins form immobile and viscoelastic interfacial films exhibiting non-Newtonian behaviour. They are also susceptible to undergo structural and conformational rearrangements *post* adsorption, which implies that the surface load, the thickness of the protein-stabilized interfaces and their physical properties may evolve during storage. Interfacial proteins generate both steric and electrostatic repulsions and can therefore form a physical barrier to droplet coalescence. However, in some cases proteins favour the physical destabilization of emulsions through droplet–droplet bridging or depletion, both of which lead to flocculation. The emulsions stabilized by proteins are also sensitive to pH and ionic strength variations as well as to thermal treatments, which can be a major inconvenience for delivery formulations.

Protein–surfactant mixtures

As already mentioned, surfactants are able to compete with protein molecules at the o/w interfaces, their higher surface activity enabling them to desorb the proteins. However, the presence at the interfaces of both proteins and small-size emulsifiers can be obtained for relatively low amounts of surfactant and in conditions allowing formation of surfactant–protein complexes (Nylander *et al.*, 1997; Bos and van Vliet, 2001).

Surface-active hydrocolloids

Polysaccharides exist in nature with a wide variety of biochemical and biomechanical functions. Polysaccharides are mostly hydrophilic with high molecular weight, and they have weak surface activity due to their strong hydrophilic character. They are currently used in emulsion stabilization as thickeners or gelling agents of the aqueous phase. However, some polysaccharides, such as gum arabic, pectin, galactomannans and modified starches, can adsorb at the interface due to the presence of either hydrophobic functions or associated amphiphilic proteins (Akhtar *et al.*, 2002; Kralova and Sjoblom, 2009; Castellani *et al.*, 2010).

Protein/polysaccharides mixtures and complexes

The emulsion stabilizing effect of different combinations of polysaccharides with proteins has been investigated, for example whey proteins/gum arabic (Klein *et al.*, 2010), β-lactoglobulin/pectin (Guzey and McClements, 2007), milk protein products/xanthan (Hemar *et al.*, 2001; Ye *et al.*, 2011). These studies demonstrate that in specific ratios and physicochemical conditions, protein–polysaccharide complexes with interfacial properties favourable to the stabilization of emulsions can be formed. However, case-by-case studies should be undertaken with such complex mixtures of biomolecules.

5.4 Emulsifiers and lipid oxidation

Prevention of lipid oxidation is one of the main technological challenges for the successful development of omega-3 enriched foods (see Jacobsen *et al.*, 2008 and also chapters 4 and 12 of this book). Because they are highly unsaturated molecules, LC PUFA are dramatically prone to oxidation. This causes formation of a wide array of lipid oxidation products. Among them, volatile compounds give rise to perceived off-flavours even at moderate levels of oxidation, because of the very low flavour thresholds of some volatiles specifically formed during oxidation of omega-3 FA. Other compounds comprising hydroperoxides and secondary compounds such as malondialdehyde and 4-hydroxy-2-hexenal (4-HHE) exhibiting potentially toxic properties are also produced, and these could prove to be a health concern (Grootveld *et al.*, 1998; Guéraud *et al.*, 2010). Recent results have accordingly shown that mice fed high fat diets containing moderately oxidized n-3 PUFA sources exhibited enhanced plasma inflammatory markers and triggered oxidative stress and inflammation in the small intestine (Awada *et al.*, 2012). It should be noted that because the sensory and toxic effects arise at very low concentrations of the molecules in food products (orders of magnitude of μg/kg), in general the oxidation of PUFA is not sufficient to affect the amount of beneficial fatty acids due to the fact that significant losses of the fatty acids concerned cannot be detected below 2–5 %, i.e. an order of magnitude of g/kg. However, significant losses may affect other beneficial molecules such as tocopherols and other antioxidants because they retard or slow down fatty acid oxidation through their own degradation. Other molecules such as proteins can also be damaged before and during lipid oxidation (Rampon *et al.*, 2001; Genot *et al.*, 2003b, 2013; Berton *et al.*, 2012).

Emulsifiers can potentially contribute to the chemical stabilization or destabilization of omega-3 PUFA oils and enriched foods through various mechanisms. Lecithins and, among phospholipids species, especially PE have been found to exert antioxidant activity in bulk oils, partly through their synergism with tocopherols and reactions between amino and carbonyl groups producing derivatives with antioxidant properties. The mechanisms involve the side-chain amino groups of the phospholipids molecules but also the cooperative effect of the hydroxy groups (Evans *et al.*, 1954; Ohshima *et al.*, 1993; Koga and Terao, 1995; Saito and Ishihara, 1997; Bandarra *et al.*, 1999; Judde *et al.*, 2003; Hidalgo *et al.*, 2005, 2008). Another mechanism involving the ability of choline and ethanolamine to break down lipid hydroperoxides into corresponding hydroxyl lipids has recently been proposed (Pan *et al.*, 2010). Interestingly, Nwosu and collaborators (1997) observed that the protective effect of phospholipids depended on the degree of unsaturation and the chain length of the fatty acids that constitute the PL. They also noticed that the phospholipids tested did not protect menhaden oil, in contrast to salmon oil (Nwosu *et al.*, 1997). These effects were assumed to result from the thermodynamic properties of the phospholipid molecules according to their fatty acid composition and from effects linked to the positional distribution of the fatty acids on the TAG structures, but there is little convincing evidence to support this.

In bulk oils, minor compounds with tensio-active properties such as free fatty acids and polar lipids are also inclined to promote oxidation (Lee and Choe, 2009; Chaiyasit *et al.*, 2007; Chen *et al.*, 2011). This has been attributed to the ability of the colloidal structures of these amphiphilic molecules such as reverse micelles to concentrate both endogenous iron and lipid hydroperoxides at the water–lipid interface, thereby increasing the ability of iron to decompose lipid hydroperoxides (Chen *et al.*, 2012).

In dispersed systems, the oxidation is generally enhanced as compared to bulk oils, whereas conflicting results can be obtained depending on the composition and physicochemical conditions of the emulsions. Several reviews present the mechanisms of lipid oxidation and the factors that are inclined to modify oxidation in these systems: see for example Frankel (2005), Genot *et al.* (2003a), Jacobsen *et al.* (2008), McClements and Decker (2000) and Waraho *et al.*, 2011. These reviews insist on the critical role of the interface in lipid oxidation. Indeed, the o/w interface area developed by the oil droplet tends to favour contacts between hydrophilic pro-oxidants and the oxidizable fatty acids and therefore to favour lipid oxidation. The emulsification step itself is also potentially pro-oxidative because of high shear stress, enhanced probabilities of contacts between PUFA, oxygen and pro-oxidative species, temperature and oxygen incorporation during homogenization (Let *et al.*, 2007; Horn *et al.*, 2012b).

Despite its critical role in the development of lipid oxidation, the interface layer can be also an effective barrier against oxygen attack and pro-oxidants, as has been observed with multilayered emulsions, or with emulsions stabilized by positively charged low molecular weight emulsifiers, the interface layers repelling metal ions. Surface-active antioxidant molecules were also found to exert very efficient protective activity against oxidation due to their location at a critical area of the system. Thus highlighting how the structural properties of the emulsifiers and their abilities to form hydrogen bonds or hydrophobic interactions with the antioxidants or to possibly segregate the antioxidant from the radicals can affect the activity of the antioxidants (Stockmann *et al.*, 2000; Heins *et al.*, 2007; Sorensen *et al.*, 2008; Conde *et al.*, 2011). Colloidal structures (micelles or vesicles) formed in the aqueous phase of the emulsions also exert a protective effect against oxidation.

In dispersed systems, lecithins (phospholipids) are inclined to exert pro- or antioxidant activities depending on their fatty acid and lipid class compositions and also on the physicochemical conditions encountered, such as pH (Cardenia *et al.*, 2011), light and interactions with other compounds. Emulsions stabilized by lecithins were less oxidizable than emulsions stabilized by sucrose esters or mono- or diacylglycerols (Fomuso *et al.*, 2002) or by Tween® 80 or citric acid ester (Haahr and Jacobsen, 2008). The presence of anionic PI and/or phosphatidic acid confers the interfacial layers a negative charge that could attract metal ions. The ability of PL to complex metal ions in their hydration sphere would also contribute to their pro-oxidant character in certain formulations (Klinkesorn *et al.*, 2005; Mozuraityte *et al.*, 2006; Horn *et al.*, 2011). On the other hand, phosphatidyl serine could improve the oxidative stability of food lipids (Terao, 2001), the same author proposing a partial hydrolysis of LC omega-3 PUFA-containing oils to form poorly oxidizable micelles of the PUFA. In the case of marine phospholipids, the presence of highly unsaturated fatty acids in the molecules could make them very sensitive to oxidative attack while PUFAs were found to be less oxidizable when located on phospholipid molecules than on TAGS (Le Grandois *et al.*, 2010).

Protein emulsifiers have repeatedly been found to exert protective activity against lipid oxidation. This is attributed to the ability of proteins to chelate metal ions and to quench free radical species, with efficiencies depending on the involved proteins and the physicochemical conditions (Villière *et al.*, 2005). Several authors have also repeatedly invoked the barrier effect of the proteins adsorbed at the interfaces. However, this explanation looks unlikely for emulsions covered by a single protein layer because the diffusion of oxygen is not retarded by a protein layer (Tikekar *et al.*, 2011). Accordingly, it has been shown that, in protein-stabilized emulsions characterized by the lowest possible amounts of unadsorbed emulsifiers, the oil droplets covered by proteins were more oxidizable than droplets of similar sizes covered by surfactants, independently of the surface charge of the droplets when emulsions were stored for a short time period (Berton *et al.*, 2011b; Tikekar *et al.*, 2011; Berton *et al.*, 2012). Interestingly, the highest oxidative stability was observed with emulsions prepared with the anionic surfactant CITREM, the mechanisms involved remaining unknown.

Indeed, as protein emulsifiers are generally present in large excess, they are present in appreciable concentrations in the aqueous phase of the emulsions. These unadsorbed fractions of protein emulsifiers efficiently protect the emulsions against oxidation through the mechanisms invoked above (Elias *et al.*, 2005; Berton *et al.*, 2011b, 2012).

5.5 The impact of emulsifiers and emulsification on flavour and texture perception

One major limitation for the incorporation of LC omega-3 PUFA in formulated foods is related to their sensory properties and, more specifically, to their flavour. Indeed, sources of omega-3 LC-PUFA such as fish oil, krill or microalgae oil often exhibit a characteristic aroma described as 'fishy', 'sea', 'sea food'. Besides these intrinsic odours, omega-3 PUFAs act as precursors of volatile compounds among which some are odorants with very potent odours (Genot *et al.*, 2003a). Incorporation of these lipids into a wide range of food products is thus a challenge for the food industry and scientists.

5.5.1 Flavour release and perception

Lipids play a dual role in flavour perception and release. Apart from their function as flavour precursors, lipids also act as solvent for lipophilic flavour compounds. Indeed, the partition of the volatile odorant compounds within the phases of the food systems and their release in the ambient atmosphere or in the mouth are key factors in how they are perceived. Volatile compounds arising from oxidation of n-3 fatty acid such as propanal, 1-penten-3-ol or 2,4-heptadienal are less lipophilic (especially propanal) than the parent volatile compounds arising from oxidation of n-6 fatty acids (hexanal, 1-octen-3-ol and 2,4-decadienal). As a consequence, an equivalent quantity of the omega-3 parent volatile compound in the lipid phase will lead to a higher concentration in the aqueous phase, which will enhance flavour perception. This partition is highly dependent on the product's fat content. Many studies have highlighted that the reduction of fat content in food causes an imbalance in the overall aroma (Widder and Fisher, 1996; Bayarri and Costell, 2009; van Aken and de Hoog, 2009). In addition, the lipid content of food affects the temporal release of aroma. Thus, in low-fat food, the flavour tends to be intense and transient when compared to the original food (Malone *et al.*, 2003). In o/w emulsions, the rate of release of lipophilic aromas increases as the oil level decreases, and the total duration of the perception is reduced. Release of hydrophilic aromas is largely unaffected by the reduction of the oil content (Malone *et al.*, 2003).

Modification of the droplet diameter gives contradictory results with regard to partition and release of aroma compounds. Nevertheless, the formation of a spherical interface appears to be a key step governing the partition behaviour of aroma compounds in emulsion. The partition coefficients of compounds exhibiting hydrophobic interactions with emulsifiers were not significantly affected by the modification of the droplet mean diameter. Conversely, the possible covalent binding of aldehydes with proteins can modify their partition behaviour when the concentration of adsorbed protein increases as in the case of droplets below 0.5 μm (Meynier *et al.*, 2005).

Encapsulation or entrapment of o/w emulsion within biopolymer gelled particles can be of interest as a means to limit the release of off-flavours from LC omega-3 PUFA enriched emulsions. Originally, oil droplet encapsulation had been proposed to offset the fat content reduction (Malone and Appelqvist, 2003).

Besides the role of lipids, proteins included in foods as emulsifier also impact on flavour release. Generally, hydrophobic interactions of lipophilic aromas with adsorbed proteins lead to an increase of the mass transfer resistance from the oil phase to the continuous phase of the emulsions, resulting in a decrease in the aroma intensity (Landy *et al.*, 1998; Rogacheva *et al.*, 1999). Incorporation of polysaccharides and hydrocolloids modifies the flavour release through their influence on the rheological and textural properties of foods (Malone *et al.*, 2003).

5.5.2 Texture perception

'Texture is the attribute of a substance resulting from a combination of physical properties and perceived by senses of touch, sight and hearing' (Jowitt, 1974). Ingredients, including thickeners, emulsifiers and fat are major determinants of the structure of products and, consequently, of their texture (Van der Bilt, 2009). The fate of a food in the mouth, in terms of aspects such as residence time, mastication requirement and saliva dilution and, consequently, its sensory perception, is conditioned by its structure. To optimize the sensory properties of food, the interaction between flavour and texture perception should be considered. In stirred yogurts, it was shown that increasing the flavouring agent concentration tended to decrease thickness and the addition of thickening agent depressed the aroma note and sweet taste, suggesting texture/flavour interactions (Paçi Kora *et al.*, 2003). Similarly, interactions between sweet taste, aroma and texture have been evidenced in model dairy desserts (Lethuaut *et al.*, 2005). All the above-mentioned aspects must be considered if omega-3 fatty acid are to be successfully added to formulated foods.

5.6 Applications of emulsifiers to stabilize delivery systems and foods enriched with omega-3 PUFA

Many food classes can be enriched in omega-3 fatty acids through the incorporation of oils containing these fatty acids. Bread and bakery products, pasta, milk and dairy products such as yogurts and cheese, infant formula, spreads, mayonnaise, poultry products, juice and soft drinks, but also chocolate, confectionery and energy bars have been accordingly fortified with liquid or encapsulated fish or linseed oils (Kolanowski and Laufenberg, 2006; Nielsen and Jacobsen, 2009; Taneja and Singh, 2012). Examples of enriched meat products, baked goods, emulsified foods, beverages and infant formula can be found in chapters 11–13.

To produce enriched food products, the edible omega-3 oils can be (i) added directly or blended with other more stable oils at any step of the process or to the final product, (ii) included in a delivery system that is then mixed with the other ingredients or added during the process. In either case, omega-3 oil systems are further processed: they are submitted to homogenization, thermal treatments, storage, etc., in conditions which are dependent on the final product.

Food products directly enriched with fish oils were found to exhibit fishy off-flavours and to oxidize rapidly (Kolanowski and Weissbrodt, 2007), whereas several delivery systems were found to provide some protection against oxidation and the appearance of the off-flavours, allowing a higher level of fortification compared to the directly incorporated oils (Kolanowski *et al.*, 2007). However, the benefits of incorporating marine oils in the form of an emulsion instead of as neat oils are highly dependent on the type of food (Let *et al.*, 2007). These authors found that the incorporation of neat oil increased the oxidative stability in the case of yogurt and dressings whereas the use of a pre-emulsion improved the stability of enriched milk.

Delivery emulsions also have the advantages of easier handling and better dispersal as compared to the original oils. The delivery system can be a liquid o/w emulsion, a spread (w/o emulsion) or a solid powder in which the oils are encapsulated (see Chapter 6). The use of other systems, such as edible microemulsions and oleogels, can be also anticipated in the coming years (Marangoni and Garti, 2011).

As compared to the original oils, delivery systems pose specific problems. For instance, liquid o/w emulsions are easy to disperse into water-based foods but, because of their high water content, storage is difficult due to their physical, chemical and possibly microbial instabilities. Their handling and storage may also increase costs. To overcome such difficulties, emulsions are often dehydrated (Taneja and Singh, 2012). Finally, the delivery system is incorporated into the final product. This means that it is blended with other ingredients. This step tends to destabilize the original delivery system, for instance due to competitive adsorption at the interface, and consequently to affect the chemical and physical stabilities of the product. Importantly, it was found that when freshly mixed emulsions of different compositions were re-homogenized together, there was a rapid exchange of oil between the droplets, the rate being faster with a surfactant emulsifier than with a protein emulsifier (Elwell *et al.*, 2004; Samtlebe *et al.*, 2012). Therefore, the initially protected sensitive molecules may be transported into an environment where their oxidation is favoured.

Emulsifiers, either naturally present in the ingredients (amphiphilic proteins, membrane lipids) or intentionally added (Table 5.1), contribute to the stabilization of the final products. As explained above, they reduce oil leakage, contribute to texture, modify lipid oxidation kinetics and impact on flavour release and perception.

In real formulations, due to the great number of surface-active molecules present, competitive adsorption phenomena and interactions between adsorbed and non-adsorbed molecules take place and modify the composition and the stabilizing properties of the interfaces (Friberg and Larsson, 1997; Nylander *et al.*, 1997). The exact composition and properties of the o/w stabilizing interfaces are often poorly understood as also is the effective partition of the emulsifiers within the different phases of the systems according to their respective solubility and phase-forming properties. It remains therefore difficult to predict their physical and chemical stabilities and to obtain formulations that fulfil all the above requirements. This is why most of the literature concerns simplified systems in which the influence or relevant parameters can be sorted out. Additionally, the know-how for real applications with commercial outcomes is generally not available.

The first applications of omega-3 delivery systems concerned cosmetics, pharmaceutics or clinical uses. They were often based on the stabilizing effects of low molecular weight emulsifiers including, to a large extent, synthetic ones. Indeed, small size surfactants are generally considered to be more effective in stabilizing small oil droplets than biopolymers (proteins) under similar conditions of emulsification because they adsorb more rapidly on the droplet surface (Qian and McClements, 2011). Additionally, they present fewer safety issues regarding allergenic potential and microbial security (proteins are subject to intensive denaturation and degradation reactions under the severe conditions of sterilization required for clinical applications). For instance, formulations containing omega-3 fatty acids emulsified by polyethylene glycol esters for cosmetic and pharmaceutical applications (dermal creams) have been described in the patent US 2011/0293755 A1 (Sigurjonsson *et al.*, 2011). In the formulation, omega-3 PUFA were protected against oxidation by a mix of antioxidants. The preparation of a parenteral emulsion in which the oil phase was composed of soy a oil and fish oil diglycerides forming droplets with mean diameters between 290 and 300 nm and stabilized by egg yolk phospholipids has also been described (Decklbaum and Carpentier, 2010). Nanoemulsions containing fish oil blended with medium-chain triglycerides and rapeseed oil stabilized by soya lecithin and Tween® 80 have also been described (Kabri *et al.*, 2011).

Proteins and lecithins are generally considered to be the emulsifiers of choice to prepare delivery systems enriched in omega-3 PUFA for food applications because of their natural origin and their good emulsifying properties. Thus o/w emulsions containing marine or omega-3 vegetable oils droplets of micrometre sizes have been formulated for delivery usages. Actual developments concern sub-micron or nanoemulsions (McClements, 2011, 2012). For instance, nanoemulsions (average droplet diameter ≅ 225 nm) containing 5–10 % (w/v) omega-3 vegetable oil were stabilized by whey protein isolate (Chalothorn and Warisnoicharoen, 2012). A fish o/w emulsion stabilized by whey proteins–caseinate complexes obtained by moderate heat treatment is also available commercially. The emulsion, which exhibits an average droplet size around 200 nm, presents good physical stability and low oxidation level (Taneja and Singh, 2012). It was used to enrich processed cheese with omega-3 PUFA (50 g kg^{-1}). The fortified cheese exhibited a lower level of oxidation and better sensory quality than the cheese directly enriched with the same amount of fish oil (Ye *et al.*, 2009). Alternatively, the technique of solvent (ethyl acetate) evaporation has been proposed to prepare corn or fish oil nanoemulsions (mean diameter around 70 nm) stabilized by whey protein isolate (Lee and McClements, 2010). The nanoemulsion was stable to salt addition, thermal treatment, freezing/thawing cycles, but less oxidatively stable to oxidation than the conventional emulsion (droplet size distribution from 50 to >1000 nm and mean diameter of 325 nm).

Lecithins from various origins have also been tentatively used to prepare food delivery emulsions, either as sole emulsifier or in combination with proteins. Fish oil emulsions prepared at neutral pH with milk phospholipids fractions or soy lecithins were found to be less oxidatively stable than emulsions prepared with milk proteins (Horn *et al.*, 2011). For acid emulsions, the authors concluded that lecithins were potentially of great interest and that further investigations were required. Marine phospholipids were used to prepare omega-3 delivery systems containing, or not containing, fish oil (Belhaj *et al.*, 2010; Lu *et al.*, 2012). The latter systems contained oil droplets covered by a single layer of phospholipids, liposomes and micelles in different proportions according to the phospholipids proportion in the blend, a minimum of 3 % of phospholipids in the oil phase being required according to the authors to ensure the stabilization of the lipid droplets. In these conditions, satisfactory physical and chemical stabilities of the emulsions were reported. Fish oil emulsions containing proteins, polysaccharides, lecithins and other low molecular weight emulsifiers, either alone or in combinations, have also been used to produce encapsulated omega-3 oils (Garg *et al.*, 2006). For instance, Klinkesorn *et al.* (2005) prepared double-layered lecithin–chitosan emulsions by electrostatic layer-by-layer deposition technique. These double-layered emulsions had a better oxidative stability than the emulsions stabilized only with lecithin.

5.7 Future trends

A broad consensus exists concerning the positive impact of the consumption of omega-3 and PUFA on human health and on the statement that merely consuming fish will not fulfil the EPA+DHA daily intake recommendation for all populations (from 190–650 mg/day for EPA+DHA depending on the national or international organization (Garg *et al.*, 2006; AFSSA, 2010; Taneja and Singh, 2012)). The growing interest in incorporating emulsified lipids into food formulations with a high amount of omega-3 LC-PUFA is strengthened by results indicating that emulsification of fish oil enhances the absorption of omega-3 PUFAs such as EPA and DHA in healthy adults (Garaiova *et al.*, 2007). Indeed, other studies have investigated the effect of the food matrix on the bioavailability of EPA and DHA from fish oil. In a study by Schram *et al.* (2007), the same amount of fish oil was incorporated into fitness bars, yogurt drink, bread and butter and oil capsules, with different rates of absorption observed for the fish-oil supplemented food products compared to when fish oil was administered in capsule form. In this study, ingestion of yoghurt led to faster absorption of lipids, particularly omega-3 fatty acids (Schram *et al.*, 2007).

The nature of the omega-3 PUFA-carrying molecule is also of importance. Up to now, conflicting results have been found regarding the most suitable source of omega-3 LC-PUFA. Bioavailability of EPA and DHA in the form of free fatty acids, ethyl esters, TAGs or phospholipids has been investigated recently (Dyerberg *et al.*, 2011). Results highlighted the higher bioavailability of EPA and DHA (124 %) from re-esterified TAGs compared with natural fish oil or free fatty acids. Ethyl esters supplies offered the lowest bioavailability of EPA and DHA (73 %) when compared to re-esterified TAGs (Dyerberg *et al.*, 2011).

In contrast, results concerning the bioavailability of EPA and/or DHA from TAGs or phospholipids gave no final and clear conclusion. Nevertheless, it has been suggested that a lower intake of EPA and DHA, as phospholipids contained in krill oil, could achieve a similar plasma concentration of EPA and DHA (Ulven *et al.*, 2011). Tou *et al.* (2011) observed significantly lower DHA digestibility and brain accretion in growing female rats fed salmon or tuna oil than when the omega-3 source was krill oil, containing n-3 PUFA as phospholipids, but they did not notice any significant increase of the oxidative stress. These nutritional aspects should now be taken into account in the design of future formulations containing omega-3 PUFA.

In these new formulations, several objectives, for which the choice of the emulsifiers can be critical, should be integrated: guarantee the physical stability of the delivery system before and after incorporation; limit the oxidation reaction during handling and storage; enhance or control the rate of lipolysis, and, *in fine*, the bioaccessibility of the targeted fatty acids. To reach these goals, it is proposed to make use of developments in nanostructured systems to increase the total o/w surface area. This means that the structure and the composition of the interface layers should be optimized to ensure long-term physical stability of the newly designed structures and to limit oxidation without inhibiting lipolysis during digestion. The potential of natural surface-active molecules from under-exploited sources to organize into new nanostructured delivery assemblies should now be investigated. Emulsifier–emulsifier interactions should also be looked for.

Last, but not least, the oxidative fate of omega-3 PUFA during digestion and the absorption of oxidized lipids is an emerging issue with possible health implications (Baynes, 2007; Kanner, 2007; Awada *et al.*, 2012). Enrichment of foods with LC omega-3 PUFA will have to deal with the issue of how to protect these beneficial nutrients against oxidation during digestion. Likewise, the question of the digestive fate of the assemblies and the emulsifying molecules should be addressed.

5.8 Sources of further information

Books cited in this chapter related to emulsifiers and emulsions

- BOCKISH M (1998) *Fats and Oil Handbook*. Champaign, IL: AOCS Press.
- FRIBERG S E and LARSSON K (eds) (1997) *Food Emulsions*. New York: Marcel Dekker.

- MCCLEMENTS D J (2005) *Food Emulsion Principles, Practices, and Technique* (2nd edn). Boca Raton, FL: CRC Press.
- MCCLEMENTS D J and DECKER E A (eds) (2009) *Designing Functional Foods. Measuring and controlling food structure breakdown and nutrient absorption*. Oxford: Woodhead.
- WHITEHURST R J (2004) *Emulsifiers in Food Technology*. Oxford: Blackwell.

Concerning the legal aspects of the use of various emulsifiers in Europe
Website of EFSA: http://www.efsa.europa.eu/fr/, see also the *EFSA Journal*: http://www.efsa.europa.eu/en/publications/efsajournal.htm and the database on food additives: https://webgate.ec.europa.eu/sanco_foods/main/?event=display.

5.9 Acknowledgements

This work was supported by the French National Research Agency (ANR); grant ANR-08-ALIA-002, AGEcaninox project. T. H. K acknowledges her PhD grant from ANR.

C. Genot and A. Meynier are participants in the FA1005 COST Action INFOGEST on food digestion.

5.10 References

AFSSA (2010) *Avis de l'agence française de sécurité sanitaire des aliments relatif à l'actualisation des apports nutritionnels conseillés pour les acides gras*. Maisons-Alfort (F), available at: http://www.anses.fr/Documents/NUT2006sa0359.pdf [accessed January 2013].

AKHTAR M, DICKINSON E, MAZOYER J and LANGENDORFF V (2002) 'Emulsion stabilizing properties of depolymerized pectin'. *Food Hydrocolloids*, 16, 249–256.

AKOH C C and MIN D B (2002) *Food Lipids Chemistry, Nutrition, and Biotechnology*. New York: Marcel Dekker.

ASTORG P, ARNAULT N, CZERNICHOW S, NOISETTE N, GALAN P and HERCBERG S (2004) 'Dietary intakes and food sources of n-6 and n-3 PUFA in French adult men and women'. *Lipids*, 39, 527–535.

AWADA M, SOULAGE C O, MEYNIER A, DEBARD C, PLAISANCIÉ P, BENOIT B, PICARD G, LOIZON E, CHAUVIN M A, ESTIENNE M, PERETTY N, GUICHARDANT M, LAGARDE M, GENOT C and MICHALSKI M C (2012) 'Dietary oxidized n-3 PUFA induce oxidative stress and inflammation: Role of intestinal absorption of 4-HHE and reactivity in intestinal cells'. *J Lipid Res*, 53, 2069–2080.

BANDARRA N M, CAMPOS R M, BATISTA I, NUNES M L and EMPIS J M (1999) 'Antioxidant synergy of alpha-tocopherol and phospholipids'. *J Am Oil Chem Soc*, 76, 905–913.

BAUCH A, LINDTNER O, MENSINK G B M and NIEMANN B (2006) 'Dietary intake and sources of long-chain n-3 PUFAs in German adults'. *Eur J Clin Nutr*, 60, 810–812.

BAYARRI S and COSTELL E (2009) 'Optimising the flavour of low-fat foods', in MCCLEMENTS D J and DECKER E A (eds), *Designing Functional Foods. Measuring and Controlling Food Structure Breakdown and Nutrient Absorption.* Cambridge: Woodhead, 431–452.

BAYNES J W (2007) 'Dietary ALES are a risk to human health – not'. *Mol Nutr Food Res*, 51, 1102–1106.

BELHAJ N, ARAB-TEHRANY E and LINDER M (2010) 'Oxidative kinetics of salmon oil in bulk and in nanoemulsion stabilized by marine lecithin'. *Process Biochem*, 45, 187–195.

BERTON C, GENOT C and ROPERS M H (2011a) 'Quantification of unadsorbed protein and surfactant emulsifiers in oil-in-water emulsions'. *J Colloid Interface Sci*, 354, 739–748.

BERTON C, ROPERS M H, VIAU M and GENOT C (2011b) 'Contribution of the interfacial layer to the protection of emulsified lipids against oxidation'. *J Agric Food Chem*, 59, 5052–5061.

BERTON C, ROPERS M-H, GUIBERT D, SOLÉ V and GENOT C (2012) 'Modifications of interfacial proteins in oil-in-water emulsions prior to and during lipid oxidation'. *J Agric Food Chem*, 60, 8659–8671.

BOCKISH M (1998) *Fats and Oil Handbook*. Champaign, IL: AOCS Press.

BOS M A and VAN VLIET T (2001) 'Interfacial rheological properties of adsorbed protein layers and surfactants: A review'. *Adv Colloid Interface Sci*, 91, 437–471.

BUESCHELBERGER H-G (2004) 'Lecithins', in WHITEHURST R J (ed.), *Emulsifiers in Food Technology.* Oxford: Blackwell, 1–39.

CAPEK I (2004) 'Degradation of kinetically-stable o/w emulsions'. *Adv Colloid Interface Sci*, 107, 125–155.

CARDENIA V, WARAHO T, RODRIGUEZ-ESTRADA M T, MCCLEMENTS D J and DECKER E A (2011) 'Antioxidant and prooxidant activity behavior of phospholipids in stripped soybean oil-in-water emulsions'. *J Am Oil Chem Soc*, 88, 1409–1416.

CASTELLANI O, GUIBERT D, AL-ASSAF S, AXELOS M, PHILLIPS G O and ANTON M (2010) 'Hydrocolloids with emulsifying capacity. Part 1 – Emulsifying properties and interfacial characteristics of conventional (*Acacia senegal* (l.) willd. var. *senegal*) and matured (Acacia (*sen*) *SUPER GUM*™) *Acacia senegal*'. *Food Hydrocolloids*, 24, 193–199.

CHAIYASIT W, ELIAS R J, MCCLEMENTS D J and DECKER E A (2007) 'Role of physical structures in bulk oils on lipid oxidation'. *Crit Rev Food Sci Nutr*, 47, 299–317.

CHALOTHORN K and WARISNOICHAROEN W (2012) 'Ultrasonic emulsification of whey protein isolate-stabilized nanoemulsions containing omega-3 oil from plant seed'. *Am J Food Technol*, 7, 532–541.

CHARALAMBOUS G and DOXASTAKIS G (eds) (1989) *Food Emulsifiers. Chemistry, Technology, Functional Properties and Applications*. Amsterdam: Elsevier Science.

CHEN L, REMONDETTO G E and SUBIRADE M (2006) 'Food protein-based materials as nutraceutical delivery systems'. *Trends Food Sci Technol*, 17, 272–283.

CHEN B C, MCCLEMENTS D J and DECKER E A (2011) 'Minor components in food oils: A critical review of their roles on lipid oxidation chemistry in bulk oils and emulsions'. *Crit Rev Food Sci Nutr*, 51, 901–916.

CHEN B C, PANYA A, MCCLEMENTS D J and DECKER E A (2012) 'New insights into the role of iron in the promotion of lipid oxidation in bulk oils containing reverse micelles'. *J Agric Food Chem*, 60, 3524–3532.

CONDE E, GORDON M H, MOURE A and DOMINGUEZ H (2011) 'Effects of caffeic acid and bovine serum albumin in reducing the rate of development of rancidity in oil-in-water and water-in-oil emulsions'. *Food Chem*, 129, 1652–1659.

COTTRELL T and VAN PEIJ J (2004) 'Sorbitan esters and polysorbates', in WHITEHURST R J (ed.), *Emulsifiers in Food Technology.* Oxford: Blackwell, 162–185.

DECKLBAUM R J and CARPENTIER Y (2010) *Omega-3 diglyceride emulsions*. US patent application 12/441,795.

DICKINSON E (2003) 'Hydrocolloids at interfaces and the influence on the properties of dispersed systems'. *Food Hydrocoll*, 17, 25–39.

DICKINSON E (2009) 'Hydrocolloids as emulsifiers and emulsion stabilizers'. *Food hydrocolloids*, 23, 1473–1482.

DYERBERG J, MADSEN P, MULLER J M, AARDESTRUP I and SCHMIDT E B (2011) 'Bioavailability of marine n-3 fatty acid formulations'. *Prostaglandins Leukot Essent Fatty Acids*, 83, 137–141.

EFSA (2010a) 'Scientific opinion on dietary reference values for fats, including saturated fatty acids, polyunsaturated fatty acids, monounsaturated fatty acids, *trans* fatty acids, and cholesterol'. *EFSA J*, 8 (3), 1461, available at: http://www.efsa.europa.eu/fr/scdocs/doc/1461.pdf [accessed February 2013].

EFSA (2010b) 'Scientific opinion on the safety of sucrose esters of fatty acids prepared from vinyl esters of fatty acids and on the extension of use of sucrose esters of fatty acids in flavourings'. *EFSA J*, 8 (3), 1512, available at: http://www.efsa.europa.eu/de/scdocs/doc/1512.pdf [accessed February 2013].

ELIAS R J, MCCLEMENTS D J and DECKER E A (2005) 'Antioxidant activity of cysteine, tryptophan, and methionine residues in continuous phase beta-lactoglobulin in oil-in-water emulsions'. *J Agric Food Chem*, 53, 10248–10253.

ELWELL M W, ROBERTS R F and COUPLAND J N (2004) 'Effect of homogenization and surfactant type on the exchange of oil between emulsion droplets'. *Food hydrocolloids*, 18, 413–418.

EVANS C D, COONEY P, SCHOLFIELD C R and DUTTON H J (1954) 'Soybean 'lecithin' and its fractions as metal-inactivating agents'. *J Am Oil Chem Soc*, 31, 295–297.

FOMUSO L B, CORREDIG M and AKOH C C (2002) 'Effect of emulsifier on oxidation properties of fish oil-based structured lipid emulsions'. *J Agric Food Chem*, 50, 2957–2961.

FRANKEL E N (ed.) (2005) *Lipid Oxidation.* Bridgwater: The Oily Press.

FRIBERG S E and LARSSON K (eds) (1997) *Food Emulsions.* New York: Marcel Dekker.

GARAIOVA I, GUSHINA I A, PLUMMER S F, TANG J, WANG D and PLUMMER N T (2007) 'A randomised cross-over trial in healthy adults indicating improved absorption of omega-3 fatty acids by pre-emulsification'. *Nutr J*, 6, 4. DOI: 1186/1475-2891-6-4

GARG M L, WOOD L G, SINGH H and MOUGHAN P J (2006) 'Means of delivering recommended levels of long chain n-3 polyunsaturated fatty acids in human diets'. *J Food Sci*, 71, R66–R71.

GARTI N (1999) 'What can nature offer from an emulsifier point of view: Trends and progress?'. *Colloids Surf, A*, 152, 125–146.

GARTI N and LESER M E (2001) 'Emulsification properties of hydrocolloids'. *Polym Adv Technol,* 12, 123–135.

GENOT C, MEYNIER A and RIAUBLANC A (2003a) 'Lipid oxidation in emulsions', in KAMAL-ELDIN A (ed.), *Lipid Oxidation Pathways.* Champaign, IL: AOCS Press, 190–244.

GENOT C, MEYNIER A, RIAUBLANC A and CHOBERT J M (2003b) 'Protein alterations due to lipid oxidation in multiphase systems', in KAMAL-ELDIN A (ed.), *Lipid Oxidation Pathways.* AOCS Press, 265–292.

GENOT C, BERTON C and ROPERS M H (2013), 'The role of the interfacial layer and emulsifying proteins proteins in the oxidation in oil-in-water emulsions', in LOGAN A, NIENABER U and PAN X M (eds), *Lipid Oxidation: Challenges in Food Systems.* Champaign, IL: AOCS Press, 177–210.

GROOTVELD M, ATHERTON M D, SHEERIN A N, HAWKES J, BLAKE D R, RICHENS T E, SILWOOD C J L, LYNCH E and CLAXSON A W D (1998) 'In vivo absorption, metabolism, and urinary excretion of α,β-unsaturated aldehydes in experimental animals – relevance to the development of cardiovascular diseases by the dietary ingestion of thermally stressed polyunsaturate-rich culinary oils'. *J Clin Invest*, 101, 1210–1218.

GUÉRAUD F, ATALAY M, BRESGEN N, CIPAK A, ECKL P M, HUC L, JOUANIN I, SIEMS W and UCHIDA K (2010) 'Chemistry and biochemistry of lipid peroxidation products'. *Free Radic Res*, 44, 1098–1124.

GUPTA R and MURALIDHARA H S (2001) 'Interfacial challenges in the food industry: A review'. *Trends Food Sci Technol*, 12, 382–391.

GUTIÉRREZ J M, GONZÁLEZ C, MAESTRO A, SOLÈ I, PEY C M and NOLLA J (2008) 'Nano-emulsions: New applications and optimization of their preparation'. *Curr Opin Colloid Interface Sci*, 13, 245–251.

GUZEY D and MCCLEMENTS D J (2007) 'Impact of electrostatic interactions on formation and stability of emulsions containing oil droplets coated by beta-lactoglobulin–pectin complexes'. *J Agric Food Chem*, 55, 475–485.

HAAHR A M and JACOBSEN C (2008) 'Emulsifier type, metal chelation and pH affect oxidative stability of *n*-3-enriched emulsions'. *Eur J Lipid Sci Technol*, 110, 949–961.

HASENHUETTL G L (2008) 'Synthesis and commercial preparation of food emulsifiers', in HASENHUETTL G L and HARTEL R W (eds), *Food Emulsifiers and Their Applications.* New York: Springer 11–37.

HAUSER H (1987) 'Spontaneous vesiculation of uncharged phospholipid dispersions consisting of lecithin and lysolecithin'. *Chem Phys Lipids*, 43, 283–299.

HEINS A, MCPHAIL D B, SOKOLOWSKI T, STOCKMANN H and SCHWARZ K (2007) 'The location of phenolic antioxidants and radicals at interfaces determines their activity'. *Lipids*, 42, 573–582.

HEMAR Y, TAMEHANA M, MUNRO P A and SINGH H (2001) 'Viscosity, microstructure and phase behavior of aqueous mixtures of commercial milk protein products and xanthan gum'. *Food hydrocolloids*, 15, 565–574.

HENNERE G, PROGNON P, BRION F, ROSILIO V and NICOLIS I (2009) 'Molecular dynamics simulation of a mixed lipid emulsion model: Influence of the triglycerides on interfacial phospholipid organization'. *J Mol Struct THEOCHEM*, 901, 174–185.

HIDALGO F J, NOGALES F and ZAMORA R (2005) 'Changes produced in the antioxidative activity of phospholipids as a consequence of their oxidation'. *J Agric Food Chem*, 53, 659–662.

HIDALGO F J, NOGALES F and ZAMORA R (2008) 'The role of amino phospholipids in the removal of the cito and geno-toxic aldehydes produced during lipid oxidation'. *Food Chem Toxicol*, 46, 43–48.

HORN A F, NIELSEN N S, ANDERSEN U, SOGAARD L H, HORSEWELL A and JACOBSEN C (2011) 'Oxidative stability of 70 % fish oil-in-water emulsions: Impact of emulsifiers and pH'. *Eur J Lipid Sci Technol*, 113, 1243–1257.

HORN A F, NIELSEN N S and JACOBSEN C (2012a) 'Iron-mediated lipid oxidation in 70 % fish oil-in-water emulsions: Effect of emulsifier type and pH'. *Int J Food Sci Technol*, 47, 1097–1108.

HORN A F, NIELSEN N S, JENSEN L S, HORSEWELL A and JACOBSEN C (2012b) 'The choice of homogenisation equipment affects lipid oxidation in emulsions'. *Food Chem*, 134, 803–810.

ISHII F and NII T (2005) 'Properties of various phospholipid mixtures as emulsifiers or dispersing agents in nanoparticle drug carrier preparations'. *Colloids Surf, B*, 41, 257–262.

ISRAELACHVILI J N (1992) *Intermolecular and Surfaces Forces*. London: Academic Press.

JACOBSEN C, LET M B, NIELSEN N S and MEYER A S (2008) 'Antioxidant strategies for preventing oxidative deterioration of food enriched with n-3 polyunsaturated lipids: A comprehensive evaluation'. *Trends Food Sci Technol*, 19, 76–93.

JAFARI S M, ASSADPOOR E, HE Y H and BHANDARI B (2008) 'Re-coalescence of emulsion droplets during high-energy emulsification'. *Food Hydrocoll*, 22, 1191–1202.

JOWITT R (1974) 'The terminology of food texture'. *J Texture Stud*, 5, 351–358.

JUDDE A, VILLENEUVE P, ROSSIGNOL-CASTERA A and LE GUILLOU A (2003) 'Antioxidant effect of soy lecithins on vegetable oil stability and their synergism with tocopherols'. *J Am Oil Chem Soc*, 80, 1209–1215.

KABRI T-H, ARAB-TEHRANY E, BELHAJ N and LINDER M (2011) 'Physico-chemical characterization of nano-emulsions in cosmetic matrix enriched on omega-3'. *J Nanobiotechnol*, 9. DOI: 10.1186/1477-3155-9-41

KANNER J (2007) 'Dietary advanced lipid oxidation endproducts are risk factors to human health'. *Mol Nutr Food Res*, 51, 1094–1101.

KLEIN M, ASERIN A, SVITOV I and GARTI N (2010) 'Enhanced stabilization of cloudy emulsions with gum arabic and whey protein isolate'. *Colloids Surf, B*, 77, 75–81.

KLINKESORN U, SOPHANODORA P, CHINACHOTI P, MCCLEMENTS D J and DECKER E A (2005) 'Increasing the oxidative stability of liquid and dried tuna oil-in-water emulsions with electrostatic layer-by-layer deposition technology'. *J Agric Food Chem*, 53, 4561–4566.

KOGA T and TERAO J (1995) 'Phospholipids increase radical-scavenging activity of vitamin-E in a bulk oil model system'. *J Agric Food Chem*, 43, 1450–1454.

KOLANOWSKI W and LAUFENBERG G (2006) 'Enrichment of food products with polyunsaturated fatty acids by fish oil addition'. *Eur Food Res Technol*, 222, 472–477.

KOLANOWSKI W and WEISSBRODT J (2007) 'Sensory quality of dairy products fortified with fish oil'. *Int Dairy J*, 17, 1248–1253.

KOLANOWSKI W, JAWORSKA D, LAUFENBERG G and WEISSBRODT J (2007) 'Evaluation of sensory quality of instant foods fortified with omega-3 PUFA by addition of fish oil powder'. *Eur Food Res Technol*, 225, 715–721.

KRALOVA I and SJOBLOM J (2009) 'Surfactants used in food industry: A review'. *J Dispers Sci Technol*, 30, 1363–1383.

KULLENBERG D, TAYLOR L A, SCHNEIDER M and MASSING U (2012) 'Health effects of dietary phospholipids'. *Lipids Health Dis*, 11. DOI: 10.1186/1476-511X-11.3

LANDY P, ROGACHEVA S, LORIENT D and VOILLEY A (1998) 'Thermodynamic and kinetic aspects of the transport of small molecules in dispersed systems'. *Colloids Surf, B*, 12, 57–65.

LARSSON K (2004) 'Molecular organization of lipids and emulsions', in SJOBLOM J (ed.), *Food Emulsions* (4 edn). New York: Marcel Dekker, 93–106.

LE GRANDOIS J, MARCHIONI E, AENNAHAR S, GUIFFRIDA F and BINDLER F (2010) 'Identification and kinetics of oxidized compounds from phosphatidylcholine molecular species'. *Food Chem*, 119, 1233–1238.

LEE J and CHOE E (2009) 'Effects of phosphatidylcholine and phosphatidylethanolamine on the photooxidation of canola oil'. *J Food Sci*, 74, C481–C486.

LEE S J and MCCLEMENTS D J (2010) 'Fabrication of protein-stabilized nanoemulsions using a combined homogenization and amphiphilic solvent dissolution/evaporation approach'. *Food hydrocolloids*, 24, 560–569.

LET M B, JACOBSEN C and MEYER A S (2007) 'Lipid oxidation in milk, yoghurt, and salad dressing enriched with neat fish oil or pre-emulsified fish oil'. *J Agric Food Chem*, 55, 7802–7809.

LETHUAUT L, BROSSARD C, MEYNIER A, ROUSSEAU F, LLAMAS G, BOUSSEAU B and GENOT C (2005) 'Sweetness and aroma perceptions in dairy desserts varying in sucrose and aroma levels and in textural agent'. *Int Dairy J*, 15, 485–493.

LU F S H, NIELSEN N S, BARON C P, JENSEN L H S and JACOBSEN C (2012) 'Physicochemical properties of marine phospholipid emulsions'. *J Am Oil Chem Soc*, 89, 2011–2024.

MALONE M E and APPELQVIST I A M (2003) 'Gelled emulsion particles for the controlled release of lipophilic volatiles during eating'. *J Control Release*, 90, 227–241.

MALONE M E, APPELQVIST I A M and NORTON I T (2003) 'Oral behaviour of food hydrocolloids and emulsions. Part 2. Taste and aroma release'. *Food hydrocolloids*, 17, 775–784.

MARANGONI A G and GARTI N (eds) (2011) *Edible Oleogels: Structure and Health Implications*. Champaign, IL: AOCS Press.

MARSZALL L and VAN VALKENBURG J W (1982) 'The effect of glycols on the hydrophile–lipophile balance and the micelle formation of nonionic surfactants'. *J Am Oil Chem Soc*, 59, 84–87.

MCCLEMENTS D J (2005) *Food Emulsion Principles, Practices, and Technique* (2nd edn) Boca Raton, FL: CRC Press.

MCCLEMENTS D J (2007) 'Critical review of techniques and methodologies for characterization of emulsion stability'. *Crit Rev Food Sci Nutr*, 47, 611–649.

MCCLEMENTS D J (2011) 'Edible nanoemulsions: Fabrication, properties, and functional performance'. *Soft Matter*, 7, 2297–2316.

MCCLEMENTS D J (2012) 'Nanoemulsions versus microemulsions: Terminology, differences, and similarities'. *Soft Matter*, 8, 1719–1729.

MCCLEMENTS D J and DECKER E A (2000) 'Lipid oxidation in oil-in-water emulsions: Impact of molecular environment on chemical reactions in heterogeneous food systems'. *J Food Sci*, 65, 1270–1282.

MEYER B J (2011) 'Are we consuming enough long chain omega-3 polyunsaturated fatty acids for optimal health?'. *Prostaglandins Leukot Essent Fatty Acids*, 85, 275–280.

MEYNIER A, LECOQ C and GENOT C (2005) 'Emulsification enhances the retention of esters and aldehydes to a greater extent than changes in the droplet size distribution of the emulsion'. *Food Chem*, 93, 153–159.

MOONEN H and BAS H (2004) 'Mono- and diglycerides', in WHITEHURST R J (ed.), *Emulsifiers in Food Technology.* Oxford: Blackwell, 40–58.

MOOTOOSINGH K S T and ROUSSEAU D (2006) 'Emulsions for the delivery of nutraceutical lipids', in SHAHIDI F (ed.), *Nutraceutical and Specialty Lipids and Their Co-products.* Boca Raton, FL: CRC Press Taylor & Francis Group, 281–300.

MOURITSEN O G (2011) 'Lipids, curvature, and nano-medicine'. *Eur J Lipid Sci Technol*, 113, 1174–1187.

MOZURAITYTE R, RUSTAD T and STORRO I (2006) 'Oxidation of cod phospholipids in liposomes: Effects of salts, pH and zeta potential'. *Eur J Lipid Sci Technol*, 108, 944–950.

NELEN B A P and COOPER J M (2004) 'Sucrose esters', in WHITEHURST R J (ed.), *Emulsifiers in Food Technology.* Oxford: Blackwell, 131–161.

NIELSEN N S and JACOBSEN C (2009) 'Methods for reducing lipid oxidation in fish-oil-enriched energy bars'. *Int J Food Sci Technol*, 44, 1536–1546.

NII T and ISHII F (2004) 'Properties of various phosphatidylcholines as emulsifiers or dispersing agents in microparticle preparations for drug carriers'. *Colloids Surf, B*, 39, 57–63.

NITSCHKE M and COSTA S G V A O (2007) 'Biosurfactants in food industry'. *Trends Food Sci Technol*, 18, 252–259.

NWOSU C V, BOYD L C and SHELDON B (1997) 'Effect of fatty acid composition of phospholipids on their antioxidant properties and activity index'. *J Am Oil Chem Soc*, 74, 293–297.

NYLANDER T, ARNEBRANT T, BOS M and WILDE P (1997) 'Protein emulsifier interactions', in HASENHUETTL G L and HARTEL R W (eds) *Food Emulsifiers and Their Applications.* New York: Springer, 89–172.

OHSHIMA T, FUJITA Y and KOIZUMI C (1993) 'Oxidative stability of sardine and mackerel lipids with reference to synergism between phospholipids and alpha-tocopherol'. *J Am Oil Chem Soc*, 70, 269–276.

OSBORN H T and AKOH C C (2002) 'Structured lipids – novel fats with medical, nutraceutical, and food applications'. *Compr Rev Food Sci Food Saf*, 1, 93–103.

PAÇI KORA E, LATRILLE E, SOUCHON I and MARTIN N (2003) 'Texture-flavor interactions in low fat stirred yogurt: How mechanical treatment, thickener concentration and aroma concentration affect perceived texture and flavor'. *J Sensory Stud*, 18, 367–390.

PAN X, IRWIN A J, LEONARD M and WELSBY D (2010) 'Choline and ethanolamine decompose lipid hydroperoxides into hydroxyl lipids'. *J Am Oil Chem Soc*, 87, 1235–1245.

PICHOT R, SPYROPOULOS F and NORTON I T (2010) 'O/W emulsions stabilised by both low molecular weight surfactants and colloidal particles: The effect of surfactant type and concentration'. *J Colloid Interface Sci*, 352, 128–135.

QIAN C and MCCLEMENTS D J (2011) 'Formation of nanoemulsions stabilized by model food-grade emulsifiers using high-pressure homogenization: Factors affecting particle size'. *Food hydrocolloids*, 25, 1000–1008.

RAMPON V, LETHUAUT L, MOUHOUS-RIOU N and GENOT C (2001) 'Interface characterization and aging of bovine serum albumin stabilized oil-in-water emulsions as revealed by front-surface fluorescence'. *J Agric Food Chem*, 49, 4046–4051.

ROGACHEVA S, ESPINOSA-DIAZ M A and VOILLEY A (1999) 'Transfer of aroma compounds in water–lipid systems: Binding tendency of β-lactoglobulin'. *J Agric Food Chem*, 47, 259–263.

RON E Z and ROSENBERG E (2001) 'Natural roles of biosurfactants'. *Environ Microbiol*, 3, 229–236.

ROSENBERG E and RON E Z (1999) 'High- and low-molecular-mass microbial surfactants'. *Appl Microbiol Biotechnol*, 52, 154–162.

SADTLER W M, GUELY M, MARCHAL P and CHOPLIN L (2004) 'Shear-induced phase transitions in sucrose ester surfactant'. *J Colloid Interface Sci*, 270, 270–275.

SAGALOWICZ L and LESER M E (2010) 'Delivery systems for liquid food products'. *Curr Opin Colloid Interface Sci*, 15, 61–72.

SAITO H and ISHIHARA K (1997) 'Antioxidant activity and active sites of phospholipids as antioxidants'. *J Am Oil Chem Soc*, 74, 1531–1536.

SALAGER J L, ANTON R, ANDÉREZ J M and AUBRY J M (2001) 'Formulation des microémulsions par la méthode du HLD'. *Techniques de l'ingénieur*, Génie des procédés, J2, 1–20.

SAMTLEBE M, YUCEL U, WEISS J and COUPLAND J N (2012) 'Stability of solid lipid nanoparticles in the presence of liquid oil emulsions'. *J Am Oil Chem Soc*, 89, 609–617.

SATHIVEL S, PRINYAWIWATKUL W, NEGULESCU I, KING J M and BASNAYAKE B F A (2003) 'Effects of purification process on rheological properties of catfish oil'. *J Am Oil Chem Soc*, 80, 829–832.

SCHRAM L B, NIELSEN C J, PORSGAARD T, NIELSEN N S, HOLM R and MU H (2007) 'Food matrices affect the bioavailability of (n-3) polyunsaturated fatty acids in a single meal study in humans'. *Food Res Int*, 40, 1062–1068.

SCHULTZ S, WAGNER G, URBAN K and ULRICH J (2004) 'High-pressure homogenization as a process for emulsion formation'. *Chem Ing Technol*, 27, 361–368.

SHINODA K (1967) 'The correlation between the dissolution state of nonionic surfactant and the type of dispersion stabilized with the surfactant'. *J Colloid Interface Sci*, 24, 4–9.

SHINODA K and SAITO H (1969) 'The stability of o/w type emulsions as functions of temperature and the HLB of emulsifiers: The emulsification by PIT-method'. *J Colloid Interface Sci*, 30, 258–263.

SIGURJONSSON F G, ILIEVSKA B and BALDURSSON B T (2011) *Stabilized formulation comprising omega-3 fatty acids and use of the fatty acids for skin care and/or wound care*. US patent application 2011/0293, 755.

SIOEN I, DEVROE J, INGHELS D, TERWECOREN R and DE HENAUW S (2010) 'The influence of n-3 PUFA supplements and n-3 PUFA enriched foods on the n-3 LC PUFA intake of Flemish women'. *Lipids*, 45, 313–320.

SORENSEN A D M, HAAHR A M, BECKER E M, SKIBSTED L H, BERGENSTAHL B, NILSSON L and JACOBSEN C (2008) 'Interactions between iron, phenolic compounds, emulsifiers, and pH in omega-3-enriched oil-in-water emulsions'. *J Agric Food Chem*, 56, 1740–1750.

STAUFFER C E (2005) 'Emulsifiers for the food industry', in SHAHIDI F (ed.), *Bailey's Industrial Oil and Fat Products* (6th edn). Hoboken, NJ: Wiley.

STOCKMANN H, SCHWARZ K and HUYNH-BA T (2000) 'The influence of various emulsifiers on the partitioning and antioxidant activity of hydroxybenzoic acids and their derivatives in oil-in-water emulsions'. *J Am Oil Chem Soc*, 77, 535–542.

SZUTS A, BUDAI-SZUCS M, EROS I, OTOMO N and SZABO-REVESZ P (2010) 'Study of gel-forming properties of sucrose esters for thermosensitive drug delivery systems'. *Int J Pharm*, 383, 132–137.

TANEJA A and SINGH H (2012) 'Challenges for the delivery of long-chain n-3 fatty acids in functional foods'. *Annu Rev Food Sci Technol*, 3, 105–123.

TERAO J (2001) 'Factors affecting the oxidative stability of emulsified oil and membranous phospholipids'. *J Oleo Sci*, 50, 393–397.

TIKEKAR R V, JOHNSON A and NITIN N (2011) 'Real-time measurement of oxygen transport across an oil–water emulsion interface'. *J Food Eng*, 103, 14–20.

TOU J C, ALTMAN S N, GIGLIOTTI J C, BENEDITO V A and CORDONIER E L (2011) 'Different sources of omega-3 polyunsaturated fatty acids affects apparent digestibility, tissue deposition, and tissue oxidative stability in growing female rats'. *Lipids Health Dis*, 10. 179. DOI: 1186/1476-511X-10-179

ULVEN S, KIRKHUS B, LAMGLAIT A, BASU S, ELIND E, HAIDER T, BERGE K, VIK H and PEDERSEN J (2011) 'Metabolic effects of krill oil are essentially similar to those of fish oil but at lower dose of EPA and DHA, in healthy volunteers'. *Lipids*, 46, 37–46.

URBAN K, WAGNER G, SCHAFFNER D, ROGLIN D and ULRICH J (2006) 'Rotor–stator and disc systems for emulsification processes'. *Chem Ing Technol*, 29, 24–31.

VAN AKEN G A and DE HOOG E H A (2009) 'Oral processing and perception of food emulsions: The relevance for fat reduction in food', in MCCLEMENTS D J and DECKER E A (eds), *Designing Functional Foods. Measuring and Controlling Food Structure Breakdown and Nutrient Absorption.* Cambridge: Woodhead, 481–501.

VAN DER BILT A (2009) 'Oral physiology, mastication and food perception', in MCCLEMENTS D J and DECKER E A (eds), *Designing Functional Foods. Measuring and Controlling Food Structure Breakdown and Nutrient Absorption.* Cambridge: Woodhead, 3–37.

VAN NIEUWENHUYZEN W and SZUHAJ B F (1998) 'Effects of lecithins and proteins on the stability of emulsions'. *Fett/Lipid*, 100, 282–291.

VILLIÈRE A, VIAU M, BRONNEC I, MOREAU N and GENOT C (2005) 'Oxidative stability of bovine serum albumin and sodium caseinate-stabilized emulsions depends on metal availability'. *J Agric Food Chem*, 53, 1514–1520.

WARAHO T, MCCLEMENTS D J and DECKER E A (2011) 'Mechanisms of lipid oxidation in food dispersions'. *Trends Food Sci Technol*, 22, 3–13.

WHITEHURST R J (2004) *Emulsifiers in Food Technology*. Oxford: Blackwell.

WIDDER S and FISHER N (1996) 'Measurement of the influence of food ingredients on flavour release by headspace chromatography–olfactometry', in TAYLOR A J and

MOTTRAM D S (eds), *Flavour Science. Recent Developments.* Cambridge: The Royal Society of Chemistry, 405–412.

WINSOR P A (1956) 'Solvent properties of amphiphilic compounds'. *Butterworths Scientific Publications*, 58, 1103–1104.

YASHODHARA B M, UMAKANTH S, PAPPACHAN J M, BHAT S K, KAMATH R and CHOO B H (2009) 'Omega-3 fatty acids: A comprehensive review of their role in health and disease'. *Postgrad Med J*, 85, 84–90.

YE A, CUI J, TANEJA A, ZHU X and SINGH H (2009) 'Evaluation of processed cheese fortified with fish oil emulsion'. *Food Res Int*, 42, 1093–1098.

YE A, GILLILAND J and SINGH H (2011) 'Thermal treatment to form a complex surface layer of sodium caseinate and gum arabic on oil–water interfaces'. *Food Hydrocoll*, 25, 1677–1686.

YIN H X, SOLVAL K M, HUANG J Q, BECHTEL P J and SATHIVEL S (2011) 'Effects of oil extraction methods on physical and chemical properties of red salmon oils (*Oncorhynchus nerka*)'. *J Am Oil Chem Soc*, 88, 1641–1648.

6

Spray drying and encapsulation of omega-3 oils

C. J. Barrow and B. Wang, Deakin University, Australia and B. Adhikari and H. Liu, University of Ballarat, Australia

DOI: 10.1533/9780857098863.2.194

Abstract: Due to strong clinical data supporting a variety of health benefits, omega-3 oils are being increasingly added to food and beverage products. However, these bioactive lipids need to be protected against autoxidation and degradation during food processing and storage. Microencapsulation technology is employed to stabilise omega-3 oils and enable their delivery into food and beverage products without impacting the taste and shelf-life of the product. In this chapter, we provide an overview of microencapsulation techniques used to encapsulate and stabilise omega-3 oils. The advantages and disadvantages of each method are described and compared. Also, important properties of the microencapsulated ingredients, such as payload, oxidative stability and bioavailability, are described. Although a variety of methods have been used to microencapsulate omega-3 oils, two methods are primarily used commercially. These are complex co-acervation and spray-dried emulsion formation. These two methods are compared and contrasted, and their future development discussed.

Key words: omega-3 oils, microencapsulation, complex co-acervation, oxidative stability.

6.1 Introduction

6.1.1 The health benefits of dietary omega-3 oils

Omega-3 fatty acids are unsaturated fatty acids that have a double bond at the third carbon atom from the end of the carbon chain. The most common omega-3 fatty acids are α-linolenic acid (ALA, 18:3), eicosapentaenoic acid (EPA, 20:5) and docosahexaenoic acid (DHA, 22:6). Among these three, EPA and DHA are the most clinically active and can be accumulated in humans by eating oily fish, taking fish oil supplements or eating foods fortified with these healthy oils. ALA is considered an essential fatty acid because it cannot be synthesized in the body, whereas EPA and DHA are sometimes termed as 'physiologically essential' as these longer chain omega-3 oils are more important functionally (Francois *et al.*, 2003; Ismail, 2005; Hibbeln *et al.*, 2006).

Omega-3 oils have significant benefits to human health since they have numerous physiological roles, including impacting cell membrane fluidity, cellular signaling, gene expression and eicosanoid metabolism. Bang and Dyerherg (1973) suggested a correlation between the diet of the Inuit containing large amounts of omega-3 oils, particularly EPA and DHA from fish and seal oil, and their low rates of coronary heart disease. Since then, numerous clinical studies have reported the beneficial effect of omega-3 fatty acids on a variety of disease including cancer (De Deckere, 1999; Hull, 2011), cardiovascular disease (Wang *et al.*, 2006; Yokoyama *et al.*, 2007), immune functions (Damsgaard *et al.*, 2007), neurology disorders (Amminger *et al.*, 2010) and inflammation (Wall *et al.*, 2010). Clinical trials using EPA and DPA supplementation of 875–1000 mg/day reported a reduced risk of sudden cardiac death and a lowering of triacylglycerol (TAG) levels, and these appear to be the most clinically proven benefits of EPA and DHA (Giannuzzi *et al.*, 2008). Fish oils such as tuna oil and anchovy/sardine oil have been shown to be beneficial for inflammatory bowel diseases such as Crohn's disease (Bulluzzi *et al.*, 1996). The wide range of health benefits described for EPA and DHA have created the perception that these oils are general wellness products. A general wellness ingredient tends to find more success as a functional food ingredient than does an ingredient targeted at a specific health indication.

Modern food habits, particularly in Western society, are characterized by the consumption of a relatively large amount of fast food and corn and soybean oils, which contain high levels of both saturated fat and omega-6 fat. A study by Ambring *et al.* (2006) suggested that a higher serum phospholipid omega-6/omega-3 ratio was linked to the higher death rate from cardiovascular disease, and there is a lower omega-6/omega-3 ratio in the Mediterranean diet.

Western diets are also characterized by relatively low consumptions of omega-3 oils. For example, for the majority of North Americans and Australians intakes of EPA and DHA are less than 200 mg/day (Raper *et al.*, 1992; Kris-Etherton *et al.*, 2000). The Japanese diet, high in oily fish, and the Mediterranean diet, high in olive oil, are both associated with a relatively low risk of inflammatory mediated diseases, supporting the importance of consumption of healthy oils in the prevention of many modern diseases (Kamei *et al.*, 2002; Ambring *et al.*, 2006). However, changing the dietary habits of Western society is very difficult and so companies strive to add healthy oils such as omega-3s to widely consumed food staples (Jafar *et al.*, 1994).

In recent years, a wide variety of commercial food products enriched with omega-3 fatty acids have been developed (Kolanowski and Laufenberg, 2006). This has been driven by the introduction of recommended consumption levels and Recommended Daily Intake (RDI) levels issued by a number of bodies. For example, the Canadian government recommended each person between 25 and 49 years old should consume 1.5 g of omega-3 oils per day. The British Nutrition Foundation recommends consumption of two oily fish meals weekly, corresponding to about 1.5 g EPA + DHA per week. According to USDA, the acceptable upper limit of EPA and DHA for adult male and female is 1600 and 1100 mg/day, respectively. The Heart Foundation in Australia also recommends 200 mg of omega-3 (including ALA) a day (Sharma, 2005). In 2006, Australia introduced Nutrient Reference Values (NRVs) with suggested daily targets for the consumption of DHA, EPA and DPA of 610 mg for men and 530 mg for women. Over the last several years in various countries, a variety of widely consumed foods such as bakery and dairy products have been fortified with omega-3 oils, as illustrated in Table 6.1.

6.1.2 The oxidative instability of omega-3 oils

There are still technical challenges in the production, transportation and storage of functional foods enriched with omega-3 oils from either fish or microbial sources, since these unsaturated lipids are extremely susceptible

Table 6.1 Examples of food products fortified with omega-3 fatty acids worldwide

Product type	Commercial examples
Bread and bakery products	Diamant Vital omega-3 Kruste (Diamant Mühle, Germany)
	Tip Top Up sliced bread and muffins (Tip Top bakeries, Australia)
	Hi Q DHA bread (Bunge Defiance, Australia)
	DHA-bread and DHA table rolls (Yamazaki Baking, Japan)
	Nutribread (William Jackson Bakery, UK)
	Nimble Heartbeat (British Bakeries, UK)
	Leva omega-3-bread (Pagen, Sweden)
Milk and dairy products	Omega-3 milk (Parmalat, USA)
	Mleko omega-3-UHT milk (SM Sudowa, Poland)
	Omi-3 yoghurt (SM Siedlece, Poland)
	Plus omega-3-latte and omega-3-yogurt (Parmalat, Italy)
Juice and soft drinks	Tidal Wave Superfood Juice (Naked Juice, California, USA)
	Bertrams Omega functional Juices (Bentrams, UK)
	My way wellness drink (Designer Foods, Germany)
	Chikara Mizu soft drink (Kirin Breweries, Japan)
Egg products	DHA Gold eggs (Omega Tech, USA)
	Oro Omega-3 eggs (Unione Cascine Vapladana, Italy)
	Eggs plus (Polgrim's Pride, USA)
Meat and poultry products	Strasburg sausage (Hans, Australia)
	Omega cool burger (Pals, Norway)
	Omega-3 Jamon Cocido cooked ham breast (Carnicas Serrano, Spain)

to oxidative deterioration. For example, DHA (with six double bonds) has been demonstrated to be over 50 times more susceptible to oxidation than oleic acid (with only one double bond), primarily due to its high number of unsaturated double bonds (Frankel, 2005). EPA and DHA can rapidly react with oxygen in a free radical reaction process known as autoxidation in which hydroperoxides (ROOHs) are formed through reaction at an allylic center (CH_2 adjacent to a double bond). These hydroperoxides then rapidly degrade to a range of volatile ketones and aldehydes. Some of these breakdown products have very low sensory threshold values, which means even small levels of oxidation can be detected by human taste and smell. For example, the aldehydes *trans,cis*-2,6-nonadienal and *trans,cis*-3,6-nonadienal formed during EPA and DHA autoxidation are known to cause an undesirable odor and taste in some food products even at a level as low as 0.01 ppm (Barrow *et al.*, 2007). Therefore, these oils need to be stabilized against oxidation before they can be successfully added to food or beverage products without negatively impacting the taste, smell or shelf-life of the product. This is primarily achieved through a combination of antioxidant addition and microencapsulation.

6.2 Microencapsulation methods for stabilizing omega-3 oils in food

Microencapsulation can be defined as a process to entrap one substance, normally an active ingredient, within another coating substance at the micro scale (Dickinson, 1992; McClements, 2005). Since the 1950s, microencapsulation has been applied in a variety of industries, particularly for pharmaceutical drug or vaccine delivery and in the printing industry. However, most recently, food ingredient manufacturers are applying microencapsulation technologies to the addition of unstable functional bioactive compounds into novel food products. Matsuno and Adachi (1993) and McClements (2005) described several advantages of lipid bioactive microencapsulation, including retarding autoxidation, enhancing stability and masking off taste of lipid ingredients. For food products, it is important that the encapsulation be at the micro scale, since ingredients with particle sizes of greater than about 100 μm create an unwanted mouthfeel as they are large enough to be sensed (Truelstrup-Hansen *et al.*, 2002).

It is well established that the oxidative stability of omega-3 oils is significantly enhanced after microencapsulation (Onuki *et al.*, 2003; Wu *et al.*, 2005; Kolanowski and Weibbrodt, 2007). For example, Borneo *et al.* (2007) have reported that DHA and EPA were microencapsulated into cookies in a matrix of starch and gelatin with good sensory outcomes. Overall, various types of food product, such as bread, instant food, yoghurts, cheeses, butter and cream, can be fortified with microencapsulated fish oil at limited levels without sensory changes (Kolanowski and Weibbrodt, 2007; Kolanowski *et al.*, 2007; Gökmen *et al.*, 2011; Borneo *et al.*, 2007).

6.2.1 Shell materials for microencapsulation

The shell materials are the protecting material coating the outside of the bioactive oils, acting as a barrier to oxidation as well as masking off-flavors. In most processes used for oil encapsulation an early step is to form an emulsion of the oil and primary shell components, as Figs. 6.1–6.3 in Section 6.3 show. An emulsifying agent is necessary for dispersing the oil phase into an aqueous phase. An emulsifier is a surface-active substance, which has a strong tendency to adsorb at oil–water (o/w) interfaces, thereby promoting the formation and rapid stabilization of emulsion droplets by interfacial action. In molecular terms, the emulsifier is an amphiphilic compound containing a hydrophilic (water-preferring) part and a lipophilic (fat-preferring) part. The primary shell-material component is normally a protein or polysaccharide, depending upon the process and desired properties of the microencapsulated ingredient (see also Section 6.3).

6.2.2 Hydrophile–lipophile balance

The most widely used system for classifying emulsifiers is the hydrophile–lipophile balance (HLB) scale, with values from 1 to 40, as firstly developed by Griffin (1949). A low HLB number indicates that the emulsifier is more lipophilic, while a high value indicates that it is hydrophilic (Dickinson, 1993). To get the desired emulsifying properties, it is normally desirable to use a blend of emulsifiers rather than a single one. An optimized blend can produce a more stable emulsion than one prepared with a single emulsifier of the same HLB value. For example, for microencapsulation efficiency and yield of DHA in corn starch, a mixture of Tween® 85 and Tween® 20 was found to be superior to either one individually (Chang, 1997).

However, although it is useful for classifying emulsifiers, the HLB values system is of little value in the formulation of food products. This is because most food emulsions are stabilized by proteins for which the simple HLB concept is not applicable (Dickinson, 1993). A low molecular weight surfactant may exhibit competitive adsorption in protein-stabilized emulsions, hence causing destabilization (Chen and Dickinson, 1995).

6.2.3 Lipid-based microencapsulation systems

One of the most useful delivery systems for lipophilic bioactive ingredients is through lipid-based encapsulation systems. Generally, lipid-based delivery systems are believed to improve bioactive wetting and dissolution properties and modulate bioactive absorption and chemical stability, as well as enable targeting of specific tissues (McClements and Li, 2010). Phospholipids are excellent emulsifiers due to their glycerol backbone, which is bound to two fatty acids (hydrophobic) and a phosphoric acid (hydrophilic). For example, lecithin is one of the most widely used emulsifiers in the food industry. Horn *et al.* (2011) compared the effects of emulsifier type on lipid oxidation stability for microencapsulated omega-3 fatty acids. Results indicated that at low pH, phospholipid-based emulsions can be a suitable delivery system for a 70% fish oil-in-water (o/w) emulsion (Horn *et al.*, 2011).

6.2.4 Protein-based microencapsulation systems

Food proteins are natural polymeric emulsifiers, which can carry an important nutritional value along with considerable functionality (Chen *et al.*, 2006). Their chemical and structural versatility makes them appropriate for encapsulation and delivery of bioactive ingredients. This is partly due to their amphoteric nature and natural abundance. Indeed, protein-based systems have been reported as being relatively simple to prepare, with low cost and offering the possibility to deliver hydrophobic bioactive compounds. However, the emulsifying properties of proteins are significantly affected by pH, ionic strength, temperature and the addition of small molecular surfactants. For example, at pH values close to their isoelectric point, proteins can become poor emulsifiers, because of the minimization of electrostatic repulsive forces.

Common proteins used in the food industry include dairy protein, gelatin and various plant proteins. Dairy protein derived from milk is the most widely used protein emulsifier. For example, β-casein, which is rich in proline residues but has no cysteine residues, is a flexible protein with little ordered secondary structure and no intramolecular cross-links (Shimada *et al.*, 1982). The coating layer formed by caseins tends to be larger and thicker, compared with those formed by globular proteins such as β-lactoglobulin. Kagami *et al.* (2003), Keogh *et al.* (2001) and Bao *et al.* (2011) reported the microencapsulation of fish oil using whey and casein proteins. These studies indicated that the oxidative stability of omega-3 oils was significantly enhanced using this method of microencapsulation. Plant proteins, such as soy protein, gliadin and glutenin (two fractions derived from gluten), can also be used for the microencapsulation of bioactive lipids, with a high yield (Yajima, 1990; Taguchi *et al.*, 1992; Lazko *et al.*, 2004; Gan *et al.*, 2008). Recently, Liao *et al.* (2012) reported the use of a cross-linked wheat gluten matrix to microencapsulate fish oil using succinic acid deamination. An additional advantage of using some proteins such as whey and soybean is that the denaturation caused by drying is able to induce thermal gelation and form cross-linking between protein coating layers to retard the oxidation of omega-3 fatty acids (Lazko *et al.*, 2004; Gan *et al.*, 2008). However, protein delivery systems also raise various concerns, particularly regarding issues of allergenicity and off-flavors resulting from protein hydrolysis and the formation of peptides with strong flavors.

6.2.5 Carbohydrate-based microencapsulation systems

Natural carbohydrates are often high molecular weight water-soluble biopolymers and have low surface activity at the o/w interface, which means they are poor at forming primary adsorbed layers in emulsion systems that include protein or surfactants. However, some carbohydrates can be used as emulsifiers even though their emulsifying properties are relatively poor. As an example, gum arabic is the mostly widely used carbohydrate emulsifier in the food industry. It is a complex blend of natural polysaccharides composed of three components: arabinogalactan-protein (about 10 wt % of total), arabinogalactan (90–99 wt % of total) and glycoprotein (about 1 wt % of total) (Phillips and Williams, 2000). Gum arabic could act as a genuine emulsifier due to the emulsifying capability of its protein-containing fractions, although its emulsifying activity is nearly one tenth that of milk protein (Dickinson, 1993). Large carbohydrates can also significantly impact solution viscosity. For example, the viscosity of the o/w emulsion stabilized by gum arabic significantly increases with increasing lipid payload or polysaccharide concentration (McNamee *et al.*, 1998; Nakauma *et al.*, 2008). Gum arabic can be an extremely effective emulsifier at low pH, at high ionic strength and in the presence of beverage coloring agents. However, the gum is expensive to use in practice because a rather high gum/oil ratio (~1:1) is required in order to prepare fine stable emulsion droplets ($d_{32} \ll 1$ μm) (McNamee *et al.*, 1998; Nakauma *et al.*, 2008).

Starch and its derivatives have also been widely used to microencapsulate unstable lipid ingredients, including omega-3 oils (Lesmes *et al.*, 2009; Zabar *et al.*, 2009, 2010). Recently, Gökmen *et al.* (2011) showed that starch encapsulated omega-3 oils can be added into breads with minimal adverse effects on the product's sensorial properties, and the coating layer was shown to retard lipid oxidation during baking, compared to controls containing non-encapsulated oils.

6.2.6 Mixed microencapsulation systems of protein and carbohydrate

Both proteins and carbohydrates have limitations when used to microencapsulate unstable oils. The use of mixed microencapsulation systems has been studied and can have advantages over single-shell material encapsulates. Carbohydrates can be incorporated to improve the drying properties of the wall matrix, by enhancing the formation of a dry outer shell around the drying droplets with protein coating layers (Sheu and Rosenberg, 1995). Meanwhile, the application of food-grade Maillard reaction products has been demonstrated to enhance the emulsion functionality. Gan *et al.* (2008) reported that the addition of ribose induced cross-linking by Maillard reaction during the drying process, which would more significantly enhance the shelf-life of the encapsulated fish oil. The Maillard reaction between a protein and carbohydrate in the shell can enhance stability and increase shell cross-links.

Complex co-acervates formed between polyanionic carbohydrates and polycationic protein could also be used to encapsulate the lipid ingredients. This process requires two oppositely charged polymers and so a combination of protein and carbohydrate materials can be applied using this method. For example, complex co-acervates of gum arabic or pectin with protein emulsifier such as gelatin and β-lactoglublin have been used for encapsulation of unstable oil ingredients (Lamprecht *et al.*, 2001; Weinbreck *et al.*, 2004). Zimet and Livney (2009) used complex co-acervation between β-lactoglublin and pectin to encapsulate DHA rich oil. The results showed that DHA degradation was significantly reduced (only 5–10 % loss) when DHA were encapsulated in β-lactoglublin-pectin co-acervates, as compared to about 80 % loss of unprotected DHA in non-encapsulated control samples.

6.3 Emulsion assemblies for omega-3 oils

The microencapsulation products for omega-3 oils could be either in liquid (emulsion) or solid (powder) state. An emulsion is a system with a smaller dispersed phase in another larger continuous phase. The omega-3 oil enriched emulsions could be added into dairy or beverage products directly, or dried into powders by different drying techniques such as spray drying and freeze drying for the further fertilization in various food matrices. The droplet size of emulsions could be in the range of nano- and micro-scales. It was demonstrated that the encapsulation of omega-3 oils into emulsion systems can significantly enhance oxidative stability (Lamprecht *et al.*, 2001; Kolanowski and Weibbrodt, 2007). Some examples of microencapsulation emulsion assemblies of omega-3 oils are shown in Table 6.2. In this section, several types of emulsion assemblies namely single- and multilayered emulsion and multiple emulsions, will be discussed, with the advantages and disadvantages of each.

6.3.1 Single-layered oil-in-water (o/w) emulsions

The single-layered o/w emulsion is also referred to as the conventional o/w emulsion. It is the simplest emulsion, with oil droplets dispersed in an aqueous continuous phase, coated by a surfactant (emulsifier) forming a thin interfacial layer (Dickinson, 1992). Generally, an o/w emulsion is prepared by emulsifying the oil phase in an aqueous continuous phase containing water-soluble emulsifier using e.g. high shear mixer, high pressure homogenizer, microfluidizer or ultrasonic homogenizer (Fig. 6.1).

The oxidative stability of omega-3 oils can be significantly improved by encapsulation into single-layered o/w emulsion-based systems, partly because interactions between the fatty acids and redox active metal ions can be minimized by controlling the interfacial charge and layer thickness (McClements and Decker, 2000). Moreover, the properties of the oil droplets in o/w emulsions can be controlled by use of the correct emulsifier. A variety of emulsifiers have been applied to the encapsulation and

Table 6.2 Several encapsulation systems utilized to encapsulate omega-3 fatty acids

Encapsulation system	Encapsulated ingredient	Shell material	Product properties	Reference
Single-layered o/w emulsion	Algal oil	Whey protein	Utilized as a direct addictive to yogurt, consumer panel could not distinguish strong fish flavor after 22 days storage	Chee *et al.* (2005)
Single-layered o/w emulsion	Tuna oil	Chitosan, maltodextrin, whey protein	Droplet size around 10 μm after 30 days storage, encapsulation efficiency > 80 %, low water activity	Klaypradit and Huang (2008)
Spray-dried single-layered o/w emulsion	Fish oil	Pectin	Droplet size < 2 μm, oxidative stability strengthened	Drusch (2007)
Spray-dried single-layered o/w emulsion	Fish oil	Barley protein	Encapsulation efficiency > 92.9 %, loading efficiency 46.5–50.1 %, omega-3 oils stable at 40 °C for 8 weeks	Wang *et al.* (2011b)
Freeze-dried single-layered o/w emulsion	Sandeel oil	Sodium caseinate, lactose, maltodextrin	Particle size < 1 μm, more oxidative stable	Heinzelmann *et al.* (2000)
Spray-dried multilayered o/w emulsion	Tuna oil	Lecithin, chitosan	Droplet size 5–30 μm, low moisture, oil retention levels > 85 %, water dispensability < 1 min, strengthened oxidative stability	Klinkesorn *et al.* (2006)
w/o/w multiple emulsion	Fish oil	Insulin, Arlatone F 127®	Excellent oxidative stability during storage at 4 °C for 6 weeks	Cournarie *et al.* (2004)

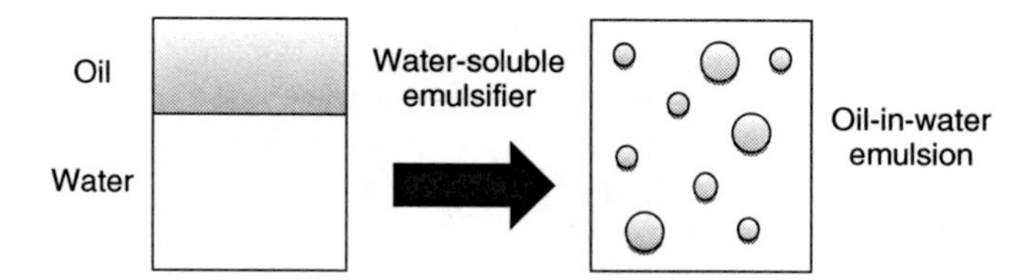

Fig. 6.1 Schematic representation of the formation of single-layered oil-in-water (o/w) emulsions.

stabilization of omega-3 oils in food products, such as milk, yogurts, ice cream and meat products (McClements and Decker, 2000; Chee *et al.*, 2005; Sharma, 2005; Lee *et al.*, 2006). In some cases, these systems provided improved oxidative stability as compared with the incorporation of omega-3 oil directly without prior emulsification (Chee *et al.*, 2005; Kolanowski and Weibbrodt, 2007).

Single-layered o/w emulsions are widely used in the modern food industry, due to ease of preparation and relatively low cost. However, there are disadvantages of single-layered o/w emulsion as a delivery system for omega-3 oils in most food products. One of these limitations is that single-layered o/w emulsions are prone to physical instability when exposed to environmental stresses such as thermal treatment, freeze/thawing, pH extremes and high mineral concentrations, resulting in the degradation of the encapsulated ingredient. A second limitation is that there are a limited number of food-grade emulsifiers that could be employed to form the interfacial layers surrounding the oil droplets while also providing some oxidative protection. It is important to continue to developed new improved emulsifier and emulsification systems (Molina *et al.*, 2001; McClements, 2004). A third limitation is that in liquid emulsion form the encapsulated material is not effectively protected from the surrounding matrix. Therefore, an emulsion that works well in one food or beverage system may work poorly in another. This means that for liquid emulsion systems in general it is necessary to optimize the emulsification system and the antioxidant protection system for each specific food or beverage product. This is a major limitation to the industrial utility of o/w liquid emulsions.

6.3.2 Multilayered o/w emulsions

Multilayered o/w emulsions are o/w emulsions with multiple emulsifier layers coating the outside of the oil droplets in a continuous aqueous phase. These are normally produced using multiple steps. For example, the double-layered o/w emulsion can be prepared using following steps: (i) a coarse o/w emulsion is firstly prepared containing a polyelectrolyte in aqueous phase at a pH where there is no strong electrostatic attraction between the droplets and the polyelectrolyte; and (ii) the pH of the coarse emulsion is

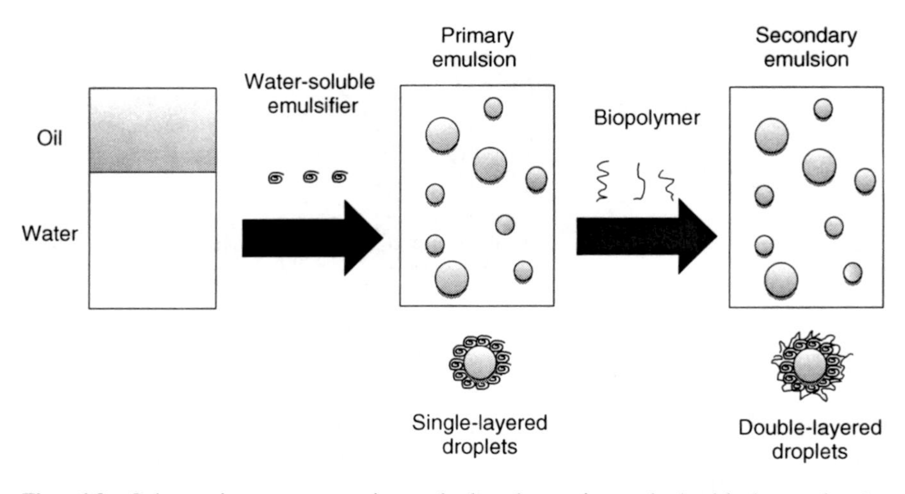

Fig. 6.2 Schematic representation of the formation of double-layered o/w emulsions.

adjusted to introduce strong electrostatic attractions between droplets and the polyelectrolyte, which leads to the adsorption of polyelectrolyte onto the droplet surface as a new coating layer. The formation of double-layered emulsions is illustrated in Fig. 6.2. The number of coating layers can be increased by adsorption of different biopolymers, repeating the same procedure.

The properties of the droplets, such as composition, surface charge, thickness and responsiveness to environmental stresses, can be optimized by the careful control of system composition and preparation conditions (Decher and Schlenoff, 2003). Compared with single-layered o/w emulsions, the oxidative stability of encapsulated omega-3 oils can be significantly improved by minimizing the interaction between the lipids and transition metals ions, by controlling the interfacial charge and thickness of the droplets (McClements and Decker, 2000). For example, multilayered o/w emulsions were reported for the encapsulation of omega-3 oils by Klinkesorn *et al.* (2005, 2006). In this study, tuna oil was encapsulated using a lecithin–chitosan double layer. Results indicated that the oxidative stability of encapsulated omega-3 oils was significantly improved, compared with single-layered emulsions.

Although the use of multilayered emulsions for the encapsulation of omega-3 oils is appealing, there are challenges to overcome for food applications. One difficulty is that there needs to be careful control of additional ingredients and procedures are relatively complex compared with single-layered o/w emulsions. Also, in multilayered o/w emulsions, droplet aggregation can occur through bridging flocculation, depletion flocculation or other effects (Guzey *et al.*, 2004; Wang *et al.*, 2011a). The oil-phase fractions must be relatively low to avoid destabilizations, which can result in relatively low payloads of bioactive ingredients.

6.3.3 Multiple emulsions

Water-in-oil-in-water ($w_1/o/w_2$) emulsions are emulsions with oil droplets (o-phase) containing smaller water droplets (w_1-phase), which are then dispersed into a larger continuous aqueous phase (w_2-phase), where w_1 and w_2 phases are the inner and outer aqueous phases, respectively. These emulsions can be prepared using the following procedure: (i) the w_1/o emulsion is prepared by emulsifying the w_1 phase in oil phase containing hydrophobic emulsifier; then (ii) the final $w_1/o/w_2$ emulsion is prepared by emulsifying the w_1/o emulsion into an aqueous phase with a water-soluble emulsifier, as illustrated in Fig. 6.3. Generally, similar equipment could be employed to prepare multiple emulsions as is used for single-layered o/w emulsions.

These $w_1/o/w_2$ emulsions are primarily employed to encapsulate hydrophilic bioactive ingredients in the inner w_1 phase, rather than hydrophobic ingredient in the intermediate oil phase. However, this method can be utilized to trap the hydrophobic ingredient as well, particularly when it is desirable to entrap both a hydrophilic bioactive ingredient and a hydrophobic one together within the same emulsion. There are a few examples of multiple emulsions containing omega-3 oils and $w_1/o/w_2$ emulsions used to encapsulate omega-3 oils were reported by Onuki *et al.* (2003) and Cournarie *et al.* (2004). Results indicated that the encapsulated fish oil

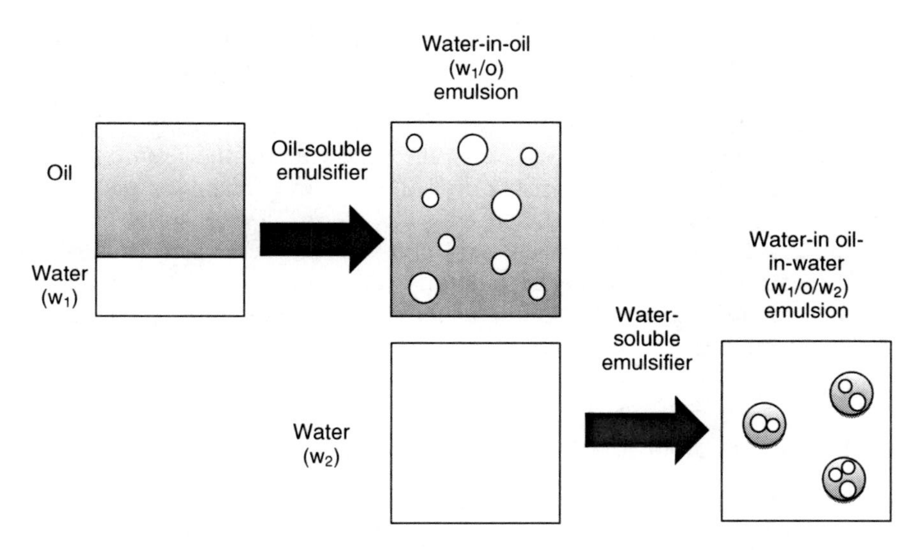

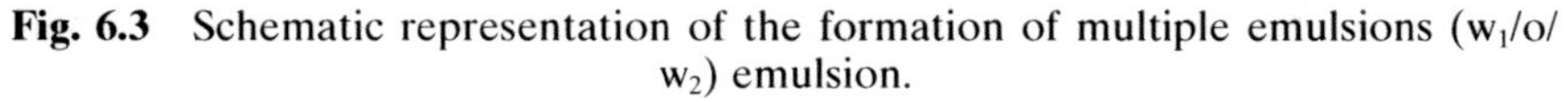

Fig. 6.3 Schematic representation of the formation of multiple emulsions ($w_1/o/w_2$) emulsion.

maintains better stability than when encapsulated in a single-layered o/w emulsion for storage at 4 °C.

Similarly, there are also $o_1/w/o_2$ emulsions, with aqueous droplets (w-phase) containing smaller oil phase (o_1-phase), dispersing in outer oil phase (o_2-phase). The preparation procedure is similar to $w_1/o/w_2$ emulsion. Cho *et al.* (2006) reported the use of an $o_1/w/o_2$ emulsion to encapsulate omega-3 oil. Results indicated that the oxidative stability of the omega-3 oil was enhanced by the cross-linking between soy protein isolate using transglutaminase. One advantage of these more complex systems for the stabilization of omega-3 oils is that they act as intermediate between simple liquid emulsions and more expensive dried powders. For example, they can help to put a stronger physical barrier between the food or beverage matrix and the unstable oil ingredient compared to conventional o/w emulsions, thereby possibly overcoming some of the need for application-specific emulsifier and antioxidant development required for simple emulsions.

Overall, for an emulsion-based encapsulation system, a stable emulsion with dispersed small oil droplets is important for a successful microencapsulation. It is therefore important to select an appropriate microencapsulation shell material as well emulsifiers. Besides spray drying and freeze drying microencapsulation techniques (i.e. spray dried- and freeze-dried emulsions, respectively), emulsification also acts as the first step in several microencapsulation techniques, including complex co-acervation, liposome entrapment and spray chilling or cooling.

6.4 Microencapsulation techniques for stabilizing omega-3 oils

There are number of techniques for microencapsulation of omega-3 oils for incorporation into food and beverage products. By the requirements of emulsification before encapsulation, the methods could be classified into emulsification-based (e.g. spray drying, freeze drying, spray cooling or chilling, liposome entrapment and complex co-acervation) and non-emulsification-based microencapsulation techniques (e.g. fluidized-bed coating, extrusion-based techniques, supercritical fluid-based techniques). These techniques will be described below.

6.4.1 Emulsification-based microencapsulation techniques

Microencapsulation using spray drying (spray-dried emulsions)

Spray drying is one of the oldest and the most widely used encapsulation techniques in the food industry, and it has also been applied commercially in the stabilization of omega-3 oil for food and infant formula.

The fine powder prepared by spray drying is in the size range 10–50 μm (Gharsallaoui *et al.*, 2007; Nedovic *et al.*, 2011), hence the spray-dried micro-encapsulated powder could be added into food matrices without significantly changing their mouthfeel. Until now, spray drying has been the mostly widely used microencapsulation technique used in the modern food industry; around 80–90 % of encapsulates in the modern food industry are spray-dried ones (Porzio, 2007).

The structure of spray-dried microcapsules usually comprises an active core ingredient entrapped in a protective polymer or matrix. The first step of the process is to emulsify the core ingredient in concentrated shell dispersion until 1–3 μm or smaller oil droplets are formed. Different emulsion systems, such as single- or multilayered o/w emulsions, have been employed to entrap and encapsulate omega-3 oils. For spray-dried emulsions, the spray drying step is particularly important since the particles form in the spray drier. Therefore, spray drying controls the particle size. Although spray drying appears relatively harsh, with inlet temperatures as high as 200–300 °C, the rapid evaporation of water from the coating keeps the encapsulated core far below these temperatures, and so flow rate and duration of exposure of the individual particles to drying are particularly important.

There are several advantages for the microencapsulation of bioactive ingredients using spray drying. The process is economical, flexible and uses readily available equipment to prepare microencapsulated powder from gram to multiple tonne scale. A key advantage is that shell material composition is flexible since a large range of protein and carbohydrate materials can form shells during spray drying. However, there are also some disadvantages. These are primarily that the process can vary greatly from one spray drier to another. Also, particle size can be difficult to control and problems can be caused by non-uniform conditions in the drying chamber (Nedovic *et al.*, 2011). The loading of encapsulated ingredient (payload) can be relatively low in spray-dried emulsions, usually around 20–30 %, but up to 50 % is possible, and surface oil content can be relatively high, which can lead to sensory problems for the microencapsulation of omega-3 oils using this method.

Microencapsulation using freeze drying (freeze-dried emulsions)

Freeze drying can be utilized for drying of sensitive ingredients, since it is a mild drying method that occurs at low temperature. Therefore, it can be a useful method for the preparation of products containing omega-3 oils (Heinzelmann *et al.*, 2000). However, the commercial cost of freeze drying is much higher than spray drying and related methods, so it is mainly employed to dry very high value ingredients such as probiotic bacteria. The powders produced by freeze drying also tend to have a more porous structure than spray-dried ones, which can decrease stability and increase the cost of transportation and storage. In addition, drying times are often very long and the method is difficult to scale to multi-tonne levels, limiting the utilization of freeze drying in the modern food industry.

Microencapsulation using spray cooling and chilling

The processes of spray cooling and chilling are similar to spray drying, since they involve an emulsification of the encapsulated core ingredient in a dissolved shell material, followed by spraying the emulsion out from nozzles. The primary differences are the temperature in the cooling chamber and the type of shell material. In spray cooling and chilling, high melting fats are usually used as the shell material. During cooling in the cool air, the fat layer will solidify and the core ingredient is immobilized inside the hardened shell.

A large amount of water-soluble bioactive ingredients, such as flavors, food acids, vitamins, enzymes or mineral salts, have been encapsulated into solid fat particles by spray cooling or chilling. These microcapsules are insoluble in water due to the lipid coatings. This method has been used for omega-3 oils encapsulation but has not been particularly successful. This is partially because the shell material can dissolve during food processing and also because dispersion in a beverage is difficult due to the highly hydrophobic natural of the shell material. Microencapsulated omega-3 oils formed using other methods, such as spray-drying or complex co-acervation, can be further coated using spray cooling. In this manner, a protein-based encapsulate can be coated with a fat layer. However, if the coating is not a complete water barrier then the microcapsules can burst as the inner protein shell expands in aqueous food or beverage products. The advantage of an additional fat coating is primarily to improve the oxygen barrier and so in dry food products, and particularly in powdered products such as protein supplement powders, this additional coating can provide a storage advantage.

Microencapsulation using liposome entrapment

Liposome-based microencapsulation techniques have been used primarily in pharmaceutical applications to achieve targeted delivery or controlled release of an encapsulated ingredient. However, in recent years this technology has evolved for use in the microencapsulation of biologically active and unstable ingredients for food industry (Gregoriadis, 1987; Kim and Baianu, 1991; Kubo *et al.*, 2003). Phospholipids are primarily used as the encapsulating agent in liposome-based microencapsulation. Once mixed with water under low shear, phospholipids arrange themselves into sheets, with the hydrophilic heads upwards and hydrophobic tails downwards. By the joining of the tails, a bilayer membrane with some aqueous phase entrapped in it can be formed, as shown in Fig. 6.4. Both water-soluble and lipid ingredients can be encapsulated at the same time. The water-soluble ingredients are entrapped within the droplets, while the wall material can hold the lipid ingredients. Large unilamellar vesicles (LUV) are used in the

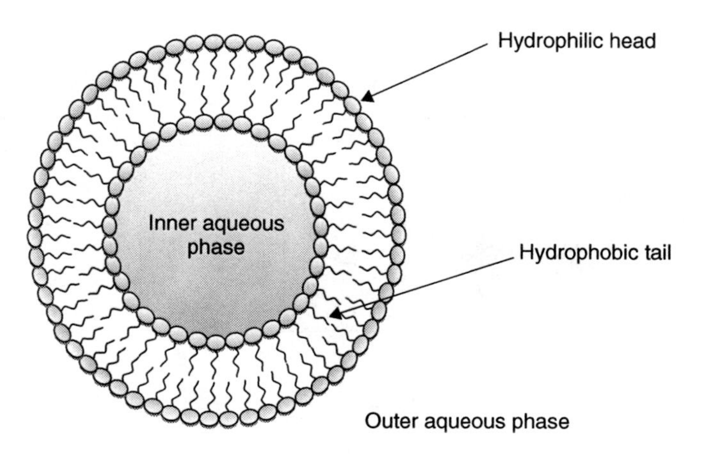

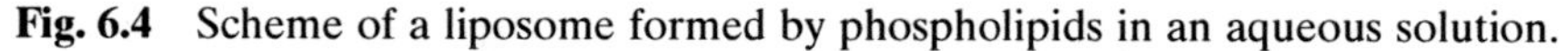
Fig. 6.4 Scheme of a liposome formed by phospholipids in an aqueous solution.

food industry, primarily due to their high encapsulation efficiency, ease of preparation and relatively good stability.

The main advantage of liposome microencapsulation systems over other microencapsulation systems is that the encapsulated ingredients within micro-capsules exhibit much higher water activity, as compared with other microencapsulation systems such as spray drying, extrusion and fluidized bed drying. Microencapsulating DHA rich oils using liposome systems can protect this unsaturated fatty acid from peroxidation (Kubo *et al.*, 2003). Another beneficial property of liposomes is that they can be targeted to specific locations within food products (Fresta and Puglisi, 1999; Lee *et al.*, 2000). Meanwhile, it has been demonstrated that the hydrophobic components could be incorporated more efficiently into the lipid membranes (Kulkarni and Vargha-Butler, 1995). For example, in the study by Marsanasco *et al.* (2011), the lipid-soluble vitamin E was encapsulated by liposomal systems at 50 mM with high encapsulation efficiency around 99 %. However, the high commercial cost and sometimes low physicochemical stability improvements result in limited application of this technology in the stabilization of omega-3 oils for food purposes.

Microencapsulation using complex co-acervation

Co-acervation, first developed in the 1950s to produce a two-component ink system for carbonless copy paper, is now promoted in modern industry for microencapsulation of bioactive ingredients. Complex co-acervation can be employed to microencapsulate a variety of liquid ingredients, including omega-3 oils. Protein–polysaccharides and protein–polyphosphate complex co-acervates are often used for the microencapsulation and delivery of omega-3 oils into a variety of food and beverage products. Examples of complex co-acervate systems include gelatin–gum arabic, β-lactoglobulin–pectin, whey protein–carrageenan and gelatin–sodium hexametaphosphate

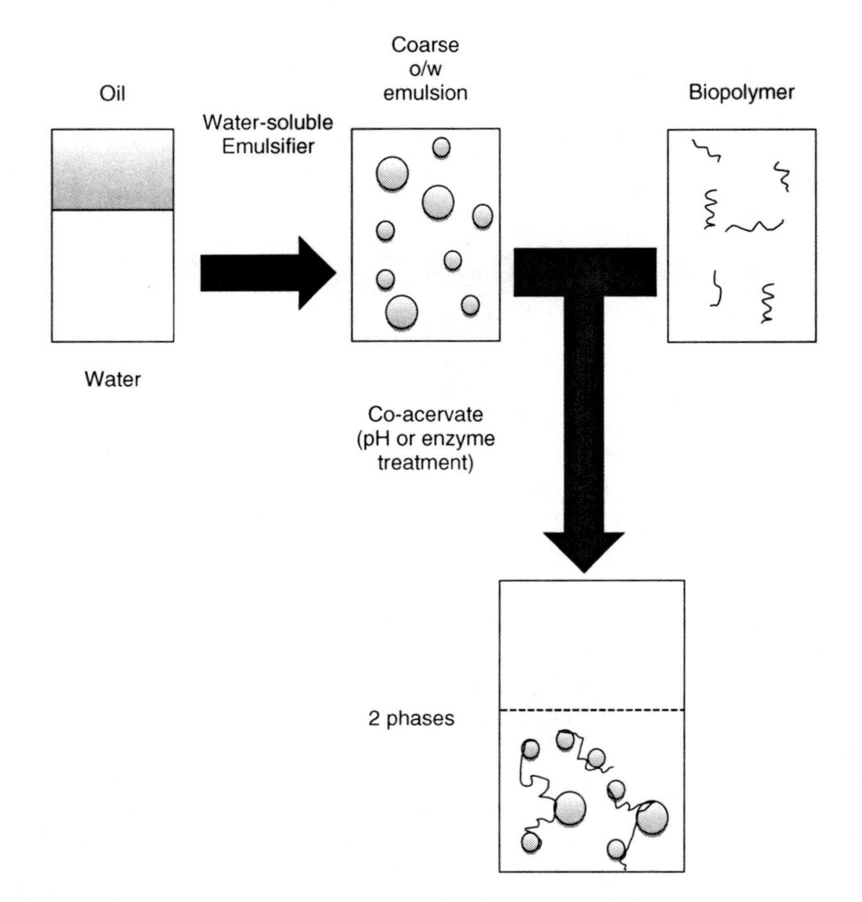

Fig. 6.5 Schematic representation of the formation of hydrogel particles by complex co-acervation.

(Fogle and Hörger, 1972; Burgess and Carless, 1984; Kazmierski *et al.*, 2003; Weinbreck *et al.*, 2004; Barrow *et al.*, 2007). Commonly, drying techniques such as spray drying were employed to dry the complex co-acervates-enriched system for final products (Barrow *et al.*, 2007; Bao *et al.*, 2011).

The formation of complex co-acervates is illustrated in Fig. 6.5. As shown in the figure, in the first process step, a coarse o/w emulsion is prepared by emulsifying the oil phase in an aqueous continuous phase containing the water-soluble emulsifier. The properties of the droplets, such as droplet size, surface charge and layer thickness, can be optimized through the selection of appropriate emulsifiers. In some cases, the protein itself can act as the emulsifier. The complex co-acervates are produced by mixing this coarse o/w emulsion with an appropriate biopolymer solution and adjusting the pH and temperature conditions to promote complex co-acervation. For example, if there are two biopolymers that have sufficiently electrostatic attractive forces between them in aqueous solution, the solution will separate into two different phases, a phase rich in both polymers and the other phase depleted in both polymers. Then the biopolymer-rich phase can either be a co-acervate or a precipitate, depending on the strength of the electrostatic attraction and the charge density of the two biopolymers. Meanwhile, several methods could be employed to enhance the stability of the microcapsules, including shell-hardening by washing with organic solvent and cross-linking by thermal or enzymatic methods (Lamprecht *et al.*, 2001; Barrow *et al.*, 2007; Bao *et al.*, 2011).

Lamprecht *et al.* (2001) prepared omega-3 enriched microcapsules using complex co-acervation with gelatin and gum acacia. In their study, besides the optimization of preparation parameters, the effects of shell-hardening and cross-linking were also studied. This work indicated that omega-3 fatty acids encapsulated in microcapsules with shell-hardened by ethanol-washing exhibited the most improved oxidative stability, followed by the microcapsules prepared by spray drying and cross-linking by dehydroascorbic acid.

Complex co-acervates also tend to form particles with good stability after cross-linking, and have been used successfully to microencapsulate omega-3 oil. Two types of complex co-acervates are used for the microencapsulation of omega-3 oil. The first is referred to as 'single-core' complex co-acervation. This is the traditional method whereby oil droplets are encapsulated with a single shell, so that each particle contains primarily one oil droplet. During complex co-acervation, particle aggregation is normally minimized through process optimization. However, a more recent form of complex co-acervation involves enhancing the particle aggregation process to form 'multi-core' complex co-acervates (Barrow *et al.*, 2007).

The multi-core method of complex co-acervation (Barrow *et al.*, 2007) involves initially dissolving the two polymers, gelatin and polyphosphate, in water at a pH where they have the same charge. This is a pH above the pI of gelatin so that it has a negative charge. The solution is homogenized to form an o/w emulsion with oil droplet size of around 1–5 μm. Gelatin acts as the emulsifier in this system. The pH is adjusted to promote complex co-acervation of gelatin and polyphosphate, which leads to the formation of essentially single-core microcapsules of approximately 5 μm average particle size. In a single pot reaction, these complex coacervates are allowed to aggregate and the aggregation is halted when the particle size reaches about 30 μm average size. The temperature is then adjusted to enable further co-acervate deposition around the aggregated agglomerations, so that a relatively thick outer shell forms. Transglutaminase is then employed to induce the cross-linking between lysines and glutamines within the gelatin so that the complex co-acervates do not redissolve. The resulting particles are very low in surface oil, probably because any residue oil sticks to the surface of the initially formed hydrophobic single-core particles before agglomeration, so that after encapsulation of the agglomerates very little oil is present to stick to the outer surface after spray drying. This low level of outer oil is a key reason why the sensory performance of these microcapsules is particularly good in a range of food products. Also contributing to the good sensory performance of these microcapsules is the fact that the outer shell is relatively thick, since it is formed as a subsequent step to initial complex co-acervation and agglomeration. The thickness of the outer shell is an important parameter for preventing oxygen from penetrating into the particles. The ability to form an outer shell as a secondary step to agglomeration also enables a relatively high payload of oil to be achieved. This is normally around 60 % but can be as high as 80 % in some food applications. A higher payload means a significantly reduced manufacturing cost, since less shell material and processing time are required per gram of oil delivered (Barrow *et al.*, 2007). Barrow *et al.* (2009) also studied the bioavailability of this gelatin–polyphosphate-based fish oil powder, which suggested that there was no difference in effect between the fish oil capsules and the microencapsulated fish oil powder.

A major advantage of the use of complex co-acervation for the microencapsulation of omega-3 oils is that the oil payload can be extremely high, up to 80 %, and the particle size can be small, well below 50 μm. Also, the thickness of the outer shell can be higher using complex co-acervation than using other methods, leading to improved sensory stability. However, there are some limitations to the utilization of complex co-acervation for the encapsulation of unstable food ingredients such as omega-3 oils. One disadvantage is that the process can be difficult to carry out since there is a narrow pH range and ionic strength range where the co-acervates are stable (Turgeon *et al.*, 2007; Bedie *et al.*, 2008). To stabilize the co-acervates it is necessary to cross-link soon after co-acervate formation to prevent dissociation. Gluteraldehyde or transglutaminase can be used to induce cross-linking between gelatin-based co-acervates (Strauss and Gibson, 2004; Barrow *et al.*, 2007). Transglutaminase is the most commonly used cross-linking method in the food industry, since it is the most acceptable cross-linking agent for food products. Dickinson (2008) reported that the linkage between the terminal or side-chain amine groups on a protein molecule with the reducing end of a glucosidic chain (monosaccharide, oligosaccharide or polysaccharide) would significantly enhance the stability of co-acervates. Cross-linking methods applied to inhibit the reversibility of complex co-acervation taking advantage of this strategy include the Maillard reaction between protein and polysaccharides and the use of polyphenolics to cross-link protein. Neither of these methods has been applied commercially. Complex co-acervation is so far the most successful method to microencapsulate omega-3 oils for stabilization and delivery into food and beverage products. The advantage of high payload and enhanced oxidative stability of omega-3 oils, compared to other methods, outweighs the shell material limitations for most commercial applications.

6.4.2 Non-emulsification-based microencapsulation techniques

Microencapsulation using fluidized-bed coating
Fluidized bed coating is used to coat solid particles. It was developed in the 1950s primarily for the pharmaceutical industry (Dewettinck and Huyghebaert, 1999). The solid core particles are suspended in air and the shell material is sprayed onto these particles to form an outer coating. A range of shell materials, such as fat, carbohydrates, emulsifiers or proteins, can be used in this process. In the nutritional supplement and food ingredient area, this methods is used for coating unstable solid ingredients such as vitamin C (Dezarn, 1995). It could potentially be employed to give an additional coating to microencapsulated omega-3 fatty acids particles, rather than for encapsulating oil droplets directly. This method has not been shown to be appropriate for the direct microencapsulation of omega-3 oils.

Microencapsulation using extrusion-based techniques
Co-extrusion and spinning disk are extrusion-based encapsulation techniques which have potential utilization in the microencapsulation of omega-3 oils. Co-extrusion begins with extruding a heated aqueous polymer solution through an outer tube and the oil to be encapsulated through an inner tube into a moving stream of a carrier fluid. One advantage of the co-extrusion over spray drying is that the core and shell can be miscible to avoid possible coalescence between them. In spinning disk processing, the encapsulation matrix passed over a rotating disk to form microparticles by centrifugal force. Finally, chilling or drying techniques are normally employed to solidify the microparticles.

The particle size of the microcapsules prepared by co-extrusion and rotating disk is 150–2000 μm and 30 μm to 2 mm, respectively (Shahidi and Han, 1993). Because particles with a size larger than 100 μm tend to change the texture and mouthfeel of food (Truelstrup-Hansen *et al.*, 2002), extrusion-based techniques have not been applied successfully to the microencapsulation of omega-3 oils for addition to food products.

Microencapsulation using supercritical fluid based techniques
Supercritical fluids could also be used for the microencapsulation of food ingredients because of their unique physical properties. The core ingredients are dispersed in shell material that is already solubilized in a supercritical fluid such as carbon dioxide. Appropriate evaporation of the supercritical fluid results in the formation of a coated particle. In rapid expansion of supercritical solutions (RESS), microencapsulation takes place when the pressurized supercritical solvent containing the coating material and the active ingredient is released through a small orifice. An abrupt pressure drop causes desolvation of the shell material and the formation of a coating layer around the active ingredient. The thickness of the shell layer formed using supercritical fluid-based encapsulation is between 100 μm and a monomolecular layer. There are literature and patents reporting the

Table 6.3 Summary of the characteristics of the techniques for microencapsulation

Encapsulation technique	Particle size	Payload (%)	Surface oil	Bioavailability
Simple coacervation	20–200 μm	<60	Lower	High
Complex co-acervation	5–200 μm	70–90	Lowest	High
Spray drying	1–50 μm	<40	High	Medium
Freeze drying	1–100 μm	<40	High	Medium
Liposome entrapment	0.1–1 μm	Low	NA	High
Spray chilling or cooling*	20–200 μm	10–20	NA	NA
Extrusion-based technique*	15–2000 μm	6–20	Low	NA
Fluidized bed coating*	>100 μm	60–90	NA	High
Supercritical fluid technique*	Monomolecular layer –100 μm	NA	NA	NA

*Indicates the technique has not been successfully applied in microencapsulation of omega-3 oils.
Sources: Madene *et al.*, 2006; Gouin, 2004.

microencapsulation of ingredients including vitamin C, xylitol and potassium chloride using various shell materials. This method has not been widely applied to the microencapsulation of omega-3 oils, but has some potential in this regard (Benoit *et al.*, 1996; Richard *et al.*, 1998).

Overall, the mostly widely commercialized microencapsulation techniques are spray drying and complex co-acervation. Table 6.3 gives a summary of the characteristics of the techniques and assemblies discussed, and their commercial industrialization characteristics are shown in Fig. 6.6 (Desobry *et al.*, 1997; Gouin, 2004; Madene *et al.*, 2006).

6.5 Characteristics and analysis of microencapsulated omega-3 oil products

After the preparation of microcapsules, it is important to be able to characterize them both physically and in terms of their performance in food and beverage products. First, all ingredients used must be food grade. Not only should the ingredients be permitted in food, but food companies and consumers prefer that all materials are natural food ingredients, rather than synthetic products. Not only does this limit the range of materials that can be used, it can also complicates the analysis since multiple complex natural products are often used, rather than synthetic single ingredients.

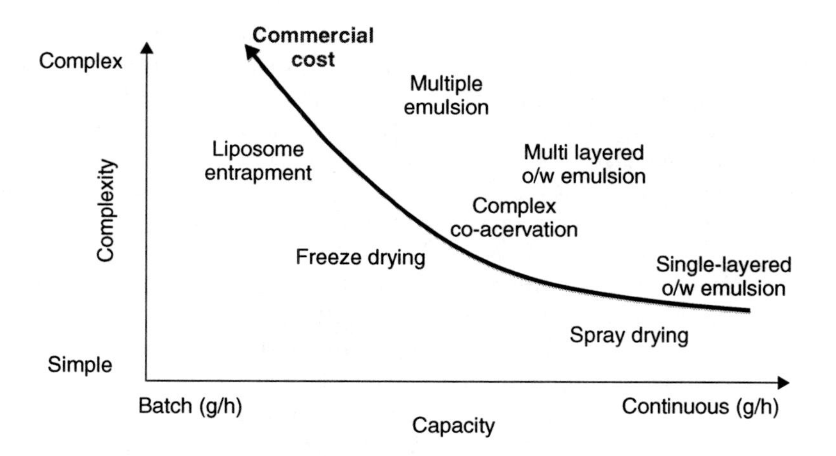

Fig. 6.6 Summary of industrialization characters of different microencapsulation techniques and assemblies for omega-3 oils.

Characterization of the microcapsule properties includes characteristics such as particle size, oil payload, surface oil levels and physical stability. Characterization of the microcapsule performance includes, in particular, sensory performance in food and beverage products, such as sensory shelf-life. But performance also includes bioavailability and physical performance in a food or beverage products, such as a low level of physical breakdown during extrusion, cooking or homogenization processes. Some of these characteristics and methods for evaluating microcapsules are discussed below.

Droplet and particle size: The particle size of microcapsules used in food should be below 100 μm to avoid the mouth detection of 'grittiness' or alteration in food texture (Truelstrup-Hansen *et al.*, 2002). Also the particle size distribution should be narrow to control the properties and consistency of the microcapsules. The particle size and thickness of shell material can be determined using an optical microscope. During the emulsification process, the droplet size can be determined using light-scattering techniques. Droplet size is an important parameter that should be measured early to indicate and optimize the effect of emulsifying parameters such as processing circle, homogenization pressure or emulsifier concentration. In the case of multicore structures, it is this droplet size that primarily defines the inner particle sizes. High-resolution imaging microscopes, e.g. for scanning electron microscopy (SEM) can also be utilized to determine the particle size (Gökmen *et al.*, 2011; Rodea-González *et al.*, 2012), but are more useful for examining the particle surface. Confocal laser scanning microscopy (CLSM) is very effective to determine various domains inside the microcapsules, such as oil–protein interfaces (Lamprecht *et al.*, 2001).

Oxidative stability of encapsulated lipid: The primary purpose of the microencapsulation is to stabilize the internally trapped oil against oxidative degradation. The physical barrier is important, since it can help prevent contact with oxygen, transition metal ions and light. The oxygen barrier in particular is a key parameter and primarily varies with shell thickness and shell material. The primary methods for examining microencapsulated powder oxidative stability include: (i) extraction of oil from powder and applying standard oil methods such as acid value, peroxide value and anisidine value; (ii) head-space analysis, or water extraction followed by gas chromatography (GC) analysis, of the volatiles from the powder directly; (iii) accelerated analysis using a Rancimat or Oxypress (Kralovec *et al.*, 2012). All three methods have been used with success, but each has drawbacks. For example: (i) extraction of encapsulated lipids out of microcapsules is a complicated procedure; (ii) the standard methods such as peroxide value are highly sensitive to the experimental conditions, and to assess whether a lipid is in the growth or decay phase of the hydroperoxide formation it is necessary to determine the amount of hydroperoxides as function of time (Shahidi and Wanasundara, 2002); (iii) the oxygen methods, such as head space analysis are limited because the oxidation of possible protein fraction also uses up oxygen (Melton, 1983); and (iv) there is still concern that the results of accelerated tests do not adequately model real lipid oxidation. Hence it is normally important to use a combination of these methods to determine oxidative stability of a microencapsulation system.

Surface oil: The surface oil, also named free oil, is the amount of non-encapsulated oil which is adsorbed onto the surface of the final product. Surface oil tends to be oxidized or degraded relatively easily and so high amounts of free oil lead to off-flavors and odors in the powder or food where the powder is incorporated. Typically, surface oil should be below 0.1 % (w/w) to result in a product with good sensory properties. However, surface oil is normally measured as solvent extractable oil, which can significantly over-estimate the amount on the surface, since oil close to the surface can also be extracted. The surface oil of the powder product is normally extracted by washing with organic solvent such as hexane, ethyl acetate or methanol, and quantification by weighing the collected lipid after drying, or using quantitative spectroscopic methods like UV-VIS or IR spectroscopy. Alternatively, surface oil can be measured through specific quantitative staining, although this has not been accomplished successfully for fish oil.

Payload: Payload represents the percentage of lipid bioactive ingredient per gram of the powder and affects both cost per active dose delivered and amount of powder added per serving of food. A higher payload indicates less coating material is required to deliver a specific dosage of encapsulated ingredients, so both cost and impact on food are minimized. Payload can be calculated by the equation $PL = M_E/M_p$ where PL stands for payload, M_E and M_T stand for the mass of the encapsulated ingredient and the total mass of the products, individually. Ideally, an encapsulation system should have as high a payload as possible. Similarly, there are other factors named loading capacity and loading efficiency that can be measured. Loading capacity is a measure of the mass of encapsulated ingredient per unit mass of the coating material, and loading efficiency is the ability of the encapsulated system to retain the encapsulated ingredient over time. The following equations can be applied: $LC = M_E/M_C$ and $LE = M_E(t)/M_E(0)*100$, where LC stands for loading capacity, LE stands for the loading efficiency, M_E and M_C stand for mass of the encapsulated ingredient and the coating material, respectively, $M_E(t)$ and $M_E(0)$ are the mass of encapsulated ingredients at time t and time 0, respectively. The LC and LE should be as high as possible for an ideal encapsulation product.

Payload can be measured gravimetrically by quantitative extraction of the oil from a known amount of microcapsules, followed by weighting of the oil. For greatest accuracy, water content should be determined using a moisture balance before extraction of oil. Nondestructive methods to determine payload have recently been developed, including the use of Fourier transform infrared (FTIR) spectroscopy (Vongsvivut *et al.*, 2012).

Sensory analysis: It is very important to evaluate the sensory properties of an encapsulating powder, since the sensory characteristics of foods will ultimately dictate their acceptability for specific applications. A large amount of sensory testing of omega-3 fatty acid fortified food products has taken place. For example, in the study of Chee *et al.* (2005), the trained panel could distinguish a strong fishy flavor in the omega-3 oils fertilized yogurt after 22 days storage. However, the consumer panel regarded it as similar to the control ones and exhibited 'moderately like'. Similarly, the sensory analysis of fish oil enriched energy bar and pâté were also studied by Nielsen and Jacobsen (2009, 2012). It was concluded that the off-flavor could be a barrier for enrichment of fish oil in these food products, but it is still possible to obtain a pâté product with good sensory properties and acceptable shelf life of eight weeks.

Although a trained sensory panel is the best way to evaluate the sensory impact of the microencapsulated powder over time on a food product, the sensory stability of the powder itself can also be measured (Serfert *et al.*, 2010). One method is again to develop a trained sensory panel that become familiar with tasting the powders that can be tasted in water, in a bland product such as gelatin, or as a dry powder. Sandgruber and Buettner (2012) developed a quantitative sensory evaluation method by means of high resolution gas chromatography–olfactometry (HRGC–O). Although it has met with some successes, in general, human sensory testing needs to be used in conjunction with analytical methods.

Bioavailability: An encapsulation system should enhance or at least not decrease the bioavailability of the encapsulated ingredient. Higgins *et al.* (1999) showed that there was no difference between the bioavailability of omega-3 fatty acids given as microencapsulated fish oil in milkshake, and that delivered as fish oil capsule. Similarly, Barrow *et al.* (2009) compared the bioavailability of microencapsulated omega-3 oils by complex coacervation with standard fish-oil soft-gel capsules through a double-blind cross-over study in 14 male subjects. The results indicated that serum phospholipid levels of long-chain omega-3 fatty acids increased equivalently in both subjects groups. The bioequivalence between microencapsulated omega-3 fatty acids in a food matrix are those in a fish-oil capsule indicated that the fortification of foodstuff with microencapsulated omega-3 fatty acids could offer the potential to increase intakes of omega-3 fatty acids with current recommendations. In general, protein shell materials are likely to be digested and therefore will provide high bioavailability. In most cases, this is also true for polysaccharide and fat coatings, with the exception of indigestible shell materials such as chitin, where bioavailability testing is particularly important.

6.6 Conclusion and future trends

Microencapsulation of omega-3 oils is technically and commercially viable for the delivery of these oils into a range of food and beverage products with minimal or no impact on the shelf-life and sensory properties of the product. There are already a large amount of functional foods fortified with omega-3 oils launched worldwide. A variety of microencapsulation techniques and systems are currently utilized, although the most successful in terms of use in a broad range of foods are complex co-acervation and spray-dried emulsion technologies. Several key properties are important for testing the quality of the microcapsule products. Payload, sensory, oxidative stability and bioavailability analysis are all required to fully test a microencapsulated ingredient. The shelf-life of microencapsulated omega-3 oil as an ingredient within the food product should be equal to or longer than the shelf-life of the food matrix itself. Payload should be as high as possible and all the ingredients used should be food grade and allowable in food for the purpose used.

This chapter has briefly reviewed various types of emulsion assemblies, namely single- and multilayered o/w emulsion and multiple emulsion for encapsulation of omega-3 oils. These liquid emulsion-based assemblies have the advantage of lower costs than powder products and are particularly applicable to direct applications that have high water content, such as milk and margarine. Emulsification also acts as the first step in different microencapsulation techniques, including spraying drying, freeze drying and complex co-acervation. Generally, liquid emulsions need to be tailored to specific applications and food formulations, and are generally less stabilizing than microencapsulated powders.

Different microencapsulation techniques for omega-3 oils were also overviewed. Spray drying and complex co-acervation are two widely commercialized techniques for microencapsulation of this bioactive lipid. Spray-dried powders in general have the advantage of low cost and high flexibility in choice of shell material. Limitations include moderate payload and relatively high surface oil. Complex co-acervation provides a relatively low cost, particularly when high payloads are taken into account. However, the primary disadvantage of complex co-acervation is the limited choice of shell materials available for successful microencapsulation.

Because of the well-reported health benefits of omega-3 fatty acids, the omega-3 functional food market is predicted to continue to expand. Although current technologies are quite good, lower cost methods and application-specific methods will continue to be developed. Also, there is still a need for increased stability of these powders, to further broaden the food application range possible for delivery of omega-3 oils, particularly in long shelf-life multi-serve dry food products such as cereal, where further improvements in both cost and stability are required.

6.7 References

AMBRING, A., JOHANSSON, M., AXELSEN, M., GAN, L. M., STRANDVIK, B. and FRIEBERG, P. (2006) Mediterranean-inspired diet lowers the ratio of serum phospholipids n–6 to n–3 fatty acids, the number of leukocytes and platelets and vascular endothelial growth factor in healthy subjects. *American Journal of Clinical Nutrition*, 83, 575–581.

AMMINGER, G. P., SCHÄFER, M., PAPAGEORGIOU, K., KLIER, C. M., COTTON, S. M., HARRIGAN, S. M., MACKINNON, A., MCGORRY, P. D. and BERGER, G. E. (2010) Long-chain ω-3 fatty acids for indicated prevention of psychotic disorders. *Archives of General Psychiatry*, 67, 146–154.

BANG, H. P. and DYERBERG, J. (1973) The composition of food consumed by Greenlandic Eskimos. *Acta Medica Scandinavica*, 200, 69–73.

BAO, S. S., HU, X., C., ZHANG, K., XU, X. K., ZHANG, H. M. and HUANG, H. (2011) Characterization of spray-dried microalgal oil encapsulated in cross-linked sodium caseinate matrix induced by microbial transglutaminase. *Journal of Food Science*, 76, E112–E118.

BARROW, C. J., NOLAN, C. and JIN, Y. L. (2007) Stabilization of highly unsaturated fatty acids and delivery into foods. *Lipid Technology*, 19, 108–111.

BARROW, C. J., NOLAN, C. and HOLUB, B. J. (2009) Bioequivalence of encapsulated and microencapsulated fish-oil supplementation. *Journal of Functional Food*, 1, 38–43.

BEDIE, G. K., TURGEON, S. L. and MAKHLOUF, J. (2008) Formation of native whey protein isolate-low methoxyl pectin complexes as a matrix for hydro-soluble food ingredient entrapment in acidic foods. *Food Hydrocolloids*, 22, 836–844.

BENOIT, J. P., ROLLAND, H., THIES, C. and VANDEVELDE, V. (1996) *Method of coating particles*. EP 0706821.

BORNEO, R., KOCER, D., GHAI, G., TEPPER, B. J. and KARWE, M. V. (2007) Stability and consumer acceptance of long-chain omega-3 fatty acids (eicosapentaenoic acid, 25:5, n-3) in cream-filled sandwich cookies. *Journal of Food Science*, 72, S50–S54.

BULLUZZI, A., BRIGNOLA, C., CAMPIERI, M., PERA, A., BOSCHI, S. and MIGLIOLI, M. (1996) Effect of an enteric-coated fish-oil preparation on relapses in Crohn's disease. *New England Journal of Medicine*, 334, 1557–1560.

BURGESS, D. J. and CARLESS, J. E. (1984) Microelectrophoretic study of gelatin and acacia for the prediction of complex coacervation. *Journal of Colloid Interface Science*, 98, 1–8.

CHANG, P. S. (1997) Microencapsulation and oxidative stability of docosahexaenoic acid, in SHAHIDI, F. and CADWALLADER, K. (eds), *Flavor and Lipid Chemistry of Seafoods.* Washington, DC: American Chemical Society, 264–273.

CHEE, C. P., GALLAHER, J. J., DJORDJEVIC, D., FARAJI, H., MCCLEMENTS, D. J., DECKER, E. A., HOLLENDER, R., PETERSON, D. G., ROBERTS, R. F. and COUPLAND, J. N. (2005) Chemical and sensory analysis of strawberry flavored yogurt supplemented with an algae oil emulsion. *Journal of Dairy Research*, 72, 311–316.

CHEN, J. and DICKINSON, E. (1995) Protein/surfactant interactions. Part 3. Competitive adsorption of protein+surfactant in emulsions. *Colloids and Surface Science A: Physicochemical and Engineering Aspects*, 101, 77–85.

CHEN, L. Y., REMONDETTO, G. E. and SUBIRADE, M. (2006) Food protein-based materials as nutraceutical delivery systems. *Trends Food Science and Technologies*, 17, 272–283.

CHO, Y. H., SHIM, H. K. and PARK, J. (2006) Encapsulation of fish oil by an enzymatic gelation process using transglutaminase cross-linked proteins. *Journal of Food Science*, 68, 2717–2723.

COURNARIE, F., SAVELLI, M. P., ROSILIO, W., BRETEZ, F., VAUTHIER, C., GROSSIORD, J. L. and SEILLER, M. (2004) Insulin-loaded w/o/w multiple emulsions: comparison of the performances of systems prepared with medium-chain-triglycerides and fish oil. *European Journal of Pharmaceutics and Biopharmaceutics*, 58, 477–482.

DAMSGAARD, C. T., LAURITZEN, L., KJÆR, T. M. R., HOLM, P. K. I., FRUEKILDE, M. B., MICHAELSEN, K. F. and FRØKIÆR, H. (2007) Fish oil supplementation modulates immune function in health infants. *Journal of Nutrition*, 137, 1031–1036.

DE DECKERE, E. A. (1999) Possible beneficial effects of fish and fish n-3 polyunsaturated fatty acids in breast and colorectal cancer. *European Journal of Cancer Prevention*, 8, 213–221.

DECHER, G. and SCHLENOFF, J. B. (2003) *Multilayer Thin Films: Sequential Assembly of Nanocomposite Materials*. Weinheim: Wiley-VCH.

DESOBRY, S. A., NETTO, F. M. and LABUZA, T. P. (1997) Comparison of spray-drying, drum-drying and freeze-drying for β-carotene encapsulation and preservation. *Journal of Food Science*, 62, 1158–1162.

DEWETTINCK, K. and HUYGHEBAERT, A. (1999) Fluidized bed coating in food technology. *Trends in Food Science & Technology*, 10, 163–168.

DEZARN, T. J. (1995) Food ingredient encapsulation, in RISCH, S. J. and REINECCIUS, G. A. (eds.) *Encapsulation and Controlled Release of Food Ingredients.* Washington DC: American Chemical Society, 74–86.

DICKINSON, E. (1992) *An Introduction to Food Colloids*. Oxford: Oxford Science Publishers.

DICKINSON, E. (1993) Towards more natural emulsifiers. *Trends in Food Science & Technology*, 4, 330–334.

DICKINSON, E. (2008) Interfacial structure and stability of food emulsions as affected by protein-polysaccharide interactions. *Soft Matter*, 4, 932–942.

DRUSCH, S. (2007) Sugar beet pectin: A novel emulsifying wall component for microencapsulation of lipophilic good ingredients by spray-drying. *Food Hydrocolloids*, 21, 1223–1228.

FOGLE, M. V. and HÖRGER, G. (1972) *Encapsulation process by complex coacervation using inorganic polyphosphates and organic hydrophilic polymeric material.* US Patent 3, 697, 437.

FRANCOIS, C. A., CONNOR, S. L., BOLEWICZ, L. C. and CONNOR, W. E. (2003) Supplementing lactating women with flaxseed oil does not increase docosahexaenoic acid in their milk. *American Journal of Clinical Nutrition*, 77, 226–233.

FRANKEL, E. (2005) *Lipid Oxidation*. Bridgwater: The Oily Press.

FRESTA, M. and PUGLISI, G. (1999) Enzyme loaded liposomes for cheese ripening. *Microspheres, Microcapsulates and Lipisomes*, 2, 639–670.

GAN, C. Y., CHENG, L. H. and EASA, A. M. (2008) Evaluation of microbial transglutaminase and ribose cross-linked soy protein isolate-based microcapsules containing fish oil. *Innovative Food Science and Emerging Technologies*, 9, 563–569.

GHARSALLAOUI, A., ROUDAUT, G., CHAMBIN, O., VOILLEY, A. and SAUREL, R. (2007) Applications of spray-drying in microencapsulation of food ingredients: an overview. *Food Research International*, 40, 1107–1121.

GIANNUZZI, P., MAGGIONI, A., CECI, V., CHIEFFO, C., GATTONE, M., GRIFFO, R., MARCHIOLI, R., SCHWEIGER, C., TAVAZZI, L., URBINATI, S., VALAGUSSA, F. and VANUZZO, D. (2008) Global secondary prevention strategies to limit event recurrence after myocardial infarction: results of the GOSPEL study. A multicenter, randomized controlled trial from the Italian cardiac rehabilitation network. *Archives of Internal Medicine*, 168, 2194–2204.

GÖKMEN, V., MOGOL, B. A., LUMAGA, R. B., FOGLIANO, V., KAPLUN, Z. and SHIMONI, E. (2011) Development of functional bread containing nanoencapsulated omega-3 fatty acids. *Journal of Food Engineering*, 105, 585–591.

GOUIN, S. (2004) Microencapsulation: industrial appraisal of existing technologies and trends. *Trends in Food Science & Technology*, 15, 330–347.

GREGORIADIS, G. (1987) Encapsulation of enzymes and other agents liposomes, in ANDREWS, A. J. (ed.) *Chemical Aspects in Food Enzymes.* London: Royal Society of Chemistry, 93–94.

GRIFFIN, W. C. (1949) Classification of surface active agents by HLB. *Journal of Society of Cosmetic Chemists*, 1, 311–326.

GUZEY, D., KIM, H. J. and MCCLEMENTS, D. J. (2004) Factors influencing the production of o/w emulsions stabilized by beta-lactoglobulin–pectin membranes. *Food Hydrocolloids*, 18, 967–975.

HEINZELMANN, K., FRANKE, K., VELASCO, J. and MÁRQUEZ-RUÍZ, G. (2000) Microencapsulation of fish oil by freeze-drying techniques and influence of process parameters on oxidative stability during storage. *European Food Research and Technology*, 211, 234–239.

HIBBELN, J. R., NIEMINEN, L. R., BLASBALG, T. L., RIGGS, J. A. and LANDS, W. E. (2006) Healthy intakes of n−3 and n−6 fatty acids: estimations considering worldwide diversity. *American Society for Clinical Nutrition*, 83, S1483–S1493.

HIGGINS, S., CARROLL, Y. L., O'BRIEN, N. M. and MORRISSEY, P. A. (1999) Use of microencapsulated fish oil as a means of increasing omega-3 polyunsaturated fatty acid intake. *Journal of Human Nutrition and Dietetics*, 12, 265–271.

HORN, A. F., NIELSEN, N. S. and JACOBSEN, C. (2011) Oxidative stability of 70 % fish oil-in-water emulsions: impact of emulsifier and pH. *European Journal of Lipid Science and Technology*, 113, 1243–1257.

HULL, M. A. (2011) Omega-3 polyunsaturated fatty acids. *Best Practice & Research Clinical Gastroenterology*, 25, 547–554.

ISMAIL, H. M. (2005) The role of omega-3 fatty acids in cardiac protection: An overview. *Frontiers in Bioscience*, 10, 1079–1088.

JAFAR, S. S., HULTIN, H. O., BOMBO, A. P., CROWTHER, J. B. and BARLOW, S. M. (1994) Stabilization by antioxidants of mayonnaise made from fish oil. *Journal of Food Lipids*, 1, 295–311.

KAGAMI, Y., SUGIMURA, S., FUJISHIMA, N., MATSUDA, K., KOMETANI, T. and MATSUMURA, Y. (2003) Oxidative stability, structure, and physical characteristics of microcapsules formed by spray drying of fish oil with protein and dextrin wall materials. *Journal of Food Science*, 68, 2248–2255.

KAMEI, M., KI, M., KAWAGOSHI, M. and KAWAI, N. (2002) Nutritional evaluation of Japanese take-out lunches compared with Western-style fast foods supplied in Japan. *Journal of Food Composition and Analysis*, 15, 35–45.

KAZMIERSKI, M., WICKER, L. and CORREDIG, M. (2003) Interactions of β-lactoglobulin and high-methoxyl pectins in acidified systems. *Journal of Food Science*, 68, 1673–1679.

KEOGH, M. K., O'KENNEDY, B. T., KELLY, J., AUTY, M. A., KELLY, P. M. and FUREBY, A. (2001) Stability to oxidation of spray-dried fish oil powder microencapsulated using milk ingredients. *Food and Chemical Toxicology*, 66, 217–224.

KIM, Y. D. and BAIANU, I. C. (1991) Novel liposome micro-encapsulation techniques for food applications. *Trends Food Science and Technology*, 2, 55–61.

KLAYPRADIT, W. and HUANG, Y. W. (2008) Fish oil encapsulation with chitosan using ultrasonic atomizer. *Lebensmittel-Wissenschaft Technologie*, 41, 1133–1139.

KLINKESORN, U., SOPHANODORA, P., CHINACHOTI, P., MCCLEMENTS, D. J. and DECKER, E. A. (2005) Stability of spray-dried tuna oil emulsions encapsulated with two-layered interfacial membranes. *Journal of Agriculture and Food Chemistry*, 53, 8365–8371.

KLINKESORN, U., SOPHANODORA, P., CHINACHOTI, P., DECKER, E. A. and MCCLEMENTS, D. J. (2006) Characterization of spray-dried tuna oil emulsified in two-layered interfacial membranes prepared using electrostatic layer-by-layer deposition. *Food Research International*, 39, 449–457.

KOLANOWSKI, W. and LAUFENBERG, G. (2006) Enrichement of food products with polyunsaturated fatty acids by fish oil addition. *European Food Research and Technology*, 222, 472–477.

KOLANOWSKI, W. and WEIBBRODT, J. (2007) Sensory quality of dairy products fortified with fish oil. *International Dairy Journal*, 17, 1248–1253.

KOLANOWSKI, W., JAWORSKA, D., LAUFENBERG, G. and WEIBBRODT, J. (2007) Evaluation of sensory quality of instant foods fortified with omega-3 PUFA by addition of fish oil powder. *European Food Research and Technology*, 225, 715–721.

KRALOVEC, J. A., ZHANG, S. C., ZHANG, W. and BARROW, C. J. (2012) A review of the progress in enzymatic concentration and microencapsulation of omega-3 rich oil from fish and microbial sources. *Food Chemistry*, 131, 639–644.

KRIS-ETHERTON, P. M., TAYLOR, D. S., YU-POTH, S., HUTH, P., MORIARTY, K., FISHELL, V., HARGROVE, R. L., ZHAO, G. and ETHERTON, T. D. (2000) Polyunsaturated fatty acids in the food chain in the United States. *American Journal of Clinical Nutrition*, 71, 179s–188s.

KUBO, K., SEKINE, S. and SAITO, M. (2003) Docosahexaenoic acid-containing phosphatidylethanolamine in the external layer of liposomes protects docosahexaenoic acid from 2, 2′-azobis(2-aminopropane) dihydrochloride-mediated lipid peroxidation. *Archives of Biochemistry and Biophysics*, 410, 141–148.

KULKARNI, S. B. and VARGHA-BUTLER, E. I. (1995) Study of liposomal drug delivery systems encapsulation efficiencies of some steroids in MLV liposomes. *Colloids and Surfaces. B, Biointerfaces*, 4, 77–85.

LAMPRECHT, A., SCHAFER, U. and LEHR, C. M. (2001) Influences of process parameters on preparation of microparticle used as a carrier system for omega-3 unsaturated fatty acid ethyl esters used in supplementary nutrition. *Journal of Microencapsulation*, 18, 347–357.

LAZKO, J., POPINEAU, Y. and LEGRAND, J. (2004) Soy glycinin microcapsules by simple coacervation method. *Colloids and Surfaces B: Biointerfaces*, 37, 1–8.

LEE, S. J., JIN, B. H., HWANG, Y. I. and LEE, S. C. (2000) Encapsulation of bromelain in liposome. *Journal of Food Science and Nutrition*, 5, 81–85.

LEE, S., FAUSTMAN, C., DJORDJEVIC, D., FARAJI, H. and DECKER, E. A. (2006) Effect of antioxidants on stabilization of meat products fortified with n-3 fatty acids. *Meat Science*, 72, 18–24.

LESMES, U., COHEN, S. H., SHENER, Y. and SHIMONI, E. (2009) Effects of long chain fatty acid unsaturation on the structure and controlled release properties of amylose complexes. *Food Hydrocolloids*, 23, 667–675

LIAO, L., LUO, Y., ZHAO, M. and WANG, Q. (2012) Preparation and characterization of succinic acid deamidated wheat gluten microspheres for encapsulation of fish oil. *Colloids and Surfaces B: Biointerfaces*, 92, 305–314.

MADENE, A., JACQUOT, M., SCHER, J. and DESOBRY, S. (2006) Flavour encapsulation and controlled release – a review. *International Journal of Food Science & Technology*, 41, 1–21.

MARSANASCO, M., MÁRQUEZ, A. L., WAGNER, J. R., ALONSO, S. D. V. and CHIARAMONI, N. S. (2011) Liposomes as vehicles for vitamins E and C: An alternative to fortify orange juice and offer vitamin C protection after heat treatment. *Food Research International*, 44, 3039–3046.

MATSUNO, R. and ADACHI, S. (1993) Lipid encapsulation technology – techniques and applications to food. *Trends in Food Science and Technology*, 4, 256–261.

MCCLEMENTS, D. J. (2004) Protein-stabilized emulsions. *Current Opinion in Colloid & Interface Science*, 9, 305–313.

MCCLEMENTS, D. J. (2005) *Food Emulsions: Principles, Practice, and Techniques* (2nd edn). Boca Raton, FL: CRC Press.

MCCLEMENTS, D. J. and DECKER, E. A. (2000) Lipid oxidation in oil-in-water emulsions: Impact of molecular environment on chemical reactions in heterogeneous food systems. *Journal of Food Science*, 65, 1270–1282.

MCCLEMENTS, D. J. and LI, Y. (2010) Structured emulsion-based delivery systems: Controlling the digestion and release of lipophilic food components. *Advances in Colloid and Interface Science*, 159, 213–228.

MCNAMEE, B. F., O'RIORDAN, E. A. and O'SULLIVAN, M. (1998) Emulsification and encapsulation properties of gum arabic. *Journal of Agricultural and Food Chemistry*, 46, 4551–4555.

MELTON, S. L. (1983) Methodology for following lipid oxidation in muscle foods. *Food Technology*, 37, 105–111.

MOLINA, E., PAPADOPOULOU, A. and LEDWARD, D. A. (2001) Emulsifying properties of high pressure treated soy protein isolate and 7S and 11S globulins. *Food Hydrocolloids*, 15, 263–269.

NAKAUMA, M., FUNAMI, T., NODA, S., ISHIHARA, S., AL-ASSAF, S., NISHINARI, K. and PHILIPS, G. O. (2008) Comparison of sugar beet pectin, soybean soluble polysaccharide and gum arabic as food emulsifiers. 1. Effect of concentration, pH, and slat on the emulsifying properties. *Food Hydrocolloids*, 22, 1254–1267.

NEDOVIC, V., KALUSEVIC, A., MANOJLOVIC, V., LEVIC, S. and BUGARSKI, B. (2011) An overview of encapsulation technologies for food applications. *Procedia Food Science*, 1, 1806–1815.

NIELSEN, N. A. and JACOBSEN, C. (2009) Methods for reducing lipid oxidation in fish-oil-enriched energy bars. *International Journal of Food Science & Technology*, 44, 1536–1546.

NIELSEN, N. A. and JACOBSEN, C. (2012) Oxidation in fish oil enriched fish pâté. *Journal of Food Biochemistry,* DOI: 10.1111/j.1745-4514.2011.00605.x.

ONUKI, Y., MORISHITA, M., WATANABE, H., CHIBA, Y., TOKIWA, S., TAKAYAMA, K. and NAGAI, T. (2003) Improved insulin enteral delivery using water-in-oil-in-water multiple emulsion incorporating highly purified docosahexaenoic acid. *STP Pharma Sciences*, 13, 231–235.

PHILLIPS, G. O. and WILLIAMS, P. A. (2000) Gum arabic, in PHILLIPS, G. O. and WILLIAMS, P. A. (eds), *Handbook of Hydrocolloids*. Cambridge: CRC Press, Woodhead, 155–168.

PORZIO, M. A. (2007) Flavour delivery and product development. *Food Technology*, 1, 22–29.

RAPER, N. R., CRONIN, F. J. and ECLER, J. (1992) Omega-3 fatty acid content of the US food supply. *Journal of the American College of Nutrition*, 11, 304–308.

RICHARD, J., THIES, C., GAJAN, V. and BENOIT, J. P. (1998) A novel solvent-free process to prepare drug delivery systems. *Proceedings of the 25th International Symposium on Controlled Release of Bioactive Materials*. St Paul, MN: Controlled Release Society, 140–141.

RODEA-GONZÁLEZ, D. A., CRUZ-OLIVARES, J., ROMÁN-GUERRERO, A., RODRÍGUEZ-HUEZO, M. E., VERNON-CARTER, E. J. and PÉREZ-ALONSO, C. (2012) Spray-dried encapsulation of chia essential oil (*Salvia hispanica* L.) in whey protein concentrate–polysaccharide matrices. *Journal of Food Engineering*, 111, 102–109.

SANDGRUBER, S. and BUETTNER, A. (2012) Comparative human-sensory evaluation and quantitative comparison of odour-active oxidation markers of encapsulated fish oil products used for supplementation during pregnancy and the breastfeeding period. *Food Chemistry*, 133, 458–466.

SERFERT, Y., DRUSCH, S. and SCHWARZ, K. (2010) Sensory odour profiling and lipid oxidation status of fish oil and microencapsulated fish oil. *Food Chemistry*, 123, 968–975.

SHAHIDI, F. and HAN, X. Q. (1993) Encapsulation of food ingredients. *Critical Reviews in Food Science and Nutrition*, 33, 501–547.

SHAHIDI, F. and WANASUNDARA, U. N. (2002) Methods for measuring oxidative rancidity in fats and oils, in AKOH, C. C and MIN, D. B. (eds), *Food Lipids: Chemistry, Nutrition and Biotechnology.* New York: Marcel Dekker.

SHARMA, R. (2005) Market trends and opportunities for functional dairy beverages. *Australian Journal of Dairy Technology*, 60, 195–198.

SHEU, T. Y. and ROSENBERG, M. (1995) Microencapsulation by spray drying ethyl caprylate in whey protein and carbohydrate wall systems. *Journal of Food Science*, 60, 98–103.

SHIMADA, A., YAZAWA, E. and ARAI, S. (1982) Preparation of proteinaceous surfactants by enzymatic modification and evaluation of their functional properties in a concentrated emulsion system. *Agricultural and Biological Chemistry*, 46, 173–182.

STRAUSS, G. and GIBSON, S. M. (2004) Plant phenolics as cross-linkers of gelatin gels and gelatin-based coacervates for use as food ingredients. *Food Hydrocolloids*, 18, 81–89.

TAGUCHI, K., IWAMI, K., IBUKI, F. and KAWABATA, M. (1992) Oxidative stability of sardine oil embedded in spray-dried egg white powder and its use for n-3 unsaturated fatty acid fortification of cookies. *Bioscience, Biotechnology and Biochemistry*, 56, 560–563.

TRUELSTRUP-HANSEN, L., ALLAN-WOJTAS, P. M., JIN, Y. L. and PAULSON, A. T. (2002) Survival of Ca-alginate microencapsulated Bifidobacterium spp. in milk and simulated gastrointestinal conditions. *Food Microbiology*, 19, 35–45.

TURGEON, S. L., SCHMITT, C. and SANCHEZ, C. (2007) Protein–polysaccharide complexes and coacervates. *Current Opinion in Colloid and Interface Science*, 12, 166–178.

VONGSVIVUT, J., HERAUD, P., ZHANG, W., KRALOVEC, J. A., MCNAUGHTON, D. and BARROW, C. J. (2012) Quantitative determination of fatty acid compositions in microencapsulated fish oil supplements using Fourier transform infrared (FTIR) spectroscopy. *Food Chemistry*, 135, 603–609.

WALL, R., ROSS, R. P., FITZGERALD, G. F. and STANTON, C. (2010) Fatty acids from fish: the anti-inflammatory potential of long-chain omega-3 fatty acids. *Nutrition Reviews*, 68, 280–289

WANG, C., HARRIS, W. S., CHUNG, M., LICHTENSTEIN, A. H., BALK, E. M., KUPELNICK, B., JORDAN, H. S. and LAU, J. (2006) N-3 fatty acids from fish or fish-oil supplements, but not alpha-linolenic acid, benefit cardiovascular disease outcomes in primary- and secondary prevention studies: a systematic review. *American Journal of Clinical Nutrition*, 84, 5–17.

WANG, B., WANG, L. J., LI, D., ADHIKARI, B. and SHI, J. (2011a) Effect of gum arabic on stability of oil-in-water emulsions stabilized by flaxseed and soybean protein. *Carbohydrate Polymers*, 86, 343–351.

WANG, R., TIAN, Z. and CHEN, L. (2011b) Nano-encapsulations liberated from barley protein microparticles for oral delivery of bioactive compounds. *International Journal of Pharmaceutics*, 406, 153–162.

WEINBRECK, F., NIEUWENHUIJSE, H., ROBIJN, G. W. and DE KRUIF, C. G. (2004) Complexation of whey proteins with carrageenan. *Journal of Agricultural Food Chemistry*, 52, 3550–3555.

WU, K. G., CHAI, X. H. and YUE, C. (2005) Microencapsulation of fish oil by simple coacervation of hydroxypropyl methylcellulose. *Chinese Journal of Chemistry*, 23, 1569–1572.

YAJIMA, M. (1990) *Stabilized oil and fat powder*. EP 372669.

YOKOYAMA, M., ORIGASA, H., MATSUZAKI, M., MATSUZAWA, Y., SAITO, Y., ISHIKAWA, Y., OIKAWA, S., SASAKI, J., HISHIDA, H., ITAKURA, H., KITA, T., KITABATAKE, A., NAKAYA, N., SAKATA, T., SHINADA, K. and SHIRATO, K. (2007) Effects of eicosapentaenoic acid on major coronary events in hypercholesterolaemic patients (JELIS): a randomized open-label, blinded endpoint analysis. *Lancet*, 369, 1090–1098.

ZABAR, S., LESMES, U., KATZ, I., SHIMONI, E. and BIANCO-PELED, H. (2009) Studying different dimensions of amylose–long chain fatty acid complexes: molecular, nano and micro level characteristics. *Food Hydrocolloids*, 23, 1918–1925.

ZABAR, S., LESMES, U., KATZ, I., SHIMONI, E. and BIANCO-PELED, H. (2010) Structural characterization of amylose-long chain fatty acid complexes produced via the acidification method. *Food Hydrocolloids*, 24, 347–357.

ZIMET, P. and LIVNEY, Y. D. (2009) Beta-lactoglobulin and its nanocomplexes with pectin as vehicles for ω-3 polyunsaturated fatty acids. *Food Hydrocolloids*, 23, 1120–1126.

7

Analysis of omega-3 fatty acids in foods and supplements

J. M. Curtis and B. A. Black, University of Alberta, Canada

DOI: 10.1533/9780857098863.2.226

Abstract: This chapter provides a background to methods commonly used for the analysis of omega-3 fatty acids in foods and supplements, with emphasis on recent literature. The range of methods for the extraction of lipids and their conversion to fatty acid methyl esters (FAME) are described. Procedures using gas–liquid chromatography with flame ionization detection (GC/FID) are reviewed in detail for omega-3 FAME along with alternative instrumental techniques.

Key words: food analysis, gas–liquid chromatography / flame-ionization detector (GC/FID) fatty acid methyl esters (FAME), omega-3 fatty acids.

7.1 Introduction

The rise in popularity of omega-3 enriched foods has resulted in a corresponding need for the analysis of these fortified or functional foods in order to ensure product consistency as well as to provide reliable nutritional analysis for consumer and regulatory acceptance. In principle, the analysis of omega-3 fatty acids should be no more complicated than any other analysis of food fatty acid composition. However, in practice this may not be the case, for a variety of reasons. These include the problem of having low levels of omega-3 fatty acids present in some foods that must be measured against a higher background of more abundant fatty acids. There are additional challenges in quantitatively extracting the omega-3 fatty acids, especially if they are encapsulated for greater stability or are matrix bound, for instance by extrusion.

Although supplements and foods mostly contain omega-3 fatty acids in the triacylglyceride (TAG) form, other esterified forms such as ethyl esters or phospholipids, or even free fatty acids are also used. Hence, care should be taken to ensure that the analytical method selected is able to quantify all of the forms of fatty acids present in the sample that make up the total bioavailable omega-3 fatty acid content. Indeed, the term 'fatty acids' is generally used to describe all of the fatty acyl moieties present and only rarely are the free acid forms of those compounds distinguished from the whole. Hence care must also be taken when considering the results of fatty acid analyses, especially for supplements, since stated omega-3 amounts may be expressed as free fatty acid, ethyl ester or triacylglyceride equivalents, even though this might not be the fatty acid form actually present. In this chapter, in common with much of the literature, the term 'fatty acid' is not meant to imply any particular form, either bound to glycerol or free.

Finally, there are special considerations for the quantification of omega-3 fatty acids themselves, including their propensity for oxidation and the need for careful control of response factors relating to them. These considerations apply equally to omega-3 fatty acids measured in foods and to those found in more concentrated forms in supplements. This chapter provides a background to some of the methods commonly used for analysis of omega-3 fatty acids in foods and supplements along with reference to recent literature and reviews for further reading on individual topics.

7.2 The analysis of omega-3 oils by gas–liquid chromatography / flame ionization detector (GC/FID)

Gas–liquid chromatography (GLC or GC) was first developed in the early 1950s (James and Martin, 1952) and rapidly became an established analytical method to separate compound mixtures containing relatively volatile organic compounds. The basic principle of the separation is based on the differential partition of analytes between a gaseous mobile phase and a liquid stationary phase coated on the inner surface of a column, giving rise to characteristic retention times. Since the 1980s, capillary GC in which the stationary phase coated on the inner surface of a fused-silica capillary has been the standard technique for determining the fatty acid composition of oils (Christie, 1989). In these methods, oils are first converted into volatile derivatives, usually the methyl or ethyl esters of fatty acids (FAME or FAEE). The separated FAME eluting from the column are usually monitored by a flame ionization detector (FID), which is a non-specific detector with a relatively uniform response to most organic compounds (Ackman and Sipos, 1964) that has been the most universally used GC detector for organic compounds for more than 40 years.

Gas chromatography with flame-ionization detection (GC/FID) remains the most robust and widely used method for the characterization of fatty acid mixtures (Ackman, 2008). This is in spite of the remarkable advances in GC combined with mass spectrometry (GC/MS). Clearly GC/MS has much higher analytical power (Christie, 1998) due to its ability to identify molecular species or even isomeric structures through techniques such as the use of 4,4-dimethyloxazoline (DMOX) derivatives (see Section 7.4). However, a major drawback of GC/MS is the wide range of response factors for different fatty acid species making it difficult to use for reliable quantification (Dodds *et al.*, 2005). In contrast, the FID detector has a relatively uniform response to most organic compounds and hence is very suitable for quantification of individual FAME or groupings of selected FAME such as total omega-3 fatty acids. Hence, for around half a century, GC/FID has been the method of choice for the analysis of fatty acids and the most important method for the quantification of omega-3 fatty acids. The practical and theoretical details of the GC/FID method are thoroughly reviewed elsewhere and selected examples are given in Table 7.1.

7.2.1 The importance of GC/FID response factors

To a first-order approximation, the measurement of omega-3 levels in dietary supplements is a relatively straightforward process. It involves the quantification of fatty acid components at percent levels by GC/FID following well-established procedures for the conversion of oils into FAME, or directly as FAEE. Thus, given that the response factors for FAME by GC/FID are similar, it should be possible to measure fatty acid profiles directly from GC/FID peak areas. This approach is indeed useful for

Table 7.1 Review papers and book chapters related to the analysis of omega-3 fatty acids

Method	Author	
GC/FID FAME general	Ackman (2002)	
	Ackman (2008)	
	Christie (1989)	
	Christie and Han (2010)	
	Cruz-Hernandez and Destaillats (2012)	
	Shantha (1992)	
GC/FID omega-3 FAME	Ruiz-Rodriquez *et al.* (2010)	
	Schreiner (2006a)	
Alternative omega-3 analytical methods	Carrapiso and García (2000)	Microwave + SFE
	Christie (1998)	GC/MS
	Christie and Han (2010)	LC; SFC; NMR
	Diehl (2001)	NMR
	Dobson and Christie (2002)	GC/MS
	Lima and Abdalla (2002)	HPLC
	Moretti and Caprino (2009)	GC/MS
	Ruiz-Rodriquez *et al.* (2010)	LC
	Standal *et al.* (2011)	NMR
Analysis of omega-3 in foods	Crews (2008)	
	Dobson (2008)	
	Stark (2012)	

Notes: HPLC = high-performance chromatography; NMR = nuclear magnetic resonance; SFC = supercritical-fluid chromatography; SFE = supercritical-fluid extraction.

qualitative measurements, but a basic premise of analytical chemistry is the need to relate absolute amounts to true weight measurements of pure standards, and hence peak areas alone cannot provide accurate quantification. As pointed out by Joseph and Ackman (1992, 489):

> Although the results of GC analyses of fatty acid methyl esters are usually reported as area percentages of eluted components, the area percentages of EPA and DHA must be converted to absolute weights per gram of sample for informative labelling of nutritional supplements. This conversion requires the use of internal or external standards, and for accuracy, correction factors of the FID response must be applied.

Thus, with growing interest in the wide-ranging beneficial effects of omega-3 fatty acids that flourished in the 1980s, and in particular the demonstrated cardiovascular benefits (Kris-Etherton *et al.*, 2003), there emerged a need to properly quantify all contributing omega-3 fatty acids in a sample. This was facilitated by the demonstration that FID response factors for different fatty acids could be calculated based on their chain lengths and number of double bonds, as reviewed earlier (Joseph and Seaborn, 1990; Curtis, 2007), once optimal GC conditions are achieved (Bannon *et al.*, 1986). This approach works well in many instances as demonstrated by interlaboratory studies of omega-3 analyses of fish oil supplements (Joseph and Ackman, 1992) for AOAC Official Method 991.39 (AOAC International, 2006). However, it later became clear that as omega-3 oils were being produced at higher omega-3 concentrations, and were further developed as pharmaceutical products containing more than 80 % by weight of omega-3 fatty acids (Breivik *et al.*, 1996), the method to quantify EPA, DHA and other omega-3 fatty acids using theoretical response factors was not sufficiently accurate. Thus, a method establishing the relationship between label claims (for omega-3 supplements or pharmaceutical product) and authentic reference standards was required (Tande *et al.*, 1992).

This method formed the basis of the European Pharmacopeia methods for the analysis of omega-3 oils. It specifically involves the determination of the response factors for EPA and DHA using reference standards of high purity, which can correct for the significant variation between the experimental GC/FID response factors of polyunsaturated fatty acids compared to those predicted based on FID responses alone. This difference was also confirmed in the development of the procedure for the determination of the fatty acid composition of marine oils and other oils containing long-chain polyunsaturated fatty acids (PUFA), known as AOCS method Ce 1i-07. This method highlights the importance of using experimental response factors for PUFA where the deviations from theoretical are at a maximum. In the method, experimental response factors for FAME are determined using a calibration solution containing 25 key compounds from C-8 to C-24 and from zero to six degrees of unsaturation.

In summary, the accurate determination of omega-3 levels in oils, supplements and foods requires the use of methods that properly correct for the experimentally observed deviations from theoretical behaviour in the GC/FID responses. These arise almost inevitably through a variety of factors related to chromatographic behaviour and sample manipulations. Debates over the best methodology will undoubtedly continue to create problems for the omega-3 industry and consumers alike. Hence, the best way forward is through the use of common analytical methods that are independently validated and widely adopted by the industry and regulatory bodies. Such methods are described below.

7.3 The measurement of omega-3 levels in foods

There is now such an abundance of data demonstrating the health benefits of consuming omega-3 fats that several countries have established recommended intakes (e.g. the UK, 0.5 % of energy from EPA and DHA) or recommended intakes expressed as ratios of omega-6 to omega-3 fatty acids (e.g. Canada 4:1–10:1). As a result, there is heightened consumer interest in fish that naturally contains omega-3 fatty acids and in foods that originally contain little or none but have been fortified with omega-3 fats in suitably stabilized forms (Hernandez and Hosokawa, 2011). In the latter case, relatively low levels of fortification are typical, in the range of 20–150 mg long-chain omega-3 per serving, so that consumption of multiple servings of omega-3 fortified functional foods is required to meet the recommended intakes. There is a clear requirement for analytical methods that accurately measure the levels omega-3 fatty acids in foods in order to justify label claims, conform to regulatory standards and allow individuals and nutritionists to be able to properly determine daily dietary intakes.

An indirect approach used to increase the omega-3 content of meat, milk and eggs is to supplement the downstream animal feed with omega-3 fatty acids (chapters 8–13). More directly, omega-3 fatty acids can be incorporated into foods in various ways, the simplest being by the direct incorporation of fish oil. However, even the incorporation of highly deodorized PUFA oils often results in products that readily form off-flavours and aromas (see, e.g. chapters 4 and 5). Such foods can only be stored for short periods of time under non-oxidative conditions, including the absence of heat, light and oxygen (Kolanowski *et al.*, 2007). Hence, in order to develop more stable functional foods containing omega-3, stabilization methods through the judicious use of antioxidants (Chapter 4), microencapsulation (Chapter 6), extrusion (Drusch *et al.*, 2012) or emulsification (Chapter 5) techniques have been developed and commercialized. The measurement of the omega-3 content of functional foods containing oils that have been protected by encapsulation or incorporation into parts of the food matrix is especially challenging. This is because, in addition to the need for the accurate determination of low levels of PUFAs that are sensitive to oxidation and may give non-ideal behaviour in the analytical techniques usually employed (such as wide deviations from theoretical GC/FID response factors), it cannot be assumed that the quantitative recovery of these fatty acids from the food matrix is always achieved.

In spite of all of the above, the general approach taken to quantify omega-3 fats from either a fortified food or a conventional food by GC/FID is still similar. An overview of the process is given in Fig. 7.1. First, an appropriate number of replicate samples must be collected from a truly homogeneous blend of the food, either before or after the food is dried. Drying, in general, facilitates lipid extraction, but it may be unnecessary for low-moisture foods. Ultimately, all omega-3 fatty acids, including free fatty acids and those bound to glycerol or to other compounds, are conventionally quantified as methyl esters (i.e. FAME) in order to take the greatest advantage of high-resolution GC.

To achieve the complete conversion of all fat in the food into FAME may first require the liberation of that fat from the food matrix, and especially carbohydrates, using digestion by strong acid or base. The fat can then be separated from the food by extraction into a lipophilic organic solvent, such as ether and, finally, transesterified by methanol using a base, acid or Lewis acid catalyst to produce FAME. A well-known and widely used example of this multistep process to produce FAME from a variety of food types is the AOAC Official Method 996.06 (AOAC International, 2006). However, some methods and foods may not use, or require, the digestion step, such as in the extraction of fat by the Bligh and Dyer method (Bligh and Dyer, 1959) using a mixture of chloroform and methanol.

An alternative approach that has been developed (Ulberth and Henninger, 1992) is to combine the digestion, extraction and derivitization steps into a single-step reaction, as indicated in Fig. 7.1. Such 'one step'/*in situ* methods (see Section 7.5) have the advantage of being considerably more efficient but lack the possibility for gravimetric determination of the total fat content and may require higher reaction temperatures, possibly making them less suitable for the determination of more volatile fatty acids. Furthermore, they do not allow the separate measurement of the recovery of extraction and the efficiency of the methylation process since these steps are combined. On the other hand, overall the 'one-step' extraction/derivitization route can be an attractive method for the analyst, saving time and unnecessary sample manipulations.

Overall, whatever process is selected for the digestion, extraction and methylation of the food prior to omega-3 quantification, it is highly advisable to first perform in-house validation of the method to demonstrate the overall accuracy, precision and reproducibility of the measurement. This requires correction for recovery of the analytes and losses during derivitization and manipulation of the extract by using appropriate internal standards, as indicated in Fig. 7.1. In addition, the validated method must take into account factors relating to the GC/FID method including the determination of response factors for omega-3 PUFAs, as discussed. Incidentally,

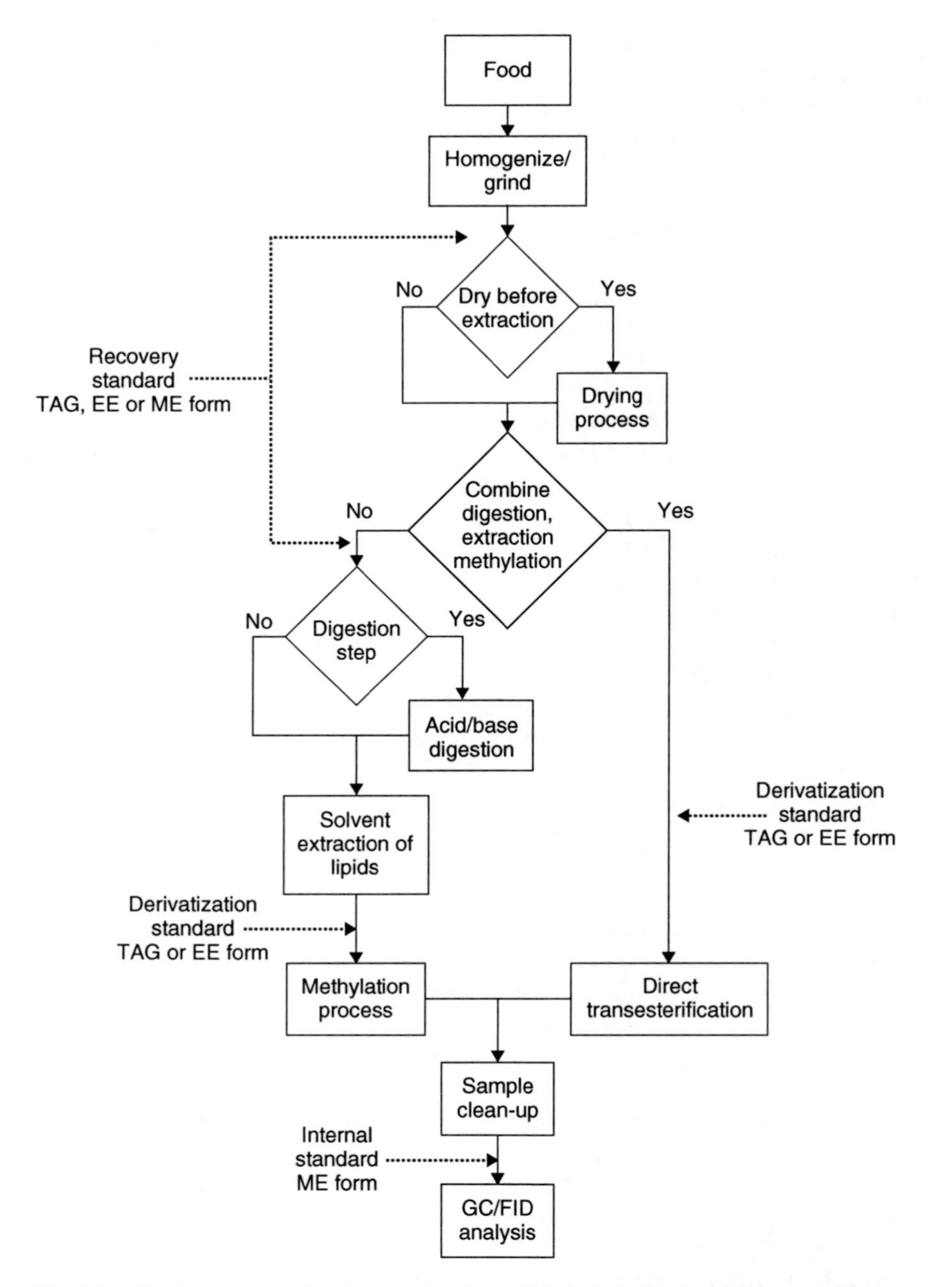

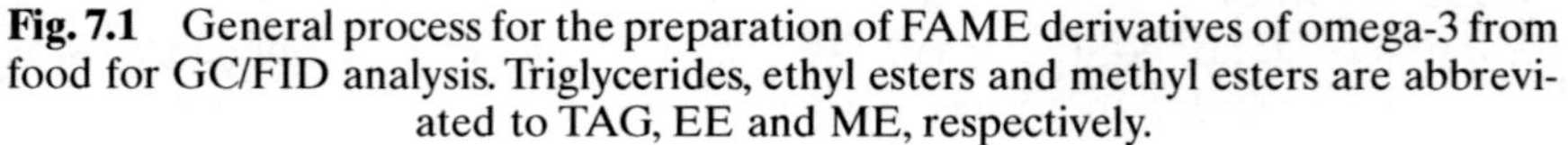

Fig. 7.1 General process for the preparation of FAME derivatives of omega-3 from food for GC/FID analysis. Triglycerides, ethyl esters and methyl esters are abbreviated to TAG, EE and ME, respectively.

Table 7.2 Selected official methods related to the analysis of omega-3 fatty acids

Method	Description
AOAC 991.39	Quantitation of fatty acids in encapsulated fish oils and fish oil methyl and ethyl esters by GC
AOAC 996.06	Quantitation of fat (total, saturated and unsaturated) in foods by GC
ISO 23065	Milk fat from enriched dairy products – determination of omega-3 and omega-6 fatty acids by GLC
AOCS Cd 1e-01	Iodine value by near infrared (NIR)
AOCS Ce 1b-89	Fatty acid composition of marine oils
AOCS Ce 1d-91	n-3 and n-6 by capillary GLC
AOCS Ce 1h-05	Fatty acid composition by capillary GC for nutrition labeling
AOCS Ce 1i-07	Fatty acids in marine and other oils containing long-chain PUFAs by GC
AOCS Ce 1k-09	Direct methylation of lipids in foods for the determination of total fat, saturated, *cis*-monounsaturated, *cis*-polyunsaturated, and *trans* fatty acids by GC
AOCS Ce 2–66	Preparation of methyl esters of fatty acids
AOCS Ce 2b-11	Direct methylation of lipids in foods by alkali hydrolysis
AOCS Ce 2c-11	Direct methylation of lipids in foods by acid–alkali hydrolysis
GOED	Monograph of standards for omega-3 fatty acid quality

such method validation should not be looked upon as a chore but rather as a golden opportunity to uncover the strengths and weaknesses of the chosen method which can save considerable time and trouble with future data.

A list of common official methods used in the analysis of omega-3 fatty acids is given in Table 7.2. The principles and advantages of particular approaches are outlined in the following section and further detail can be found in the reviews listed in Table 7.1.

7.3.1 Overview of methods separating the extraction, digestion and derivatization steps

In conventional foods, omega-3 fatty acids are mainly present in esterified forms as triacylglycerols or phospholipids. In functional foods, the fatty acids may still remain in these forms, or they may have been converted into alkyl esters, free fatty acids or microencapsulated oils. These differences in chemical constitution will influence the best choice of analytical approach although, in general, similar methods of extraction and conversion to FAME for GC/FID still apply.

For an omega-3 supplement in oil form, such as a fish or algal oil gelatin capsule, no lipid extraction is necessary and one can directly proceed to the methylation process. For a food sample, sometimes the total omega-3 component can be extracted directly by organic solvents, but often solvent extraction alone is not sufficient for quantitative extraction. In such food samples, especially where oil is tightly associated with the carbohydrate matrix (for example a food having passed through an extruder), or for food in which the lipid is protected by microencapsulation or in a dairy emulsion, it is necessary to first digest the sample with strong acid or base to liberate the lipid. These methods can also liberate lipids bound as lipoproteins or glycolipids. They are described in commonly applied methods like AOAC Official Method 996.06 (AOAC International, 2006) and should ideally be performed in the presence of an internal standard (e.g. triundecanoin) to correct for any losses.

As pointed out by Ackman (2008), hydrochloric acid digestion does not hydrolyse all glycerides completely to free fatty acids. Furthermore, alkali digestion may produce ester side-products rather than alkali salts (or soaps) if alcohols are present. However, these problems can be overcome by the subsequent derivatization method so that all fatty acids are extracted and converted to methyl esters. In some, but not all cases, hydrolysis with alkaline may give a higher recovery of free fatty acids from foods with lipids with high association to other components, such as certain types of powdered products (Dobson, 2008), and this approach is fairly standard for dairy products. Usually the procedure will involve treatment with dilute acid to convert the soaps to free fatty acids. Finally, after either acid or alkali digestion, fatty acids are extracted with organic solvents such as petroleum either, diethyl ether or hexane.

Often, lipids are defined as being soluble in organic solvents and immiscible in water. However, it is important to keep in mind that polarities differ considerably between lipid classes and, to a lesser extent, between individual fatty acids such as between omega-3 PUFA and saturates. In addition, food systems may contain high or low amounts of water making them hard to wet with some lipophilic solvents. This problem can be overcome by gently drying the food prior to solvent extraction (e.g. by freeze drying) or by judicious choice of solvent systems as below. Solvent extraction is well described elsewhere (e.g. Ackman, 2008; Dobson, 2008) so only a few common methods will be described here in outline.

The extraction of intact total lipids, including the omega-3 component, from food products can be achieved by the Folch method (Folch *et al.*, 1957). This uses a 2:1 chloroform–methanol mixture where the water present in the food dissolves in methanol so that the chloroform layer containing the lipid separates easily. The famous variation developed by Bligh and Dyer (1959) was to incorporate enough water to result in a monophasic system for extraction of tissue. Subsequently, dilution with water and/or chloroform results in a biphasic system with the lipid in the chloroform layer. It has been reported that the Bligh and Dyer method under-estimates lipid content for very high fat samples (Iverson *et al.*, 2001), which could be a concern for some foods, but this is also dependent on the solvent/sample ratio used. As a general rule, the Bligh and Dyer method may be preferred for high moisture samples or those with low lipid content, but overall the Folch method is still considered one of the most reliable extraction methods for the quantification of lipids (Iverson *et al.*, 2001; Manirakiza *et al.*, 2001). If a gravimetric determination of total fat is required, then the Soxhlet and Goldfisch methods (see, e.g. Min and Ellefson, 2010) or automated versions of them can be used. However, because of the long extraction times using excess solvents and prolonged heating, these methods are not suitable for extracting omega-3 PUFA for subsequent analysis. The extraction efficiencies of several versions of the Soxhlet method were compared to the Bligh and Dyer method and a modified version of it for the extraction of fat from a wide range of foods (Manirakiza *et al.*, 2001). The conclusion reached was that, although good precision could be achieved using many methods, the actual fat recoveries varied significantly depending on the extraction used. This conclusion applies equally well to the extraction of total omega-3 content of a food.

7.3.2 Less conventional extraction methods

A wide range of fatty acid extraction techniques have been recently reviewed by Ruiz-Rodriguez *et al.* (2010). It is evident that while some of the less 'standard' methods described in that review can have advantages over the more conventional methods described above, in general these extraction methods have not yet been subjected to the same level of critical review and hence care is needed to ensure that extractions proceed with high recovery and without bias.

Supercritical-fluid extraction (SFE) is a method that operates under mild conditions by using CO_2 with low concentrations of solvent modifiers as the extraction fluid at low temperatures. An investigation of the use of SFE for the measurement of the total fat content in food and animal feed was recently described (Ivanov *et al.*, 2011). By careful optimization of the extraction parameters, such as the level of ethanol co-solvent and amount of adsorbent, SFE was optimized for food or feed materials using regression analysis such that there were no significant differences between total fat measured by SFE compared to exhaustive Soxhlet extractions using petroleum ether. Hence these authors concluded that SFE can be recommended for the determination of total fat content in place of Soxhlet or other exhaustive extraction method. However, an important advantage of the SFE method is that it does not require toxic solvents or other chemicals, using CO_2 and ethanol only.

Another major advantage compared to the reported Soxhlet method is that the measured levels of PUFA were dramatically higher using SFE extraction (Ivanov *et al.*, 2011). For example, the proportion of PUFA (including omega-3 PUFA) measured in the SFE lipid extracts of ten feed samples was in the range 63–72 % compared to 24–48 % in the Soxhlet extract. This was explained by the degradation of the sample during the Soxhlet extraction so that, for example, linoleic acid was converted largely into monounsaturates, the mechanism of which was not given. Such degradation did not occur for SFE, where extraction is at low temperature in an inert atmosphere. Hence, fatty acid compositions of samples obtained by SFE were more representative than those from Soxhlet extracts even though the total fat measured gravimetrically by either method was the same.

A further example of this effect was reported (Arnáiz *et al.*, 2011) for SFE compared to Soxhlet extraction of lipids from broccoli leaves. SFE extracts were found to have higher percentages of unsaturated fatty acids, especially of the omega-3 linolenic acid. However, it should be pointed out that the fatty acid degradation described in these two studies would not be expected to occur during extraction by the Folch or Bligh and Dyer methods. Nonetheless, where the specialized equipment is available and the method is properly optimized, SFE is an excellent alternative to solvent extraction methods, widely promoted as being more 'environmentally friendly'. It is quite possible that SFE will become a more widely accepted and standardized method for omega-3 and total fat analysis in the future.

Microwave-assisted extraction (MAE), ultrasound-assisted extraction (UAE) (Adam *et al.*, 2012) and accelerated solvent extraction (ASE) are all accelerated processes that require less solvent than traditional extraction methods. MAE, involving the irradiation of a sample in the presence of a small volume of solvent, can be performed on samples that contain water, meaning that no drying step is required. Although the use of microwaves can result in lipid oxidation and can be used to accelerate chemical reactions, conditions typically used for MAE do not alter the fatty acid composition of a sample and are milder than solvent extraction techniques involving prolonged heating (Carrapiso and García, 2000). MAE has recently been compared to other solvent extraction methods for measuring the total lipid content of frozen fish (Ramalhosa *et al.*, 2012). It was concluded that MAE had high extraction efficiency and repeatability, is convenient, rapid with low solvent use, can be readily automated and is amenable to extraction of multiple samples in parallel. Although omega-3 measurement was not discussed in this study, if the unsaturated fatty acid content is not changed by the MAE method, as described above, this would provide a very attractive method using equipment that is becoming more common in many laboratories.

ASE is a rapid automated procedure that makes use of pressurized solvents and elevated temperatures. The usefulness of ASE for lipid extractions was demonstrated (Dodds *et al.*, 2004) for 100 mg fish (a NIST standard reference material (SRM)) samples rather than the large sample sizes used previously). Comparable, though not identical, values were obtained for the SRM and the authors pointed out the discrepancies that occur when considering gravimetric fatty acid determination rather than using GC/FID data to demonstrate fatty acid composition. An important advance in the use of ASE for total lipid extraction from food samples has recently been reported (Ullah *et al.*, 2011). In this work, ASE extraction was preceded by acid or base treatment, and ion exchange resins were used in conjunction with the ASE to remove residual reagents. Using this method, excellent fat recoveries were measured both gravimetrically and via FAME analyses. These were obtained for a range of foods from low fat content (e.g. milk) to high fat content (e.g. mayonnaise) and for two NIST food SRMs. The ASE method is fully automated, although the reported procedure for acid/base digestion and preparation of the sample prior to ASE was not. As with SFE, the equipment required for ASE is relatively expensive but with some real advantages over solvent extraction methods performed using glassware.

It is worth pointing out here that whatever method of lipid extraction is used, great care must be taken to minimize oxidation of the lipid extract. Samples should be stored at freezer temperatures and the oxygen-containing atmosphere surrounding the lipid fraction should be replaced with an inert gas such as nitrogen or argon. The use of an antioxidant such as butylated hydroxytoluene (BHT) is specified in many methods. This can be an advantage to maintain the integrity of the lipid sample, especially in the case of omega-3 or other PUFA. However, peaks arising from the addition of antioxidants must be identified in subsequent GC or other chromatographic measurements.

7.4 Methyl esters and other fatty acid derivatives

The standard methods for determination of omega-3 fatty acids by GC/FID (see Table 7.2) require that lipid samples be first converted from the form of triacylglycerides, phospholipids or other naturally present form into methyl esters (i.e. FAME). The only exception to this rule is that some supplements are available as ethyl esters, which can be analysed by GC/FID directly (Tande *et al.*, 1992). However, it should be noted that methods for the direct quantification of ethyl esters exclude fatty acids that may be present bound in residual glycerides or other compounds not fully converted to ethyl esters.

FAME are easily prepared and are the most common derivatives to be analysed by GC (Christie and Han, 2010). The established methylation methods suitable for lipid extracts are reviewed elsewhere (see Table 7.1); the combined extraction and derivatization methods that are suitable for omega-3 containing foods are discussed in Section 7.5. The important omega-3 fatty acids that are usually quantified include:

- α-linolenic acid – 9*cis*,12*cis*,15*cis*–18:3
- stearidonic acid – 6*cis*,9*cis*,12*cis*,15*cis*–18:4
- eicosatetraenoic acid – 8*cis*,11*cis*,14*cis*,17*cis*–20:4
- eicosapentaenoic acid (EPA) – 5*cis*,8*cis*,11*cis*,14*cis*,17*cis*–20:5

- docosapentaenoic acid (DPA) – 7*cis*,10*cis*,13*cis*,16*cis*,19*cis*–22:5
- docosahexaenoic acid (DHA) – 4*cis*,7*cis*,10*cis*,13*cis*,16*cis*,19*cis*–22:6

In addition, the omega-3 fatty acid heneicosapentaenoic acid 6*c*, 9*c*, 12*c*, 15*c*, 18*c*–21:5, present in small amounts in lipids from fish and most other marine organisms (Mayzaud and Ackman, 1978), can be included in the determination of total omega-3.

Since the above omega-3 fatty acids can be readily identified by comparison to available FAME standards or mixtures of standards, identification of unknown peaks in the chromatogram is generally not necessary in omega-3 analysis provided that sufficient resolution is achieved. However, it is worth pointing out that other derivatives of fatty acids are often used for the structural analysis of fatty acids (see Fig. 7.2) using GC/MS (Dobson and Christie, 2002). These derivatives can also be used to confirm the identity of an omega-3 or other unsaturated fatty acid. For example, both 4,4-dimethyloxazoline (DMOX) and 3-pyridylcarbinol esters (picolinyl esters) are well-known derivatives which replace the carboxyl group on the fatty acid chain. Each of these derivatives contains a nitrogen atom within a ring structure, which localizes the charge from ionization and gives rise to the characteristic fragmentation, remote from the localized charge, along the fatty acid hydrocarbon chain. Interpretation of the diagnostic ions resulting from fragmentation allows for the determination of double bond position relative to the carboxyl group (Christie, 1998). Both DMOX and picolinyl esters can be separated by GC although DMOX derivatives have

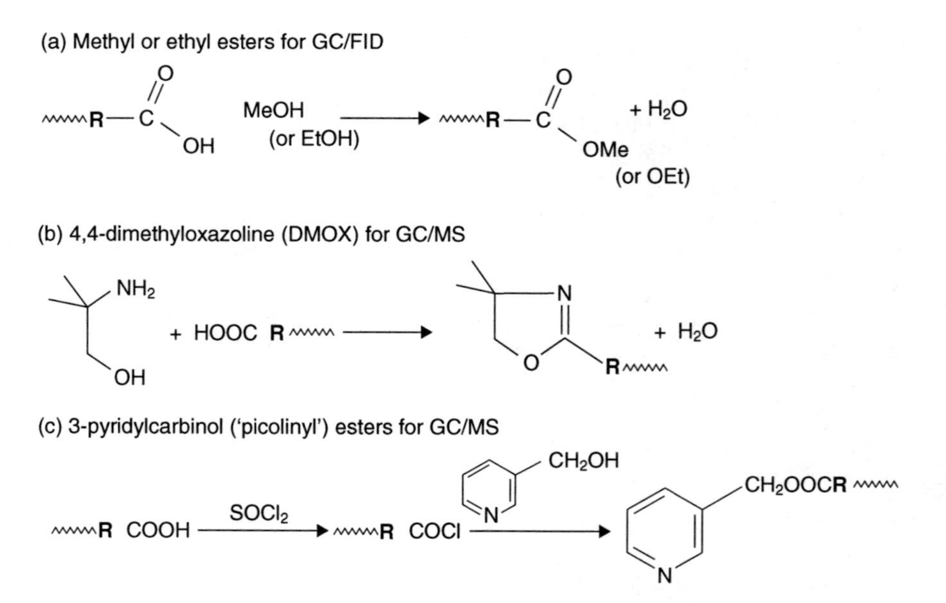

Fig. 7.2 (a–c) Comparison of fatty acid derivatives for GC and GC/MS analyses.

the advantage of being only slightly less volatile than methyl esters (Christie *et al.*, 1986; Zhang *et al.*, 1988).

7.4.1 GC columns to resolve omega-3 FAME

A requirement of all chromatographic procedures is that the system is able to separate components to be quantified from other components and to produce repeatable peak areas, retention times and peak widths within an acceptable run-time. Hence, in principle, the GC/FID analysis of omega-3 fatty acids only requires the separation of the seven omega-3 FAME mentioned above, along with any internal standards used. However, for food analysis it is more common practice to use GC methods that also separate other FAME relevant to health and nutrition, as well as the omega-3 FAME, so that total saturated, monounsaturated and polyunsaturated fat can be quantified.

In principle, it is possible to specify in a method a particular column, injector liner, carrier gas and all flow rates and temperatures. However, in practice the actual chromatogram obtained will vary between laboratories, makes of gas chromatograph, days and even between column batches. A more practical approach is to define a system performance check that ensures that a system is able to separate important components that are most likely to co-elute. For example, in AOCS Official Method Ce 1i-07 (Determination of saturated, *cis*-monounsaturated and *cis*-polyunsaturated fatty acids in marine and other oils containing long-chain polyunsaturated fatty acids by capillary GLC), a general description of the column type is given: '*the capillary GC column should be of fused silica capillary 30 m in length, and 0.25 mm i.d., 0.25 μm coating of polyethylene glycol (PEG)*' followed by a list of examples from six suppliers. Then, the system suitability check specifies that the chromatography is such that authentic FAME standards of heneicosapentaenoic acid (n-3 21:5) should be baseline separated from the internal standard tricosanoic acid (23:0), and lignoceric acid (24:0) should be baseline separated from DHA (n-3 22:6) which should be baseline resolved from the 24:1 isomers. If these critical separations are achieved on a similar phase to that specified in the method, then it is likely that all of the separations required for omega-3 analysis are achieved.

However, this does not mean that all GC/FID peaks are, in reality, single components. For example, PUFA components such as EPA and DHA are assumed to be in the *all-cis* configuration but, following heat treatment during processing of an omega-3 containing supplement or food, it is highly likely that a small percentage of these PUFA components are isomerized to the many possible geometrical isomers containing one or more *trans* double bonds, even assuming no bond migration. The *trans* isomers of monounsaturates, and especially 18:1 fatty acids, have been studied in detail and GC methods developed to separate many of the possible isomers using 100–200 m long columns and long run-times (Kramer *et al.*, 2002). However, there is such a large increase in the number of possible isomers as the number of double bonds increase that it becomes impossible to separate all positional and geometrical isomers of PUFA. In summary, the assumed *all-cis* peaks for PUFA such as EPA may in reality co-elute with low abundance isomers of *all-cis* EPA. Such complex co-elutions can be revealed by using silver ion chromatography prior to GC (Fournier *et al.*, 2006) but usually remain hidden in PUFA quantification by GC/FID.

Since any column used must be qualified by the user as 'fit for purpose', meeting the requirements of the separation and the analyst, it is not particularly useful to describe in detail the exact columns that have been used in published analyses, but rather we give a brief overview that could be helpful in column selection. As indicated above, methods specifically designed for fish oil analysis tend to favour the polar 'wax' columns containing polyethylene glycol or Carbowax™, such as Supelcowax™ or Omegawax™ (Supelco) or Famewax (Restek) which are especially successful in resolving long-chain omega-3 fatty acids whilst keeping run-times in the 20–45 min range for standard bore columns. The performance of these columns (and others) should be monitored over time since critical pairs that are readily separated with a new column may co-elute after a number of runs.

Methods aiming at more universal fatty acid separations including resolving some *cis/trans* isomers of monounsaturates would typically use a longer column (60–200 m) and most frequently make use of columns having a high percentage of cyanopropyl polysiloxane phase. Examples of the latter include BPX-70 and BPX-90 (SGE), CP-Sil 88 (Varian) DB-23 (Agilent) and SP-2560 (Supelco) (see Cruz-Hernandez and Destaillats, 2012). Many studies have looked at the elution patterns of these phases in detail to understand the effect of phase composition (Harynuk *et al.*, 2006), predict the fatty acid elutions (Mjøs, 2003) and optimize their performance for food lipid analysis including omega-3s (Petrović *et al.*, 2010). Recently, a comparison of the use of 30 m wax columns with the 100 m cyanopropyl colum SP-2560 (Santercole *et al.*, 2012) concluded that whilst the wax columns are valuable in identifying PUFA and are specified in standard methods for marine oils (e.g. AOCS Ce1i-07), they are not effective in separating unsaturated geometric isomers, as mentioned above. In order to even partially identify these *trans* isomers, both pre-fractionation using silver ion solid-phase extraction and analysis by both columns is necessary. This will not be practical for most food analyses.

In addition to the above GC column methods, there are some newer developments that are beneficial in omega-3 analyses. Firstly, most standard methods have been developed using conventional GC columns used under moderate conditions and hence have relatively long run-times. However, much work has been done in optimizing equivalent separations at high speed using microbore columns and other instrumental techniques. The separation of the important omega-3 fatty acids in less than 5 min has been demonstrated in a number of studies as described in a recent review (Cruz-Hernandez and Destaillats, 2009). Such high throughput analysis is desirable to allow routine omega-3 measurements in food lipids. Another important advance in GC analysis is the use of two-dimensional (2D) GC for the analysis of FAME (Western *et al.*, 2002). In comprehensive 2D GC, components eluting from a conventional first column are 'modulated' onto a second short column of different phase and with a fast cycle time. The combination of two orthogonal separations means that much greater separating power can be achieved overall. Although specialized equipment is required, there is considerable potential for 2D-GC to be used in solving some of the challenges in complex FAME analysis.

7.5 'One-step' methods combining extraction, digestion and derivatization

In order to reduce the number of steps of sample manipulation, the amount of solvent used and the overall time and efficiency for derivitization and analysis, *in situ* derivitization methods, also known as 'one-step extraction' (OSE) methods, have been developed. As indicated in Fig. 7.1, these methods allow a suitably homogeneous sample containing fatty acids within a food or tissue to undergo lipid extraction and transesterification to FAME in a single step. The need for a homogeneous sample cannot be overemphasized given the inhomogeneity of many foods containing, or fortified with, omega-3s and the small sample size typical for these methods. However, the simplicity of the OSE approach allows for replicates to be readily performed.

The principles of OSE are not new, having been proposed in the 1960s (Abel *et al.*, 1963) for the extraction of lipids from bacteria with transesterification using BCl_3, in the 1980s (Lepage and Roy, 1984) using methanolic HCl prepared by the addition of acetyl chloride to methanol for adipose tissue and (Sukhija and Palmquist, 1988) for feed. The OSE method of Sukhija and Palmquist, who also used methanolic HCl but added benzene at the start of extraction, was later used for processed foods (Ulberth and Henninger, 1992) and it was shown that the total fat content of a BCR® food reference material, determined by GC/FID of FAME produced by the OSE method, matched exactly the reference values. The Ulberth and Henninger method (1992) was used to quantify freeze-dried egg yolk lipids which contain small but significant amounts of DHA (Schreiner, 2006b). This method was also later adapted for use with microencapsulated fish oil powder (MEG-3®, Ocean Nutrition Canada) incorporated into omega-3 fortified functional foods (Curtis *et al.*, 2008). This encapsulated powder is a challenging matrix since it comprises an enzymatically cross-linked protein shell, which remains at least partially intact with the typical organic solvents used for lipid extraction. The reported OSE method involves heating a dry sample with methanolic HCl, prepared from acetyl chloride, along with the toluene extraction solvent. At the end of the reaction period, the FAME appear in the toluene phase. It is essential to carefully monitor recoveries through the OSE process, as described by Curtis *et al.* (2008). In the latter study, the internal standard trinonadecanoin is used both to correct for derivitization efficiency, since it is added as a triacylglyceride but measured as a FAME, and for losses due to sample handling. In addition, as for all accurate omega-3 analyses, an internal standard (methyl tricosanoate) is added prior to GC analysis and external standards of pure EPA- and DHA-FAME are used to determine experimental response factors.

A drawback of this acid-catalysed OSE procedure, also pointed out by Stark (2012), is that it is only suitable for low-moisture foods. Therefore, the first step must always be to dry the sample by a gentle procedure, ideally lyophilization. A useful refinement to the acid-catalysed OSE method has been reported (Xu *et al.*, 2010) in which the sample with methanol–benzene mixture is cooled in a dry ice bath prior to addition of acetyl chloride directly into the cold mixture. This reduces the hazards to the analyst due to the exothermic reaction with acetyl chloride. Then, the authors found that instead of carrying out the methylation at 100 °C (which is a higher temperature than suggested in other OSE methods) they were able to leave the reaction in the dark at room temperature for 24 h. The recovery of the omega-3 PUFA standard of DHA was close to 100 % using this method whereas, with the other two methods which involved high-temperature methylation, lower values were obtained. Similar results were seen for DHA levels in some commercial emulsions. Additional fatty acid peaks were formed under the high-temperature methylation conditions, but these were not seen for room-temperature methylation. More work is still required to see if this low-temperature methylation could be effective in food analysis but, nonetheless, the possibility of minimizing thermal damage to omega-3 PUFA merits further investigation.

It is well known that the conversion of lipids into FAME can be catalysed by acidic or basic conditions (Carrapiso and García, 2000). The advantage of the acidic conditions described above is that both free fatty acids and those bound in other lipids, such as triacylglycerides or phospholipids, are converted to FAME. A disadvantage is that long reaction times and elevated temperatures are required – typically for most OSE procedures 1–2 h at 60–80 °C. The use of base-catalysed OSE procedures, on the other hand, may have the advantage of being faster and requiring lower temperatures, but they catalyse transesterification reactions, not esterification reactions, so that free fatty acids and certain other minor classes of lipids do not get converted to FAME. A solution to this problem widely used in the analysis of omega-3 oils is to use both base- and acid-catalysed procedures to ensure complete methylation (Ackman, 1998). A variation on this general idea has been described in the 'direct' method of O'Fallen *et al.* (2007). They showed the effectiveness of a method conducted in up to 33 % water for the extraction/methylation of wet meat tissues, oils including fish oil, and feedstuffs. The procedure is to first saponify the wet sample using KOH in methanol at 55 °C for 1.5 h. Then, the sample is neutralized and the free fatty acids are converted to FAME by H_2SO_4-catalysed esterification in the same tube at 55 °C for a further 1.5 h. It is significant that this procedure is conducted on wet samples – indeed the authors point out that this is of course required for hydrolysis – and, like all *in situ* methods, requires no separate lipid extraction step.

Zhu *et al.* (2011) compared the use of acid- and base-catalysed OSE methods with solvent extraction or acid hydrolysis/solvent extraction followed by acid catalysed methylation for the analysis of EPA and DHA in fortified cereal-based foods – flaked breakfast cereal, snack bar, bread and muffins. The omega-3 fortification of the foods used an 'encapsulated fish oil emulsion' formed by passing fish oil and a protein solution through a high-pressure homogenizer. They used a similar acid catalysed OSE method to that described above (Curtis *et al.*, 2008) except for the use of methanolic HCl with dimethoxypropane in place of methanolic HCl from acetyl chloride, and they used a saponification/acid catalysed esterification method similar to O'Fallon *et al.* (2007). All four methods they studied were found to be suitable for analysis of fish oil whereas, in the foods they tested, the acid catalysed OSE method was overall the best for determination of EPA and DHA and the saponification method was especially suitable for bread. Their concluding words of warning were that it may still be necessary to determine the optimal extraction method for each food type. Clearly, the extraction of the fish oil emulsion was not effective using Soxhlet solvent extraction alone as had been observed in the earlier report on microencapsulated oil (Curtis *et al.*, 2008).

In summary, the various manifestations of one-step or *in situ* extraction/methylation procedures are readily adaptable to omega-3 analysis of foods and supplements. They offer the potential for higher throughput (Stark, 2012), lower cost and potentially more accurate and precise results. However, currently there is not one standardized method suitable for all food types, so method optimization and validation for individual food types remains essential.

7.6 Examples in literature of the analysis of omega-3 containing foods

7.6.1 Dairy products

Dairy products are a promising food class for the incorporation of omega-3 fatty acids because of their high usage in many cultures and their storage under refrigerated conditions. Incorporation into the milk can be achieved to some extent via omega-3 supplementation of the feed of the lactating animals (Or-Rashid *et al.*, 2009). In this case, omega-3 analysis could be performed following standard official methods of extraction and methylation procedures for dairy products usually using base hydrolysis, such as ISO-IDF (2001, 2002) or AOAC 996.06 (AOAC International, 2006), which specifies extraction of fat from dairy products except cheese using ammonium hydroxide (in ethanol/water at 70–80 °C with shaking in a Mojonnier flask) followed by extraction into ether. For cheese, AOAC 996.06 specifies hydrolysis using ammonium hydroxide followed by hydrochloric acid on a steam bath. In all cases, as discussed earlier in this chapter, for accurate omega-3 analysis consideration should be given to use of appropriate columns, standards and response factors. This is especially important since dairy fat contains a high amount of short-chain fatty acids and hence methods are not optimized for long-chain PUFA such as DHA. In particular, triundecanoin (C11:0 triglyceride) can be used as an internal standard for dairy fat analysis and in AOAC 996.06, but short-chain fatty acids may not be the most suitable for measurement of omega-3 PUFA. To measure the DHA content of milk 'naturally enhanced' with DHA, Or-Rashid *et al.* (2009) used a modified Bligh and Dyer extraction followed by acidification, then methylation of the lipid extract in benzene with sodium methoxide at room temperature for 25 min and, finally, treatment with methanolic sulfuric acid at 50 °C for 15 min. This multistep procedure, which separates extraction from base-catalysed methylation and acid-catalysed esterification steps, is in contrast to OSE procedures or the direct procedure described by O'Fallon *et al.* (2007) that is directly applicable to milk without fat extraction, and has also been applied to several cheeses.

Omega-3 fatty acids may also be incorporated into the food by the addition of fish or algal oils or encapsulated oils (Bermúdez-Aguirre and Barbosa-Cánovas, 2011). In the latter case, any method to measure omega-3 fatty acids must fully release the microencapsulated fat. The direct method of O'Fallon *et al.* (2007) was used, starting with hydrolysis by KOH, which appeared to be effective in liberating fatty acids from encapsulated oils in milk products, although the recovery of omega-3 was not stated (Bermúdez-Aguirre and Barbosa-Cánovas, 2011).

7.6.2 Meat

Meat can provide significant quantities of long-chain omega-3 fatty acids with a high amount of docosapentaenoic acid (DPA, 20:5 n-3) relative to marine sources (Howe *et al.*, 2007). One method proposed to measure total fatty acids in adipose tissue (Aldai *et al.*, 2006) makes use of direct saponification of the sample by KOH in methanol followed by methylation using trimethylsilyl diazomethane (TMS-DM), a source of diazomethane said to be safer to handle and more stable with fewer side reactions. The emphasis of that report was measurement of conjugated linoleic acid (CLA), but the validation included EPA in the list of fatty acids selected for validation measurements. Good linearity was achieved for EPA with a limit of quantitation (LOQ) of 0.033 mg for standards. However, the reported response factors relative to the C21:0 internal standard were far from the theoretical values for the FID detector and the coefficients of variance for fatty acid measurements on meat samples, including the omega-3s, were relatively high.

A subsequent comparison of four methods for extraction and methylation of fat from meat (Juárez *et al.*, 2008) also concluded that the use of TMS-DM, in that case following Folch extraction, also showed higher variation than other methods. As described in Section 7.5, the method of O'Fallon was developed with meat tissue samples in mind and provides a one-reaction vessel procedure for extraction and methylation. However, care must be taken to use an appropriate internal standard for omega-3 PUFA and to use response factors. The method described (O'Fallon, 2007) uses C13:0 methyl ester as internal standard, selected because it is soluble in methanol, but this not ideal for quantifying long-chain PUFA and is not in the triglyceride form so complete conversion of sample to methyl esters must be assumed. Since most fatty acid methods are designed to quantitatively convert all fatty acids into FAME, information on the distribution of fatty acids amongst lipid classes is generally lost.

Although fractionation into lipid classes is beyond the scope of this chapter (but see, e.g. Ruiz *et al.*, 2004), it is worth pointing out that FAME analysis of specific lipid fractions is readily achieved. For example, using simple procedures, lipids from fish (European perch) and reindeer meat were fractionated into polar and neutral lipids by solid-phase extraction or into triacylglycerides and phospholipids by thin-layer chromatography (Sampels and Pickova, 2011). It was found that the omega-3 content of the polar lipid content of the reindeer meat was 11 % (mostly DPA and EPA) but only 3 % in the neutral lipid fraction; the corresponding results for perch lipids were 51 % (mostly DHA) and 23 %. Some differences between the fractionation methods were noted (Sampels and Pickova, 2011).

7.7 Alternative analytical methods for omega-3 analysis

Although GC/FID analysis of FAME accounts for the overwhelming majority of omega-3 fatty acid determinations, other methods of analysis are possible and can be used to confirm GC/FID results or impart additional information or functionality as described in outline below.

7.7.1 GC/MS and LC/MS

The success of the FID detector comes from it being a universal detector for organic compounds that are amenable to GC analysis, providing a highly reproducible and fairly uniform response over a wide dynamic range. It is therefore ideal for the quantification of FAME components. The drawback of the FID is that it does not provide any further structural information over what can be indirectly inferred from the GC retention times. In contrast, mass spectrometry coupled to gas chromatography (GC/MS) still provides retention time data but, in addition, provides a wealth of information that can relate to the true identity of the compound. For instance, electron impact mass spectra can be matched to compounds in extensive libraries for identification; chemical ionization mass spectra can confirm the molecular weight of a FAME and, hence, chain length and number of double bonds; and high-resolution exact mass measurements that are becoming increasingly routine can be used to confirm the elemental composition. Derivatives of fatty acids other than FAME can be chosen to enhance fragmentation.

However, the major factor limiting the use GC/MS in place of GC/FID for quantitative FAME analysis is that response factors for different compounds vary considerably, so the concept of achieving approximate quantification using peak areas does not hold. Instead, each individual fatty acid should have its own calibration curve. Despite this, some authors have recently presented methods that do allow quantification by GC/MS, especially when using selected ion monitoring (SIM) mode (Dodds *et al.*, 2005). Particularly encouraging is the proposal (Thurnhofer and Vetter, 2006) to use d_3-FAME as internal standards for GC/MS in SIM mode. These would have to be added after transesterification but, where pure standards of the fatty acids are available – as is the case for the omega-3 fatty acids – they provide ideal internal standards having the identical properties to the analytes but separated by three *m/z* units in the mass spectra. However, to date there are very few reports of the use of GC/MS in quantitative FAME analysis.

In contrast, there are now many reports of lipid analyses by LC/MS as reviewed by Christie and Han (2010). In general, such data falling into the general category of 'lipidomics' is not suitable for the accurate determination of omega-3 contents even where intact molecular species are identified as containing omega-3 fatty acids. Rather, these lipidomic experiments are most suitable for elucidation of differences in lipid profiles between individual samples that differ in biological state or between specimens. They do not, in general, rigorously quantify individual lipid species. LC methods for the analysis of fatty acids and various derivatives of fatty acids, in combination with MS and other detectors have been reviewed by Lima and Abdalla (2002).

7.7.2 Nuclear magnetic resonance (NMR)

As one of the most widely used methods for the elucidation of organic molecules (Capozzi and Cremonini, 2008), nuclear magnetic resonance (NMR) using ^{1}H, ^{13}C and ^{31}P nuclei also plays an important role in lipid analyses (Diehl, 2001). High resolution ^{1}H NMR has been used to quantify DHA and the molar concentration of total omega-3 fatty acids in fish oils (Igarashi *et al.*, 2000) and to quantify EPA and DHA (Guillén *et al.*, 2008). This has been extended to some extent into multicomponent analyses (Siddiqui *et al.*, 2003). An advance with great potential in food science is the quantitative analysis of total omega-3, EPA and DHA in the intact muscles of fish using high-resolution magic angle spinning ^{1}H NMR spectroscopy (Nestor *et al.*, 2010).

These studies are of great importance since the development of fundamental methods for omega-3 analysis allows for rigorous cross-validation of analytical measurements. Although there is no likelihood of significant displacement of GC/FID as the standard method for omega-3 analysis in the near future, such cross-validation of results is particularly important where the primary method involves several steps of sample handling, derivitization and the use of multiple standards, giving considerable scope for inaccuracies to occur. Probably the most important aspect of the use of ^{13}C NMR in omega-3 analysis comes from its ability to elucidate the regioisomeric distribution of omega-3 fatty acids in triacylglycerides (Suárez *et al.*, 2010). For example, it was shown that, in the reconstituted triacylglycerides prepared by *Candida antarctica* lipase-B glycerolysis of the ethyl ester or free fatty acid forms of anchovy/sardine fish oil, DHA was preferentially attached to the sn-1,3 positions while EPA was equally distributed, amongst sn- positions. The sn-2 substitution pattern determined by ^{13}C NMR has also been used to authenticate fish oil samples (Standal *et al.*, 2011) since the distribution between EPA, DHA and other saturated and monounsaturated fatty acids is unique for each fish species. Obtaining information on the positional distribution of fatty acids is impossible by GC/FID alone, although it is possible in combination with regiospecific enzymatic methods (Amate *et al.*, 1999). However, the ^{13}C NMR experiment has a higher information content and can also identify minor lipid components such as mono- or diglycerides or other esters (Standal *et al.*, 2011).

In addition to omega-3 quantification, ^{1}H NMR has also been used to study several chemical and physical properties of matrices containing omega-3. For instance, the oxidation of omega-3 fatty acids in fish oil samples was measured by ^{1}H NMR (Tyl *et al.*, 2008) and results were found to agree with GC measurements, except at high levels of oxidation. ^{1}H NMR techniques were also used to investigate fish oil emulsions via measurements of the transverse relaxation time (T_2) (Shen *et al.*, 2005). This provided some evidence that the unsaturated parts of the fatty acid chains within an oil droplet tend to stay in the core of the oil droplets, as previously suggested by McClements and Decker (2000).

7.7.3 Infrared (IR) spectroscopy

Infrared (IR) spectroscopy has been used in a number of areas relevant to food and oils containing omega-3 fatty acids. Fourier transform-near infrared (FT-NIR) has been adopted as an AOCS Official Method Cd

1e-01(Li *et al.*, 2000; AOCS, 2009) to measure iodine values of edible oils. FT-IR combined with GC allows separation and identification of *cis* and *trans* geometric isomers at sub-nanogram levels in edible oil samples (Mossoba *et al.*, 2001). Chemometric approaches have been implemented to develop FT-NIR calibration models based on GC/FID data to measure fatty acids in edible oils (Azizian and Kramer, 2005). These ideas were extended to allow the rapid quantification of all of the omega-3 fish oil fatty acids by FT-NIR (Azizian *et al.*, 2010). It should be remembered that these secondary measurements are only valid if samples fall within the calibration model, so their application is limited by the model developed. The study by Azizian *et al.* (2010) found that certain discrepancies in the data could only be explained by limitations in the resolution of the original GC/FID data obtained using a 30 m wax capillary GC column. The model was significantly improved when using GC/FID data obtained using a 100 m cyanopropyl column that could resolve many more geometric isomers.

FT-IR in the near-IR or mid-IR regions has been used to characterize the fatty acid composition of foodstuffs such as margarine (Hernández-Martínez *et al.*, 2010), milk (Ferrand *et al.*, 2011) and seed oil content (Kim *et al.*, 2007). The simplicity of these FT-IR measurements taken directly on the food item makes development of IR models attractive where high throughput sample analysis is required, such as in quality control, plant breeding or stability studies. Total omega-3 fatty acid content, including DHA and EPA, was quantified by FT-IR from microencapsulated fish oil without pretreatment (Vongsvivut *et al.*, 2012). Reasonable agreement was achieved between a sample test set measured using the FT-IR model or the standard GC/FID method.

7.8 Future trends

Currently, GC/FID analysis of omega-3 fatty acids as FAME is the standard method and is likely to be so for the foreseeable future. Advances in the automation of extraction and derivitization methods are underway, especially in the field of blood lipid analysis. It is likely that these will be applied in the food area but, since omega-3 fatty acids can be present in a wide range of food matrices, automation of one extraction/derivitization method for one food will not necessarily directly translate to another food. Supercritical fluid and microwave-assisted extraction methods may become more common, although growth in the use of SFE especially may be limited by the capital cost of the equipment. It would be desirable to have more standardization in OSE and similar methods of omega-3 analyses. This will require interlaboratory studies and would allow the development of new official methods for omega-3 analysis in foods. GC methods are expected to continue to advance with more emphasis on fast GC for higher throughput. It is hoped that many other valid analytical techniques will continue to be developed, such as further advances in NMR methods and 2D-GC methods. These will be essential to elucidate novel components in lipids, in more in-depth structural analyses than can be achieved by GC/FID of FAME alone, and as orthogonal techniques used in method validation. It seems highly likely that FT-IR, a rapid and inexpensive technique requiring little or no sample preparation, may play an increasingly important role in omega-3 measurements in the future. However, FT-IR measurements are most applicable where repetitive measurements on a well-defined range of food or oil samples is involved.

7.9 Sources of further information and advice

For an all encompassing review of GC and lipid analysis the reader is referred to *Gas Chromatography and Lipids: A Practical Guide* by W. W. Christie (1989). For a general review of GC and more recent methods of lipid analysis, *Lipid Analysis – Isolation, Separation, Identification and Lipidomic Analysis* (4th edition) written by Christie and Han (2010). Small selections of both books and a comprehensive review of lipid analysis are available on www.lipidlibrary.co.uk, a website developed by W. W. Christie. The Cyberlipid Center at www.cyberlipid.org is an alternative website covering many techniques for lipid analyses. Recommended reviews specific to the analysis of omega-3 fatty acids are 'Analysis of fatty acids in functional foods with emphasis on omega-3 fatty acids and conjugated linoleic acid' (Dobson, 2008) and 'Omega 3 and omega 6 fatty acids' (Stark, 2012). For more sources of information see Table 7.1.

Selected official methods specific to omega-3 analysis are as outlined in Table 7.2. These and other descriptions of lipid analysis can be found at American Oil Chemists Society – www.aocs.org; Association of Official Analytical Chemists International – www.aoac.org; and International Organization for Standardization – www.iso.org.

7.10 References

ABEL K, DESCHMERTZING H and PETERSON J I (1963) 'Classification of microorganisms by analysis of chemical composition I', *J Bacteriol*, 85, 1039–1044.

ACKMAN R G (1998) 'Remarks on official methods employing boron trifluoride in the preparation of methyl esters of the fatty acids of fish oils', *J Am Oil Chem Soc*, 75, 541–545.

ACKMAN R G (2002) 'The gas chromatograph in practical analysis of common and uncommon fatty acids for the 21st century', *Anal Chim Acta*, 465, 175–192.

ACKMAN R G (2008) 'Application of gas-liquid chromatography to lipid separation and analysis: qualitative and quantitative analysis', in CHOW C K (ed.), *Fatty Acids in Foods and Their Health Implications* (3rd edn). Boca Raton, FL: CRC Press, 47–65.

ACKMAN R G and SIPOS J C (1964) 'Application of specific response factors in the gas chromatographic analysis of methyl esters of fatty acids with flame ionization detectors', *J Am Oil Chem Soc*, 41, 377–378.

ADAM F, ABERT-VIAN M, PELTIER G and CHEMAT F (2012) '"Solvent-free" ultrasound-assisted extraction of lipids from fresh microalgae cells: a green, clean and scalable process', *Bioresour Technol*, 114, 457–465.

ALDAI N, OSORO K, BARRÓN L J R, NÁJERA A I (2006) 'Gas-liquid chromatographic method for analysing complex mixtures of fatty acids including conjugated linoleic acids (*cis*9*trans*11 and *trans*10*cis*12 isomers) and long-chain (n-3 or n-6) polyunsaturated fatty acids application to the intramuscular fat of beef meat', *J Chromatogr A*, 1110, 133–139.

AMATE L, RAMÍREZ M and GIL A (1999) 'Positional analysis of triglycerides and phospholipids rich in long-chain polyunsaturated fatty acids', *Lipids*, 34, 865–871.

AOAC INTERNATIONAL (2006) *Official Methods of Analysis of AOAC International (OMA)* (18th edn). Arlington, VA: AOAC International.

AOCS (2009) *Official Methods and the Recommended Practices of the AOCS* (6th edn). Urbana, IL: AOCS Press.

ARNÁIZ E, BERNAL J, MARTIN M T, GARCÍA-VIGUERA C, BERNAL J L and TORIBIO L (2011) 'Supercritical fluid extraction of lipids from broccoli leaves', *Eur J Lipid Sci Technol*, 113, 479–486.

AZIZIAN H and KRAMER J K G (2005) 'A rapid method for the quantification of fatty acids in fats and oils with emphasis on trans fatty acids using fourier transform near infrared spectroscopy (FT-NIR)', *Lipids*, 40, 855–867.

AZIZIAN H, KRAMER J K G, EHLER S and CURTIS J M (2010) 'Rapid quantitation of fish oil fatty acids and their ethyl esters by FT-NIR models', *Eur J Lipid Sci Technol*, 112, 452–462.

BANNON C D, CRASKE J D and HILLIKER A E (1986) 'Analysis of fatty acid methyl esters with high accuracy and reliability. V. validation of theoretical relative response factors of unsaturated esters in the flame ionization detector', *J Am Oil Chem Soc*, 63, 105–110.

BERMÚDEZ-AGUIRRE D and BARBOSA-CÁNOVAS G V (2011) 'Quality of selected cheeses fortified with vegetable and animal sources of omega-3', *LWT Food Sci Technol*, 44, 1577–1584.

BLIGH E G and DYER W J (1959) 'A rapid method of total lipid extraction and purification', *Can J Biochem Physiol*, 37, 911–917.

BREIVIK H R, BIRRETZEN B, DAH K H, KROKAN H E and BONAA K H (1996) *Fatty acid composition*, US Patent 5,502,077.

CAPOZZI R and CREMONINI M A (2008) 'Nuclear magnetic resonance spectroscopy in food analysis', in ÖTLEŞ S (ed.), *Handbook of Food Analysis Instruments*. Boca Raton, FL: CRC Press, 282–311.

CARRAPISO A I and GARCÍA C (2000) 'Development in lipid analysis: some new extraction techniques and in situ transesterification', *Lipids*, 35, 1167–1177.

CHRISTIE W W (1989) *Gas Chromatography and Lipids: a Practical Guide*. Dundee: The Oily Press.

CHRISTIE W W (1998) 'Gas chromatography–mass spectrometry methods for structural analysis of fatty acids', *Lipids*, 33, 343–353.

CHRISTIE W W and HAN X (2010) *Lipid analysis – Isolation, Separation, Identification and Lipidomic Analysis* (4th edn). Bridgwater: The Oily Press.

CHRISTIE W W, BRECHANY E Y, JOHNSON S B and HOLMAN R T (1986) 'A comparison of pyrrolidide and picolinyl ester derivatives for the identification of fatty acids in natural samples by gas chromatography–mass spectrometry', *Lipids*, 21, 657–661.

CREWS C (2008) 'Analysis of fatty acids in fortified foods', in OTTAWAY P B (ed.), *Food Fortification and Supplementation*. Boca Raton, FL: CRC Press, 153–174.

CRUZ-HERNANDEZ C and DESTAILLATS F (2009) 'Recent advances in fast gas-chromatography: application to the separation of fatty acid methyl esters', *J Liq Chromatogr Relat Technol*, 32, 1672–1688.

CRUZ-HERNANDEZ C and DESTAILLATS F (2012) 'Analysis of lipids by gas chromatography', in POOLE C (ed.), *Gas Chromatography*. Waltham: Elsevier, 529–544.

CURTIS J M (2007) 'Analysis of oils and concentrates', in BREIVIK H (ed.), *Long-Chain Omega-3 Specialty Oils*. Bridgwater: The Oily Press, 219–241.

CURTIS J M, BERRIGAN N and DAUPHINEE P (2008) 'The determination of n-3 fatty acid levels in food products containing microencapsulated fish oil using the one-step extraction method. Part 1: measurement in a raw ingredient and in dry powdered foods', *J Am Oil Chem Soc*, 85, 297–305.

DIEHL B W K (2001) 'High resolution NMR spectroscopy', *Eur J Lipid Sci Technol*, 103, 830–834.

DOBSON G (2008) 'Analysis of fatty acids in functional foods with emphasis on n-3 fatty acids and conjugated linoleic acid', in HURST W J (ed.), *Methods of Analysis for Functional Foods and Nutraceuticals* (2nd edn). Boca Raton, FL: CRC Press, 86–147.

DOBSON G and CHRISTIE W W (2002) 'Spectroscopy and spectrometry of lipids – Part 2', *Eur J Lipid Sci Technol*, 104, 36–43.

DODDS E D, MCCOY M R, GELDENHUYS A, REA L D and KENNISH J M (2004) 'Microscale recovery of total lipids from fish tissue by accelerated solvent extraction', *J Am Oil Chem Soc*, 81, 835–840.

DODDS E D, MCCOY M R, REA L D and KENNISH J M (2005) 'Gas chromatographic quantification of fatty acid methyl esters: flame ionization detection vs. electron impact mass spectrometry', *Lipids*, 40, 419–428.

DRUSCH S, REGIER M and BRUHN M (2012) 'Recent advances in the microencapsulation of oils high in polyunsaturated fatty acids', in MCELHATTON A and SORBRAL P J (eds), *Novel Technologies in Food Science*. New York: Springer, 159–182.

FERRAND M, HUQUET B, BARBEY S, BARILLET F, FAUCON F, LARROQUE H, LERAY O, TROMMENSCHLAGER J M and BROCHARD M (2011) 'Determination of fatty acid profile in cow's milk using mid-infrared spectrometry: interest of applying a variable selection by genetic algorithms before a PLS regression', *Chemometr Intell Lab*, 106, 183–189.

FOLCH J, LEES M and STANLEY G H S (1957) 'A simple method for the isolation and purification of total lipides from animal tissues', *J Biol Chem*, 226, 497–509.

FOURNIER V, JUANÉDA P, DESTAILLATS F, DIONISI F, LAMBELET P, SÉBÉDIO J and BERDEAUX O (2006) 'Analysis of eicosapentaenoic and docosahexaenoic acid geometrical isomers formed during fish oil deodorization', *J Chromatogr A*, 1129, 21–28.

GOED (2012) *GOED Voluntary Monograph (v. 4). Omega-3 EPA, Omega-3 DHA, Omega-3 EPA & DHA*. Salt Lake City, UT: Global Organization for EPA and DHA Omega-3, available at: http://www.goedomega3.com/images/stories/files/goedmonograph.pdf [accessed February 2013].

GUILLÉN M D, CARTON I, GOICOECHEA E and URIARTE P S (2008) 'Characterization of cod liver oil by spectroscopic techniques. New approaches for the determination of compositional parameters, acyl groups, and cholesterol from ^{1}H nuclear magnetic resonance and Fourier transform infrared spectral data', *J Agric Food Chem*, 56, 9072–9079.

HARYNUK J, WYNNE P M and MARRIOTT P J (2006) 'Evaluation of new stationary phases for the separation of fatty acid methyl esters', *Chromatographia*, 63, S61–S66.

HERNANDEZ E M and HOSOKAWA M (2011) *Omega-3 Oils: Applications in Functional Foods*. Urbana, IL: AOCS Press.

HERNÁNDEZ-MARTÍNEZ M, GALLARDO-VELÁZQUEZ T and OSORIO-REVILLA G (2010) 'Rapid characterization and identification of fatty acids in margarines using horizontal attenuated total reflectance Fourier transform infrared spectroscopy (HATR-FTIR)', *Eur Food Res Technol*, 231, 321–329.

HOWE P, BUCKLEY J and MEYER B (2007) 'Long-chain omega-3 fatty acids in red meat', *Nutr Diet*, 64, S135–S139.

IGARASHI T, AURSAND M, HIRATA Y, GIBBESTAD I S, WADA S and NONAKA M (2000) 'Non-destructive quantitative determination of docosahexaenoic acid and n-3 fatty acids in fish oils by high-resolution ^{1}H nuclear magnetic resonance spectroscopy', *J Am Oil Chem Soc*, 77, 737–748.

ISO-IDF (2001) *Milk and milk products – extraction methods for lipids and liposoluble compounds*, International Standard ISO 14156-IDF 172:2001. Brussels: International Dairy Federation.

ISO-IDF (2002) *Milk fat – preparation of fatty acid methyl esters*, International Standard ISO 15884-IDF 182:2002. Brussels: International Dairy Federation.

IVANOV D, ČOLOVIČ R, BERA O, LEVIČ J and SREDANOVIČ S (2011) 'Supercritical fluid extraction as a method for fat content determination and preparative technique for fatty acid analysis in mesh feed for pigs', *Eur Food Res Technol*, 233, 343–350.

IVERSON S J, LANG S L C and COOPER M H (2001) 'Comparison of the Bligh and Dyer and Folch methods for total lipid determination in a broad range of marine tissue', *Lipids*, 36, 1283–1287.

JAMES A T and MARTIN A J P (1952) 'Gas–liquid partition chromatography: the separation and micro-estimation of volatile fatty acids from formic acid to dodecanoic acid', *Biochem J*, 50, 679–690.

JOSEPH J D and ACKMAN R G (1992) 'Capillary column gas chromatographic method for analysis of encapsulated fish oils and fish oil ethyl esters: collaborative study', *J AOAC Int*, 75, 488–506.

JOSEPH J D and SEABORN G T (1990) 'The analysis of marine fatty acids', in STANSBY M E (ed.), *Fish Oils in Nutrition*. New York: Springer, 40–72.

JUÁREZ M, POLVILLO O, CONTÒ M, FICCO A, BALLICO S and FAILLA S (2008) 'Comparison of four extraction/methylation analytical methods to measure fatty acid composition by gas chromatography in meat', *J Chromatogr A*, 1190, 327–332.

KIM K S, PARK S H and CHOUNG M G (2007) 'Nondestructive determination of oil content and fatty acid composition in perilla seeds by near-infrared spectroscopy', *J Agric Food Chem*, 55, 1679–1685.

KOLANOWSKI W, JAWORSKA D, LAUFENBERG G and WEISSBRODT J (2007) 'Evaluation of sensory quality of instant foods fortified with omega-3 PUFA by addition of fish oil powder', *Eur Food Res Technol*, 225, 715–721.

KRAMER J K G, BLACKADAR C B and ZHOU J (2002) 'Evaluation of two GC columns (60-m SUPELCOWAX 10 and 100-m CP Sil 88) for analysis of milkfat with emphasis on CLA, 18:1, 18:2 and 18:3 isomers, and short- and long-chain FA', *Lipids*, 37, 823–835.

KRIS-ETHERTON P M, HARRIS W S and APPEL L J (2003) 'Fish consumption, fish oil, omega-3 fatty acids, and cardiovascular disease', *Arterioscler Thromb Vasc Biol*, 23, 20–30.

LEPAGE G and ROY C C (1984) 'Improved recovery of fatty acid through direct transesterification without prior extraction or purification', *J Lipid Res*, 25, 1391–1396.

LI H, VAN DE VOORT F R, ISMAIL A A, SEDMAN J, COX R, SIMARD C and BUIJS H (2000) 'Discrimination of edible oil products and quantitative determination of their iodine value by Fourier transform near-infrared spectroscopy', *J Am Oil Chem Soc*, 77, 29–36.

LIMA E S and ABDALLA D S P (2002) 'High-performance liquid chromatography of fatty acids in biological samples', *Anal Chim Acta*, 465, 81–92.

MANIRAKIZA P, COVACI A and SCHEPENS P (2001) 'Comparative study on total lipid determination using Soxhlet, Roese-Gottlieb, Bligh & Dyer, and modified Bligh & Dyer extraction methods', *J Food Compos Anal*, 14, 93–100.

MAYZAUD P and ACKMAN R G (1978) 'The 6,9,12,15,18-heneicosapentaenoic acid of seal oil', *Lipids*, 13, 24–28.

MCCLEMENTS D J and DECKER E A (2000) 'Lipid oxidation in oil-in-water emulsions: impact of molecular environment on chemical reactions in heterogeneous food systems', *J Food Sci*, 65, 1270–1282.

MIN D B and ELLEFSON W C (2010) 'Fat analysis', in NIELSON S S (ed.), *Food Analysis* (4th edn). New York: Springer, 117–132.

MJØS S A (2003) 'Identification of fatty acids in gas chromatography by application of different temperature and pressure programs on a single capillary column', *J Chromatogr A*, 1015, 151–161.

MORETTI V M and CAPRINO F (2009) 'Analysis of n-3 and n-6 fatty acids', in NOLLET L M L and TOLDRA F (eds), *Handbook of Seafood and Seafood Products Analysis*. Boca Raton, FL: CRC Press, 377–392.

MOSSOBA M M, MCDONALD R E, YURAWECZ M P and KRAMER J K G (2001) 'Application of on-line capillary GC-FTIR spectroscopy to lipid analysis', *Eur J Lipid Sci Technol*, 103, 826–829.

NESTOR G, BANKEFORS J, SCHLECHTRIEM C, BRÄNNÄS E, PICKOVA J and SANDSTRÖM C (2010) 'High-resolution ^{1}H magic angle spinning NMR spectroscopy of intact arctic char (*Salvelinus alpines*) muscle, quantitative analysis of n-3 fatty acids, EPA and DHA', *J Agric Food Chem*, 58, 10799–10803.

O'FALLON J V, BUSBOOM J R, NELSON M L and GASKINS C T (2007) 'A direct method for fatty acid methyl ester synthesis: application to wet meat tissues, oils, and feed-stuffs', *J Anim Sci*, 85, 1511–1521.

OR-RASHID M, ODONGO N E, WRIGHT T C and MCBRIDE B W (2009) 'Fatty acid profile of bovine milk naturally enhanced with docosahexaenoic acid', *J Agric Food Chem*, 57, 1366–1371.

PETROVIĆ M, KEZIĆ N and BOLANČA V (2010) 'Optimization of the GC method for routine analysis of the fatty acid profile in several food samples', *Food Chem*, 122, 285–291.

RAMALHOSA M J, PAÍGA P, MORAIS S, ALVES M R, DELERUE-MATOS C and OLIVEIRA M B P P (2012) 'Lipid content of frozen fish: comparison of different extraction methods and variability during freezing storage', *Food Chem*, 131, 328–336.

RUIZ J, ANTEQUERA T, ANDRES A I, PETRON M J and MURIEL E (2004) 'Improvement of a solid phase extraction method for analysis of lipid fractions in muscle foods' *Anal Chim Acta*, 520, 201–205

RUIZ-RODRIGUEZ A, REGLERO G and IBAÑEZ E (2010) 'Recent trends in the advanced analysis of bioactive fatty acids', *J Pharm Biomed Anal*, 51, 305–326.

SAMPELS S and PICKOVA J (2011) 'Comparison of two different methods for the separation of lipid classes and fatty acid methylation in reindeer and fish muscle', *Food Chem*, 128, 811–819.

SANTERCOLE V, DELMONTE P and KRAMER J K (2012) 'Comparison of separations of fatty acids from fish products using a 30-m Supelcowax-10 and a 100-m SP-2560 column', *Lipids*, 47, 329–344.

SCHREINER M (2006a) 'Principles for the analysis of omega-3 fatty acids', in TEALE M C (ed.), *Omega 3 Fatty Acid Research*. New York: Nova Science Publishers Inc, 1–25.

SCHREINER M (2006b) 'Optimisation of solvent extraction and direct transmethylation methods for the analysis of egg yolk lipids', *Int J Food Properties*, 9, 573–581.

SHANTHA N C (1992) 'Gas chromatography of fatty acids', *J Chromatogr*, 624, 37–51.

SHEN Z, UDABAGE P, BURGAR I and AUGUSTIN M A (2005) 'Characterization of fish oil-in-water emulsions using light-scattering, nuclear magnetic resonance, and gas chromatography–headspace analyses', *J Am Oil Chem Soc*, 82, 797–802.

SIDDIQUI N, SIM J, SILWOOD C J L, TOMS H, ILES R A and GROOTVELD M (2003) 'Multicomponent analysis of encapsulated marine oil supplements using high-resolution ^{1}H and ^{13}C NMR techniques', *J Lipid Res*, 44, 2406–2427.

STANDAL I B, AXELSON D E and AURSAND M (2011) 'Authentication of marine oils using ^{13}C NMR spectroscopy', *Lipid Technol*, 23, 152–154.

STARK K D (2012) 'Omega 3 and omega 6 fatty acids', in NOLLET F and TOLDRA L M L (eds), *Handbook of Analysis of Active Compounds in Functional Foods*. Boca Raton, FL: CRC Press, 725–746.

SUÁREZ E R, MUGFORD P F, ROLLE A J, BURTON I W and WALTER J A (2010) '^{13}C-NMR regioisomeric analysis of EPA and DHA in fish oil derived triacylglycerol concentrates', *J Am Oil Chem Soc*, 87, 1425–1433.

SUKHIJA P S and PALMQUIST D L (1988) 'Rapid method for determination of total fatty acid content and composition of feedstuffs and feces', *J Agric Food Chem*, 36, 1202–1206.

TANDE T, BREIVIK H and AASOLDSEN T (1992) 'Validation of a method for gas chromatographic analysis of eicosapentaenoic acid and docosahexenoic acid as active ingredients in medicinal products', *J Am Oil Chem Soc*, 69, 1124–1130.

THURNHOFER S and VETTER W (2006) 'Application of ethyl esters and d_3-methyl esters as internal standards for the gas chromatographic quantification of transesterified fatty acid methyl esters in food', *J Agric Food Chem*, 54, 3209–3214.

TYL C E, BRECKER L and WAGNER K (2008) '1H NMR spectroscopy as tool to follow changes in the fatty acids of fish oils', *Eur J Lipid Sci Technol*, 110, 141–148.

ULBERTH F and HENNINGER M (1992) 'One-step extraction/methylation method for determining the fatty acid composition of processed foods', *J Am Oil Chem Soc*, 69, 174–177.

ULLAH S M R, MURPHY B, DORICH B, RICHTER B and SRINIVASAN K (2011) 'Fat extraction from acid- and base-hydrolyzed food samples using accelerated solvent extraction', *J Agric Food Chem*, 59, 2169–2174.

VONGSVIVUT J, HERAUD P, ZHANG W and KRALOVEC J A (2012) 'Quantitative determination of fatty acid compositions in micro-encapsulated fish-oil supplements using Fourier transform infrared (FTIR) spectroscopy', *Food Chem*, 135, 603–609.

WESTERN R J, LAU S S, MARRIOTT P J and NICHOLS P D (2002) 'Positional and geometric isomer separation of FAME by comprehensive 2-D GC', *Lipids*, 37, 715–724.

XU Z, HARVEY K, PAVLINA T, DUTOT G, ZALOGA G and SIDDIQUI R (2010) 'An improved method for determining medium- and long-chain FAMEs using gas chromatography', *Lipids*, 45, 199–208.

ZHANG J Y, YU Q T, LIU B N and HUANG Z H (1988) 'Chemical modification in mass spectrometry. IV. 2-Alkenyl-4,4-dimethyloxazolines as derivatives for the double bond location of long-chain olefinic acids', *Biomed Environ Mass Spectrom*, 15, 33–44.

ZHU X, SVENDSEN C, JAEPELT K B, MOUGHAN P J and RUTHERFURD S M (2011) 'A comparison of selected methods for determining eicosapentaenoic acid and docosahexaenoic acid in cereal-based foods', *Food Chem*, 125, 1320–1327.

Part III

Food enrichment with omega-3 fatty acids

8

Modification of animal diets for the enrichment of dairy and meat products with omega-3 fatty acids

R. J. Dewhurst and A. P. Moloney, Teagasc, Animal & Grassland Research and Innovation Centre, Ireland

DOI: 10.1533/9780857098863.3.257

Abstract: Plants are the primary source of omega-3 polyunsaturated fatty acids (PUFA) in the land and marine food chains and provide the basis to produce milk and meat with enhanced nutritional attributes. This chapter describes the range of omega-3 PUFA sources used in animal feeding – including forages, oilseeds and fish oils – and identifies the factors controlling the incorporation of omega-3 PUFA into milk and meat. There is a particular focus on the challenges of increasing omega-3 PUFA in ruminant products as a consequence of rumen biohydrogenation, as well as limitations on elongation/desaturation of omega-3 PUFA and on incorporation of the longer chain omega-3 PUFA into triacylglycerols. The chapter also considers the implications of seeking to modify omega-3 PUFA in products for livestock health and fertility, as well as for product quality attributes such as flavour and shelf-life.

Key words: omega-3 fatty acids, milk, beef, linseed, fish oil.

8.1 Introduction

This chapter focuses on enhancing omega-3 fatty acids in ruminant milk and meat, whereas Chapter 9 deals with enhancing omega-3 fatty acids in eggs. There are two major differences between monogastrics and ruminants in relation to transfer of dietary omega-3 fatty acids into milk and meat and these are discussed in more detail in subsequent sections. Fatty acid deposition in monogastrics largely reflects dietary fatty acid composition (Wood and Enser, 1997). The process of rumen biohydrogenation in ruminants results in extensive transformation of omega-3 fatty acids to produce a range of more saturated fatty acids (SFA). A further important difference between monogastrics and ruminants is that incorporation of the long-chain omega-3 polyunsaturated fatty acids (PUFA), including 20:5 and 22:6, into triacylglycerols is limited in ruminants. They are incorporated mainly into membrane phospholipids and, therefore, are found predominantly in muscle (Enser *et al.*, 1996). This provides the opportunity to manipulate intramuscular fatty acid composition of ruminant meat without large increases in fatness *per se*.

According to the Ministry of Agriculture, Fisheries and Food (MAFF, 1998), the concentration of 18:3 in meat is in the range 30–80 mg/100 g for beef, 90–300 mg/100 g for lamb and 50–200 mg/100 g for pork. Concentrations of 20:5 are in the range 0–10 mg/100 g for beef, 30–60 mg/100 g for lamb and up to 10 mg/100 g for pork. Concentrations of 22:6 were up to 10 mg/100 g for pork, with only traces reported in lamb and no values reported for beef. Retailed milk fat, whether as milk or butter, is usually a mixture drawn from many farms and feeding systems and so variation is less than has been observed for individual experiments and diets (reported later). The normal range for retailed milk fat is between 0.3 and 0.6 % omega-3 fatty acids (Jensen, 2002), with most of this present as α-linolenic acid (18:3 n-3). Summer milk is usually at the higher end of that range (French butter: Wolff *et al.*, 1995; German milk: Precht *et al.*, 1999).

8.2 Sources of omega-3 fatty acids

8.2.1 Ruminant feedstuffs

Plants are the primary source of omega-3 fatty acids, whether in the terrestrial or marine ecosystem, the starting point being α-linolenic acid (18:3 n-3). Long-chain omega-3 fatty acids are produced in marine algae and are concentrated in the marine food chain so that fish oils are particularly rich sources of these long-chain omega-3 fatty acids, eicosapentaenoic acid (EPA; 20:5 n-3) and docosahexaenoic acid (DHA; 22:6 n-3). Concerns about overexploitation of fisheries, as well as concentration of fat-soluble pollutants in the marine ecosystem (Jacobs *et al.*, 2004; Sayanova and Napier, 2004) have led to renewed interest in plants as sources of omega-3 fatty acids for animal feeding.

α-Linolenic acid is the predominant fatty acid in grasses, representing 50–75 % of total fatty acids; there are much lower levels of the other two main herbage fatty acids (18:2 n-6 and 16:0). The main factors affecting fatty acid levels in fresh herbage are season, regrowth interval and nitrogen fertiliser use (Dewhurst *et al.*, 2001, 2006; Boufaïed *et al.*, 2003a; Elgersma *et al.*, 2005). In general, managements that increase the ratio of leaf to stem (leaf blade %) in herbage will increase total fatty acids, as well as the proportion of 18:3 n-3 (Witkowska *et al.*, 2008). The positive effect of nitrogen fertilizer on herbage fatty acids is anticipated since they are most abundant in the thylakoid membranes of chloroplasts, which are more abundant in fertilized grass. Fatty acid concentrations are lowest during summer months and particularly high in late autumn (Dewhurst *et al.*, 2001; Witkowska *et al.*, 2008) which has led to the suggestion that solar radiation and/or temperatures affect fatty acid levels in vegetative herbage (Witkowska *et al.*, 2008). Early studies found only small effects of grass cultivar or cultivar × management regime on herbage fatty acids (Dewhurst *et al.*, 2006), although Palladino *et al.* (2009) suggest a slightly higher fatty acid content in late-heading perennial ryegrasses.

Revello-Chion *et al.* (2011) showed that levels of 18:3 n-3 declined in Alpine herbage as herbage matured from vegetative stage (May) through to seed-ripening (July). There was some variation between species in the rate of decline, being more marked for the grasses (meadow grasses, cocksfoot and fescue) than legumes (red clover and sainfoin) and some herbs.

Herbage fatty acids start to be lost immediately after mowing as part of a natural plant defence mechanism. Once free fatty acids are released by lipolysis, they are acted on by the lipoxygenase/hydroperoxide lyase system that produces compounds such as *trans*-2-hexenal that are part of the plants' defence against insect herbivory and microbial colonizers. The so-called 'green odour' that is produced when herbage is mown includes these compounds derived from fatty acids. Around 25–50 % of herbage fatty acids could be lost over the course of field wilting lasting several days (Dewhurst and King, 1998). However, a recent survey of commercial grass silages in the Netherlands showed that most of the variation in 18:3 n-3 is related to stage of maturity at harvest rather than wilting or the type of silage fermentation achieved (Khan *et al.*, 2012). For example, there was a strong association between silage 18:3 n-3 and crude protein, which relates back to the co-location of many plant lipids and proteins in chloroplasts. The lack of effect of wilting is in agreement with the observation of Noci *et al.* (2007) that wilting of grass silage did not affect the fatty acid composition of beef muscle.

Linseed (*Linum usitatissimum*) is the major oilseed plant that has been used as a source of n-3 PUFA in animal feeding. Linseeds contain around 40 % oil; European linseed oil contains 56–71 % 18:3 n-3, with the remainder comprising mainly 18:2 (12–18 %) and 18:1 (10–22 %; Deutsche Gesellschaft für Fettwissenschaft, 2011). Whilst the main plant fatty acid is 18:3, there has been recent interest in sources of longer chain or more unsaturated n-3 PUFA because these might be better precursors of long-chain n-3 PUFA. Plants in the primula and borage families contain some of the necessary desaturases (Sayanova and Napier, 2004). Echium oil is extracted from the seeds of purple viper's burgloss (*Echium plantagineum*) and contains around 10 % stearidonic acid (18:4 n-3) in addition to 18:3 n-3, 18:3 n-6, 18:2 n-6 and 18:1 n-9 (Kitessa and Young, 2011). Qi *et al.* (2004) demonstrated the potential for genetic modification to increase synthesis of 20:5 n-3 in higher plants. Fish oil and marine algae are the main sources of long-chain omega-3 PUFA that have been used in animal feeding (Woods and Fearon,

2009). Microalgae are rich sources of longer chain n-3 PUFA, with different species rich in the different n-3 PUFA (Givens *et al.*, 2000). Cooper *et al.* (2004) used a marine algae from the class Dinophyceae to increase the content of 22:6 n-3 in lamb muscle phospholipids.

8.2.2 Synthesis of lipids in muscle and milk

Most of the lipids are stored in adipose tissue, and are present as glycerol esters, but there are also considerable quantities of phospholipids in the muscle membrane. An important difference between monogastric animals and ruminants is that dietary omega-3 PUFA, including 20:5 and 22:6, are not incorporated into triacylglycerols to any important extent in ruminants and are incorporated mainly into membrane phospholipids (Enser *et al.*, 1996, see Demeyer and Doreau (1999) for possible biochemical explanations). Since the amount of triacylglycerol increases as fat is deposited in muscle while the muscle membrane fraction is relatively constant in size, this provides an opportunity to increase the concentration of omega-3 fatty acids in ruminant meat without large increases in fatness *per se*, but restricts the potential size of the increase compared to that in monogastric animals. There is a limit to the amount of omega-3 fatty acids that can be deposited in phospholipids irrespective of diet, and knowledge of this limit might allow us to increase omega-3 fatty acids without increasing fat deposition *per se*.

The increase in the triacylglycerol fraction is generally accompanied by an increase in the monounsaturated fatty acid (MUFA) proportion of that fraction. Consequently, an increase in fat deposition results in an increase in the MUFA proportion and a decrease in the saturated fatty acid (SFA) and PUFA proportions of total muscle. This is illustrated by the results of Moreno *et al.* (2008), a study by dairy steers from medium maturing breed, in which sires (Holstein/Friesian) and late maturing breed sires (Belgian Blue) were slaughtered at two weights and the fatty acid composition of the longissimus muscle examined. On average, the total fatty acid concentration was higher for the earlier maturing breed and, for both breeds, increasing slaughter weight increased the concentration of fatty acids in muscle. The increase in intramuscular fat was accompanied by a decrease in the SFA and PUFA proportions and an increase in the MUFA proportion in both breeds. Comparisons between dietary treatments are often confounded by differences in fatty acid composition that result from such differences in intramuscular fat. Breed differences and effects of maturity or growth stage on the subcutaneous or intramuscular fatty acid composition of beef have been reviewed by de Smet *et al.* (2004), who concluded that much of the differences in fatty acid composition apparently due to genotype could be explained by variation in intramuscular fat concentration and that effects of genotype were, in general, much smaller than effects due to diet. One strategy to increase the omega-3 PUFA content in meat animals is to use late maturing breeds and slaughter them at lighter weights. This may not be economically attractive in many production environments.

An analogous situation pertains with bovine milk, with the longer chain and highly unsaturated omega-3 fatty acids (20:5 and 22:6) found mainly in the milk fat globule membrane (Jensen and Nielsen, 1996), which makes up only a small proportion of total milk fat (Jensen, 2002). Whilst the proportion of 18:3 in cream (triacylglycerol) was less than in the milk fat globule membrane (phospholipids), 18:3 that is not biohydrogenated in the rumen can be incorporated at high levels in bovine milk (13.9 % of milk fatty acids; Petit *et al.*, 2002).

8.3 Feeds that increase omega-3 fatty acids in ruminant milk and meat

The most common strategy to enhance meat and milk omega-3 PUFA is dietary supplementation with linseeds, linseed oil, marine oil or marine algae. Since dietary inclusion of fatty acids must be restricted to around 60 g/kg dry matter consumed, to avoid impairment of rumen function, the capacity to manipulate the fatty acid composition by use of ruminally-available fatty acids is limited.

8.3.1 Rumen-protected linseed products

Rumen biohydrogenation of fatty acids is extensive with typically only 3–7 % of supplemented omega-3 fatty acids flowing out of the rumen and available for incorporation into milk fat (Gonthier *et al.*, 2004; Shingfield *et al.*, 2011). Duodenal infusion of linseed oil has been used as an experimental approach to avoid biohydrogenation and resulted in milk fat containing 13.9 % 18:3 n-3 (Petit *et al.*, 2002).

Despite rumen biohydrogenation, a proportion of dietary PUFA bypasses the rumen intact. However, the inclusion of untreated linseed oil or untreated marine oils in the diet has only small effects on levels of omega-3 fatty acids in milk (Donovan *et al.*, 2000; Chouinard *et al.*, 2001; Abu-Ghazaleh *et al.*, 2002; Offer, 2002; Loor *et al.*, 2003; Shingfield *et al.*, 2003; Rego *et al.*, 2005). Feeding high levels of oil (600 g/day) only increased 18:3 n-3 from 0.73 to 1.13 % of milk fatty acids in the case of linseed oil (Loor *et al.*, 2003) and 20:5 n-3 from 0.05 to 0.40 % of milk fatty acids in the case of menhaden fish oil (Donovan *et al.*, 2000). Similarly, feeding linseed oil had no effect on 18:3 n-3 in subcutaneous or intramuscular fat when supplemented to moderate quality grass (Noci *et al.*, 2007).

Feeding untreated whole linseeds offers little protection from rumen biohydrogenation and only resulted in a small increase in milk 18:3 n-3 with levels still below 1 % (Petit, 2002; Petit *et al.*, 2004; Cavalieri *et al.*, 2005). A variety of procedures have been explored including the use of intact oilseeds, heat/chemical treatment of intact processed oilseeds, chemical treatment of oils to form calcium soaps or amides, emulsification/encapsulation of oils with protein and subsequent chemical protection. The most effective treatment to protect 18:3 n-3 in linseed from rumen biohydrogenation is to treat a mixture of linseed (70.8 %) with casein (10 %) and soyabeans (19.2 %) with formaldehyde (Scott and Ashes, 1993), though this is a costly process and there are concerns about the use of formaldehyde in the food chain. This product was calculated to provide around 80 % protection from rumen biohydrogenation and resulted in milk containing 3.5–6.4 % 18:3 n-3 (in comparison with control milk at 0.3–0.8 %) in the studies reported by Tymchuk *et al.* (1998) and Goodridge *et al.* (2001).

A number of workers have evaluated simpler treatments of linseeds without the inclusion of casein and soyabean. Petit *et al.* (2002) treated linseeds with formaldehyde, but only increased milk 18:3 n-3 from 1 to 2 % of milk fat. Micronized linseeds, which are cooked using infrared radiation and ground, led to small increases in milk 18:3 n-3, but no greater than was achieved with untreated linseeds (Mustafa *et al.*, 2003; Gonthier *et al.*, 2005). Extrusion of linseeds increased rumen biohydrogenation of 18:3 n-3 (96.6 % for diet including extruded linseeds vs 93.8 % for diet including untreated linseeds; Gonthier *et al.*, 2004), and the increase in milk 18:3 n-3 (0.7 %) was less than for micronized or untreated linseeds (1.3 % in both cases; the control milk fat contained 0.4 % 18:3 n-3). Moallem (2009) used a different extrusion procedure and increased milk 18:3 n-3 from 0.3 to 0.9 %. Although the transfer of 18:3 n-3 from linseed to milk was only 6.2 %, these authors suggest that there is some potential for further optimization of treatments.

The effects of feeding a range of products based on linseed, with or without processing, on fatty acid profiles of muscle and adipose tissue from beef cattle and lambs are presented in Tables 8.1 and 8.2. Studies with linseed feeding to beef cattle and lambs have led to two- to four-fold increases in proportions of 18:3 n-3 in muscle (Table 8.1). The largest increase was achieved by Berthelot *et al.* (2010) who included linseeds that had been extruded along with wheat or maize in diets for intensively-reared lambs. Although the 18:3 n-3 proportion in adipose tissue is less than in muscle/muscle phospholipid, the proportional increases in response to feeding linseed products were similar (Table 8.2).

8.3.2 Fresh herbage

Table 8.3 summarizes the results of studies in which milk fatty acid profiles were compared for cows fed fresh or ensiled forages. Fresh herbage leads to increased levels of 18:3 n-3 in milk in comparison with milk from conserved forages (Table 8.3). Most of these comparisons were between fresh herbages and silage and, as will be seen later, hays can also lead to increased 18:3 n-3 in milk. Increasing the proportion of fresh herbage in diets for cows

Table 8.1 Effects of supplementary linseed products on n-3 PUFA proportions (% of total fatty acids) in muscle or muscle phospholipids (PL) from steers and lambs

Reference	Animal type	Form of linseed		% 18:3 (control)	% increase in fatty acid (in comparison with control)			
					18:3 n-3	20:5 n-3	22:5 n-3	22:6 n-3
Scollan *et al.* (2001)	Charolais steers	Whole linseed	Muscle PL	2.13	203	154	109	115
Wachira *et al.* (2002)	Male lambs	Whole linseed	Muscle	1.44	236	151	114	144
Scollan *et al.* (2003)	Charolais steers	Protected linseed/ sunflower*	Muscle PL	2.49	128	91	80	84
Demirel *et al.* (2004)	Male lambs	Formaldehyde treated linseed	Muscle PL	4.62	178	138	131	92
Scollan *et al.* (2004a)	Charolais steers	Protected linseed/ sunflower[†]	Muscle PL	2.39	218	119	79	83
Maddock *et al.* (2006)	Crossbred heifers	Ground linseed	Muscle PL	1.37	328	154	119	113
Bas *et al.* (2007)	Mixed lambs	Extruded linseed	Muscle	0.48	278	142	124	108
Kitessa *et al.* (2009)	Lambs	Protected linseed/ sunflower*	Muscle	0.92	182	115	137	325
Berthelot *et al.* (2010)	Male lambs	Extruded linseed	Muscle	0.56	417	236	125	142
Kronberg *et al.* (2011)	Angus steers	Ground linseed	Muscle	0.69	162	127	110	NR

*Formulated to contain a 2:1 ratio of 18:2 n-6 to 18:3 n-3. [†]Formulated to contain equal amounts of 18:2 n-6 and 18:3 n-3.
NR = not recorded.

Table 8.2 Effect of supplementary linseed products on 18:3 proportions (% of total fatty acids) for adipose tissue from steers and lambs

Reference	Animal type	Form of linseed	% 18:3 (control)	% increase in 18:3 n-3
Scollan *et al.* (2001)	Charolais steers	Whole linseed	0.37	176
Wachira *et al.* (2002)	Male lambs	Whole linseed	1.27	206
Demirel *et al.* (2004)	Male lambs	Formaldehyde treated linseed	1.18	215
Bas *et al.* (2007)	Male and female lambs	Extruded linseed	0.45	366
Berthelot *et al.* (2010)	Male lambs	Extruded linseed	0.38	411

Table 8.3 Comparison of the effects of fresh pasture and conserved forages on 18:3 n-3 as a percentage of total milk fatty acids

Reference	Conserved forage	Fresh herbage	Conserved forage	Significance
Timmen and Patton (1988)	Grass or wheat silage	0.84	0.36	Not stated
Aii *et al.* (1988)	Grass hay	1.65	1.29	$P < 0.01$
Kelly *et al.* (1998)	Maize silage/ legume silage/ legume hay	0.95	0.25	$P < 0.01$
White *et al.* (2001)	Maize silage/ lucerne silage	0.71	0.38	$P < 0.01$
Offer (2002)	Grass silage	0.76	0.41	Not stated
Schroeder *et al.* (2003)	Maize silage	0.57	0.07	$P < 0.01$
Kay *et al.* (2004)	Maize silage/grass silage/grass hay	0.95	0.32	$P < 0.01$
Mohammed *et al.* (2009)	Grass silage	0.82	0.34	$P < 0.01$

also offered a total mixed ration increased levels of 18:3 n-3 in milk, whether this was achieved by restricting grazing (Morales-Almaráz *et al.*, 2010) or total mixed ration (Vibart *et al.*, 2008). The effect of fresh grass, linked to its seasonal availability, was confirmed in a survey of 19 conventional and 17 organic herds conducted by Ellis *et al.* (2006). Decaen and Ghadaki (1970) reported up to 2.4 % 18:3 n-3 in milk fat from cows grazing fresh pasture. Liu (2007) reported a mean 1.74 % 18:3 n-3 in milk from cows grazing high-quality spring pasture in New Zealand (range 1.42–2.12 %).

As has already been mentioned, the 18:3 n-3 content of herbage is highest during spring and autumn and declines during summer. This leads to a reduction in the 18:3 content of milk from grazing cows (Auldist *et al.*, 1998; Mackle *et al.*, 1999; Thomson and Van der Poel, 2000; Lock and Garnsworthy, 2003; Liu, 2007) and sheep (Nudda *et al.*, 2005). Ward *et al.* (2003) showed an increase in milk 18:3 n-3 from 0.37 to 0.52 % as the proportion of fresh pasture increased from 50 to 80 % of the diet; levels and responses were quite low, probably because pasture quality was low (neutral detergent fibre 60 % of dry matter). Pasture allowance had no effect on milk 18:3 n-3 in the studies reported by Stanton *et al.* (1997), Wales *et al.* (1999) and Stockdale *et al.* (2003). Petersen *et al.* (2011) noted an increase in 18:3 n-3 when cows were zero grazed a mixture of sown herbs (chicory, plantain, birdsfoot trefoil, white melilot and others) in comparison with zero-grazing white clover/perennial ryegrass. It is not clear which species and mechanisms were involved in this effect.

The impact of pasture in the ration of beef cattle on the fatty acid composition of muscle has been widely studied (see reviews by Scollan *et al.*, 2006 and Daley *et al.*, 2010), and selected examples are given in Table 8.4. As far as possible, studies were chosen where there was no significant difference between treatments in intramuscular fat content so that the possible confounding discussed earlier could be avoided. In general, at constant

Table 8.4 Influence of grazed grass on the fatty acid composition (mg/100 g) of beef *longissimus* muscle

(i) Proportion of grass in the diet (adapted from French et al., *2000)*

Fatty acids	Grass (g/kg dry matter)				SED*	Significance
	0	510	770	1000		
Total	3410	4490	4020	4360	650.5	Not significant
18:2n-6	120.5	105.8	94.4	85.9	6.05	$P < 0.01$ (linear)
18:3n-3	29.3	35.4	41.1	46.0	1.78	$P < 0.01$ (linear)
20:5n-3	4.9	11.0	9.8	9.4	1.32	$P < 0.05$ (quadratic)
22:6n-3†	–	–	–	–		

(ii) Length of grass feeding (days) (adapted from Noci et al., *2005a)*

Fatty acids	0	40	99	158	SED*	Significance
Total	2461	2329	2754	2515	177.5	Not significant
18:2n-6	62.1	63.7	59.4	59.0	3.32	Not significant
18:3n-3	19.6	25.4	30.9	34.4	1.86	$P < 0.001$ (linear)
20:5n-3	5.6	5.5	6.4	7.7	0.50	$P < 0.001$ (linear)
22:6n-3	3.22	2.86	2.78	2.72	0.606	Not significant

*Standard error of difference.
†Not identified on chromatogram.

intramuscular fat content, grass-fed beef has a lower proportion of SFA and a higher proportion of PUFA in intramuscular lipids. An increase in the proportion of grass in the diet of finishing steers and an increase in the duration of grazing increased the omega-3 PUFA concentration (French *et al.*, 2000; Noci *et al.*, 2005a). Dannenberger *et al.* (2004) reported EPA concentrations of 20.3 and 4.4 mg/100 g and DHA concentrations of 6.8 and 2.5 mg/100 g in muscle from grass- and concentrate-fed bulls, respectively. Argentine beef was reported to contain 15 and 4 mg/100 g EPA and 12 and 6 mg/100 g DHA for pasture and feedlot beef, respectively (Garcia *et al.*, 2008), while beef from the USA was reported to contain 8 and 4 mg/100 g EPA and 1.49 and 1.46 mg/100 g DHA for pasture and concentrate-fed steers, respectively (Leheska *et al.*, 2008). Higher concentrations of omega-3 PUFA in grass-fed beef compared to grain-fed beef have also been reported by Ponnampalam *et al.* (2006) in Australia.

8.3.3 Clover silages

Red and white clover silages led to increased levels of 18:3 n-3 in comparison with animals offered grass silages. This effect has been observed in bovine milk in a number of studies comparing diets based solely on grass silage or clover silage (Dewhurst *et al.*, 2003a; Al-Mabuk *et al.*, 2004; Moorby *et al.*, 2009; summarized in Table 8.5) and beef muscle (Lee *et al.*, 2003, 2006),

Table 8.5 Effects of clover silages (in comparison with grass silages) on 18:3 n-3 as a % of total milk fatty acids

Reference	Clover species	Concentrates (kg/day)	Grass silage	Clover silage	Significance
Dewhurst *et al.* (2003a)	White clover	8	0.43	0.91	$P < 0.001$
Dewhurst *et al.* (2003a)	White clover	8	0.40	0.96	$P < 0.001$
Dewhurst *et al.* (2003a)	Red clover	8	0.43	0.81	$P < 0.001$
Dewhurst *et al.* (2003a)	Red clover	8	0.40	1.28	$P < 0.001$
Dewhurst *et al.* (2003a)	Red clover	4	0.48	1.51	$P < 0.001$
Al-Mabuk *et al.* (2004)	Red clover	8	0.48	0.92	$P < 0.05$
Vanhatalo *et al.* (2007) (early cut)	Red clover	9	0.41	1.34	$P < 0.05$
Vanhatalo *et al.* (2007) (late cut)	Red clover	9	0.37	0.88	$P < 0.05$
Moorby *et al.* (2009)	Red clover	4	0.56	1.49	$P < 0.001$

including beef from cull cows offered red clover silage for 12 weeks prior to slaughter (Lee *et al.*, 2009). There was a three-fold increase in this fatty acid when red clover silage made up a high proportion of the diet (concentrate level was 4 kg/day) in the studies reported by Dewhurst *et al.* (2003b) and Moorby *et al.* (2009). Van Dorland *et al.* (2008) included red clover silage or white clover silage at 40 % of forage dry matter and only increased the 18:3 n-3 proportion from 0.9 % of milk fatty acids (grass silage control) to 1.04 % (red clover silage) and 1.14 % (white clover silage). The proportionally lower increase in milk 18:3 n-3 proportion when clover silages were mixed with grass silages was also observed by Dewhurst *et al.* (2003a) and Moorby *et al.* (2009) (Fig. 8.1).

The increased 18:3 n-3 in products is linked to a reduction in rumen biohydrogenation of this fatty acid (Dewhurst *et al.*, 2003b). In the case of red clover silage, some of this reduction is probably related to the action of polyphenol oxidase during ensiling that results in complexing of protein with quionones (Lee *et al.*, 2008), reducing lipolysis and consequently limiting potential for biohydrogenation. In the case of white clover silage, the reduction in biohydrogenation is related to reduced rumen retention time (increased passage rates from the rumen).

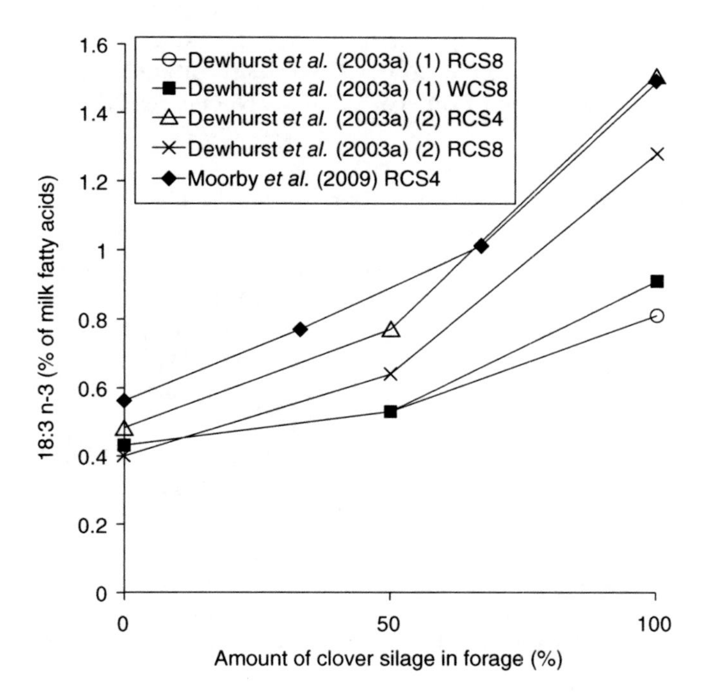

Fig. 8.1 Effects of replacing grass silage with red clover silage on 18:3 n-3 proportion in milk fat.

8.3.4 Hays

Contrary to effects with silages, a number of studies showed increased recovery of 18:3 n-3 from the diet into milk for hays in comparison with silages (Decaen and Adda, 1970; Bartsch *et al.*, 1979; Aii *et al.*, 1988). Working with mountain pastures and hays, Ferlay *et al.* (2006) noted an increased recovery of 18:3 n-3 between diet and milk with hays in comparison with fresh herbage. This resulted in milks with average 18:3 n-3 of 1.26 and 0.84 % for hay and fresh pasture treatments, respectively. This effect appears related to reduced biohydrogenation of 18:3 n-3 from hays (Boufaïed *et al.*, 2003b), although it is not clear if this is a consequence of the hay-making process itself, the later harvesting stage or lower levels of 18:3 n-3 in hays.

8.3.5 Grass silage

Warren *et al.* (2008) evaluated the effects of long-term feeding of diets divergent in n-3 and n-6 PUFA. Beef steers were grown at the same rate on either concentrates and barley straw or grass silage (with 15 % inclusion of molassed sugar beet pulp) from around seven months of age. By their first slaughter point (14 months), levels of 18:3 n-3 (3.6 vs 0.7 % of total fatty acids in muscle phospholipids), 20:5 n-3 (3.4 vs 0.8 %), 22:5 (4.6 vs 2.2 %) and 22:6 n-3 (0.93 vs 0.25 %) were all elevated for animals offered grass silage. The difference in 18:3 n-3 was similar for the animals slaughtered at 19 and 24 months (3.6 vs 0.6 % and 3.6 vs 0.5 % of 18:3, respectively). Feeding cattle whole crop wheat silage rather than grass silage decreased the deposition of omega-3 PUFA (Noci *et al.*, 2005b).

8.3.6 Tanniniferous, Alpine and other botanically diverse herbages

Ruminants grazing birdsfoot trefoil (Turner *et al.*, 2005) or sulla (Piredda *et al.*, 2002; Addis *et al.*, 2005) produce milk containing higher levels of 18:3 n-3 than cows grazing grasses and other non-tanniniferous herbages. It appears that this effect is related to reduced biohydrogenation of 18:3 n-3 in the rumen as a consequence of the action of tannins. It is not clear if this is a specific antimicrobial action of tannins or is a consequence of binding to enzymes involved in biohydrogenation.

Several studies have shown elevated levels of 18:3 n-3 in milk and dairy products from cattle grazing Alpine pastures (Dewhurst *et al.*, 2006; summarized in Table 8.6). Leiber *et al.* (2005) showed an increase in milk 18:3 despite a reduction in dietary 18:3, which was most likely a consequence of reduced rumen biohydrogenation. The Alpine meadows include legumes that are rich in condensed tannins, as well as red clover, which have already been noted to reduce rumen biohydrogenation and increase levels of 18:3 n-3 in milk.

There is a paucity of information on the effect of grazing botanically diverse pastures on the fatty acid composition of beef. Fraser *et al.* (2007)

Table 8.6 Effects of Alpine pasture on 18:3 n-3 as a percentage of total milk fatty acids

Reference	Sample type	Lowland milk	Alpine milk	Significance
Hebeisen *et al.* (1993)	Milk	0.45	2.31	$P < 0.01$
Collomb *et al.* (2001, 2002)	Milk	0.79	1.15	$P < 0.05$
Innocente *et al.* (2002)	Cheese	0.50	1.10	$P < 0.001$
Kraft *et al.* (2003)	Milk	0.33	1.17	$P < 0.05$
Hauswirth *et al.* (2004)	Cheese	0.6	1.5	$P < 0.001$
Leiber *et al.* (2005)	Milk	0.54	1.15	$P < 0.001$

reported that inclusion of a period of grazing a *Molina caerulea*-dominated semi-natural pasture increased the proportion of omega-3 PUFA in muscle lipids. A review of Moloney *et al.* (2008) considered studies that compared grazing of an English ryegrass pasture with unimproved saltmarsh pasture (Whittington *et al.*, 2006) or a botanically diverse pasture (Lourenço *et al.*, 2007a) or lowland vs mountain pastures on the west coast of Norway (Ådnøy *et al.*, 2005). Further, stable feeding of at least 70 % ryegrass silage was compared with botanically diverse silage from a natural, unfertilized grassland (Lourenço *et al.*, 2007b). A general tendency for an increase in omega-3 and total PUFA proportions in intramuscular fat is observed. For a comprehensive review of this topic, the reader is referred to Lourenço *et al.* (2008).

8.3.7 Organic production systems

Increased levels of 18:3 n-3 have been recorded for organic milk in comparison with conventionally produced milk. This observation was made both in experimental comparisons (Jahreis *et al.*, 1996) and in more recent surveys of multiple herds (Dewhurst, 2003; Ellis *et al.*, 2006) and retail milk (Butler *et al.*, 2011). The results of these studies are summarized in Table 8.7. It seems likely that this effect is related to the effects of clover silages noted above, since organic systems in the UK depend on white and red clover for nitrogen fixation.

8.3.8 Echium oil

Echium oil is a natural source of stearidonic acid (18:4 n-3). It was suggested that the greater initial desaturation may make this a better precursor of long-chain omega-3 fatty acids in milk and meat. Kitessa and Young (2011) fed a product based on echium oil protected with a protein/aldehyde complex (Scott and Ashes, 1993; see above).The high cost of this oil has meant that preliminary work has involved only small groups of cows. Whilst the product did increase levels of 18:4 n-3 and 20:5 n-3 and 22:5 n-3 in milk,

Table 8.7 Comparisons of n-3 PUFA as a percentage of total milk fatty acids in organic and conventional milk

Reference	Conventional milk	Organic milk	Significance
Jahreis *et al.* (1996) (18:3 n-3)	0.27 (indoors); 0.43 (pasture)	0.89	$P < 0.001$
Dewhurst (2003) (18:3 n-3)	0.42	0.74	$P < 0.001$
Ellis *et al.* (2006) (total n-3)	0.66	1.11	$P < 0.01$
Butler *et al.* (2011) (18:3 n-3)	0.44	0.69	$P < 0.001$
Butler *et al.* (2011) (total n-3)	0.55	0.88	$P < 0.001$

there was no increase in 22:6 n-3, confirming the limited scope to increase this fatty acid by feeding plant oils.

8.3.9 Fish oils

Fish oil fatty acids are highly unsaturated and fish oils are known to disrupt rumen function, for example leading to milk fat depression. Consequently, levels of inclusion of fish oil are limited and rumen biohydrogenation is invariably extensive (Chilliard *et al.*, 2001; Chikunya *et al.*, 2004). Nonetheless, feeding fish oils has led to incorporation of low levels of 20:5 n-3 and 22:6 n-3 in milk (Petit *et al.*, 2002), beef (Scollan *et al.*, 2001) and lamb (Wachira *et al.*, 2002; Demirel *et al.*, 2004). The highest levels of the longer chain n-3 PUFA, 20:5 and 22:6, in milk have been achieved using post-rumen infusions of fish oil (3.3 and 1.5 %; Hagemeister *et al.*, 1988) or fish oil protected from rumen biohydrogenation by the formaldehyde-treated protein method mentioned previously (1.3 and 2.2 %, respectively; Gulati *et al.*, 2003). An increase in muscle EPA and DHA concentrations was also observed by Wistuba *et al.* (2007) due to the inclusion of fish oil in feedlot rations for cattle.

More recent work has investigated the potential of combinations of linseed oil and fish oil to increase both 18:3 as well as 20:5 and 22:6. A linseed oil–fish oil treatment increased the EPA and DHA concentrations in muscle illustrating the potential of fish oil (rich in both the long-chain n-3 PUFA) to increase their concentration in beef (Scollan *et al.*, 2001), and the increase was dependent on the level of dietary inclusion (Noci *et al.*, 2007). Cooper *et al.* (2004) achieved higher incorporation of 20:5 and 22:6 into lamb muscle when they fed a mixture of fish oil and marine algae (179.1 mg/100 g muscle) in comparison with fish oil alone (74.1 mg/100 g muscle).

8.3.10 Rumen-protected fish oils

A number of researchers have investigated the potential to increase incorporation of 20:5 and 22:6 into beef and lamb using rumen protection technology. Concentrations of 20:5 were increased three-fold in lamb muscle (Kitessa *et al.* (2001) and 1.5-fold in bovine muscle (Richardson *et al.*, 2004) when the protein/formaldehyde technology was used. An alternative technology, in which fish oil was encapsulated in a pH-sensitive matrix which remained intact at rumen pH but which was broken down at the lower pH in the abomasum, thereby releasing the fish oil for digestion, was used by Dunne *et al.* (2011). This strategy also achieved a three-fold increase in 20:5, but a smaller (two-fold) increase in 22:6 in comparison to the 3.5-fold increases observed by Kitessa *et al.* (2001) and Richardson *et al.* (2004), probably because their fish oil contained relatively less 22:6.

8.4 Increasing omega-3 fatty acids in animal diets

8.4.1 Chain elongation and desaturation to increase longer-chain omega-3 fatty acids

The literature is equivocal on the effects of dietary treatments that increase milk 18:3 n-3 relative to milk 20:5 n-3 and 22:6 n-3. It appears that there is potential for small increases, but only when control levels are low. The three-fold increase in milk 18:3 n-3 obtained with extruded linseed (Moallem, 2009) was associated with small increases in 20:5 n-3 (from 0.03 to 0.06 % of milk fat) and 22:6 n-3 (from 0.037 to 0.076 % of milk fat). The dramatic increase in milk 18:3 n-3 obtained following duodenal infusion of linseed oil did not increase milk 20:5 n-3 above control levels (0.14 % of milk fat). This limitation results from the fact that the longer chain omega-3 fatty acids are mainly found in the milk fat globule membrane (Jensen and Nielsen, 1996), which makes up only a small proportion of total milk fat (Jensen, 2002).

The more than doubling of 18:3 n-3 in beef muscle as a result of feeding red clover silage to cull dairy cows for 12 weeks (1.54 % vs 0.71 % of fatty acids) was associated with smaller increases in 20:5 n-3 (0.44 vs 0.31 %) and 22:5 n-3 (0.74 vs 0.55 %) (Lee *et al.*, 2009). Similarly, the increased 18:3 n-3 in beef and lamb from animals fed linseed products has been associated with increased levels of 20:5 n-3, which is the elongation/desaturation product of 18:3 n-3 (Table 8.1). Levels of 22:6 n-3 were increased in muscle from animals fed linseeds in the studies of Wachira *et al.* (2002), Maddock *et al.* (2006) and Berthelot *et al.* (2010), but not in most studies (Table 8.1). Warren *et al.* (2008) observed significant elongation/desaturation with increases in 20:5 n-3, 22:5 n-3 and 22:6 n-3 alongside the more than five-fold increase in 18:3 n-3 obtained by feeding grass silage (n-3 PUFA rich diet) in comparison with concentrates/straw (n-6 PUFA rich diet).

8.4.2 Effects on animals receiving diets designed to increase omega-3 fatty acids in milk and meat

Whilst attempting to alter the fatty acid composition of milk and meat to have effects on the health of consumers, it should not be surprising that manipulations may influence the health and fertility of the animals receiving these diets. Supplementary fat in dairy cow diets has typically been used to address fertility and health issues associated with negative energy balance in early lactation. However, this has not been successful because fat supplements usually stimulate milk production and so have little effect on energy balance (Staples *et al.*, 1998), whilst dietary fat can also reduce circulating insulin, which has been linked to impaired fertility (Garnsworthy *et al.*, 2008).

In addition to effects of fat as an energy source, there has been recent interest in effects of dietary fatty acids on fertility and immune function, particularly in dairy cows. Fatty acids are precursors of many compounds ('eicosanoids' such as prostaglandins and leukotrienes) that are highly active in animal tissues. Whilst there have been dramatic effects on components of fertility (e.g. Petit *et al.*, 2002), the effects of dietary fatty acids on fertility are complex and not all modes of action are understood (Staples and Thatcher, 2005). Two major modes of action involve effects on levels of progesterone and prostaglandins. Fat supplements tend to increase blood cholesterol (a precursor for prostaglandin), increase the size of corpora lutea (the site of synthesis of progesterone) and may reduce the rate of clearance of progesterone – all leading to elevated progesterone, which will benefit fertility. Omega-3 fatty acids (18:3 and 20:5) may suppress the synthesis of prostaglandin F2α, and thereby increase embryo survival. These fatty acids exert their effect by competing for the enzyme prostaglandin endoperoxidase synthase (which also produces the less active prostaglandin F3α) and by displacing arachidonic acid (20:4 n-6), the precursor of prostaglandin F2α, from cell membranes.

The n-6 fatty acids lead to production of prostaglandin E2 and leukotriene B4, whilst the n-3 fatty acids produce prostaglandin E3 and leukotriene B5 which result in less severe inflammations (Calder, 2002). Whilst these effects have been studied extensively in humans, there is some evidence for effects of dietary fatty acids on immune responses during the transition period when given to dry cows (Lessard *et al.*, 2004), as well as in lactating dairy cows (Lessard *et al.*, 2003).

8.4.3 Characteristics of omega-3 PUFA enriched products

The influence of forage feeding on the fatty acid composition, processing characteristics and sensory quality of milk and meat has been regularly reviewed (e.g. Coulon and Priolo, 2002; Scollan *et al.*, 2005, 2006; Elgersma *et al.*, 2006). The sensory quality of food can be defined by the texture, the flavour, including the odour (smell attributes) and the aroma (sensations perceived by the retro-nasal airway), and the taste, perceived in particular on the tongue. The sensory quality of dairy products can be influenced by animal diet (reviewed by Coulon *et al.,* 2004; Martin *et al.,* 2005). In particular, the fatty acid composition of milk may play a role in flavour, e.g. oxidized milk and milk products are characterized by metallic, cardboard or stale flavours, and production of oxidized flavour at eight days post sampling was positively correlated with levels of 18:2n-6, 18:3n-3 and total PUFA in milk fat (Timmons *et al.*, 2001).

The fatty acid composition of milk can also influence processing characteristics whereby milk with a high PUFA concentration is more susceptible to oxidation (Murphy, 2000) and therefore has a shorter shelf-life. Milk from cows fed on red clover compared to grass silage contained more 18:2n-6 and 18:3n-3 PUFA, which also resulted in increased oxidative deterioration of milk (Al-Mabuk *et al.*, 2004). Whilst this suggests that milk with increased omega-3 PUFA is less stable, this is not necessarily the case since antioxidant compounds in the ration can protect PUFA against oxidation. While Havemose *et al.* (2004) observed that milk from cows fed grass silage had higher concentrations of the antioxidants β-carotene, lutein, zeaxanthin and α-tocopherol, than cows fed maize silage, the levels were not sufficient to prevent higher lipid oxidation in the former. In contrast, milk from dairy cows supplemented with fish oil had no oxidized favours compared with a control ration (Ramaswamy *et al.*, 2001; Nelson and Martin, 2009); this is likely due to the effects of antioxidants supplied by the herbage. Similarly, Kitessa *et al.* (2004) reported that milk from cows fed ruminally protected fish oil had similar organoleptic properties to that of a non-lipid supplemented control ration. High PUFA milk generally results in softer butter and cheese (Ryhanen *et al.*, 2005; Bobe *et al.*, 2007) while Jones *et al.* (2005) found no differences in flavour of butter or cheese manufactured from milk with a three-fold increase in 20:5 + 22:6 compared to control milk.

Characteristics important to consumer perception of the quality or eating experience of meat may also be influenced by the fatty acid composition. The colour of muscle, which greatly influences consumer decision to purchase, largely reflects the concentration (and oxidation state) of myoglobin. The bright red, oxidized myoglobin colour of beef slowly changes to brown because of conversion of myoglobin to metmyoglobin when it is exposed to air. This loss of desirable colour is linked to the oxidation of meat lipids, the rate of which is a function of the concentration and their degree of unsaturation. Thus, increasing the concentration of PUFA in meat increases the susceptibility of muscle lipids to oxidative breakdown during conditioning and retail display (Wood *et al.*, 2003). Despite the increased concentrations of PUFA in muscles compared with beef from grain-fed cattle, pasture-fed beef is generally more resistant to lipid oxidation than grain-fed beef (O'Sullivan *et al.*, 2003). This observation generally holds for fresh or aged meat (Yang *et al.*, 2002) and meat that has undergone long-term frozen storage (Farouk and Wieliczko, 2003). This reflects higher deposition of plant-derived antioxidants, in particular vitamin E, in meat from pasture-fed cattle but also increased activity of some antioxidant enzymes (Gatellier *et al.*, 2004). However, Realini *et al.* (2004) reported that while fresh steaks from pasture-fed cattle had greater lipid stability than concentrate-fed cattle, when the meat was minced the opposite was the case. The authors suggest that mincing, by disrupting cellular integrity, exposes more of the PUFA to oxidation, i.e. it provides a greater test of antioxidative protection of the omega-3 PUFA in grass-fed beef. Similarly, Yang *et al.* (2002) reported that at similar vitamin E concentrations, pasture-fed beef was less stable than concentrate beef, again highlighting the influence of the fatty acid composition of pasture-fed beef.

Wood *et al.* (2003) concluded, based on studies with monogastrics, that only when concentrations of 18:3 approach 3 % of lipids are there any adverse effects on lipid or colour stability (or flavour, below), in particular if processing conditions accelerate lipid oxidation. In support of this conclusion, when the concentration of 18:3 in beef was increased from 0.7 to 1.2 % of total lipids by feeding linseeds (Vatansever *et al.*, 2000; Kronberg *et al.*, 2011) or to 1.9 % by use of a ruminally-protected lipid supplement (Scollan *et al.*, 2003; Kitessa *et al.*, 2009), little effect on lipid stability was observed. When 18:3 was increased to 3.5 % of total fatty acids (Scollan *et al.*, 2004a), the value of thiobarbituric reactive substances (TBARS; a measure of lipid oxidation) after meat was displayed for 10 days increased considerably above the level of 2 mg malonaldehyde per kg meat at which rancidity may be detected by consumers. Colour saturation or intensity was also affected, declining fastest with the highest level of inclusion of the lipid supplement.

Long-chain PUFA are more susceptible to oxidation. When 20:5 + 22:6 increased from 17 to 30 mg/100 mg muscle due to inclusion of protected fish oil in the diet of steers, there was a small effect on colour stability, but the TBARS was increased resulting in a loss of shelf-life (Richardson *et al.*, 2004). A similar observation was made by Dunne *et al.* (2011) indicating that to maintain acceptable shelf-life of 20:5 + 22:6 enriched muscle beyond at least five days, (more) antioxidant protection is required. Nute *et al.* (2007) examined meat quality aspects of the lambs reported by Cooper *et al.* (2004), above. Beef from the combined unprotected fish oil/marine algae treatment had a higher level of long-chain omega-3 and lower colour and lipid stability compared to the unprotected fish oil alone. The appropriate ratio of vitamin E (and other antioxidants) to omega-3 PUFA in meat to ensure lipid and colour stability during processing remains to be determined.

The flavour of red meat, which develops during cooking, derives from the Maillard reaction between amino acids and reducing sugars and the thermal degradation of lipid. As some oxidation is necessary for optimum flavour development, diets which alter the fatty acid composition of the lipid fraction of meat could also alter the amount and type of volatiles produced and hence its aroma and flavour (Elmore and Mottram, 2009). The products of heat-induced oxidation of fatty acids, particularly PUFA, such as aliphatic aldehydes, ketones and alcohols, may have intrinsic flavours and they may also react further with Maillard products to give other compounds that contribute to flavour (Elmore and Mottram, 2009). Individual fatty acids have been associated with specific flavours. Larick and Turner (1990) showed that as the concentration of 18:2 in phospholipids declined and that of 18:3 increased, flavours identified as 'sweet' and 'gamey' declined whereas 'sour', 'bloody' and 'cooked beef fat' increased. Besides altering the flavour of fresh meat, PUFA are susceptible to the development of 'off-flavours' or rancidity during ageing of meat post-mortem. Beef from grass-fed cattle developed 'off-flavours' more rapidly during ageing than beef from grain-fed cattle, while fishy flavours are often detected in beef from grass-fed cattle after prolonged storage (Moore and Harbord, 1977; Xiong *et al.*, 1996).

In the European Union many consumers feel that meat from less intensively-fed animals has a better taste whilst in the USA, grass-finished beef is less acceptable (Melton, 1990). Raes *et al.* (2003) compared the fatty acid composition and flavour of retail beef from Limousin and Belgium Blue carcasses, which was produced locally in Belgium, with imported Argentinean and Irish beef. The fatty acid profiles suggested that the former meat was derived from cereal-fed animals and the latter were predominantly grass-fed. Sensory analysis and flavour volatile analysis showed that the grass-fed animals had higher flavour intensity with higher contents of low molecular weight unsaturated aldehydes derived from oxidation of long chain PUFA. In a study by Warren *et al.* (2008), loin joints from steers fed grass silage or fresh grass had higher scores for beef flavour and lower scores for abnormal flavour when compared to concentrate diets (restricted to the growth rate of the silage-fed animals). They also scored higher for 'overall liking' than the concentrate group. In a US study, steers finished on white clover had a higher 'grassy' flavour than those fed grass, and grass-fed animals produced meat which was not only higher in PUFA but was also prone to oxidation (rancidity; Larick and Turner, 1990). The authors attributed these differences in flavour to both the increased content of PUFA, particularly 18:3, its lower oxidative stability, and to odoriferous compounds stored in the depot fats.

As described above for shelf-life of meat, alterations in sensory characteristics are generally only seen when lipid oxidation is increased (Wood *et al.*, 2003). Elevating the levels of 18:3 through a ruminally protected PUFA-rich supplement increased the scores for sensory attributes such as 'abnormal' and 'rancid' (Scollan *et al.*, 2004a). There were few effects of unprotected fish oil in the study of Vatansever *et al.* (2000) while Wistuba *et al.* (2007) concluded that the differences found by a trained sensory panel due to fish oil inclusion in the diet of cattle were 'relatively small and would probably not be discernible to the average consumer'. Ponnampalam *et al.* (2002) similarly reported that sensory characteristics of lamb were not affected by dietary inclusion of fish meal or fish oil. This likely reflects the relatively small change in muscle PUFA in these studies. The increase in the concentration of 20:5 + 22:6 in muscle due to use of ruminally protected fish oil by Richardson *et al.* (2004) increased the sensory score for 'abnormal', but overall liking was not affected. Similarly, the combined unprotected fish oil/marine algae treatment had higher sensory scores for 'abnormal' and 'rancid' compared to the unprotected fish oil treatment, but overall liking was not affected (Nute *et al.*, 2007). While some of these descriptors seem negative, they contribute to the strength of the overall flavour and may in fact contribute to the acceptability of the meat. Whilst trained panellists can detect flavours that in themselves may be unpleasant, provided they are not dominant, they contribute to the overall flavour sensation.

Muscle with increased concentrations of omega-3 PUFA may therefore provide challenges to the processing sector to maintain the shelf-life and flavour required in particular markets. However, it also provides opportunities to develop new markets for nutritionally enhanced milk and meat.

8.5 Future trends

Whilst there is considerable variation in the omega-3 content of ruminant milk and meat, and we have described many of the sources of variation, levels are well short of levels regarded as beneficial in the human diet (EFSA, 2009). Rumen biohydrogenation means that it is much more costly to alter omega-3 PUFA content of ruminant products than is the case for monogastric products, although the potential to deliver omega-3 PUFA from grasses and clovers offers a lower cost solution in ruminants. Research must continue to address ways to reduce rumen biohydrogenation of omega-3 PUFA, particularly in forages; current 'natural' approaches such as physical processing and the effect of polyphenol oxidase in red clover deliver only relatively modest increases in product omega-3 PUFA. The fact that omega-3 PUFA are almost confined to the muscle phospholipids puts a further limit on increasing levels in beef and lamb, although there is more potential in milk triacylglycerols, at least for 18:3.

The relatively low levels of desaturation and chain elongation in ruminant tissues present a further problem to increasing levels of the long-chain omega-3 PUFA in ruminant products. However, there is an increasing suggestion that 18:3 omega-3 may be more beneficial in the human diet than was previously suggested and so attempts to deliver high levels of this fatty acid through milk are warranted. The study by Petit *et al.* (2002) showed that it is possible to produce milk with over 10% 18:3 omega-3, if rumen biohydrogenation can be avoided. A further challenge that must be addressed by research is the increased incidence of reduced shelf-life and taints in milk and meat with high levels of omega-3 PUFA. In particular, there is a need to define the optimal balance of omega-3 PUFA and antioxidants in ruminant products.

8.6 Conclusion

Ruminant milk and meat can make significant contributions to intakes of 18:3 omega-3, but contribute only small amounts of long-chain omega-3 PUFA in the human diet. Whilst a number of ruminant feedstuffs contain omega-3 PUFA, extensive rumen biohydrogenation means that only a small proportion of dietary 18:3 omega-3 passes from the rumen and is available to be incorporated into milk and meat. Unfortunately, animal feeds that are rich in omega-3 PUFA (such as linseed and fish oil), as well as methods for processing feeds to reduce rumen biohydrogenation are expensive, so there would have to be a significant price premium for milk or meat produced in this way. Plants are the primary source of omega-3 in the food chain, and altering levels of 18:3 omega-3 in forages for ruminants offers the lowest cost approach to increase inputs of omega-3 PUFA to the food chain. Further research should be directed to reduce rumen biohydrogenation of herbage PUFA and increase the activities of enzymes involved in synthesis of long-chain omega-3 PUFA in muscle and the mammary gland.

8.7 Sources of further information and advice

Related review papers are available as follows:

- all aspects of the composition of milk fat and fatty acids: Jensen (2002)
- fatty acid composition of beef muscle: Daley *et al.* (2010)
- genetic effects on meat fatty acids: de Smet *et al.* (2004)
- diet effects on milk fatty acids: Dewhurst *et al.* (2006), Lourenço *et al.* (2008)
- effects of botanically diverse pastures: Moloney *et al.* (2008)
- diet effect on milk quality: Martin *et al.* (2005)
- diet effects on meat quality: Scollan *et al.* (2006)

8.8 References

ABUGHAZALEH, A.A, SCHINGOETHE, D.J., HIPPEN, A.R., KALSCHEUR, K.F. and WHITLOCK, L.A. (2002) 'Fatty acid profiles of milk and rumen digesta from cows fed fish oil, extruded soybeans or their blend', *J Dairy Sci*, 85, 2266–2276.

ADDIS, M., CABIDDU, A., PINNA, G., DECANDIA, M., PIREDDA, G., PIRSI, A. and MOLLE, G. (2005) 'Milk and cheese fatty acid composition in sheep fed Mediterranean forages with reference to conjugated linoleic acid cis-9, trans-11', *J Dairy Sci*, 88, 3443–3454.

ADNØY, T., HAUG, A., SORHEIM, O., THOMASSON, M.S., VARSEGI, Z. and EIK, L.O. (2005) 'Grazing on mountain pastures – does it affect meat quality in lambs?', *Livest Prod Sci*, 94, 25–31.

AII, T., TAKAHASHI, S., KURIHARA, M. and KUME, S. (1988) 'The effects of Italian ryegrass hay, haylage and fresh Italian ryegrass on the fatty acid composition of cows' milk', *Jap J Zootech Sci*, 59, 718–724.

AL-MABUK, R.M., BECK, N.F.G. and DEWHURST, R.J. (2004) 'Effects of silage species and supplemental vitamin E on the oxidative stability of milk', *J Dairy Sci*, 87, 406–412.

AULDIST, M.J., WALSH, B.J. and THOMSON, N.A. (1998) 'Seasonal and lactational influences on bovine milk composition in New Zealand', *J Dairy Res*, 65, 401–411.

BARTSCH, B.D., GRAHAM, E.R.B. and MCLEAN, D.M. (1979) 'Protein and fat composition and some manufacturing properties of milk from dairy cows fed on hay and concentrates in various ratios', *Aust J Agric Res*, 30, 191–199.

BAS, P., BERTHELOT, V., POTTIER, E. and NORMAND, J. (2007) 'Effect of level of linseed on fatty acid composition of muscles and adipose tissues of lambs with emphasis on *trans* fatty acids', *Meat Sci*, 77, 678–688.

BERTHELOT, V., BAS, P. and SCHMIDELY, P. (2010) 'Utilization of extruded linseed to modify fatty acid composition of intensively-reared lamb meat: Effect of associated cereals (wheat vs. corn) and linoleic acid content of the diet', *Meat Sci*, 84, 114–124.

BOBE, G., ZIMMERMAN, S., HAMMOND, E.G., FREEMAN, A.E., PORTER, P.A., LUHMAN, C. M. and BEITZ, D.C. (2007) 'Butter composition and texture from cows with different milk fatty acid compositions fed fish oil or roasted soybeans', *J Dairy Sci*, 90, 2596–2603.

BOUFAÏED, H., CHOUINARD, P.Y., TREMBLAY, G.F., PETIT, H.V., MICHAUD, R. and BÉLANGER, G. (2003a) 'Fatty acids in forages. I. Factors affecting concentrations', *Can J Anim Sci*, 83, 501–511.

BOUFAÏED, H., CHOUINARD, P.Y., TREMBLAY, G.F., PETIT, H.V., MICHAUD, R. and BÉLANGER, G. (2003b) 'Fatty acids in forages. II. In vitro ruminal biohydrogenation of linolenic and linoleic acids from timothy', *Can J Anim Sci*, 83, 513–522.

BUTLER, G., STERGIADIS, S., SEAL, C., EYRE, M. and LEIFERT, C. (2011) 'Fat composition of organic and conventional retail milk in northeast England', *J Dairy Sci*, 94, 24–36.

CALDER, P.C. (2002) 'Dietary modification of inflammation with lipids', *Proc Nutr Soc*, 61, 345–358.

CAVALIERI, F.B., SANTOS, G.T., MATSUSHITA, M., PETIT, H.V., RIGOLON, L.P., SILVA, D., HORST, J.A., CAPOVILLA, L.C. and RAMOS, F.S. (2005) 'Milk production and milk composition of dairy cows fed Lac100® or whole flaxseed', *Can J Anim Sci*, 85, 413–416.

CHIKUNYA, S., DEMIREL, G., ENSER, M., WOOD, J.D., WILKINSON, R.G. and SINCLAIR, L.A. (2004) 'Biohydrogenation of dietary n-3 PUFA and stability of ingested vitamin E in the rumen, and their effects on microbial activity in sheep', *Brit J Nutr*, 91, 539–550.

CHILLIARD, Y., FERLAY, A. and DOREAU, M. (2001) 'Effect of different types of forages, animal fat or marine oils in cow's diet on milk fat secretion and composition, especially conjugated linoleic acid (CLA) and polyunsaturated fatty acids', *Livest Prod Sci*, 70, 31–48.

CHOUINARD, P.Y., CORNEAU, L., BUTLER, W.R., CHILLIARD, Y., DRACKLEY, J.K. and BAUMAN, D.E. (2001) 'Effect of dietary lipid source on conjugated linoleic acid concentrations in milk fat', *J Dairy Sci*, 84, 680–690.

COLLOMB, M., BÜTIKOFER, U., SIEBER, R., BOSSET, J-O. and JEANGROS, B. (2001) 'Conjugated linoleic acid and trans fatty acid composition of cows' milk fat produced in lowlands and highlands', *J Dairy Res*, 68, 519–523.

COLLOMB, M., BÜTIKOFER, U., SIEBER, R., JEANGROS, B. and BOSSET, J.O. (2002) 'Composition of fatty acids in cow's milk fat produced in the lowlands, mountains and highlands of Switzerland using high-resolution gas chromatography', *Int Dairy J*, 12, 649–659.

COOPER, S.L., SINCLAIR, L.A., WILKINSON, R.G., HALLETT, K.G., ENSER, M. and WOOD, J.D. (2004) 'Manipulation of the n-3 polyunsaturated fatty acid content of muscle and adipose tissue in lamb', *J Anim Sci*, 82, 1461–1470.

COULON, J.B. and PRIOLO, A. (2002) 'Influence of forage feeding on the composition and organoleptic properties of meat and dairy products, bases for a 'terroir' effect', *Grassland Sci Eur,* 7, 513–524.

COULON, J.-B., DELACROIX-BUCHET, A., MARTIN, B. and PIRISI, A. (2004) 'Relationships between ruminant management and sensory characteristics of cheeses: a review', *Lait*, 84, 221–241.

DALEY, C.A., ABBOTT, A., DOYLE, P.S., NADER, G.A. and LARSON, S. (2010) 'A review of fatty acid profiles and antioxidant content in grass-fed and grain-fed beef', *Nutr J*, 9, 10–12.

DANNENBERGER, D., NUERNBERG, G., SCOLLAN, N.D., SCHABBEL, W., STEINHART, H., ENDER, K. and NUERNBERG, K. (2004) 'Effect of diet on the deposition of n-3 fatty acids, conjugated linoleic and C18:1 trans fatty acids isomers in muscle lipids of German Holstein bulls', *J Agric Food Chem*, 52, 6607–6615.

DE SMET, S., RAES, K. and DEMEYER, D. (2004) 'Meat fatty acid composition as affected by genetics: a review', *Anim Res,* 53, 81–98.

DECAEN, C. and ADDA, J. (1970) 'Evolution de la secretion des acides gras des matieres grasses du lait au cours de la lactation de la vache', *Ann Biol Anim Biochem Biophys*, 10, 659–677.

DECAEN, C. and GHADAKI, M.B. (1970) 'Variation de la secretion des acides gras des matières grasses du lait de vache à l'herbe et au cours des six premières semaines d'exploitation du fourrage vert', *Ann Zootech*, 19, 399–411.

DEMEYER, D. and DOREAU, M. (1999) 'Targets and procedures for altering ruminant meat and milk lipids', *Proc Nutr Soc*, 58, 593–607.

DEMIREL, G., WACHIRA, A.M., SINCLAIR, L.A., WILKINSON, R.G., WOOD, J.D. and ENSER, M. (2004) 'Effects of dietary n-3 polyunsaturated fatty acids, breed and dietary vitamin E on the fatty acids of lamb muscle, liver and adipose tissue', *Brit J Nutr*, 91, 551–565.

DEUTSCHE GESELLESCHAFT FÜR FETTWISSENSCHAFT (2011) *Fettsäurezusammensetzung wichtiger pflanzlicher und tierischer Speisefette und –öle*, available at: http://www.dgfett.de/material/fszus.php [accessed February 2013].

DEWHURST, R.J. (2003) 'Fatty acids in milk fat from organic dairy farms', in *Elm Farm Research Centre Bulletin*, October 11.

DEWHURST, R.J. and KING, P.J. (1998) 'Effects of extended wilting, shading and chemical additives on the fatty acids in laboratory grass silages', *Grass Forage Sci*, 53, 219–224.

DEWHURST, R.J., SCOLLAN, N.D., YOUELL, S.J., TWEED, J.K.S. and HUMPHREYS, M.O. (2001) 'Influence of species, cutting date and cutting interval on the fatty acid composition of grasses', *Grass Forage Sci*, 56, 68–74.

DEWHURST, R.J., FISHER, W.J., TWEED, J.K.S. and WILKINS, R.J. (2003a) 'Comparison of grass and legume silages for milk production. 1. Production responses with different levels of concentrate', *J Dairy Sci*, 86, 2598–2611.

DEWHURST, R.J., EVANS, R.T., SCOLLAN, N.D., MOORBY, J.M., MERRY, R.J. and WILKINS, R.J. (2003b) 'Comparisons of grass and legume silages for milk production. 2. In vivo and in sacco evaluations of rumen function', *J Dairy Sci*, 86, 2612–2621.

DEWHURST, R.J., SHINGFIELD, K.J., LEE, M.R.F. and SCOLLAN, N.D. (2006) 'Increasing the concentrations of beneficial polyunsaturated fatty acids in milk produced by dairy cows in high-forage systems', *Anim Feed Sci Technol,* 13, 168–206.

DONOVAN, D.C., SCHINGOETHE, D.J., BAER, R.J., RYALI, J., HIPPEN, A.R. and FRANKLIN, S.T. (2000) 'Influence of dietary fish oil on conjugated linoleic acid and other fatty acids in milk fat from lactating dairy cows', *J Dairy Sci*, 83, 2620–2628.

DUNNE, P., ROGALSKI, J., CHILOS, S., MONAHAN, F.J., KENNY, D.A. and MOLONEY, A.P. (2011) 'Long chain n-3 polyunsaturated fatty acid concentration and colour and lipid stability of muscle from heifers offered a ruminally protected fish oil supplement', *J Agric Food Chem*, 59, 5015–5025.

EFSA (2009) 'Scientific opinion: Labeling reference intake values for n-3 and n-6 polyunsaturated fatty acids', *EFSA J*, 1176, 1–11, available at: http://www.efsa.europa.eu/fr/scdocs/doc/1176.pdf [accessed February 2013].

ELGERSMA, A., MAUDET, P., WITKOWSKA, I.M. and WEVER, A.C. (2005) 'Effects of nitrogen fertilisation and regrowth period on fatty acid concentrations in perennial ryegrass (*Lolium perenne* L.)', *Ann Appl Biol*, 147, 145–152.

ELGERSMA, A., TAMMINGA, S. and ELLEN, G. (2006) 'Modifying milk composition through forage', *Anim Feed Sci Technol*, 131, 207–225.

ELLIS, K.A., INNOCENT, G., GROVE-WHITE, D., CRIPPS, P., MCLEAN, W.G., HOWARD, C.V. and MIHM, M. (2006) 'Comparing fatty acid composition of organic and conventional milk', *J Dairy Sci*, 89, 1938–1950.

ELMORE, J.S. and MOTTRAM, D.S. (2009) 'Flavour development in meat', in KERRY J.P. and LEDWARD, D. (eds), *Improving the Sensory and Nutritional Quality of Fresh Meat*. Cambridge: Woodhead, 111–146.

ENSER, M., HALLETT, K., HEWETT, B., FURSEY, G.A.J. and WOOD, J.D. (1996) 'Fatty acid content and composition of English beef, lamb and pork at retail', *Meat Sci*, 44, 443–458.

FAROUK, M.M. and WIELICZKO, K.J. (2003) 'Effect of diet and fat content on the functional properties of thawed beef', *Meat Sci*, 64, 451–458.

FERLAY, A., MARTIN, B., PRADEL, P., COULON, J.B. and CHILLIARD, Y. (2006) 'Influence of grass-based diets on milk fatty acid composition and milk lipolytic system in tarentaise and Montbeliarde cow breeds', *J Dairy Sci*, 89, 4026–4041.

FRASER, M.D., DAVIES, D.A., WRIGHT, I.A., VALE, J.E., NUTE, G.R., HALLETT, K.G. and RICHARDSON, R.I. (2007) 'Effect on upland finishing systems of incorporating winter feeding of red clover and summer grazing of *Molinia*-dominated semi-natural rough pastures', *Grass Forage Sci*, 62, 284–300.

FRENCH, P., STANTON, C., LAWLESS, F., O'RIORDAN, E.G., MONAHAN, F.J., CAFFREY, P.J. and MOLONEY, A.P. (2000) 'Fatty acid composition, including conjugated linoleic acid, of intramuscular fat from steers offered grazed grass, grass silage or concentrate-based diets', *J Anim Sci*, 78, 2849–2855.

GARCÍA, P.T., PENSEL, N.A., SANCHO, A.M., LATIMORI, N.J., KLOSTER, A.M., AMIGONE, M.A. and CASAL, J.J. (2008) 'Beef lipids in relation to animal breed and nutrition in Argentina', *Meat Sci*, 79, 500–508.

GARNSWORTHY, P.C., LOCK, A., MANN, G.E., SINCLAIR, K.D. and WEBB, R. (2008) 'Nutrition, metabolism, and fertility in dairy cows: 2. Dietary fatty acids and ovarian function', *J Dairy Sci*, 91, 3824–3833.

GATELLIER, P., MERCIER, Y. and RENERRE, M. (2004) 'Effect of diet finishing mode (pasture or mixed diet) on antioxidant status of Charolais bovine meat', *Meat Sci*, 67, 385–394.

GIVENS, D.I., COTTRILL, B.R., DAVIES, M., LEE, P.A., MANSBRIDGE, R.J. and MOSS, A.R. (2000) 'Sources of *n*-3 polyunsaturated fatty acids additional to fish oil for livestock diets: A review', *Nutr Abstr Rev Series B*, 70, 3–19.

GOODRIDGE, J., INGALLS, J.R. and CROW, G.H. (2001) 'Transfer of omega-3 linolenic acid and linoleic acid to milk fat from flaxseed or Linola protected with formaldehyde', *Can J Anim Sci*, 81, 525–532.

GONTHIER, C., MUSTAFA, A.F., BERTHIAUME, R., PETIT, H.V., MARTINEAU, R. and OUELLET, D.R. (2004) 'Effects of feeding micronized and extruded flaxseed on ruminal fermentation and nutrient utilization by dairy cows', *J Dairy Sci*, 87,1854–1863.

GONTHIER, C., MUSTAFA, A.F., OULLET, D.R., CHOUINARD, P.Y., BERTHIAUME, R. and PETIT, H.V. (2005) 'Feeding micronized and extruded flaxseed to dairy cows: Effects on blood parameters and milk fatty acid composition', *J Dairy Sci*, 88, 748–756.

GULATI, S.K., MCGRATH, S., WYN, P.C. and SCOTT, T.W. (2003) 'Preliminary results on the relative incorporation of docosahexaenoic and eicosapentaenoic acids into cows milk from two types of rumen protected fish oil', *Int Dairy J*, 13, 339–343.

HAGEMEISTER, H., PRECHT, D. and BARTH, C.A. (1988) 'Zum transfer von omega-3-fettsäuren in das milchfett bei kühen', *Michwissenschaft*, 43, 153–158.

HAUSWIRTH, C.B., SCHEEDER, M.R.L. and BEER, J.H. (2004) 'High ω-3 fatty acid content in alpine cheese. The basis for an alpine paradox', *Circulation*, 109, 103–107.

HAVEMOSE, M.S., WEISBERG, M.R., BRADIE, W.C.P. and NIELSEN, J.H. (2004) 'Influence of feeding different types of roughage on the oxidative stability of milk', *Int Dairy J*, 14, 563–570.

HEBEISEN, D.F., HOEFLIN, F., REUSCH, H.P., JUNKER, E. and LAUTERBURG, B.H. (1993) 'Increased concentrations of omega-3 fatty acids in milk and platelet rich plasma of grass-fed cows', *Int J Vitaminol Nutr Res*, 63, 229–233.

INNOCENTE, N., PRATURLON, D. and CORRADINI, C. (2002) 'Fatty acid profile of cheese produced with milk from cows grazing on mountain pastures', *Ital J Food Sci*, 14, 217–224.

JACOBS, M.N., COVACI, A., GHERGHE, A. and SCHEPEN, P. (2004) 'Time trend investigation of PCBs, PBDEs and organochlorine pesticides in selected n-3 polyunsaturated fatty acid rich dietary fish oil and vegetable oil supplements; nutritional relevance for human essential n-3 fatty acid requirements', *J Agric Food Chem*, 52, 1780–1788.

JAHREIS, G., FRITSCHE, J. and STEINHART, H. (1996) 'Monthly variations of milk composition with special regard to fatty acids depending on season and farm management system – Conventional versus ecological', *Fett/Lipids*, 98, 356–369.

JENSEN, R.G. (2002) 'The composition of bovine milk lipids: January 1995 to December 2000', *J Dairy Sci*, 85, 295–350.

JENSEN, S.K. and NIELSEN, K.N. (1996) 'Tocopherols, retionol, β-carotene, and fatty acis in the globule membrane and fat globule core in cows' milk', *J Dairy Res*, 63, 566–574.

JONES, E.L., SHINGFIELD, K.J., KOHEN, C., JONES, A.K., LUPOLI, B., GRANDISON, A.S., BEEVER, D.E., WILLIAMS, C.M., CALDER, P.C. and YAQOOB, P. (2005) 'Chemical, physical, and sensory properties of dairy products enriched with conjugated linoleic acid', *J Dairy Sci*, 88, 2923–2937.

KAY, J.K., ROCHE, J.R., KOLVER, E.S., THOMSON, N.A. and BAUMGARD, L.H. (2004) 'A comparison between feeding systems (pasture and TMR) and the effect of vitamin E supplementation on plasma and milk fatty acid profiles in dairy cows', *J Dairy Res*, 72, 322–332.

KELLY, M.L., KOLVER, E.S., BAUMAN, D.E., VAN AMBURGH, M.E. and MULLER, L.D. (1998) 'Effect of pasture on concentrations of conjugated linoleic acid in milk of lactating cows', *J Dairy Sci*, 81,1630–1626.

KHAN, N.A., CONE, J.S., FIEVEZ, V. and HENDRIKS, W.H. (2012) 'Causes of variation in fatty acid content and composition in grass and maize silages', *Anim Feed Sci Technol*, 174, 36–45.

KITESSA, S.M. and YOUNG, P. (2011) 'Enriching milk fat with n–3 polyunsaturated fatty acids by supplementing grazing dairy cows with ruminally protected Echium oil', *Anim Feed Sci Technol*, 170, 35–44.

KITESSA, S.M., GULATI, S.K., ASHES, J.R., SCOTT, T.W. and FLECK, E. (2001) 'Effect of feeding tuna oil supplement protected against hydrogenation in the rumen on growth and n-3 fatty acid content of lamb fat and muscle', *Aust J Agric Res*, 52, 433–437.

KITESSA, S.M., GULATI, S.K., SIMOS, G.C., ASHES, J.R., SCOTT, T.W., FLECK, E. and WYNN, P.C. (2004) 'Supplementation of grazing dairy cows with rumen-protected tuna oil enriches milk fat with n-3 fatty acids without affecting milk production or sensory characteristics', *Brit J Nutr*, 91, 271–277.

KITESSA, S.M, WILLIAMS A., GULATI, S., BOGHOSSIAN, V., REYNOLDS, J. and PEARCE, K.L. (2009) 'Influence of duration of supplementation with ruminally protected linseed oil on the fatty acid composition of feedlot lambs', *Anim Feed Sci Technol,* 151, 228–239.

KRAFT, J., COLLOMB, M., MÖCKEL, P., SIEBER, R. and JAHREIS, G. (2003) 'Differences in CLA isomer distribution of cow's milk lipids', *Lipids*, 38, 657–664.

KRONBERG, S.L., SCHOLLJEGERDES, E.J., LEPPER, A.N. and BERG, E.P. (2011) 'The effect of flaxseed supplementation on growth, carcass characteristics, fatty acid profile, retail shelf life, and sensory characteristics of beef steers finished on grasslands of the Northern Great Plains', *J Anim Sci*, 89, 2892–2903.

LARICK, D.K. and TURNER, B.E. (1990) 'Flavor characteristics of forage- and grain-fed beef as influenced by phospholipid and fatty acid compositional differences', *J Food Sci*, 55, 312–317.

LEE, M.R.F., HARRIS, L.J., DEWHURST, R.J., MERRY, R.J. and SCOLLAN, N.D. (2003) 'The effect of clover silages on long chain fatty acid transformations and digestion in beef steers', *Anim Sci*, 76, 491–501.

LEE, M.R.F., CONNELLY, P.L., TWEED, J.K.S., DEWHURST, R.J., MERRY, R.J. and SCOLLAN, N.D. (2006) 'Effects of high sugar ryegrass and mixtures with red clover silage on rumen function. 2. Lipid metabolism', *J Anim Sci*, 84, 3061–3070.

LEE, M.R.F., SCOTT, M.B., TWEED, J.K.S., MINCHINJ, F.R. and DAVIES, D.R. (2008) 'Effects of polyphenol oxidase on lipolysis and proteolysis of red clover silage with and without a silage inoculant (*Lactobacillus plantarum* L54)', *Anim Feed Sci Technol*, 144, 125–136.

LEE, M.R.F., EVANS, P.R., NUTE, G.R., RICHARDSON, R.I. and SCOLLAN, N.D. (2009) 'A comparison between red clover and grass silage feeding on fatty acid composition, meat stability and sensory quality of the *M. longissimus* muscle of dairy cull cows', *Meat Sci*, 81, 738–744.

LEHESKA, J.M., THOMPSON, L.D., HOWE, J.C., HENTGES, E., BOYCE, J., BROOKS, J.C., SHRIVER, B., HOOVER, L. and MILLER, M.K. (2008) 'Effects of conventional and grass-feeding systems on the nutrient composition of beef', *J Anim Sci*, 86, 3575–3585.

LEIBER, F., KREUZER, M., NIGG, D., WETTSTEIN, H.R. and SCHEEDER, M.R.L. (2005) 'A study on the causes for the elevated n-3 fatty acids in cow's milk of alpine origin', *Lipids*, 40, 191–202.

LESSARD, M., GAGNON, M. and PETIT, H.V. (2003) 'Immune response of postpartum dairy cows fed flaxseed', *J Dairy Sci*, 86, 2647–2657.

LESSARD, M., GAGNON, M., GODSON, G.L. and PETIT, H.V. (2004) 'Influence of parturition and diets enriched in n-3 or n-6 polyunsaturated fatty acids on immune response of dairy cows during the transition period', *J Dairy Sci*, 87, 2197–2210.

LIU, Y. (2007) *Rumen biohydrogenation of polyunsaturated fatty acids in high quality pasture*, M Agr Sc Thesis, Lincoln University, New Zealand.

LOCK, A.L. and GARNSWORTHY, P.C. (2003) 'Seasonal variation in milk conjugated linoleic acid and Δ(9)-desaturase activity in dairy cows', *Livest Prod Sci*, 79, 47–59.

LOOR, J.J., SORIANO, F.D., LIN, X., HERBEIN, J.H. and POLAN, C.E. (2003) 'Grazing allowance after the morning or afternoon milking for lactating cows fed a total mixed ration (TMR) enhances trans11–18:1 and cis9,trans11–18:2 (rumenic acid) in milk fat to different extents', *Anim Feed Sci Technol*, 109, 105–119.

LOURENÇO, M., VAN RANST, G., DE SMET, S., RAES, K. and FIEVEZ, V. (2007a) 'Effect of grazing pastures with different botanical composition by lambs on rumen fatty acid metabolism and fatty acid pattern of Longissimus muscle and subcutaneous fat', *Animal*, 1, 537–545.

LOURENÇO, M., DE SMET, S., RAES, K. and FIEVEZ, V. (2007b) 'Effect of botanical composition of silages on rumen fatty acid metabolism and fatty acid composition in *Longissimus* muscle and subcutaneous fat of lambs', *Animal*, 1, 911–921.

LOURENÇO, M., VAN RANST, G., VLAEMINCK, B., DE SMET, S. and FIEVEZ, V. (2008) 'Influence of different dietary forages on the fatty acid composition of rumen digesta as well as ruminant meat and milk', *Anim Feed Sci Technol*, 145, 418–437.

MACKLE, T.R., BRYANT, A.M., PETCH, S.F., HILL, J.P. and AULDIST, M.J. (1999) 'Nutritional influences on the composition of milk from cows of different protein phenotypes in New Zealand', *J Dairy Sci*, 82, 172–180.

MADDOCK, T.D., BAUER, F.L., KOCH, K.B., ANDERSON, V.L., MADDOCK, R.J., BARCELO-COBLIJN, G., MURPHY, E.J. and LARDY, G.P. (2006) 'Effect of processing flax in beef feedlot diets on performance, carcass characteristics, and trained sensory panel ratings', *J Anim Sci*, 84, 1544–1551.

MAFF (1998) *Food Fatty Acids Supplement to McCance and Widdowsons The Composition of foods*. London: Ministry of Agriculture, Fisheries and Food.

MARTIN, B., VERDIER-METZ, I., BUCHIN, S., HURTAUD, C. and COULON, J.B. (2005) 'How do the nature of forages and pasture diversity influence the sensory quality of dairy livestock products?', *Anim Sci*, 81, 205–212.

MELTON, S.L. (1990) 'Effects of feeds on flavour of red meats: A review', *J Anim Sci*, 68, 4421–4435.

MOALLEM, U. (2009) 'The effects of extruded flaxseed supplementation to high-yielding dairy cows on milk production and milk fatty acid composition', *Anim Feed Sci Technol*, 152, 232–242.

MOHAMMED, R., STANTON, C.S., KENNELLY, J.J., KRAMER, J.K.G., MEE, J.F., GLIMM, D.R. and O'DONOVAN, M. (2009) 'Grazing cows are more efficient than zero-grazed and grass silage-fed cows in milk rumenic acid production', *J Dairy Sci*, 92, 3874–3893.

MOLONEY, A.P., FIEVEZ, V., MARTIN, B., NUTE, G.R. and RICHARDSON, R.I. (2008) 'Botanically diverse forage-based rations for cattle: implications for product composition and quality and consumer health', *Grassland Sci Eur*, 13, 361–374.

MOORBY, J.M., LEE, M.R.F., DAVIES, D.R., KIM, E.J., NUTE, G.R., ELLIS, N.M. and SCOLLAN, N.D. (2009) 'Assessment of dietary ratios of red clover and grass silages on milk production and milk quality in dairy cows', *J Dairy Sci*, 92, 1148–1160.

MOORE, V.J. and HARBORD, M.W. (1977) 'Palatability of beef from cattle fed maize silage and pasture', *NZ J Agric Res*, 20, 279–281.

MORALES-ALMARZ, E., SOLDADO, A., GONZÁLEZ, A., MARTÍNEZ-FERNÁNDEZ, A., DOMÍNGUEZ-VARA, I., DE LA ROZA-DELGADO, B. and VICENTE, F. (2010) 'Improving the fatty acid profile of dairy cow milk by combining grazing with feeding of total mixed ration', *J Dairy Res*, 77, 225–230.

MORENO, T., KEANE, M.G., NOCI, F. and MOLONEY, A.P. (2008) 'Fatty acid composition of muscle from Holstein-Friesian steers of New Zealand and European/American descent and from Belgian Blue x Holstein-Friesian steers, slaughtered at two weights', *Meat Sci*, 80, 157–169.

MURPHY, J.J. (2000) 'Synthesis of milk fat and opportunities for nutritional manipulation', in AGNEW, R.E., AGNEW, K.W. and FEARON, A.M. (eds), *Milk Composition, Occasional Publication No. 25*. Penicuik: British Society of Animal Science, 201–222.

MUSTAFA, A.F., CHOUINARD, P.Y. and CHRISTENSEN, D.A. (2003) 'Effects of feeding micronized flaxseed on yield and composition of milk from Holstein cows', *J Sci Food Agric*, 83, 920–926.

NELSON, K.A.S. and MARTIN, S. (2009) 'Increasing omega fatty acid content in cow's milk through diet manipulation: Effect on milk flavour', *J Dairy Sci*, 92, 1378–1386.

NOCI, F., FRENCH, P., MONAHAN, F.J. and MOLONEY, A.P. (2005a) 'The fatty acid composition of muscle fat and subcutaneous adipose tissue of pasture-fed beef heifers: Influence of duration of grazing', *J Anim Sci*, 83, 1167–1178.

NOCI, F., O'KIELY, P., MONAHAN, F.J., STANTON, C. and MOLONEY, A.P. (2005b) 'Conjugated linoleic acid concentration in M. Longissimus dorsi from heifers offered sunflower oil-based concentrates and conserved forages', *Meat Sci*, 69, 509–518.

NOCI, F., MONAHAN, F.J., SCOLLAN, N.D. and MOLONEY, A.P. (2007) 'The fatty acid composition of muscle adipose tissue of steers offered unwilted or wilted grass silage supplemented with sunflower oil and fish oil', *Brit J Nutr*, 97, 502–513.

NUDDA, A., MCGUIRE, M.A., BATTACONE, G. and PULINA, G. (2005) 'Seasonal variation in conjugated linoleic acid and vaccenic acid in milkfat of sheep and its transfer to cheeses and ricotta', *J Dairy Sci*, 88, 1311–1319.

NUTE, G.R., RICHARDSON, R.I., WOOD, J.D., HUGHES, S.I., WILKINSON, R.G., COOPER, S.L. and SINCLAIR, L.A. (2007) 'Effect of dietary oil source on the flavour and the colour and lipid stability of lamb meat', *Meat Sci*, 77, 547–555.

OFFER, N.W. (2002) 'Effects of cutting and ensiling grass on levels of CLA in bovine milk', in GECHIE, L.M. and THOMAS, C. (eds), *XIIIth International Silage Conference*, 11–13 September, Scottish Agricultural College, Auchincruive, 16–17.

O'SULLIVAN, A., GALVIN, K., MOLONEY, A.P., TROY, D.J., O'SULLIVAN, K. and KERRY, J.P. (2003) 'Effect of pre-slaughter ratios of forages and or concentrates on the composition and quality of retail packaged beef', *Meat Sci*, 63, 279–286.

PALLADINO, R.A., O'DONOVAN, M., KENNEDY, E., MURPHY, J.J., BOLAND, T.M. and KENNY, D.A. (2009) 'Fatty acid composition and nutritive value of twelve cultivars of perennial ryegrass', *Grass Forage Sci*, 64, 219–226.

PETERSEN, M.B., SØEGAARD, K. and JENSEN, S.K. (2011) 'Herb feeding increases n-3 and n-6 fatty acids in cow milk', *Livest Sci*, 141, 90–94.

PETIT, H.V. (2002) 'Digestion, milk production, milk composition, and blood composition of dairy cows fed whole flaxseed', *J Dairy Sci*, 85, 1482–1490.

PETIT, H.V., DEWHURST, R.J., SCOLLAN, N.D., PROULX, J.G., KHALID, M., HARESIGN, W., TWAGIRAMUNGU, H. and MANN, G.E. (2002) 'Milk production and composition, ovarian function, and prostaglandin secretion of dairy cows fed omega-3 fats', *J Dairy Sci*, 85, 889–899.

PETIT, H.V., GERMIQUET, C. and LEBEL, D. (2004) 'Effect of feeding whole, unprocessed sunflower seeds and flaxseed on milk production, milk composition, and prostaglandin secretion in dairy cows', *J Dairy Sci*, 87, 3889–3898.

PIREDDA, G., BANNI, S., CARTA, G., PIRISI, A., ADDIS, M. and MOLLE, G. (2002) 'Influenza dell'alimentazione al pascolo sui livelli di acido rumenico in latte e formaggio ovino', *Prog Nutr*, 4, 231–235 (Abstract in English).

PONNAMPALAM, E.N., SINCLAIR, A.J., EGAN, A.R., FERRIER, G.R. and LEURY, B.J. (2002) 'Dietary manipulation of muscle long chain omega-3 and omega-6 fatty acids and sensory properties of lamb meat', *Meat Sci*, 60, 125–132.

PONNAMPALAM, E.N., MANN, N.J. and SINCLAIR, A.J. (2006) 'Effect of feeding systems on omega-3 fatty acids, conjugated linoleic acid and trans fatty acids in Australian beef cuts: potential impact on human health', *Asia Pac J Clin Nutr*, 15, 21–29.

PRECHT, D. and MOLKENTIN, J. (1997) 'Effect of feeding on conjugated cisΔ9,transΔ11,-octadecadienoic acid and other isomers of linoleic acid in bovine milk fats', *Nahrung*, 41, 330–335.

PRECHT, D., MOLKENTIN, J. and VAHLENDIECK, M. (1999) 'Influence of the heating temperature on the fat composition of milk fat with emphasis on *cis–trans* isomerisation', *Nahrung*, 43, 25–33.

QI, B.X., FRASER, T., MUGFORD, S., DOBSON, G., SAYANOVA, O., BUTLER, J., NAPIER, J.A., STOBART, A.K. and LAZARUS, C.M. (2004) 'Production of very long chain polyunsaturated omega-3 and omega-6 fatty acids in plants', *Nat Biotechnol*, 22, 739–745.

RAES, K., BALCAEN, A., DIRINCK, P., DE WINNE, A., CLAEYS, E., DEMEYER, D. and DE SMET, S. (2003) 'Meat quality, fatty acid composition and flavour analysis in Belgian retail beef', *Meat Sci*, 65, 1237–1246.

RAMASWAMY, N., BAER, R.J., SCHINGOETHE, D.J., HIPPEN, A.R., KASPERSON, K.M. and WHITLOCK, L.A. (2001) 'Composition and flavour of milk and butter from cows fed fishoil, extruded soybeans, or their combination', *J Dairy Sci*, 84, 2144–2151.

REALINI, C.E., DUCKETT, S.K., BRITO, G.W., DALLA RIZZA, M. and DE MATTOS, D. (2004) 'Effect of pasture vs. concentrate feeding with or without antioxidants on carcass characteristics, fatty acid composition, and quality of Uruguayan beef', *Meat Sci*, 66, 567–577.

REGO, O.A., ROSA, H.J.D., PORTUGAL, P., CORDEIRO, R., BORBA, A.E.S., VOULEZA, C.M. and BESSA, R.J.B. (2005) 'Influence of dietary fish oil on conjugated linoleic acid, omega-3 and other fatty acids in milk fat from grazing dairy cows', *Livest Prod Sci*, 95, 27–33.

REVELLO-CHION, A., TABACCO, E., PEIRETTI, P.G. and BORREANI, G. (2011) 'Variation in the fatty acid composition of alpine grassland during spring and summer', *Agron J*, 103, 1072–1080.

RICHARDSON, R.I., HALLETT, K.G., BALL, R., ROBINSON, A.M., NUTE, G.R., ENSER, M., WOOD, J.D. and SCOLLAN, N.D. (2004) 'Effect of free and ruminally-protected fish oils on fatty acid composition, sensory and oxidative characteristics of beef loin muscle', *Proc 50th Int Conf Meat Sci Technol*, Helsinki, 2.43.

RYHANEN, E.L., TALLAVAARA, K., GRIINARI, J.M., JAAKOLA, S., MANTERE-ALHONEN, S. and SHINGFIELD, K.J. (2005) 'Production of conjugated linoleic acid enriched milk and dairy products from cows receiving grass silage supplemented with a cereal-based concentrate containing rapeseed oil', *Int Dairy J*, 15, 207–217.

SAYANOVA, O.V. and NAPIER, J.A. (2004) 'Eicosapentaenoic acid: biosynthetic routes and the potential for synthesis in transgenic plants', *Phytochem*, 65, 147–158.

SCHROEDER, G.F., DELAHOY, J.E., VIDAURRETA, I., BARGO, F., GAGLIOSTRO, G.A. and MULLER, L.D. (2003) 'Milk fatty acid composition of cows fed a total mixed ration or pasture plus concentrates replacing corn with fat', *J Dairy Sci*, 86, 337–3248.

SCOTT, T.W. and ASHES, J.R. (1993) 'Dietary lipids for ruminants: protection, utilization, and effects on remodelling of skeletal muscle phospholipids', *Aust J Agric Res*, 44, 495–508.

SCOLLAN, N.D., CHOI, N.J., KURT, E., FISHER, A.V., ENSER, M. and WOOD, J.D. (2001) 'Manipulating the fatty acid composition of muscle and adipose tissue in beef cattle', *Brit J Nutr*, 85, 115–124.

SCOLLAN, N.D., ENSER, M., GULATI, S., RICHARDSON, R.I. and WOOD, J.D. (2003) 'Effect of including a ruminally protected lipid supplement in the diet on the fatty acid composition of beef muscle in Charolais steer', *Brit J Nutr*, 90, 709–716.

SCOLLAN, N., ENSER, M., RICHARDSON, R.I., GULATI, S., HALLETT, K.G., NUTE, G.R. and WOOD, J.D. (2004a) 'The effects of ruminally-protected dietary lipid on the lipid composition and quality of beef muscle', *Proc 50th Int Conf Meat Sci Technol*, Helsinki, 2.50.

SCOLLAN, N.D., ENSER, M., RICHARDSON, I., GULATI, S., HALLETT, K.G. and WOOD, J.D. (2004b) 'The effects of including ruminally protected lipid in the diet of Charolais steers on animal performance, carcass quality and the fatty acid composition of longissimus dorsi muscle', *Proc Brit Soc Anim Sci Meeting*, 5–7 April, York, 87.

SCOLLAN, N.D., DEWHURST, R.J., MOLONEY, A.P. and MURPHY, J.J. (2005) 'Improving the quality of products from grassland', in MCGILLOWAY, D.A. (ed.) *Grassland: a Global Resource*. Wageningen: Wageningen Academic Publishers, 41–56.

SCOLLAN, N., HOCQUETTE, J.F., NUERNBERG, K., DANNENBERGER, D., RICHARDSON, I. and MOLONEY, A. (2006) 'Innovations in beef production systems that enhance the nutritional and health value of beef lipids and their relationship with meat quality', *Meat Sci*, 74, 17–33.

SHINGFIELD, K.J., AHVENJÄRVI, S., TOIVONEN, V., ÄRÖLÄ, A., NURMELA, K.V.V., HUHTANEN, P. and GRIINARI, J.M. (2003) 'Effect of fish oil on biohydrogenation of fatty acids and milk fatty acid content in cows', *Anim Sci*, 77, 165–179.

SHINGFIELD, K.J., LEE, M.R.F., HUMPHRIES, D.J., SCOLLAN, N.D., TOIVONEN, V., BEEVER, D.E. and REYNOLDS, C.K. (2011) 'Effect of linseed oil and fish oil alone or as an equal mixture on ruminal fatty acid metabolism in growing steers fed maize silage-based diets', *J Anim Sci*, 89, 3728–3741.

STANTON, C., LAWLESS, F., KJELLMER, G., HARRINGTON, D., DEVERY, R., CONNOLLY, J.F. and MURPHY, J. (1997) 'Dietary influences on bovine milk cis-9, trans-11-conjugated linoleic acid content', *J Food Sci*, 62, 1083–1086.

STAPLES, C.R. and THATCHER, W.W. (2005) 'Effects of fatty acids on reproduction of dairy cows', in GARNSWORTHY, P.C. and WISEMAN, J. (eds), *Recent Advances in Animal Nutrition*. Nottingham: Nottingham University Press, 229–256.

STAPLES, C.R., BURKE, J.M. and THATCHER, W.W. (1998) 'Influence of supplemental fats on reproductive tissues and performance of lactating cows', *J Dairy Sci*, 81, 856–871.

STOCKDALE, C.R., WALKER, G.P., WALES, W.J., DALLEY, D.E., BIRKETT, A., SHEN, Z. and DOYLE, P.T. (2003) 'Influence of pasture and concentrates in the diet of grazing dairy cows on the fatty acid composition of milk', *J Dairy Res*, 70, 267–276.

THOMSON, N.A. and VAN DER POEL, W. (2000) 'Seasonal variation of the fatty acid composition of milk fat from Friesian cows grazing pasture', *Proc NZ Soc Anim Prod*, 60, 314–317.

TIMMEN, H. and PATTON, S. (1988) 'Milk fat globules: fatty acid composition, size and in vivo regulation of fat liquidity', *Lipids*, 23, 685–689.

TIMMONS, J.S., WEISS W.P., PALMQUIST D.L. and HARPER W.J. (2001) 'Relationship among roasted soybeans, milk components, and spontaneous oxidized flavour of milk', *J Dairy Sci*, 84, 2440–2449.

TURNER, S.-A., WAGHORN, G.C., WOODWARD, S.L. and THOMSON, N.A. (2005) 'Condensed tannins in birdsfoot trefoil (*Lotus corniculatus*) affect the detailed composition of milk from dairy cows', *Proc NZ Soc Anim Prod*, 65, 283–289.

TYMCHUK, S.M., KHORASANI, G.R. and KENNELLY, J.J. (1998) 'Effect of feeding formaldehyde and heat-treated oil seed on milk yield and composition', *Can J Anim Sci*, 78, 793–800.

VAN DORLAND, H.A., KREUZER, M., LEUENBERGER, H. and WETTSTEIN, H.-R. (2008) 'Comparative potential of white and red clover to modify the milk fatty acid profile of cows fed ryegrass-based diets from zero-grazing and silage systems', *J Sci Food Agric*, 88, 77–85.

VANHATALO, A., KUOPPALA, K., TOIVONEN, V. and SHINGFIELD, K.J. (2007) 'Effects of forage species and stage of maturity on bovine milk fatty acid composition', *Eur J Lipid Sci Technol*, 109, 856–867.

VATANSEVER, L., KURT, E., ENSER, M., NUTE, G.R., SCOLLAN, N.D., WOOD, J.D. and RICHARDSON, R.I. (2000) 'Shelf life and eating quality of beef from cattle of different breeds given diets differing in n-3 polyunsaturated fatty acid composition', *Anim Sci*, 71, 471–482.

VIBART, R.E., FELLNER, V., BURNS, J.C., HUNTINGTON, G.B. and GREEN, J.T.JR. (2008) 'Performance of lactating dairy cows fed varying levels of total mixed ration and pasture', *J Dairy Res*, 75, 471–480.

WACHIRA, A.M., SINCLAIR, L.A., WILKINSON, R.G., ENSER, M., WOOD, J.D. and FISHER, A.V. (2002) 'Effects of dietary fat source and breed on the carcass composition, n-3 polyunsaturated fatty acid and conjugated linoleic acid content of sheep meat and adipose tissue', *Brit J Nutr*, 88, 697–709.

WALES, W.J., DOYLE, P.T., STOCKDALE, C.R. and DELLOW, D.W. (1999) 'Effects of variation in herbage mass, allowance, and level of supplementation on nutrient intake and milk production of dairy cows in spring and summer', *Aust J Exp Agric*, 39, 119–131.

WARD, A.T., WITTENBERG, K.M., FROEBE, H.M., PRZYBYLSKI, R. and MALCOLMSON, L. (2003) 'Fresh forage and solin supplementation on conjugated linoleic acid levels in plasma and milk', *J Dairy Sci*, 86, 1742–1750.

WARREN, H.E., SCOLLAN N.D., NUTE G.R., HUGHES S.I., WOOD J.D. and RICHARDSON R.I. (2008) 'Effects of breed and a concentrate or grass silage diet on beef quality in cattle of 3 ages. II. Meat stability and flavour', *Meat Sci*, 78, 270–278.

WHITE, S.L., BERTRAND, J.A., WADE, M.R., WASHBURN, S.P., GREEN, J.T. and JENKINS, T.C. (2001) 'Comparison of fatty acid content of milk from Jersey and Holstein cows consuming pasture or a total mixed ration', *J Dairy Sci*, 84, 2295–2301.

WHITTINGTON, F.W., DUNN, R., NUTE, G.R., RICHARDSON, R.I. and WOOD, J.D. (2006) 'Effect of pasture type on lamb product quality', in WOOD, J.D. (ed.) *New developments in sheep meat quality, Proc 9th Ann Langford Food Ind Conf.* Edinburgh: BSAS, 27–32.

WISTUBA, T.J., KEGLEY, E.B., APPLE, J.K. and RULE, D.C. (2007) 'Feeding feedlot steers fish oil alters the fatty acid composition of adipose and muscle tissue', *Meat Sci*, 77, 196–203.

WITKOWSKA, I.M., WEVER, C., GORT, G. and ELGERSMA, A. (2008) 'Effects of nitrogen rate and regrowth interval on perennial ryegrass fatty acid content during the growing season', *Agron J*, 100, 1371–1379.

WOLFF, R.L., BAYARD, C.C. and FABIEN, R.J. (1995) 'Evaluation of sequential methods for the determination of butterfat composition with emphasis on trans-18:1 acids: Application to the study of seasonal variations in French butter', *J Amer Oil Chem Soc*, 72, 1471–1483.

WHO (2003) *Diet, nutrition and the prevention of chronic diseases*, Report of a joint WHO/FAO expert consultation, WHO Technical Report Series 916. Geneva: World Health Organization.

WOOD, J.D. and ENSER, M. (1997) 'Factors influencing fatty acids in meat and the role of antioxidants in improving meat quality', *Brit J Nutr*, 78, S49–S60.

WOOD, J.D., RICHARDSON, R.I., NUTE, G.R., FISHER, A.V., CAMPO, M.M., KASAPIDOU, E., SHREAD, P.R. and ENSER, M. (2003) 'Effects of fatty acids on meat quality: a review', *Meat Sci*, 66, 21–32.

WOODS, V.B. and FEARON, A.M. (2009) 'Dietary sources of unsaturated fatty acids for animals and their transfer into meat, milk and eggs: a review', *Livest Sci*, 126, 1–20.

XIONG, Y.L., MOODY, W.G., BLANCHARD, S.P., LIU, G. and BURRIS, W.R. (1996) 'Postmortem proteolytic and organoleptic changes in hot-boned muscle from grass-fed and grain-fed and zeranol implanted cattle', *Food Res Int*, 29, 27–34.

YANG, A., LANARI, M.C., BREWSTER, M. and TUME, R.K. (2002) 'Lipid stability and meat colour of beef from pasture- and grain-fed cattle with or without vitamin E supplement', *Meat Sci*, 60, 41–50.

9

Egg enrichment with omega-3 fatty acids

G. Cherian, Oregon State University, USA

DOI: 10.1533/9780857098863.3.288

Abstract: Consumer awareness of the beneficial effects of omega-3 fatty acids has led to a demand for economical and easily available sources of these nutrients as an alternative to marine foods. In response to this, the poultry industry has launched several brands of omega-3 enriched eggs, consumption of which could contribute over 50% of the recommended daily intake of omega-3 fatty acids. However, problems relating to lipid oxidation and consequent decreased shelf-life, loss of omega-3 fatty acids during storage and decreased sensory qualities remain as problems. The use of feed additives such as vitamin E and other types of antioxidants is under consideration to resolve these issues.

Key words: eggs, omega-3 fatty acids, lipid oxidation, antioxidant, human health.

9.1 Introduction

In the years since 2000, a wide variety of foods containing health-promoting nutrients have been launched into the market as 'functional foods.' Eggs are no exception to the category of functional foods. Among the different nutrients targeted for enrichment in eggs, fatty acids belonging to the omega-3 family have been explored in detail by several researchers.[1,2] The current chapter describes briefly the composition of egg lipids with emphasis on omega-3 fatty acids, the physiological and dietary factors affecting egg lipid composition, omega-3 fatty acid enrichment and egg quality, nutritional evaluation of omega-3 fatty acid-modified eggs, and the challenges associated with omega-3 fatty acid enrichment in chicken eggs.

9.2 Egg lipid composition, formation and deposition

9.2.1 Composition

An average chicken egg weighs about 55 g and is composed of approximately 9.5 % shell, 63 % egg white and 27.5 % yolk. The yolk or the 'oocyte' is a single massive cell and constitutes about 16 g in an average chicken egg. The yolk comprises 51–52 % water, 16–17 % protein and 31–33 % fat, including cholesterol, fat-soluble vitamins, pigments and some minerals. Lipids or fats are the major components in yolk, representing 60 % of the yolk on a dry weight basis. The main constituents of yolk lipids are very low and high density lipoproteins. Trace levels of lipids have been observed in the whites (<0.1 %). Egg yolk lipids are made up mainly of triacylglycerol, phospholipids, free cholesterol and some other minor lipids (e.g. cerebroside). Triacylglycerol and phospholipids comprise up to 65–68 and 29–32 %, respectively, of yolk lipids. The cholesterol content of an average egg may vary from 210 to 215 mg. Fatty acids are the most prevalent components of triglycerides and phospholipids and constitute up to >4 g in an average egg. The fatty acids in eggs are mainly of medium to long chain length, that is, they have 14- to 22-carbon atoms with different degrees of saturation as well as configurations. Commercially, in the USA, table eggs are produced from white or brown leghorn hens fed diets predominantly based on corn and soybean. Eggs laid by hens fed such diets consist of about 2 g saturated fatty acids, 2.5 g monounsaturated fatty acids, and 1–1.1 g polyunsaturated fatty acids (PUFA), of which omega-6 and omega-3 fatty acids may constitute 0.9 and 0.2 mg, respectively.

9.2.2 Egg yolk lipid formation and deposition

To understand egg lipid composition, it is essential to understand the physiological and dietary factors involved in lipid synthesis in the laying hen. Egg lipid formation is a finely tuned process orchestrated through action of the hen's hormones and liver tissue.[3] At hatch, pullets have a finite number of ovarian follicles present which, at sexual maturity, increase in size to form an array of small follicles as well as a hierarchy of large follicles that vary in size. Yolk is deposited into follicles as they proceed through the hierarchy to become mature through a process called vitellogenesis.

Physiological factors

In chickens, the liver is the primary organ for fat synthesis. In response to an increase in oestrogen concentration at sexual maturity, the hen liver synthesizes triacylglycerol and several apolipoproteins such as $apoB_{100}$, apo VLDL-II (very low density lipoporotein) and vitellogenin.[4] At the onset of egg laying, triacylglycerol synthesis in the hen liver increases over four-fold in association with concurrent increases in plasma VLDL content.[4] Similarly, plasma concentrations of vitellogenin also increase at the onset of egg laying. The lipoproteins that are targeted towards the yolk are smaller in size than regular VLDL and are called VLDLy.[5] Binding of VLDLy particles to receptors on the oocyte plasma membrane is through receptor-mediated endocytosis.[6] The lipids of VLDLy and vitellogenin are delivered to the oocyte without much alteration.

Triacylglycerol is the major component contributing over two-thirds of VLDLy lipids. Substantial amounts of phospholipids are also present, and free cholesterol constitutes about 5 % of VLDLy lipids. Within the oocyte, the endocytotic vesicles that are packed with yolk precursor undergo a series of fusions to form large yolk spheres. Thus the efficient uptake of VLDLy particles together with other lipoproteins is responsible for the dramatic expansion of the oocyte to form the yolk.[6,7] The majority of yellow yolk and lipids are deposited in the final phase (7–11 days before ovulation) of follicle maturity.

Nutritional factors: role of hen diet

In a typical layer hen diet, fats constitute 3–5 % and are from plant (e.g. vegetable oils, oil seeds) or animal (marine oils, rendered fat) sources. Fat in the hen's diet serves as a source of energy and essential fatty acids that cannot be synthesized by the hen. Fat synthesis in the liver comes *de novo* from the diet, re-utilizing fatty acids obtained as components of portomicron (chylomicron) remnants, or from free fatty acids that are released from adipose tissue. The saturated fatty acids of yolk lipids are synthesized in the hen liver and are transported to the yolk through lipoproteins. Therefore palmitic acid (16:0) is the predominant saturated fatty acid followed by stearic acid (18:0). Minor amounts of 20:0 are also found in eggs. The total saturated fatty acids constitute 30–33 % in regular commercial table eggs, of which palmitic acid is the predominant fatty acid.

The steroyl CoA desaturase (Δ^9-desaturase) is a key enzyme involved in fatty acid synthesis and facilitates the induction of one double bond to saturated fatty acids to form monounsaturated fatty acids.[8] The conversion of stearic acid (18:0) to oleic acid (18:1 n-9) and palmitic acid (16:0) to palmitoleic acid (18:1 n-7) occurs by Δ^9-desaturase enzyme. Birds lack the enzymes that introduce double bonds beyond carbon 9, counting from the carboxyl group, in the acyl chain. Because these include the Δ^{12}- and Δ^{15}-desaturases, birds cannot synthesize linoleic (18:2 n-6) and α-linolenic acids (18:3 n-3). These essential fatty acids are required by the avian cells and should be included in the hen diet. Linoleic and α-linolenic acid are also known as omega-6 and omega-3 fatty acids, respectively (based on the position of the first double bond from the CH_3 end). Although avian cells cannot synthesize linoleic and α-linolenic acids, they can metabolize them by further desaturation and elongation to form longer chain 20- and 22-carbon omega-3 and omega-6 fatty acids such as eicosapentaenoic acid (EPA), arachidonic acid, docosapentaenoic acid (DPA) and docosahexaenoic acid (DHA). A list of the omega-6 and omega-3 fatty acids and their concentrations reported in eggs is shown in Table 9.1. For example, feeding hens diets containing omega-3 fats such as fish oil or flax seeds leads to deposition of EPA, DPA and DHA into yolk lipids while including high n-6 oils such as sunflower leads to significant increases in the deposition of linoleic and arachidonic acids into the egg yolk.[9] Thus egg yolk PUFA

Table 9.1 Some of the common omega-6 and omega-3 fatty acids and their concentrations in chicken eggs

Omega-6 fatty acid	mg/egg	Omega-3 fatty acid	mg/egg
Linoleic acid (18:2 n-6)	780.0	α-Linolenic acid (18:3 n-3)	35.0
Arachidonic acid (20:4 n-6)	98.0	Eicosapentaenoic acid (20:5 n-3)	5.0
Docosatetraenoic (22:4 n-6)	5.2	Docosapentaenoic acid (22:5 n-3)	9.0
Docosapentaenoic acid (22:5 n-6)	6.8	Docosahexaenoic acid (22:6 n-3)	60.0

Notes: Concentration reported as mg/egg based on an average egg weighing 16 g yolk and 5 g fat. Values are subject to change based on hen's diet, strain or age.

content mirrors dietary fat as a result of the efficient uptake of VLDLy and other yolk precursors from the hen's serum into the growing oocyte. Such abrupt changes in yolk PUFA composition upon feeding omega-3 fatty acid rich specialty diets have led to the success in production and marketing of omega-3 PUFA-modified chicken eggs worldwide. Overall, final yolk fatty acid composition is influenced by a combination of factors including dietary supply, rate of fatty acid synthesis and transport from the liver, and deposition to yolk.

9.3 Modifying egg lipid composition

9.3.1 Egg and cholesterol controversy

Eggs, due to their low cost, excellent nutrient profile, ease of availability and versatility in food preparation, are a popular food item for all cultures. However, per capita consumption of eggs has seen a dramatic reduction over the past decades, especially in Western countries.[10] One of the major concerns associated with egg consumption is high cholesterol and saturated fat content. Thus eggs have been considered as blood cholesterol-raising foods and have been taken out of menu. Efforts to reduce egg cholesterol through genetic, dietary and pharmacological means have been attempted, but with limited success.[11] Several clinical studies have been conducted to examine the effect of egg consumption on serum cholesterol. [12,13] Although no direct effect of egg consumption on serum cholesterol has been observed from these studies, the results have not helped to revert the decline in egg consumption or reduce consumer-phobia about eggs as a food to avoid. Minimal progress in the area of egg yolk cholesterol reduction has prompted researchers to investigate alternative methods to improve the nutritional quality of the egg. Consequently, extensive research on reducing saturated fatty acids and increasing omega-3 fatty acids in chicken eggs, thereby increasing their nutritional quality, has been conducted. Researchers have been successful in achieving their goal and the results from such studies have been the subject of many peer-reviewed articles, reviews and book chapters.[14,15,16]

9.3.2 Reasons for increasing omega-3 fatty acids in chicken eggs

The pioneering studies by Dyerberg and Bang[17] suggesting the protective role of omega-3 PUFA against cardiovascular disease has led to an incredible amount of research concerning the relationship between dietary fats and human health. Subsequently, other epidemiological and clinical studies have documented that increased consumption of omega-3 PUFA offers potential in reducing the risk of coronary heart disease, atherosclerosis, hypertension and other cardiovascular diseases.[18,19] In addition, long-chain omega-3 PUFA such as DHA are components of the central nervous system and are considered 'essential' for normal growth, maturation and development of central nervous system.[20,21] Diets deficient in these fatty acids can result in impairments in functions of the cardiovascular, central nervous and immune systems.[19,22,23] The reported health effects of omega-3 PUFA have invoked considerable efforts for including different sources of omega-3 fatty acids in the diet. Traditionally, omega-3 fatty acids in the human diet come from terrestrial (e.g. green leafy vegetables, oil seeds such as flax) or marine (e.g. fatty fish) sources. α-Linolenic acid is the plant form of omega-3 fatty acid while longer chain fatty acids such as EPA, DPA, and DHA come from marine oils and fatty fish foods. The dietary supply of omega-3 fatty acids does not meet the required amounts due to limited fish intake and also due to high levels of omega-6 fatty acids in the foods produced through modern-day intensive production systems. This has led to a vast imbalance in the ratio of omega-6:omega-3 fatty acids in the current diet. For example, in Western countries dietary omega-6:omega-3 fatty acid ratios may range from 10:1 to 20:1, compared to a ratio of 1:1 in early hunter gatherer diets.[24]

9.3.3 Egg omega-3 fatty acid enrichment through hen's diet

Manipulating the hen's diet has been a successful way to enrich eggs with omega-3 fatty acids.[9,14,15] Both plant and marine oils are used in poultry diets for omega-3 fatty acid enrichment in eggs. In nature, omega-3 fatty acids are predominantly seen in the chloroplast of green leafy vegetables and also in seed oils such as flax (*Linum usitatissimum*), canola (*Brassica napus*), chia (*Salvia hispanica*) and *Camelina sativa*. Table 9.2 lists some of the feed sources and their omega-3 fatty acid content. Among the different plant-based sources, flaxseed is the most common ingredient used for omega-3 fatty acid enriched egg production due to its availability and high omega-3 fatty acid content and other nutritive value such as energy and protein.[9,14] Different marine sources (fish meal, fish oil, algae) are also used to increase the omega-3 fatty acids in eggs. Use of menhaden oil in hen feed to increase

Table 9.2 Omega-3 fatty acid content in some of the commonly reported feed sources for hens

Common name	α-Linolenic (18:3 n-3) (g/100 g)	Long-chain omega-3 fatty acid* (g/100 g)
Flaxseed	22.8	0
Perilla	58.0	0
Chia seed	17.6	0
Fish oil	1.5	36.0
Marine algae	0.0	11.0

*EPA+DPA+DHA.
Note: Results varied with batch, cultivars, or processing methods used.

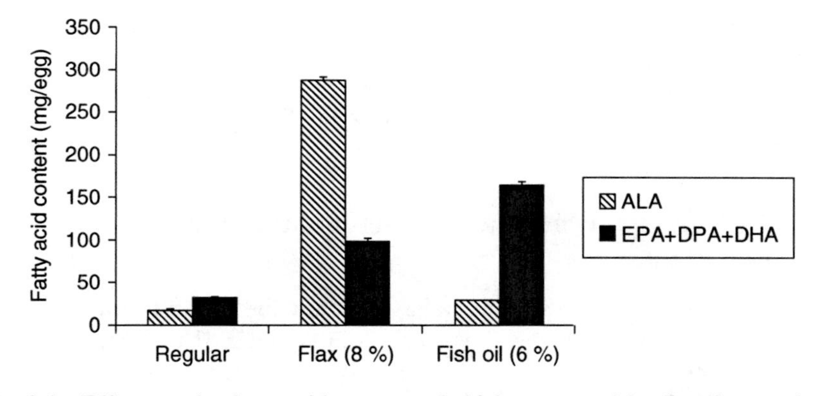

Fig. 9.1 Effect on the fatty acid content of chicken eggs of feeding flax seeds or fish oil to laying hens.

omega-3 fatty acids in eggs has been widely reported. Incorporation of marine fats results in an increase in the content of 20- and 22-C long chain omega-3 fatty acids such as EPA, DPA, DHA while addition of plant-based omega-3 fatty acids leads to enrichment of predominantly α-linolenic acid in eggs. Due to the limited ability of humans to convert α-linolenic acid into EPA and DHA, which are metabolically more active and important than α-linolenic acid, eggs from fish oil-fed birds may provide more health-promoting omega-3 fatty acids. Figure 9.1 shows the omega-3 fatty acid content of eggs from hens fed diets containing fish oil or flaxseeds.

9.3.4 Feeding omega-3 fats: hen production performance and egg quality aspects

Several authors reported different levels and forms of flax in laying hen diets and inclusion levels anywhere from 5 to 30 % of has been reported.[9,25,26]

However, discrepancies in the content of omega-3 fatty acids per egg, egg weight and shell quality, and production performances upon feeding flax to layer birds exist in the literature. Among the different factors that contributed to the disparity in the results are: form (ground, whole seed, processed) and amount of flax fed to hens, amount of other n-6 fatty acids in the diet, duration of feeding, age and strain of the hen. When summarizing the effects of feeding flax to egg laying hens, several trends on hen performance and egg quality are obvious. These include: (i) reduction in egg weight and yolk weight upon increase in dietary flax; (ii) decrease in body weight of birds, reduction in egg shell quality when fed for a longer time (over two months), and decrease in feed consumption. Most of the negative effects were observed when flax comprised over 10 % of the diet. However, it should be mentioned that several authors found no negative effects of including flax, while some authors reported an increase in egg production upon including flax in layer diets. Some of the negative effects associated with flax feeding on feed consumption and egg quality were due to the presence of anti-nutritional factors such as mucilage, phytic acid, antipyridoxin, trypsin inhibitors and hydrocyanic acid content in flax.[27]

9.4 Egg omega-3 fatty acid enrichment: consequences and challenges

Since the 1990s, several studies have reported the role of hens's diet in enriching egg yolk lipids with omega-3 fatty acids. These studies have reported over 300–500 mg of omega-3 fatty acids such as α-linolenic acid, EPA and DHA in eggs. Higher levels of omega-3 PUFA in eggs lead to increase in lipid oxidation products affecting the overall quality of eggs, including flavor, taste and nutritional value. This phenomenon is aggravated during storage which affects overall organoleptic aspects as well as nutrient content of enriched eggs. Thus, increasing the omega-3 fatty acid of eggs while maintaining satisfactory sensory qualities has been a challenge to food animal scientists. A great variety of substances and conditions have been studied to control lipid oxidation in prepared feeds to enhance egg sensory quality. The major strategy for the prevention of lipid oxidation is the use of phenolic antioxidants (e.g. butylated hydroxytoluene (BHT), butylated hydroxyanisole, tocopherols). Due to the limited number of antioxidants available, the major challenge for the feed industry is to optimize the concentration and combinations of available antioxidants more efficiently.

Much interest has developed in recent years in naturally occurring antioxidants because of the worldwide trend towards the usage of natural additives in feed mixes. α-Tocopheryl acetate is used as a natural antioxidant extensively in laying hens used for omega-3 egg production. In a recent study, we investigated the inclusion of α-tocopheryl acetate (50 vs 150 IU)

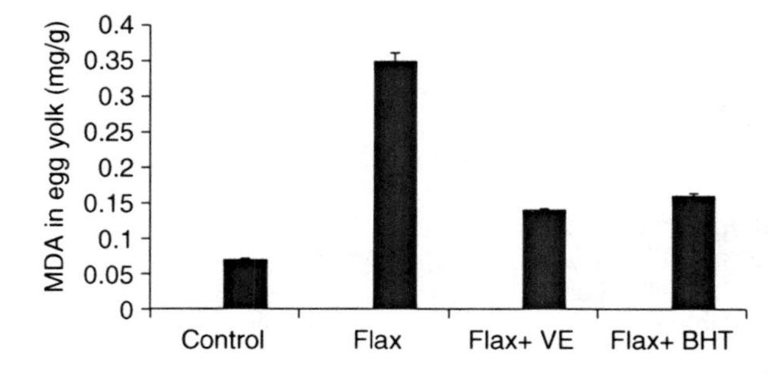

Fig. 9.2 Lipid oxidation products in eggs from hens fed flax seeds with vitamin E (VE) or BHT. (Source: adapted from Hayat *et al.*[29]) Note: MDA = malondialdehyde.

and BHT (50 vs 150 mg/kg) in hen diets containing 10 % flax on egg quality during storage. It was observed that α-tocopherol was better in preventing lipid oxidation than BHT in fresh eggs. However, neither had a significant effect on egg thiobarbituric acid (TBAR) reactive substances upon long-term storage (>60 day) or in enhancing the acceptability of n-3 fatty acid rich eggs by panelists (Fig. 9.2).[28,29]

9.4.1 Sensory characteristics and consumer acceptance of omega-3 enriched eggs

Sensory attributes and overall acceptability of omega-3 enriched eggs are very important for consumer acceptance. Flavor is consistently rated as the most important factor in determining consumption and repeat purchase of foods.[30] Therefore, maintaining egg aroma, flavor, taste and other organoleptic aspects is very important for success in the marketplace. While conducting taste panel studies on omega-3 fatty acid enriched eggs with trained and untrained panelists, it was observed that a majority (75–80 %) of the untrained panelists could not distinguish omega-3 enriched vs control eggs for aroma and flavor.[28] However, trained panelists could detect the difference and noted the eggs were 'different' from control eggs containing no omega-3 fatty acids. In general, the main off-flavor in eggs produced by feeding flax or marine oil to hens has been reported as 'fishy' by most panelists.[28]

9.4.2 Human studies with omega-3 fatty acid enriched eggs

The health effect of consuming omega-3 fatty acid enriched eggs has been well documented by several researchers. Most studies report significant increases in serum α-linolenic, EPA and DHA with omega-3 egg consumption.[31,32] The effect on total or LDL cholesterol was minimal or negligible in most studies. Interestingly, several researchers have reported higher levels of high-density lipoprotein (HDL) cholesterol with the consumption

Table 9.3 Omega-3 fatty acid-rich egg consumption and reported health effects in humans

- Increase in plasma HDL-cholesterol
- Increase in α-linoleic, docosahexaenoic and other long-chain omega-3 fatty acids
- Reduction in linoleic, arachidonic and other omega-6 fatty acids
- Increase in DHA content of platelet phospholipids
- Decrease in platelet aggregation in adults
- No or negligible effect on total cholesterol or LDL-cholesterol
- Reduction in serum triglycerides, and systolic and diastolic blood pressure

of omega-3 fatty acid enriched eggs. Other benefits of omega-3 fatty acid enriched egg consumption include reduction in blood triglyceride, decrease in both systolic and diastolic blood pressure, and reduction in plasma omega-6 fatty acids. Incorporating omega-3 enriched eggs in the diet of nursing women has been reported to increase breast milk content of α-linolenic acid and DHA.[33] Some of the most reported effects of omega-3 fatty acid enriched egg consumption in humans are summarized in Table 9.3.

9.5 Conclusion and future trends

Consumer awareness about the beneficial effects of omega-3 fats has led them to look for alternative, affordable and easily available sources of these nutrients other than the traditional marine foods. Chicken eggs, due to their high nutrient content, low cost and ease of availability have always been a popular food for all ages and cultures. The digestive physiological features in laying chickens enable nutritionists to enrich the omega-3 PUFA content in eggs through the hen diet in a natural and sustainable manner. This technology primarily utilizes the incorporation of oils (e.g. marine oils) or oil seeds (e.g. flaxseed, chia) in the laying hen diet. In the years since 2000, the poultry industry globally has adopted this technology to successfully launch several brands of specialty omega-3 fatty acid enriched eggs. Consumption of such eggs could contribute to over 50 % of the daily recommended omega-3 fatty acid need. This can be considered a significant achievement for fulfiling current recommendations of increasing omega-3 fatty acid intakes. However, increased levels of these PUFA in eggs may perpetuate lipid oxidation resulting in decreased shelf-life and other organoleptic attributes of egg. To overcome this, further enrichment with vitamin E and other types of antioxidants has been considered. Despite this achievement, fishy taste, loss of omega-3 PUFA during storage and increased lipid oxidation products still remain a pitfall of this strategy.

The market demand for foods with nutrient composition adjusted to optimize human health and life expectancy is growing. To achieve the desirable effect of increasing bioactive compounds such as omega-3 PUFA in eggs, one must also take into account of the costs of production, availability of feed sources and egg quality, as well as sustainability aspects. Therefore, future research should aim at developing low cost feed sources, improved methods for feed processing and use of metabolically efficient hens capable of synthesizing 20- and 22-C PUFA from 18-C precursors. Such strategies will lead to the production of omega-3 enriched eggs in an economical and sustainable way. In addition, greater understanding of other factors such as nutrient labeling and long-term health effects of n-3 fatty acid enriched egg consumption in different age groups is needed to provide consumer confidence in the product.

9.6 References

1. LESKANICH CO and NOBLE RC, 'Manipulation of the n-3 polyunsaturated fatty acid composition of avian eggs and meat'. *World's Poultry Sci. J.* 1996, 53–55.
2. CHERIAN G (2009) 'Eggs and health: nutrient sources and supplement carriers', in WATSON RR (ed.), *Complementary and Alternative Therapies and the Aging Population*. San Diego, CA: Academic Press, 333–346.
3. ETCHES RJ (1984) 'Maturation of ovarian follicles', in CUNNINGHAM PE, LAKE D and HEWITT FJ (eds), *Reproductive Biology of Poultry*. Edinburgh: British Poultry Science Ltd, 51–73.
4. SPEAKE BK, MURRAY AMB and NOBLE RC, 'Transport and transformation of yolk lipids during development of the avian embryo'. *Prog. Lipid Res.* 1998, 37, 1–32.
5. WALZEM RL, HANSEN RJ, WILLIAMS DL and HAMILTON RL, 'Estrogen induction of VLDLy assembly in egg-laying hens'. *J. Nutr.* 1999, 129, 467S–472S.
6. SCHNEIDER WJ, 'Receptor-mediated mechanisms in ovarian follicle and oocyte development'. *Gen. Comp. Endocrinol.* 2009, 163, 18–23.
7. WALZEM RL, 'Lipoproteins and the laying hen: form follows function'. *Poultry and Avian Biol. Rev.* 1996, 7, 31–64.
8. NTAMBI JM and MIYAZAKI M, 'Regulation of stearoyl-CoA desaturases and role in metabolism'. *Prog. Lipid Res.* 2004, 43, 91–104.
9. CHERIAN G (2008) 'Omega-3 fatty acids: studies in avians', in DE MEESTER F and WATSON RR (eds), *Wild-Type Food in Health Promotion and Disease Prevention: The Columbus® Concept*. Totowa, NJ: Humana Press, 169–178.
10. USDA (2010) *Agricultural statistics*. Washington, DC: Government Printing Office.
11. ELKIN RG, 'Reducing shell egg cholesterol content. II. Review of approaches utilizing non-nutritive dietary factors or pharmacological agents and an examination of emerging strategies'. *Worlds Poult. Sci. J.* 2007, 63, 5–31.
12. HU FB, STAMPFER MJ, RIMM EB, MANSON JE, ASCHERIO A, COLDITZ GA, ROSNER BA, SPIEGELMAN D, SPEIZER FE, SACKS FR, HENNEKENS CH and WILLETT WC, 'A prospective study of egg consumption and risk of cardiovascular disease in men and women'. *J. Am. Med. Assoc.* 1999, 281(15), 1387–1394.
13. SCRAFFORD C, NGA T and LEILA B, 'The impact of egg consumption on heart health using the NHANES III follow-up survey'. *FASEB J.* 2009, 23, 551–557.
14. RYMER C and GIVENS DI, 'N-3 Fatty acid enrichment of edible tissue of poultry: A review'. *Lipids* 2005, 40, 121–130.
15. PALMQUIST DL, 'Omega-3 fatty acids in metabolism, health, and nutrition and for modified animal product foods'. *Prof. Anim. Sci.* 2009, 25, 207–249.

16. CHERIAN G (2011) 'Dietary manipulation of poultry to develop value-added functional foods for humans', in GUPTA L and SINGHAL KK (eds), *Animal Nutrition: Advancements in Feeds and Feeding of Livestock*. Jodhpur: Agrobios, 339–356.
17. DYERBERG J and BANG HO, 'Haemostatic function and platelet polyunsaturated fatty acids in Eskimos'. *Lancet* 1979, 314, 433–435.
18. HU FB, MANSON JE and WILLETT WC, 'Types of dietary fat and risk of coronary heart disease: A critical review'. *J. Am. Coll. Nutr.* 2001, 20(1), 5–19.
19. YASHODHARA BM, UMAKANTH S, PAPPACHAN JM, BHAT SK, KAMATH R and CHOO BH, 'Omega-3 fatty acids: a comprehensive review of their role in health and disease'. *Postgrad. Med. J.* 2009, 85, 84–90.
20. CLANDININ MT, CHAPPELL JE, LEONG S, HEIM T, SWYER PR and CHANCE GW, 'Intrauterine fatty acid accretion rates in human brain: implications for fatty acid requirements'. *Early Hum. Dev.* 1980, 4, 121–129.
21. RAMAKRISHNAN U, IMHOFF-KUNSCH B and DIGIROLAMO AM, 'Role of docosahexaenoic acid in maternal and child mental health'. *Am. J. Clin. Nutr.* 2009, 89, 958S–962S.
22. INNIS SM, 'Dietary lipids in early development: relevance to obesity, immune and inflammatory disorders'. *Curr. Opin. Endocrinol, Diabetes Obes.* 2007, 14 (5), 359–364.
23. HOLMAN RT, JOHNSON SB and HATCH TF, 'A case of human linolenic acid deficiency involving neurological abnormalities'. *Am. J. Clin. Nutr.* 1982, 35, 617–623.
24. SIMOPOULOS AP, 'Human requirement for n-3 polyunsaturated fatty acids'. *Poult. Sci.* 2000, 79, 961–970.
25. CASTON LJ, SQUIRES EJ and LEESON S, 'Hen performance, egg quality and the sensory evaluation of eggs from SCWL hens fed flax'. *Can. J. Anim. Sci.* 1994, 74, 347–353.
26. GONZALEZ-ESQUERRA R and LEESON S, 'Alternatives for enrichment of eggs and chicken meat with omega-3 fatty acids'. *Can. J. Anim. Sci.* 2001, 81, 295–305.
27. MADHUSUDHAN KI, RAMESH HP, OGAWA T, SASAOKA K and SINGH N, 'Detoxification of commercial linseed meal for use in broiler rations'. *Poult. Sci.* 1986, 65, 164–171.
28. HAYAT Z, CHERIAN G, PASHA TN, KHATTAK FM and JABBAR MA, 'Sensory evaluation and consumer acceptance of eggs from hens fed flax seed and 2 different type of antioxidants'. *Poult. Sci.* 2010, 88, 2293–2298.
29. HAYAT Z, CHERIAN G, PASHA TN, KHATTAK FM and JABBAR MA, 'Oxidative stability and lipid components of eggs from flax-fed hens: Effect of dietary antioxidants and storage'. *Poult. Sci.* 2010, 89, 1285–1292.
30. CORDELL A, SCHUTZ HG and LESBER LL, 'Consumer perceptions of foods processed by innovative and emerging technologies: A conjoint analytic study'. *Innov. Food Sci. Emerg. Technol.* 2007, 8, 73–83.
31. FARRELL DJ, 'Enrichment of hen eggs with n-3 fatty acids and evaluation of enriched eggs in humans'. *Am. J. Clin. Nutr.* 1998, 68, 538–544.
32. FERRIER LK, CASTON LJ, LEESON S, SQUIRES J, WEAVER BJ and HOLUB BJ, 'α-Linolenic acid and docosahexaenoic acid enriched eggs from hens fed flaxseed: influence on blood lipids and platelet phospholipids fatty acids in humans'. *Am. J. Clin. Nutr.* 1995, 62, 81–86.
33. CHERIAN G and SIM JS, 'Changes in the breast milk fatty acids and plasma lipids of nursing mothers following consumption of n-3 polyunsaturated fatty acid enriched eggs'. *Int. J. Appl. Basic Nutr. Sci.* 1996, 12, 8–12.

10

Enrichment of meat products with omega-3 fatty acids by methods other than modification of animal diet

D. Ansorena and I. Astiasarán, University of Navarra, Spain

DOI: 10.1533/9780857098863.3.299

Abstract: This chapter looks at research into methods of modifying the formulations of fresh, cooked and fermented meat products in order to increase their content of omega-3 fatty acids (FA). Walnut, vegetable oils rich in alpha-linoleic acid and fish and algae oils rich in long-chain omega-3 FA have traditionally been the main ingredients used for that purpose. More recently, pre-emulsified oils have been added to products along with an antioxidant supply sufficient to control lipid oxidation. Most of the products developed showed good technological and sensory properties and achieved significant omega-3 FA amounts and better omega-6/omega-3 ratios. Microencapsulation of bioactive compounds is being studied with a view to improving the stability and the bioavailability of the omega-3 supplied by the meat products.

Key words: microencapsulation, fortified meat products, pre-emulsified oils, omega-3 fatty acids, antioxidant capacity.

10.1 Introduction

Current nutritional recommendations and dietary guidelines for consumers recommend a moderate intake of meat products based on their nutritional composition. A wide range of meat products is available, with great variation in nutritional composition depending on the formulation of the product. However, in most cases meat products have some common characteristics, such as their relatively high content of salt and animal fat and the presence of curing salts (nitrites and nitrates). Products with these attributes are not always among the healthier dietary choices, particularly for people who are prone to cardiovascular diseases or obesity. Methods of improving the nutritional profile of meat products have therefore been widely studied in order to contribute to a healthier diet (Jiménez-Colmenero, 2007;

Vandendriessche, 2008; Decker and Park, 2010; Weiss *et al.*, 2010; Zhang *et al.*, 2010; Toldrá and Reig, 2011; Ansorena and Astiasarán, 2012). These modifications have involved either adding beneficial compounds to the newly developed products or removing or decreasing the amount of unhealthy ones.

The amount and composition of fat in a meat product depends on the formulation of the product and on the type and part of the animal used in its preparation. For instance, in cured ham the amount of fat can be quite low (around 4 %), whereas in dry fermented sausages it could be very high (around 40 %). Differences in the lipid profiles of the different meat types used in preparing meat products can also lead to some variability in the final amounts of cholesterol, saturated fatty acids (SFA), monounsaturated fatty acids (MUFA) and polyunsaturated fatty acids (PUFA). For instance, the PUFA/SFA and omega-6/omega-3 ratios in muscle fat are 0.11 and 2.11 for lamb, 0.15 and 1.32 for beef and 0.58 and 7.22 for pork, respectively (Wood *et al.*, 2004). It should be noted that the low omega-6/omega-3 ratio shown in ruminant meats is due to the high levels of 18:3 fatty acid in grass. In fact, the levels of PUFA in meat are dependent on the diet of the animal, as has been described in Chapter 8.

On the other hand, the recommended PUFA/SFA ratio is established between 0.4 and 1 (Wood *et al.*, 2004) and the omega-6/omega-3 ratio is established between 1 and 4 (WHO, 2003). Moreover, different health organizations have proposed dietary recommendations for the daily intakes of fatty acids for adults. EFSA has recently established an Adequate Intake (AI) of 0.5 % of energy for α-linolenic acid (ALA) and 250 mg for eicosapentaenoic acid plus docosahexaenoic acid (EPA + DHA) (based on considerations of cardiovascular health) (EFSA, 2010). In the USA, the recommendation is 0.6–1.2 % of energy for α-linolenic acid (USDA, 2010). The specific recommendations for omega-3 fatty acids, and especially long-chain omega-3 PUFA, are linked to evidence for some beneficial health effects, such as contribution to the development of infant brain and liver and decrease in the risk of tumors (Funahashi *et al.*, 2006, Kim *et al.*, 2009), cardiovascular diseases (Coates *et al.*, 2009), inflammatory disorders (Calder, 2006) and neurological disorders (Assisi *et al.*, 2006).

10.2 Enrichment of meat products with omega-3 fatty acids

Increasing the supply of omega-3 FA in foodstuffs can be performed by means of two potential strategies: feeding animals with omega-3 enriched diets in order to enhance the natural omega-3 content in eggs, fish, meat, etc., or including ingredients rich in omega-3 in the formulation of processed foods. In the case of processed meats, this second strategy has been widely investigated since 2000, using different ingredients and several different techniques.

The main technological approaches are the direct addition of omega-3 rich vegetables (walnuts) or oils (vegetable, fish and algae oils) and, especially in the last few years, the use of pre-emulsified oils which has become a good technological alternative. Usually the novel ingredients provide a partial substitute for the traditional animal fat in processed meat formulations, but sometimes the objective is partial substitution of the fat along with fat reduction. Also, antioxidants have been used to stabilize the potential oxidative process related to the increase in the PUFA content, as the higher susceptibility of PUFA to lipid oxidation compared to SFA and MUFA is widely known. In this sense, although synthetic antioxidants have been successfully used, current trends are focused on the search for natural antioxidants obtained mainly from vegetable sources.

When emulsions are used, they usually are oil-in-water (o/w) emulsions containing the omega-3 FA rich oil, water in different proportions and a protein (usually whey protein, egg proteins, sodium caseinate or soy protein isolate) as emulsifier. Microbial transglutaminase has also been used to catalyse the cross-linking between them. The protein used determines the different physicochemical properties of the systems obtained and their suitability for use as backfat replacers in the different types of meat products (Delgado-Pando *et al.*, 2010a). Proteins can also act as antioxidants, helping to stabilize the systems (Pennisi Forell *et al.*, 2010). In other cases, natural antioxidants have been used to minimize oxidation (García-Iñiguez de Ciriano *et al.*, 2010a).

The main results demonstrated by research dealing with the incorporation of omega-3 fatty acids into meat products are described in this chapter. Table 10.1 summarizes the amounts of omega-3 fatty acids (g/100 g product) and omega-6/omega-3 ratios achieved in several types of enriched meat products (fresh, cooked and dry fermented sausages). Table 10.2 summarizes work that includes the addition of antioxidants to fortified products.

10.2.1 Fresh meat products

Fresh meat products based on a mix of ground meat have been fortified with omega-3 fatty acids in different ways (Tables 10.1 and 10.2). The addition of walnut as a partial substitute for raw meat (20 % walnut instead of the same amount of raw meat material), using transglutaminase as binding agent (Serrano *et al.*, 2004), has been used in restructured beef steak (Serrano *et al.*, 2005), resulting in a significant reduction of the omega-6/omega-3 ratio. The amounts of omega-3 were 2116 and 23.40 mg/100 g in the products with and without walnuts, respectively. The products developed had a greater fat content (14.52 % compared to 1.57 % in the control) and omega-6/omega-3 ratio (3.79 compared to 10.23 in the control). As walnuts are very rich in MUFAs, a significant increase in the ratio of UFA/SFA was also achieved. Moreover, the authors reported a significant decrease in the atherogenic and thrombogenic indexes and a decrease in

Table 10.1 Amounts of omega-3 fatty acids and omega-6/omega-3 ratios in several types of enriched meat products (fresh, cooked and dry fermented sausages)

	Type of product	ALA (g/100 g)	EPA (g/100 g)	DHA (g/100 g)	Total omega-3 (g/100 g)	Omega-6/ omega-3	Reference
Fresh products							
Addition of fish oil	Ground beef patties	–	–	–	0.4	–	Lee *et al.* (2005)
Addition of walnut (20 %)	Restructured beef steak	2.07	0.41	0.07	2.11	3.79	Serrano *et al.* (2005)
Addition of emulsion of algae oil	Ground turkey patties	–	–	0.4	–	–	Lee *et al.* (2006)
Addition of emulsion of algae oil	Fresh pork sausages	–	–	0.4	–	–	Lee *et al.* (2006)
Addition of emulsion of algae oil	Restructured ham	–	–	0.32	–	–	Lee *et al.* (2006)
Pre-emulsified linseed oil – fat replacer (15 % substitution) – with antioxidants	Fresh pork sausages	2.68	0.01	0.01	2.72	1.31	Valencia *et al.* (2008)
Pre-emulsified fish oil – fat replacer (15 % substitution) – with antioxidants	Fresh pork sausages	0.27	0.70	0.44	1.55	1.91	Valencia *et al.* (2008)
Addition of linseed oil (3 %)	Low fat chicken meat patties	1.16	–	–	1.16	2.02	Singh *et al.* (2011)
Cooked products							
Walnut – fat replacer	Frankfurters	2.17	–	0.01	2.18	4.89	Ayo *et al.* (2007)
Pre-emulsified fish oil (6 % in formulation)	High fat mortadella	–	0.66	0.40	1.49	2.54	Cáceres *et al.* (2008)
Pre-emulsified fish oil (6 % in formulation)	Low fat mortadella	–	0.66	0.46	1.37	1.79	Cáceres *et al.* (2008)

Deodorized salmon oil + vitamin E+ rosemary extract – incorporated into products in brine (16.6 %)	Frankfurt sausages, cooked ham and cooked turkey breast	–	–	–	–	0.5–2.8	Reglero *et al.* (2008)
Olive oil + algae oil + seaweed – fat replacer	Low fat-frankfurters	0.06	–	0.33	0.44	1.95	López-López *et al.* (2009)
Pre-emulsified olive + linseed + fish oil – fat replacer (100 % substitution)	Low-fat frankfurters	2.03	0.29	0.20	2.62	0.47	Delgado Pando *et al.* (2010b)
Pre-emulsified linseed oil – fat replacer (25 % substitution)	Mortadella	2.4	–	–	2.4	1.9	Berasategi *et al.* (2011)
Olive + linseed + fish oil + konjac gel–fat replacer (100 % substitution)	Pâté	2.7	0.42	0.28	3.72	0.48	Delgado-Pando *et al.* (2011b)
Fermented products							
Addition of fish oil extract	Chorizo	–	0.15	0.13	0.28		Muguerza *et al.* (2004)
Pre-emulsified linseed oil – fat replacer (25 % substitution) – synthetic antioxidants (BHA + BHT)	Chorizo	2.8	–	0.02	2.82	1.93	Valencia *et al.* (2006b)
Pre-emulsified deodorized fish oil (Lysi) – fat replacer (25 % substitution)	Chorizo	0.31	0.64	0.46	1.41		Valencia *et al.* (2006a)
Pre-emulsified algae oil (DHASCO®-S) – fat replacer (15 % substitution)	Chorizo	0.27	0.04	1.30	1.71	2.62	Valencia *et al.* (2007)

(Continued)

Table 10.1 *Continued*

	Type of product	ALA (g/100 g)	EPA (g/100 g)	DHA (g/100 g)	Total omega-3 (g/100 g)	Omega-6/ omega-3	Reference
Pre-emulsified algae oil (DHASCO®-S) – fat replacer (25 % substitution)	Chorizo	0.28	0.05	1.68	2.13	2.35	Valencia *et al.* (2007)
Flaxseed encapsulated oil – fat replacer (20 % substitution)	Dutch style sausage	4.96	–	–	4.96	1.05	Pelser *et al.* (2007)
Pre-emulsified linseed oil – fat replacer (25 % substitution) – natural antioxidant (*Borago officinalis*)	Chorizo	2.5	0.01	0.03	2.5	1.85	García Iñiguez de Ciriano *et al.* (2009)
Pre-emulsified linseed + algae oil (3:2) – fat replacer (25 % substitution)	Chorizo	1.6	0.02	0.66	2.26	1.96	García Iñiguez de Ciriano *et al.* (2010b)
Walnut – fat replacer (45 % substitution)	Sucuk	1.39	0.03	–	1.42	4.13	Ercoskun and Dermici-Ercoskun (2010)

– no data available in the original paper.

Table 10.2 Summary of the use of synthetic and natural antioxidants in omega-3 enriched meat products

	Product	Lipid modification	Antioxidants and their effects	Reference
Fresh	Ground beef patties	Fish oil (n-3: 500 mg/110 g meat)	A combination of citrate, erythorbate and rosemary extract was the most effective	Lee *et al.* (2005)
	Fresh ground turkey and fresh pork sausage	Algal oil (n-3: 500 mg/110 g meat)	A combination of citrate (0.5 %), erythorbate (0.1 %) and rosemary extract (0.2 %) was effective	Lee *et al.* (2006)
	Fresh pork sausages	Linseed oil or fish oil as fat replacers (15 % substitution)	Green tea catechins (200 mg/kg) reduced lipid oxidation in raw fish sausages and improved their sensory scores after being cooked	Valencia *et al.* (2008)
Cooked	Bologna type	Pre-emulsified linseed oil as fat replacer (25 % substitution)	Lyophilized aqueous ethanol extract of *Melissa officinalis* (965 mg/kg) or BHA (200 mg/kg) controlled lipid oxidation	Berasategi *et al.* (2011)
	Frankfurters	Mixture of olive, linseed and fish oil as fat replacer (100 % substitution)	Hydroxytyrosol (100 mg/kg) was more effective antioxidant than BHT + BHA (100 + 100 mg/kg) during chilling storage	Cofrades *et al.* (2011)
	Frankfurters	Canola oil or canola + olive oil as backfat replacers (100 % substitution)	Walnut paste (2 g/100 g) contributed to a decrease in TBAR	Álvarez *et al.* (2011)
Fermented	Chorizo	Pre-emulsified deodorized fish oil as fat replacer (25 % substitution)	BHT + BHA (100 + 100 mg/kg) controlled lipid oxidation	Valencia *et al.* (2006a)
	Chorizo	Pre-emulsified linseed oil as fat replacer (25 % substitution)	BHT + BHA (100 + 100 mg/kg) controlled lipid oxidation during storage	Valencia *et al.* (2006b)
	Chorizo	Pre-emulsified algae oil as fat replacer (15 % substitution)	BHT + BHA (100 + 100 mg/kg) controlled lipid oxidation	Valencia *et al.* (2007)
	Chorizo	Pre-emulsified linseed oil as fat replacer (25 % substitution)	Lyophilized aqueous extract of *Borago officinalis* (340 mg/kg) or BHA (200 mg/kg) controlled lipid oxidation	García-Iñiguez de Ciriano *et al.* (2009)
	Chorizo	Pre-emulsified linseed + algae oil (3:2) as fat replacer (25 % substitution)	Lyophilized aqueous extract of *Melissa officinalis* (686 mg/kg) controlled lipid oxidation	García-Iñiguez de Ciriano *et al.* (2010b)

the total cholesterol supply. The stability of these products during frozen storage was also demonstrated without major adverse effects on quality characteristics, apart from discoloring (enhanced lightness and yellowness and reduced redness) (Serrano *et al.*, 2006). Although adding walnut produced certain changes in the matrix, the resulting products presented acceptable physicochemical and sensory characteristics (Cofrades *et al.*, 2004; Serrano *et al.*, 2004). A more detailed discussion on these aspects can be found in a review published by Jiménez-Colmenero *et al.* (2010).

Lee *et al.* (2005) developed omega-3 fortified ground beef patties (with 15 % fat) by adding fish oil directly (500 mg/110 g meat). They recognized the need to add an effective antioxidant to protect the product against lipid oxidation. Among different chelators (sodium tripolyphosphate, sodium citrate), radical scavengers (butylated hydroxyanisole – BHA, mixed tocopherols, rosemary extract) and reductants (sodium erythorbate), they concluded that the most effective for stabilizing color and delaying lipid oxidation was a combination of sodium citrate, sodium erythorbate and rosemary. Moreover, a similar combination of antioxidants was shown to be effective in minimizing lipid oxidation in ground turkey patties and fresh pork sausages to which an o/w emulsion containing algal oil (25 %w/w, with 40–42 % of DHA) had been added in amounts sufficient to achieve a concentration of 500 mg DHA/110 g meat (Lee *et al.*, 2006).

Fresh pork sausages enriched with pre-emulsified omega-3 rich oils were also successfully developed by Valencia *et al.* (2008) when antioxidants were used. Linseed and fish oils were substituted for 15 % of traditional pork backfat in ready-to-eat (cooked) products in an emulsion, resulting in increases in omega-3 PUFA from 1.66 to 1.86 % in the control to 9.37 and 6.49 % in products with added linseed and fish oils, respectively. When natural antioxidants (green tea catechins or green coffee antioxidant, both at 200 ppm) were added to the formulation, higher amounts of omega-3 were obtained in cooked products (11.60–11.62 % for products with linseed oil and 6.50–6.71 % for products with fish oil) compared to the corresponding omega-3 enriched batches without antioxidant, demonstrating the benefits of using an antioxidant to protect the PUFA from oxidation. The omega-6/omega-3 ratios reached values of less than 2 in every sausage developed (in contrast to 8.7–8.9 in the control products). Moreover, green tea catechins were shown to be more efficient than green coffee in reducing lipid oxidation in raw sausages containing fish oil after seven days storage.

Low-fat chicken meat patties (<10 % fat) with different levels of linseed oil (0–4 %) added directly to the formulation (as a partial substitute for the refined soybean oil used as source of added fat in the product) have been developed by Singh *et al.* (2011). They found that the products with added linseed oil (3 %) had increased omega-3 (1.163 g/100 g compared to 0.374 g/100 g in the control products) and a lower omega-3/omega-6 ratio (2.02 compared to 7.36 in the control products). Also the products were stable and microbiologically safe during refrigerated aerobic storage for 25 days, indicating that they could be commercially exploited.

10.2.2 Cooked meat products

The great variety in existing cooked meat products means that, from a technological point of view, different strategies need to be applied for the development of omega-3 PUFA enriched products (see Tables 10.1 and 10.2). The higher susceptibility of cooked meat products to lipid oxidation, resulting from heat treatment, is taken into account in traditional formulations where their antioxidant capacity to control lipid oxidation is usually assessed (Pie *et al.*, 1991; Decker and Crum, 1993). Although some studies have found similar reductions in SFA, MUFA and PUFA content as a consequence of cooking (Cortinas *et al.*, 2004), it seems logical to hypothesize an increase in susceptibility to cooking treatment when products are enriched with omega-3 PUFA.

In this regard, Lee *et al.* (2006) found that a combination of antioxidants (0.5 % citrate, 0.1 % erythorbate, 0.2 % rosemary) was able to protect against lipid oxidation in cooked products enriched with 25 % algal oil (500 mg omega-3 PUFA/110 g meat) incorporated as an emulsion. It was noted by Lee *et al.* that cooking resulted in some losses of omega-3 PUFA used to fortify meat products and that the losses were directly related to the applied temperature (ground turkey patties or fresh pork sausages showed higher loss of omega-3 PUFA than restructured hams as a consequence of the high temperature applied in the grilling process of those products). Those authors also observed that for restructured ham, nitrite curing appeared to delay lipid oxidation, so that antioxidant treatment effects were unobservable.

Enzymatic interesterified blends of lard and rapeseed oil have also been used in the production of cooked pork sausages, resulting in acceptable sensory attributes, no apparent fat excretion, PUFA/SFA ratios of 1.47–2.84 and significant amounts of α-linolenic acid (Cheong *et al.*, 2010).

Bologna-type sausages

The enrichment of Bologna-type sausages with omega-3 PUFA has been tried in different experiments (Cáceres *et al.*, 2008; Berasategi *et al.*, 2011). Fish oil added at different concentrations gave good results in traditional formulations and also in those with a 30 % lower energy value. Those formulations were adequate from a sensory point of view, increasing the omega-3 PUFA and achieving omega-6/omega-3 ratios close to 2 (in formulations with 6 % of fish oil). When the stability of the products was assessed by measurement of thiobarbituric acid reactants (TBARs), no problems with oxidation were found. When the enrichment was performed with linseed oil at 4.6 % (8.75 % emulsion), similar omega-6/omega-3 ratios were obtained (1.9). In both cases, the oils were added pre-emulsified with water and caseinate (in the case of fish oil) or soya protein (in the case of linseed oil). The increase in PUFA did not give rise to oxidation problems in either experiment. Where linseed oil was used the addition of an extra amount of antioxidants was necessary to control the oxidation process. The addition of BHA or an aqueous–ethanolic extract of *Melissa officinalis* significantly decreased the values for peroxides and TBARs before and after cooking and also showed significant increase in the potential antioxidant activities (measured through ABTS assay) of the final products (Berasategi *et al.*, 2011). When fish oil was added, no oxidative problems were found after 90 days of storage under refrigeration (Cáceres *et al.*, 2008).

Frankfurter-type sausages

The popularity of frankfurters with consumers and their technological characteristics offer a great opportunity for the development of a successful dietary omega-3 enrichment strategy. There is some evidence that walnut exercises a protective effect with regard to coronary heart disease which has led the US FDA to issue a 'qualified health claim' about walnuts and a reduced risk of heart disease (USDA, 2010). In light of this, some research has been undertaken to include walnut paste in frankfurter formulations as a source of MUFA (oleic acid) and PUFA (linoleic acid and linolenic acids) good results were obtained (Ayo *et al.*, 2007). The inclusion of 25 % walnut (total substitution for pork backfat) in frankfurters gave rise to omega-6/omega-3 ratios around 5 in contrast to 13.7 in control products (containing 20 % pork backfat) and 16.6 in traditional low fat products (containing 4 % pork backfat) and significant lower index as of atherogenicity (AI) and trombogenicity (TI). The atherogenicity index is defined as $AI = (C12{:}0 + C14{:}0 + C16{:}0) / (\omega{-}3\ PUFA + \omega{-}6\ PUFA + MUFA)$ and the thrombogenicity index is defined as $TI = (C14{:}0 + C16{:}0 + C18{:}0) / [0.5MUFA + 0.5(\omega{-}6)\ PUFA + 3(\omega{-}3)\ PUFA) + (\omega{-}3)/(\omega{-}6)]$ (Ulbricht and Southgate, 1991). These formulations also showed other nutritional advantages due to enrichment with minerals (Fe, Cu, K, Mg) and other bioactive components such as tocopherol, fibre, polyphenols and tannins (Ayo *et al.*, 2007).

Walnut paste has also been used in combination with vegetable oils (canola oil and olive oil) as backfat substitutes, showing that it could be useful for preventing lipid oxidation attributed to the presence of antioxidant vitamins (tocopherols) and antioxidant substances such as phytosterols and polyphenols (Álvarez *et al.*, 2011).

Low-fat frankfurters (12 % fat) enriched with omega-3 PUFA using algae oil (1.14 %) have been developed using a combination of seaweed (5.5 %) and a partial substitution of animal fat by olive oil or a mixture of olive oil and seaweed (López-López *et al.*, 2009). The products obtained had energy values in the range 185–195 kcal/100 g and omega-6/omega-3 ratios around 2. Furthermore, the addition of seaweed had been proved to constitute an alternative means to produce low-sodium products with significant dietary fibre content, better Na/K ratios and rich in Ca.

In other work, low-fat frankfurters (12 %) enriched with omega-3 PUFA were developed using a combination of olive, linseed and fish oils pre-emulsified with different protein systems. The products obtained had total energy values in the range 180–190 kcal/100 g and omega-6/omega-3 ratios around 0.47 (Delgado-Pando *et al.*, 2010b). Although the lipid oxidation levels attained were low, replacement of animal fat by healthier oil combinations in frankfurter formulations did promote a slight increase in lipid oxidation (Delgado-Pando *et al.*, 2011a). The same authors (Delgado-Pando *et al.*, 2011b) obtained low-fat pork liver paté with an omega-6/omega-3 ratio around 0.79 and 0.48 when partial and total pork backfat, respectively, was replaced by a combination of olive, linseed and fish oils stabilized with konjac gel (6.78 in control products). The sensory characteristics of the developed products were similar to the control samples, and no microbiological problems were detected in the new formulation.

The enrichment of frankfurters and other cooked meat products with omega-3 fatty acids gave rise not only to technological and sensory issues but also to problems related to stability. Potential functional frankfurters with low fat (11 %) and including an o/w emulsion enriched with olive, linseed and fish oils and hydroxytyrosol as antioxidant were evaluated in relation to their stability to lipid oxidation during 56 days of storage at 2 °C (Cofrades *et al.*, 2011). Hydroxytyrosol has been proved to be a powerful antioxidant in different types of foods (Pazos *et al.*, 2008; Dejong and Lanari, 2009; Medina *et al.*, 2009), having varying degrees of efficiency depending on the type of product (frankfurters, cooked meat batter, o/w emulsions) and showing greater inhibitory capacity than BHA/BHT (butylated hydroxytoluene). Reglero *et al.* (2008) used a supercritical rosemary extract and vitamin E to control the oxidation of enriched frankfurters by deodorized salmon oil, all of them incorporated through a brine.

10.2.3 Fermented products

The incorporation of sources of omega-3 fatty acids into dry fermented sausages (see Tables 10.1 and 10.2) has been less studied, probably as a consequence of their particular production process. The first experiments incorporated fish oil extracts (Muguerza *et al.*, 2004) and deodorized fish oil (Valencia *et al.*, 2006a) as sources of long-chain omega-3 fatty acids. The direct addition of a minimum amount (5.3 g/kg) carried out in the first study resulted in excellent nutritional properties, but the products did not show adequate sensory properties. This defect was solved when using the deodorized fish oil, pre-emulsified with soy protein and used as a partial substitute for pork backfat (25 %). These products supplied 0.64 g EPA/100 g product and 0.46 g DHA/100 g product, qualifying as 'high omega-3 fatty acids' products, according to European legislation, Commission Regulation (EU) 116/2010.

A specific enrichment in DHA was attempted by using microalgae oil from *Schizochytrium* sp. also substituting part of the pork backfat by an emulsion (Valencia *et al.*, 2007). Due to the high DHA content in this type of oil, a low amount of oil permits the achievement of significant DHA levels in the final product. Thus, two substitution levels were tested in that experiment, 15 and 25 %, the latter being discarded due to sensory problems. Substituting for 15 % of pork backfat gave a DHA concentration of 1.30 g/100 g, with an interesting omega-6/omega-3 ratio and good stability of products stored under vacuum for 30 days. Aerobic storage of these sausages was not viable due to the high oxidation susceptibility of the new formulation, despite the use of antioxidants. In this case, a mixture of the synthetic antioxidants BHT (100 ppm) and BHA (100 ppm) was used.

A mixture of algae oil and linseed oil (2:3) has also been used as partial fat replacer (25 %) to formulate healthier dry fermented sausages in which selenium yeast, iodized salt and a lyophilized extract of *M. officinalis* were added to complete a combination of healthier ingredients (García-Iñiguez de Ciriano *et al.*, 2010b). The resulting formulation gave rise to a sensorially acceptable and nutritionally improved product. Thus, a 50 g portion of this product would give 100 % of the recommended intake for Se, 70 % of dietary reference intake (DRI) for iodine, and 40 and 100 % of the DRI for α-linolenic and EPA+DHA, respectively. No oxidation signs were detected despite the high PUFA content, pointing to the effectiveness of the natural antioxidant added.

The need to use antioxidants in omega-3 enriched dry fermented sausages has already been pointed out when using linseed oil as a fat replacer (25 % substitution level) to increase ALA in particular (Valencia *et al.*, 2006b). In that work, a mixture of BHT and BHA was added (200 ppm). Similar antioxidant effectiveness was reached by using a lyophilized water extract of leaves obtained from *Borago officinalis* in a similar product (García-Iñiguez de Ciriano *et al.*, 2009). All these products reached the omega-3 values needed for the nutrition claim 'high omega-3', according to the European Commission Regulation 116/2010.

Sucuk is a typical dry fermented sausage popular in Turkey that contains beef fat as the main lipid source in the traditional formulation. Ercoskun and Dermici-Ercoskun (2010) improved its lipid profile by replacing part of the beef fat with walnut paste (substitution levels from 15–45 %), obtaining a lower omega-6/omega-3 ratio, cholesterol content, atherogenicity index and thrombogenicity index, without affecting the sensory properties. However, higher oxidation susceptibility was noticed in the new products.

Other strategies used for enriching dry fermented sausages in omega-3 fatty acids involved the partial replacement of pork backfat in Dutch-style fermented sausages with commercial encapsulated flaxseed oil (Pelser *et al.*, 2007) and fish oil (Josquin *et al.*, 2012). The later work compared this new approach to the addition of pure or pre-emulsified fish oil, concluding that encapsulation seemed to be the best strategy for retaining overall quality of the products.

10.3 Future trends

The functional and physiological impact of these new formulations needs to be tested in intervention studies in order to demonstrate genuine beneficial effects. Whereas 'nutrition claims' correspond to the amount of a compound in the food, 'health claims' must be scientifically substantiated in order to probe the cause–effect relationship between the food and the claimed benefit.

In this regard, some nutrition intervention studies have been conducted in order to test the beneficial health effects of certain modified meat products (Tapola *et al.*, 2004; Olmedilla *et al.*, 2006, 2008). Metcalf *et al.* (2003) demonstrated the benefits of incorporating fish oil into a range of novel commercial foods, including omega-3 enriched sausages and luncheon meat among the fortified new foods. They concluded that having a wide range of omega-3 PUFA enriched products enables those people who do not eat fish habitually or who never eat fish to benefit from the increased intake of omega-3 PUFA without radical modification of their normal dietary habits. Furthermore, from the physiological point of view, it has been demonstrated that the bioavailability of omega-3 fatty acids from enriched foods is as powerful as that from fish oil capsule supplements (Kolanowski, 2005). Nevertheless, this author pointed out the importance of the application of special types of packaging and storage conditions for avoiding the deterioration and oxidation of these foods.

As described in this chapter, the main strategy to develop omega-3 enriched meat products up to now has been the incorporation of pre-emulsified omega-3 rich oils. In the last few years, research has been focused on the development of efficient encapsulation and delivery technologies in order to increase the stability of the fatty acids against oxidation and also to improve their bioavailability in the organism. Some years ago, Baik *et al.* (2004) proved that the microencapsulation process applied to fish oil provided high encapsulation efficiency (88 % of extractable fish oil), this encapsulated fat being 10 times more stable against oxidation than the surface fat (without antioxidant addition). Barrett *et al.* (2011) have observed that encapsulation increased the stability of fish and flaxseed oils, this stability being improved when antioxidants were added. Venkateshwarlu *et al.* (2010) have investigated the oxidative stability and lipid digestibility offered by multilayer encapsulation of fish oil. They found a remarkable oxidative stability using common food ingredients such as Citrem and chitosan. Moreover, the results of the study indicated that the multilayer encapsulation approach could be an excellent alternative for delivering bioactive lipids such as omega-3 fatty acids into functional foods, such as omega-3 enriched meat products.

The evolution of nanosciences and nanotechnologies for the development of new mechanisms, such as nanodispersions, nanocapsules or biopolymeric nanoparticles for the delivery of functional ingredients seems to offer a wide range of opportunities for the food and the meat industry for innovation and formulation of new products (Huang *et al.*, 2010; Ozimek *et al.* 2010).

10.4 Conclusion

The enrichment of meat products with omega-3 by methods other than modification of the animal diet has mainly been developed through the use of vegetable ingredients, such as walnuts, the direct addition of oils rich in omega-3 and, the most usual strategy, the addition of pre-emulsified oils. In this case, o/w emulsions have been prepared and used as partial substitutes for the traditional fat present in the product. There are two important variables to be taken into account: the nature of the oil (vegetable oils rich in ALA; fish oil or algae oil rich in long-chain PUFA omega-3) and the protein source chosen for the stabilization of the emulsion. The type of emulsifier determines the microstructure of the system, affecting the physicochemical properties of the product and also having a potential antioxidant effect contributing to the stabilization of the product against lipid oxidation. The amount of emulsion which is added to the meat product and the amount of fat which is removed from the traditional formulation will determine the final fatty acid profile of the new meat product. This strategy enables significant decreases of SFA and increases of omega-3 PUFA to be achieved, with a corresponding decrease in the omega-6/omega-3 ratio. The addition of an efficient antioxidant to stabilize omega-3 enriched meat products is necessary. Encapsulation technologies are being developed to improve the oxidation stability and bioavailability of omega-3 fatty acids added to the meat products.

10.5 Sources of further information and advice

The information presented in this chapter has been mainly obtained from scientific literature published by groups worldwide. The authors have recently participated in the project CONSOLIDER INGENIO CARNISENUSA (CSD2007–00016), within the work package FUNCIOCA, that deals specifically with the development of functional meat products. More information on this topic can be found at http://www.carnisenusa.org/. In addition, Table 10.3 reports different types of omega-3 enriched meat products which are currently commercially available in different countries. This information has been obtained from the cited websites.

Table 10.3 Commercial meat products enriched in omega-3 fatty acids and a commercial mixture for enriching cooked products (data reported on websites consulted in December 2011)

Company	Product	Website
Meat products		
Zakłady Mięsne NOWAK (Poland)	Turky potted ham Omega 3	http://www.zmnowak.pl/
Zakłady Mięsne NOWAK (Poland)	Hot-dogs Omega 3	http://www.zmnowak.pl/
Famous Fritz (Canada)	Hot dogs reduced in cholesterol and enriched in omega-3	http://www.famousfritz.ca/omega3.html
Embutidos Cerrillo Fontecha (Spain)	Chorizo (dry fermented sausage)	http://www.cerrillofontecha.com/es/
Nematekas (Lithuania)	Boiled sausages and frankfurters made with linseed oil	http://www.pliusomega3.lt/
Serrano (Spain)	Cooked ham	http://www.cserrano.es/
Mixture for meat products		
Wiberg (Austria)	Omega-3 mixture with fibre for cooked sausages: combines a reduction in fat content (enabled via the fibre) with the addition of valuable omega-3 fatty acids	http://en.wiberg.eu/

10.6 References

ANSORENA, D. and ASTIASARÁN, I. (2012) Formulations for fermented sausages with health attributes, in HUI YH, OZGUL EVRANUZ E, TOLDRA F, MEUNIER-GODDIK L and CHANDAN RC (eds), *Handbook of Animal-based Fermented Food and Beverage Technology* (2nd edn). London: Taylor and Francis, CRC Press, 625–638.

ÁLVAREZ, D., DELLES, R.M., XIONG, Y.L., CASTILLO, M., PAYNE, F.A. and LAENCINA, J. (2011) Influence of canola-olive oils, rice bran and walnut on functionality and emulsion stability of frankfurters. *LWT – Food Science and Technology*, **44**(6), 1435–1442.

ASSISI, A., BANZI, R., BUONOCORE, C., CAPASSO, F., DI MUZIO, V., MICHELACCI, F., RENZO, D., TAFURI, G., TROTTA, F., VITOCOLONNA, M. and GARATTINI, S. (2006) Fish oil and mental health: the role of n-3 long-chain polyunsaturated fatty acids in cognitive development and neurological disorders. *International Clinical Psychopharmacology*, **21**(6), 319–336.

AYO, J., CARBALLO, J., SERRANO, J., OLMEDILLA-ALONSO, B., RUIZ-CAPILLAS, C. and JIMÉNEZ-COLMENERO, F. (2007) Effect of total replacement of pork backfat with walnut on the nutritional profile of frankfurters. *Meat Science*, **77**(2), 173–181.

BAIK, M., SUHENDRO, E., NAWAR, W., MCCLEMENTS, D., DECKER, E. and CHINACHOTI, P. (2004) Effects of antioxidants and humidity on the oxidative stability of microencapsulated fish oil. *Journal of the American Oil Chemists Society*, **81**(4), 355–360.

BARRETT, A.H., PORTER, W.L., MARANDO, G. and CHINACHOTI, P. (2011) Effect of various antioxidants, antioxidant levels, and encapsulation on the stability of fish and flaxseed oils: assessment by fluorometric analysis. *Journal of Food Processing and Preservation*, **35**(3), 349–358.

BERASATEGI, I., LEGARRA, S., GARCIÁ-IÑIGUEZ DE CIRIANO, M., REHECHO, S., CALVO, M.I., CAVERO, R.Y., NAVARRO-BLASCO, I., ANSORENA, D. and ASTIASARÁN, I. (2011) 'High in omega-3 fatty acids' bologna-type sausages stabilized with an aqueous-ethanol extract of *Melissa officinalis*. *Meat Science*, **88**(4), 705–711.

CÁCERES, E., GARCIA, M.L. and SELGAS, M.D. (2008) Effect of pre-emulsified fish oil – as source of PUFA n-3 – on microstructure and sensory properties of mortadella, a Spanish bologna-type sausage. *Meat Science*, **80**(2), 183–193.

CALDER, P. (2006) N-3 polyunsaturated fatty acids, inflammation, and inflammatory diseases. *American Journal of Clinical Nutrition*, **83**(6), 1505S–1519S.

CHEONG, L., ZHANG, H., NERSTING, L., JENSEN, K., HAAGENSEN, J.A.J. and XU, X. (2010) Physical and sensory characteristics of pork sausages from enzymatically modified blends of lard and rapeseed oil during storage. *Meat Science*, **85**(4), 691–699.

COATES, A.M., SIOUTIS, S., BUCKLEY, J.D. and HOWE, P.R.C. (2009) Regular consumption of n-3 fatty acid-enriched pork modifies cardiovascular risk factors. *British Journal of Nutrition*, **101**(4), 592–597.

COFRADES, S., SERRANO, A., AYO, J., SOLAS, M., CARBALLO, J. and COLMENERO, F. (2004) Restructured beef with different proportions of walnut as affected by meat particle size. *European Food Research and Technology*, **218**(3), 230–236.

COFRADES, S., SALCEDO SANDOVAL, L., DELGADO PANDO, G., LÓPEZ-LÓPEZ, I. and RUIZ-CAPILLAS, C. (2011) Antioxidant activity of hydroxytyrosol in frankfurters enriched with n-3 polyunsaturated fatty acids. *Food Chemistry*, **129**(2), 429–436.

COMMISSION REGULATION (EU) No 116/2010 of 9 February 2010 amending Regulation (EC) No 1924/2006 of the European Parliament and of the Council with regard to the list of nutrition claims. OJ, L 37/16.

CORTINAS, L., VILLAVERDE, C., GALOBART, J., BAUCELLS, M., CODONY, R., BAUCELLS, M.D. and BARROETA, A.C. (2004) Fatty acid content in chicken thigh and breast as affected by dietary polyunsaturation level. *Poultry Science*, **83**(7), 1155–1164.

DECKER, E. and CRUM, A. (1993) Antioxidant activity of carnosine in cooked ground pork. *Meat Science*, **34**(2), 245–253.

DECKER, E. and PARK, Y. (2010) Healthier meat products as functional foods. *Meat Science*, **86**(1), 49–55.

DEJONG, S. and LANARI, M.C. (2009) Extracts of olive polyphenols improve lipid stability in cooked beef and pork: Contribution of individual phenolics to the antioxidant activity of the extract. *Food Chemistry*, **116**(4), 892–897.

DELGADO-PANDO, G., COFRADES, S., RUIZ-CAPILLAS, C., TERESA SOLAS, M. and JIMÉNEZ-COLMENERO, F. (2010a) Healthier lipid combination oil-in-water emulsions prepared with various protein systems: an approach for development of functional meat products. *European Journal of Lipid Science and Technology*, **112**(7), 791–801.

DELGADO-PANDO, G., COFRADES, S., RODRIGUEZ SALAS, L. and JIMÉNEZ-COLMENERO, F. (2011b) A healthier oil combination and konjac gel as functional ingredients in low-fat pork liver pâté. *Meat Science*, **88**(2), 241–248.

DELGADO-PANDO, G., COFRADES, S., RUIZ-CAPILLAS, C., SOLAS, M.T., TRIKI, M. and JIMÉNEZ-COLMENERO, F. (2011a) Low-fat frankfurters formulated with a healthier lipid combination as functional ingredient: Microstructure, lipid oxidation, nitrite content, microbiological changes and biogenic amine formation. *Meat Science*, **89**(1), 65–71.

DELGADO-PANDO, G., COFRADES, S., RUIZ-CAPILLAS, C. and JIMÉNEZ-COLMENERO, F. (2010b) Healthier lipid combination as functional ingredient influencing sensory and technological properties of low-fat frankfurters. *European Journal of Lipid Science and Technology*, **112**(8), 859–870.

EFSA (2010) Scientific Opinion on Dietary Reference Values for fats, including saturated fatty acids, polyunsaturated fatty acids, monounsaturated fatty acids, *trans* fatty acids, and cholesterol. *EFSA Journal*, **8**(3), 1461, available at: http://www.efsa.europa.eu/fr/scdocs/doc/1461.pdf [accessed February 2013].

ERCOSKUN, H. and DEMIRCI ERCOSKUN, T. (2010) Walnut as fat replacer and functional component in sucuk. *Journal of Food Quality*, **33**(5), 646–659.

FUNAHASHI, H., SATAKE, M., HASAN, S., SAWAI, H., REBER, H.A., HINES, O.J. and EIBL, G. (2006) The n-3 polyunsaturated fatty acid EPA decreases pancreatic cancer cell growth in vitro. *Pancreas*, **33**(4), 462–462.

GARCÍA-IÑIGUEZ DE CIRIANO, M., GARCIA HERREROS, C., LAREQUI, E., VALENCIA, I. ANSORENA, D. and ASTIASARÁN, I. (2009) Use of natural antioxidants from lyophilized water extracts of *Borago officinalis* in dry fermented sausages enriched in omega-3 PUFA. *Meat Science*, **83**(2), 271–277.

GARCÍA IÑIGUEZ DE CIRIANO, M., REHECHO, S., ISABEL CALVO, M., YOLANDA CAVERO, R., NAVARRO, I., CALVO, M., CAVERO, R., NAVARRO, I., ASTIASARÁN, I. and ANSORENA, D. (2010a) Effect of lyophilized water extracts of *Melissa officinalis* on the stability of algae and linseed oil-in-water emulsion to be used as a functional ingredient in meat products. *Meat Science*, **85**(2), 373–377.

GARCÍA-IÑIGUEZ DE CIRIANO, M., LAREQUI, E., REHECHO, S., CALVO, M.I., CAVERO, R.Y., NAVARRO-BLASCO, I., ASTIASARÁN, I. and ANSORENA, D. (2010b) Selenium, iodine, omega-3 PUFA and natural antioxidant from *Melissa officinalis* L.: A combination of components from healthier dry fermented sausages formulation. *Meat Science*, **85**(2), 274–279.

HUANG, Q., YU, H. and RU, Q. (2010) Bioavailability and delivery of nutraceuticals using nanotechnology. *Journal of Food Science*, **75**(1), R50–R57.

JIMÉNEZ-COLMENERO, F. (2007) Healthier lipid formulation approaches in meat-based functional foods. Technological options for replacement of meat fats by non-meat fats. *Trends in Food Science & Technology*, **18**(11), 567–578.

JIMÉNEZ-COLMENERO, F., SÁNCHEZ-MUNIZ, F.J. and OLMEDILLA-ALONSO, B. (2010) Design and development of meat-based functional foods with walnut: Technological, nutritional and health impact. *Food Chemistry*, **123**(4), 959–967.

JOSQUIN, N.M., LINSSEN, J.P. and HOUBEN, J.H. (2012) Quality characteristics of Dutch-style fermented sausages manufactured with partial replacement of pork back-fat with pure, pre-emulsified or encapsulated fish oil. *Meat Science*, **90**(1), 81–86.

KIM, J., PARK, H.D., PARK, E., CHON, J. and PARK, Y.K. (2009) Growth-inhibitory and proapoptotic effects of alpha-linolenic acid on estrogen-positive breast cancer cells second look at n-3 fatty acid. *Natural Compounds and their Role in Apoptotic Cell Signaling Pathways*, **1171**, 190–195.

KOLANOWSKI, W. (2005) Bioavailability of omega-3 PUFA from foods enriched with fish oil – A mini review. *Polish Journal of Food and Nutrition Sciences*, **14**(4), 335–340.

LEE, S., DECKER, E., FAUSTMAN, C. and MANCINI, R. (2005) The effects of antioxidant combinations on color and lipid oxidation in n-3 oil fortified ground beef patties. *Meat Science*, **70**(4), 683–689.

LEE, S., HERNANDEZ, P., DJORDJEVIC, D., FARAJI, H. and HOLLENDER, R. (2006) Effect of antioxidants and cooking on stability of n-3 fatty acids in fortified meat products. *Journal of Food Science*, **71**(3), C233–C238.

LÓPEZ-LÓPEZ, I., BASTIDA, S., RUIZ-CAPILLAS, C., BRAVO, L., LARREA, M.T., SANCHEZ-MUNIZ, F., COFRADES, S. and JIMÉNEZ-COLMENERO, F. (2009) Composition and antioxidant capacity of low-salt meat emulsion model systems containing edible seaweeds. *Meat Science*, **83**(3), 492–498.

MEDINA, I., LOIS, S., ALCANTARA, D., LUCAS, R. and MORALES, J.C. (2009) Effect of lipophilization of hydroxytyrosol on its antioxidant activity in fish oils and fish oil-in-water emulsions. *Journal of Agricultural and Food Chemistry*, **57**(20), 9773–9779.

METCALF, R., JAMES, M., MANTZIORIS, E. and CLELAND, L. (2003) A practical approach to increasing intakes of n-3 polyunsaturated fatty acids: use of novel foods enriched with n-3 fats RID G-8681-2011. *European Journal of Clinical Nutrition*, **57**(12), 1605–1612.

MUGUERZA, E., ANSORENA, D. and ASTIASARÁN, I. (2004) Functional dry fermented sausages manufactured with high levels of n-3 fatty acids: nutritional benefits and evaluation of oxidation. *Journal of the Science of Food and Agriculture*, **84**(9), 1061–1068.

OLMEDILLA-ALONSO, B., GRANADO-LORENCIO, F., HERRERO-BARBUDO, C. and BLANCO-NAVARRO, I. (2006) Nutritional approach for designing meat-based functional food products with nuts. *Critical Reviews in Food Science and Nutrition*, **46**(7), 537–542.

OLMEDILLA-ALONSO, B., GRANADO-LORENCIO, F., HERRERO-BARBUDO, C., BLANCO-NAVARRO, I., BLAZQUEZ-GARCIA, S. and PEREZ-SACRISTAN, B. (2008) Consumption of restructured meat products with added walnuts has a cholesterol-lowering effect in subjects at high cardiovascular risk: A randomised, crossover, placebo-controlled study. *Journal of the American College of Nutrition*, **27**(2), 342–348.

OZIMEK, L., POSPIECH, E. and NARINE, S. (2010) Nanotechnologies in food and meat processing. *Acta Scientiarum Polonorum – Technologia Alimentaria*, **9**(4), 401–412.

PAZOS, M., ALONSO, A., SANCHEZ, I. and MEDINA, I. (2008) Hydroxytyrosol prevents oxidative deterioration in foodstuffs rich in fish lipids. *Journal of Agricultural and Food Chemistry*, **56**(9), 3334–3340.

PELSER, W.M., LINSSEN, J.P.H., LEGGER, A. and HOUBEN, J. (2007) Lipid oxidation in n-3 fatty acid enriched Dutch style fermented sausages. *Meat Science*, **75**(1), 1–11.

PENNISI FORELL, S.C., RANALLI, N., ZARITZKY, N.E., ANDRÉS, S.C. and CALIFANO, A.N. (2010) Effect of type of emulsifiers and antioxidants on oxidative stability, colour and fatty acid profile of low-fat beef burgers enriched with unsaturated fatty acids and phytosterols. *Meat Science*, **86**(2), 364–370.

PIE, J., SPAHIS, K. and SEILLAN, C. (1991) Cholesterol oxidation in meat-products during cooking and frozen storage. *Journal of Agricultural and Food Chemistry*, **39**(2), 250–254.

REGLERO, G., FRIAL, P., CIFUENTES, A., GARCÍA-RISCO, M.R., JAIME, L., MARIN, F.R., PALANCA, V., RUIZ-RODRÍGUEZ, A., SANTOYO, S., SEÑORÁNS, F.J., SOLER-RIVAS, C., TORRES, C. and IBAÑEZ, E. (2008) Meat-based functional foods for dietary equilibrium omega-6/omega-3. *Molecular Nutrition & Food Research*, **52**(10), 1153–1161.

SERRANO, A., COFRADES, S. and JIMÉNEZ-COLMENERO, F. (2004) Transglutaminase as binding agent in fresh restructured beef steak with added walnuts. *Food Chemistry*, **85**(3), 423–429.

SERRANO, A., COFRADES, S., RUIZ-CAPILLAS, C., OLMEDILLA-ALONSO, B., HERRERO-BARBUDO, C. and JIMÉNEZ-COLMENERO, F. (2005) Nutritional profile of restructured beef steak with added walnuts. *Meat Science*, **70**(4), 647–654.

SERRANO, A., COFRADES, S. and JIMÉNEZ-COLMENERO, F. (2006) Characteristics of restructured beef steak with different proportions of walnut during frozen storage. *Meat Science*, **72**(1), 108–115.

SINGH, R., KUMAR CHATLI, M., KUMAR BISWAS, A. and SAHOO, J. (2011) Quality and storage stability of chicken meat patties incorporated with linseed oil. *Journal of Food Quality*, **34**(5), 352–362.

TAPOLA, N., LYYRA, M., KARVONEN, H., UUSITUPA, M. and SARKKINEN, E. (2004) The effect of meat products enriched with plant sterols and minerals on serum lipids and blood pressure. *International Journal of Food Sciences and Nutrition*, **55**(5), 389–397.

TOLDRÁ, F. and REIG, M. (2011) Innovations for healthier processed meats. *Trends in Food Science & Technology*, **22**(9), 517–522.

ULBRITCH, T.L.V. and SOUTHGATE, D.A.T. (1991) Coronary heart disease: seven dietary factors. *Lancet*, **338**, 985–992.

USDA (2010) *Dietary Guidelines for Americans*. Washington DC: US Department of Health and Human Services/US Department of Agriculture, available at: http://www.cnpp.usda.gov/Publications/DietaryGuidelines/2010/PolicyDoc/PolicyDoc.pdf [accessed February 2013].

VALENCIA, I., ANSORENA, D. and ASTIASARÁN, I. (2006a) Nutritional and sensory properties of dry fermented sausages enriched with n-3 PUFAs. *Meat Science*, **72**(4), 727–733.

VALENCIA, I., ANSORENA, D. and ASTIASARÁN, I. (2006b) Stability of linseed oil and antioxidants containing dry fermented sausages: A study of the lipid fraction during different storage conditions. *Meat Science*, **73**(2), 269–277.

VALENCIA, I., ANSORENA, D. and ASTIASARÁN, I. (2007) Development of dry fermented sausages rich in docosahexaenoic acid with oil from the microalgae *Schizochytrium* sp.: Influence on nutritional properties, sensorial quality and oxidation stability. *Food Chemistry*, **104**(3), 1087–1096.

VALENCIA, I., O'GRADY, M.N., ANSORENA, D., ASTIASARÁN, I. and KERRY, J.P. (2008) Enhancement of the nutritional status and quality of fresh pork sausages following the addition of linseed oil, fish oil and natural antioxidants. *Meat Science*, **80**(4), 1046–1054.

VANDENDRIESSCHE, F. (2008) Meat products in the past, today and in the future. *Meat Science*, **78**(1–2), 104–113.

VENKATESHWARLU, G., SANDRA, S., MCCLEMENTS, D.J. and DECKER, E.A. (2010) Oxidative stability and in vitro digestibility of fish oil-in-water emulsions containing multilayered membranes. *Journal of Agricultural and Food Chemistry*, **58**(13), 8093–8099.

WEISS, J., GIBIS, M., SCHUH, V. and SALMINEN, H. (2010) Advances in ingredient and processing systems for meat and meat products. *Meat Science*, **86**(1), 196–213.

WHO (2003) *Diet, Nutrition and the Prevention of Chronic Diseases.* Technical report series 916. Geneva: World Health Organization.

WOOD, J., RICHARDSON, R., NUTE, G., FISHER, A., CAMPO, M., KASAPIDOU, E., SHEARD, P. and ENSER, M. (2004) Effects of fatty acids on meat quality: a review. *Meat Science*, **66**(1), 21–32.

ZHANG, W., XIAO, S., SAMARAWEERA, H., LEE, E.J. and AHN, D.U. (2010) Improving functional value of meat products. *Meat Science*, **86**(1), 15–31.

11

Enrichment of baked goods with omega-3 fatty acids

E. M. Hernandez, Omega Protein Inc., USA

DOI: 10.1533/9780857098863.3.319

Abstract: This chapter examines different applications of omega-3 fatty acids in baked products using novel methods in the protection of the oil against oxidation, such as the use of stable blends, new antioxidants and microencapsulation systems. It also addresses methods of incorporation of omega-3s into bakery products and discusses new products such as omega-3 nutritional bars now available in the market. This chapter also discusses analytical techniques for evaluation of omega-3 fats in baked goods.

Key words: omega-3 fatty acids, baked goods, nutritional bars, omega-3 analysis, omega 3 bread.

11.1 Introduction

Lipids play important roles in food processing and food quality. Fats and oils define the organoleptic and texture properties of many food products as well as their shelf-life (Kinsella, 1988). This is particularly true for baked food products. More importantly, lipids, especially omega-3 fatty acids, play essential roles in many biological and metabolic processes (Dupont, 1996). In general, there is an increasing awareness of the health benefits of omega-3 fatty acids which is reflected by the growth in consumption of omega-3 fats either as dietary supplements or in fortified foods. Omega-3 fatty acids, particularly the longer chain fatty acids eicosapentaenoic acid (EPA) and docosahexaenoic acid (DHA), have been more studied for their health promotion and disease prevention properties (Simopoulos, 1997; Shahidi, 2011).

EPA and DHA cannot be synthesized by the human body so they have to be consumed directly through diet or derived from α-linolenic acid (ALA) through metabolic reactions. The conversion of ALA to EPA and DHA has been reported as being limited. As a result, the fortification of many foods and supplements favors the use of omega-3 oils with EPA and DHA.

Omega-3 fatty acids can be obtained from vegetable oils and marine products. Vegetable oils like soybean and canola and other seeds like flaxseed, walnut and chia are common sources of the shorter chain omega-3 ALA. Flaxseed and flaxseed oil are often used in baked food products as a source of omega-3s. The longer chain omega-3 fatty acids, EPA and DHA, used in food fortification and food supplements, are obtained mainly from cold-water fish oils. Long-chain omega-3 as DHA can also be obtained from microalgae oil which is widely used commercially as an infant formula ingredient and in some fortified foods and supplements (Carlson *et al.*, 1993; Jensen *et al.*, 2000; Cheatham *et al.*, 2006; Drover *et al.*, 2009). A relatively new source of long-chain omega-3s is krill oil (Massrieh, 2008), but the use of it has not been reported in any food applications yet.

The current trend in the industry is to introduce healthier fats into food products, especially in foods that are traditionally high in fat. As mentioned above, fats and oils in general can have a positive effect in food formulations for processing, quality, organoleptic and texture properties. They can also have a negative effect when oxidized, particularly in the case of omega-3s. Fats and oils in general have to be extracted and processed through a series of preset steps in order to ensure that they meet the minimum specifications for human consumption (Hernandez, 2005).

Until recently, the food industry used fats that were more stable against oxidation such as hydrogenated oils and saturated fats. Hydrogenated oils are used in some food applications, such as frying and baking, in order to ensure longer shelf-life and provide adequate rheological properties for the final products. However, since it was reported that high intake of *trans* fats can increase the risk of cardiovascular disease, the use of hydrogenated oils is decreasing and changes are taking place in the food industry to reformulate with healthier fats and oils. The implementation of these changes was accelerated in 2006 when some governments started requiring food companies to include the amounts of *trans* fats in the food facts labels. Another consequence of these changes is that oils high in saturated fat, such as palm oil, are being commonly used to replace hydrogenated oil. Also, oils high in linoleic acid (omega-6), such as corn oil and sunflower oil, and high in oleic acid, such as modified sunflower and canola oil, are being used to replace high-in-*trans* partially hydrogenated oils, used also in fried and baked products. Table 11.1 shows the fatty acid composition of the main oils and fats used by the bakery industry.

In light of recent consumer demand for foods and food products containing healthier oils, manufacturers have introduced several foods fortified with omega-3 fatty acids. The main categories of foods being fortified with omega-3s are dairy products, nutritional beverages and baked goods. Clinical/ enteral nutrition products come next, followed by prescription omega-3 products and infant formulas (Frost and Sullivan, 2010).

Table 11.1 Approximate fatty acid composition of major vegetable oils used in bakery foods

Fatty acid	Soybean[1]	Canola[2]	Corn[3]	Sunflower[3]	High oleic sunflower[4]	Palm[3]
Lauric (C12:0) (%)	0.1	–	–	0.5	–	0.4
Myristic (C14:0) (%)	0.2	–	–	0.1	–	1.1
Palmitic (C16:0) (%)	10.7	3.7	12.3	6.4	3.6	43.8
Stearic (C18:0) (%)	3.9	2.1	1.9	4.5	4.4	4.4
Oleic (C18:1) (%)	22.8	66.9	27.7	22.1	81.1	39.1
Linoleic (C18:2) (%)	50.8	16.9	56.1	65.6	8.4	10.2
Linolenic (C18:3) (%)	6.8	7.9	1.0	0.5	–	–

Sources: [1]Erickson, 1995. [2]Jenab *et al.*, 2006. [3]Dubois *et al.*, 2007. [4]Purdy, 1986.

Menhaden oil was the first fish oil approved as a food ingredient (GRAS, generally recognized as safe) (CFR 184.1472) by the US government in 1997. Later on, several other fish oils from salmon, tuna, anchovy and mackerel, as well as oils from microalgae were granted self-affirmed GRAS status by the FDA. This has allowed the development of foods fortified with fish oil omega-3s from several sources and approved for use in a wide variety of foods. However, limits were set by the FDA that the combined intake of EPA and DHA from these oil sources must not exceed 3 g/day. Table 11.2 shows the general composition of omega-3 oils for fortification of foods.

11.2 Omega-3 fatty acids in baked goods

Omega-3 fatty acids can be effectively delivered through a variety of baked goods, such as several types of breads, nutritional bars, cereals and cookies. Some baked goods are relatively low in water activity and this makes them good candidates for omega-3 fortification. Baked products have been widely studied as food products that can also be effectively fortified with other bioactive compounds. For example, breads and flours have been reported to be good carriers of nutraceuticals, such as omega-3 fatty acids, phenolic glucosides, lignans, phytosterols, fructo oligosaccharides, inulin and other dietary fibers (Hayta and Ozugur, 2011). Highly purified and deodorized omega-3 oils from flaxseed, fish and microalgae oils, paired with effective antioxidants, are now been successfully used in several commercial baked products (see Table 11.3).

Table 11.2 Approximate composition of omega-3 oils used in foods

Fatty acid	Menhaden[1]	Anchovy[2]	Cod liver[3]	Tuna[4]	Microalgae[5]	Flax[6]
Lauric (C12:0) (%)	–	–	–		2.8	–
Myristic (C14:0) (%)	7.9	8.1	4.8	3.4	12.7	
Palmitic (C16:0) (%)	19.8	16.7	14.2	15.8	13.4	5.1
Palmitoleic (C16:1) (%)	9.8	11.6	8.3	6.1	1.4	–
Stearic (C18:0) (%)	3.4	4.1	2.6	4.5	–	3.3
Oleic (C18:1) (%)	12.6	9.3	16.9	19.3	21.8	18.1
Linoleic (C18:2) (%)	1.3	1.6	2.4	1.8	1.3	15.3
Linolenic (C18:3) (%)	1.2	0.8	0.9	0.4	–	58.2
Eicosapentaenoic (C20:5) (%)	12.7	22.1	9.8	7.6	0.2	–
Docosahexaenoic (C22:6) (%)	11.2	10.7	10.3	22.9	42.3	–

Sources: [1]McGill and Moffat, 1992; [2]Standal *et al.*, 2012; [3]Indarti *et al.*, 2005; [4]Koriyama *et al.*, 2002; [5]Arterburn *et al.*, 2007; [6]Ciftci *et al.*, 2012.

Bread is also a convenient vehicle for introducing omega-3 fatty acids into the diet because it is a food that is universally consumed; it presents in general it offers a stable environment for polyunsaturated fatty acids (PUFA) as it is relatively low in moisture and has a short shelf-life. Furthermore, the plastic shortenings commonly used in bread formulations are usually very stable and can be used to incorporate omega-3 oils as a more stable matrix.

In general, one of the main challenges for incorporation of omega-3 fats into foods, particularly in baked goods, is that the products are subjected to high temperatures and exposed to air during processing. Also, extended shelf-life is required, sometimes over a year, for some of the baked goods. In the case of bread, this is not as much an issue since normally the shelf-life required is only a few weeks. Another challenge in fortifying baked goods is to have the ability to handle and store refrigerated or frozen ingredients, as is required for most fish oils. Although it contains ALA and not long-chain omega-3s, flax has, so far, been the most widely used omega-3 source to fortify a variety of baked goods, cereals and snack bars (Chang *et al.*, 1991; Chen *et al.*, 1992; Aliani *et al.*, 2011, 2012). However, because of the growing awareness that EPA and DHA are more bioactive, a number of baked products fortified with fish and microalgae oil have been introduced into the market.

In the case of flaxseed, both the oil and the flour can be utilized to fortify baked products. Flax meal has the added advantage that it can be

Table 11.3 Examples of baked products fortified with omega-3 fats

Brand	Serving size	ALA (mg)	EPA (mg)	DHA (mg)	Sources (accessed February 2013)
Wonder + Headstart 100 % whole wheat bread (USA)	75 g (2 slices)	–	–	15	http://wonderbread.ca/products/breads/4
Healthy Life Flaxseed bread (USA)	41 g (2 slices)	90	–	–	http://www.healthylifebread.com/pages/original/flaxseed-with-omega-3-bread.php
Bürgen® Soy-Lin® bread (Germany)	83 g (2 slices)	1500	–	–	http://www.burgen.com.au/range/soylin.aspx
Tip Top bread (Australia)	74 g (2 slices)	83.6	5900	26.6	http://www.tiptop.com.au/up/white-omega-3dha-sandwich
Diego's Omega 3 wraps (Australia)	43 g (1 wrap)	219	6.8	29.5	http://www.sandiego.com.au/pages/nutrition.php
Mission flax seed and blue com tortillas (USA)	1 tortilla (36 g)	120	–	–	http://www.missionmenus.com/Pantry.aspx
Omega Smart bars (USA)	63 g (1/bar)	2000	–	–	http://www.omegasmartbar.com/nutrition-health-bars.htm
Detour Lean Muscle Bar (USA)	90 g (1/bar)	1000–2000	–	–	http://www.detourbar.com/cookie-dough-caramel-crisp.html
Omega Cookie (USA)	60 g (1 cookie)	–	2000 (EPA + DHA)		http://www.omega3innovations.com/index.php/omega-cookie.html

used to substitute for flour in several bakery formulations. Besides containing carbohydrates, flax meal contains soluble fiber, gums and lignans that can act as stabilizers to improve the texture and quality of finished baked products. It has been reported to improve loaf volume and oven spring and, in general, to improve bread texture and nutritional characteristics. Milled flax was also reported to be able to replace 10–15 % of the flour used in yeast-bread formulations. However, the amount of yeast added had to be increased by 25 % to maintain the same proof time, texture and consistency (Shearer and Davies, 2005).

Flaxseed flour was used commercially in breads by several bakeries in the USA and Canada in the late 1980s. It was also used commercially in muffins, cookies and other bakery mixes. It was reported that flaxseed flour not only improved the nutritional properties of baked goods but also improved the general quality of the finished product. The gums and lignans in flaxseed were reported to act as stabilizers and dough enhancers (Carter, 1993). Omega-3 fortified breads from flaxseed oil are now consumed worldwide. They are especially popular in Japan, Canada, the USA and now Latin America.

Pohjanheimo *et al.* (2006) conducted a more formal evaluation of bread rolls containing flaxseed and flaxseed oil including sensory, instrumental texture measurement and chemical analysis of the various components including fatty acids, fiber, secoisolariciresinol diglycoside and cadmium. They reported that the flaxseed rolls retained moisture and softness more efficiently than the control rolls that did not contain flaxseed. No off-odors were detected during the storage period up to six days at room temperature, although flaxseed rolls and cinnamon rolls were higher in unsaturated fats. The flaxseed rolls were also high in fiber, thus further increasing the nutrition value of the fortified breads. Koca and Anil (2007) also reported on the rheological and baking properties of flaxseed/wheat composites used in the preparation of breads. Wheat flour was replaced with flaxseed flour at several levels and the farinographic water absorption, dough development time and mixing tolerance index increased with the amount of flaxseed added to the flour, whereas dough stability decreased at 100, 150 and 200 g/kg of flaxseed flour substitution. The extensographic energy of dough also decreased at 150 and 200 g/kg flaxseed substitution. The specific volume of flaxseed flour breads was similar to that of control bread.

The replacement of soybean oil with flaxseed oil in the preparation of whole wheat flaxseed bread enriched with omega-3 was reported by De Aguiar *et al.* (2011). They reported that the partial substitution of soybean oil with flaxseed oil, at 25, 50 and 75 % levels in bread formulations, resulted in an increased ALA content and the gradual reduction of the n-6/n-3 ratio, without negative effects on bread quality or sensorial attributes.

When higher amounts of flaxseed are required for supplementation, flavor of the final product may be negatively affected. Aliani *et al.* (2011) evaluated the flavor profile of various muffins and snack bars formulated with higher amounts of flaxseed required for clinical trials. Each snack bar and muffin was formulated to contain 30g of fine milled brown flaxseed; one snack bar or muffin was the amount participants were required to ingest each day, equivalent to 6g of ALA. They reported that muffin formulations with flaxseed had significantly lower sweetness and significantly higher flax aroma and flavor, as well as bitter taste compared with the non-flax muffin. They report on the need to use flavorings such as orange cranberry, gingerbread raisin and cappuccino chocolate chip in snack bar formulations to mask the intensities for the flax aroma and flavor. Similar conclusions were reached for flaxseed-fortified bagels (Aliani *et al.*, 2011, 2012).

Encapsulated flaxseed oil has also been used to protect against oxidation and to prevent the formation of acrylamide and hydroxyl methyl furfural (HMF) in breads (Gökmen *et al.*, 2011). They reported that, comparing with its free form, addition of nanoencapsulated flaxseed oil increased final product quality and safety by lowering lipid oxidation and formation of harmful compounds in breads during baking.

Fish oil in both liquid or powder forms has also been successfully used in baked goods. These include breads, muffins, buns, pastries, bagels, cookies and pizza dough. Bread is one of the first foods fortified commercially with omega-3 fish oil. Breads fortified with long-chain omega-3 fats were introduced commercially in Denmark in the early 1990s as a white bread enriched with microencapsulated fish oil, under the name of 'Omega Bread'. This bread was a significant source of long-chain omega-3s and contained 40–55mg of omega-3 fatty acids per 100g. It was reported that by eating 200g daily of this bread, the consumer would get 25–30% of the amount of higher omega-3 PUFA present in 30g of mixed fish (Nielsen, 1992).

Encapsulated fish oil is preferred because it adds protection against oxidation and makes it easier to incorporate into the dry fraction of bakery formulations. Yep *et al.* (2002) reported the use of microencapsulated tuna oil to enrich bread with DHA to study the effect of low doses (100mg per day) on plasma long-chain omega-3 PUFA levels. They found that the DHA in the enriched bread was bioavailable in low doses and improved plasma long-chain omega-3 PUFA status in both the acute and the chronic study. For this study, they used bread containing microencapsulated tuna oil at approximately 20mg of long-chain omega-3 PUFA per slice. They reported that after three weeks of daily consumption of bread enriched with low-dose microencapsulated tuna oil (60mg long-chain omega-3 PUFA/day), there was an increase in long-chain omega-3 PUFA content in the plasma total lipids (18% rise) as well as the phospholipid fraction (12% rise). One major disadvantage is that the process of encapsulation can more than double the cost of the omega-3 ingredient.

Liu *et al.* (2001) also reported on the effects of a daily intake of of fish oil in bread; 36 subjects with hyperlipidemia were randomly divided into three groups: stable fish oil with oat fiber, control with oat fiber and control with wheat fiber. Plasma levels of EPA and DHA and total omega-3 fatty acids were increased after two and four weeks of daily intake of 93g bread containing 1.3g of stable fish oil. Triglycerides were decreased and high density lipoprotein (HDL)-cholesterol increased after intake of the bread containing stable fish oil. No significant changes occurred in the control groups. Furthermore, intake of the bread containing stable fish oil did not induce any signs of lipid peroxidation, as measured by analysis of malondialdehyde, one of the most frequently used biomarkers for lipid peroxidation.

Fortification of breads with DHA-rich microalgae oil was reported at levels containing 50 mg DHA/slice (32 g per slice) (Serna-Saldivar *et al.*, 2006; Serna-Saldivar and Abril, 2011). They added the algae oil to the formulations as straight oil, as an emulsion and in microencapsulated powder form. The results indicated that the straight algae oil source yielded breads with textural properties almost identical to those of the control. They also used flaxseed and fish oils in the bread as a comparison. Bread prepared with flax showed acceptable results while fish oil bread had adequate baking properties but lost flavor and overall acceptability during the last stages of storage. They also reported that the breads with the lowest acceptability were the ones fortified with microencapsulated oils. These breads absorbed less water, had lower baking properties and tended to have higher firmness during the last days of storage. They suggested that the encapsulation and the carrier ingredients used to protect the oil might adversely affect the physical characteristics of the bread dough.

Costa de Conto *et al.* (2012) also conducted studies on the fortification of bread with microencapsulated omega-3 and compared texture and organoleptic effect with breads prepared with rosemary extracts. The results obtained showed that the addition of microencapsulated omega-3 affected the texture characteristics (specific volume, firmness, color) of white pan breads. The bread had good sensory acceptance (scores > 5), even at the maximum dosage of omega-3 (5 g/100 g total mass). It was suggested that the addition of microcapsules could dilute the gluten and cause interference with the retention of gases during the baking process. On the other hand, the addition of rosemary extract had almost no influence on the textural and sensory characteristics of white pan bread, within the ranges studied.

Lu and Norziah (2010) reported positive results in the preparation of wholemeal bread and white bread prepared by substituting shortening with liquid-refined menhaden fish oil at levels of 0.5, 1.0 and 1.5 % (w/w). The EPA and DHA in breads after baking were reported as 68.7–72.8 % of the added level with no further significant changes during storage for both types of breads. Results from gas chromatography (GC) analyses correlated well with peroxide and anisidine value analyses, which showed relatively low values throughout the storage time.

11.3 Omega-3 fatty acids in nutrition bars

Nutrition bars are not just a concentrated source of calories but can also be used as delivery systems for several types of specialized nutrients and bioactive compounds (Hallund *et al.*, 2006; Miller *et al.*, 2006; Egert *et al.*, 2012). This is reflected by the sharp growth of the market share of nutritional and energy bars in the last few years. US retail sales of cereal/granola bars and energy/nutrition bars reached $5.7 billion in 2011 (Packaged Facts, 2012). Nutrition and energy bars were initially targeted to high performance athletes as a source of extra fuel calories. More recently, nutrition bars are being marketed to a more diverse population with more diverse nutritional needs. There are several types of nutrition bars currently being sold: (i) protein bars; (ii) meal replacement bars; (iii) energy bars; (iv) diet bars; and (v) nutraceutical bars. Protein bars contain higher amounts of protein, usually about 10–30 g, and many of them also contain vitamins and/or minerals. Meal replacement bars contain the necessary amount of protein, carbohydrates, vitamins and minerals that are typically found in a healthy meal. An energy bar is a dietary supplement for athletes who need to maintain a high caloric intake due to high physical activity. Regarding omega-3 fortification of nutrition bars, flaxseed is still the most widely used ingredient (Aliani *et al.*, 2011).

Use of fish oil as a source of the longer chain length omega-3 fatty acids, EPA and DHA, in nutrition bars is still challenging due to the long shelf-life required for this product, sometimes over a year. Thus microencapsulated fish oil seems to be the most viable delivery system for long-chain omega-3s in nutrition bars (Nielsen and Jacobsen, 2009). Table 11.3 shows examples of different baked products fortified with omega-3 at different dose levels and with different types of omega-3 fatty acids.

11.4 Application techniques for adding omega-3 fatty acids to foods

In recent years, manufacturers have overcome many of the challenges that previously limited omega-3 application in food products. Technological advances, such as microencapsulation, and the development of new antioxidants to protect polyunsaturated oils have been major contributors to the increase in omega-3 fortified foods because they help reduce or eliminate the fishy odors and taste that tend to arise as omega-3 fatty acids oxidize (Venkateshwarlu *et al.*, 2004; Kolanowski *et al.*, 2007; Shahidi and Zhong, 2010).

When effective antioxidant systems are used, straight fish oil can also be formulated in fortified foods including baked products. These antioxidant blends can be natural and/or synthetic. Common synthetic antioxidants widely used in foods include butylated hydroxyanisole (BHA), butylated hydroxytoluene (BHT), propyl gallate (PG) and tertbutylhydroquinone (TBHQ). However, there are some concerns regarding their safety at high levels; therefore, their use in foods is limited, typically to less than 200 ppm. Their use is also generally discouraged in nutraceutical products.

New effective natural antioxidants have been developed from plant and herb extracts, such as rosemary and oregano, that have been found to be as effective antioxidants as some synthetic ones. Rosemary extracts are reported to be particularly effective, in combination with other antioxidants such as tocopherols, in the protection of PUFA (Xin and Shun, 1993; Shahidi and Zhong, 2010). The active compounds in rosemary extract are reported to be phenols, such as carnosol, rosmanol, rosmaridiphenol, and phenolic acids, such as carnosic acid and rosmarinic acid. These extracts have been used effectively to prevent oxidation specifically in fish oils. Rosemary compounds have also been reported to inhibit the formation of products of oxidation such as conjugated dienes and pentenal in fish oil emulsions (Frankel *et al.*, 1996).

Antioxidant systems sometimes work more efficiently when used in combination with other antioxidants and other chelating agents (Shahidi and Zhong, 2010). Nielsen and Jacobsen (2009) and Horn *et al.* (2009) reported on the oxidation stability of energy bars fortified with fish oil. They showed that pre-emulsification of the fish oil with antioxidants showed some protection, but using microencapsulated fish oil provided the best results. They also reported that the addition of the metal chelator ethylene diamine tetraacetic acid (EDTA) (100–2000 ppm) to emulsified fish oil decreased the oxidative stability of the energy bars compared with the energy bars with emulsified fish oil but without EDTA (Horn *et al.*, 2009 and Nielsen and Jacobsen, 2009).

Horn *et al.* (2009) observed, in energy bars fortified with fish oil, that at certain concentrations, pro-oxidative effects can take place in the presence of antioxidants such as tocopherols, caffeic acid and ascorbyl palmitate. They suggested that this effect might be due to the reduction of transition metals to their most active state. This further illustrates the need to use microencapsulated fish oil when fortifying supplements that contain other nutrients such as minerals and vitamins.

Microencapsulation is widely used in the food and supplements industries to protect omega-3s against oxidation and also to facilitate their incorporation into foods. Fish oil in powder form, microencapsulated or co-acervated, is used to protect against oxidation and is also especially convenient for manufacturers with limited frozen or refrigerated storage capacity for ease of storage and handling (Brazel, 1999; Kolanowski *et al.*, 2002, 2007; Jónsdóttir *et al.*, 2005). However, before omega-3 oils can be stabilized and protected against oxidation, they have to be properly treated to remove impurities and potentially harmful contaminants using processing techniques such as specialized refining and molecular distillation (Hernandez, 2005). Tables 11.4 and 11.5 show some of the parameters the industry uses to assess the quality of edible oils used in food, including shortenings used in bakery products and omega-3 oils used to fortify foods.

Table 11.4 Quality parameters for fish oils

Acid value	≤3 mg KOH/g
Peroxide value	≤5 meq/kg
Anisidine value	≤20
TOTOX	≤26
PCDDs and PCDFs	≤2 ppt
Dioxin-like PCBs	≤3 ppt
Marker PCBs	≤90 ppb
Mercury	≤0.1 ppm
Cadmium	≤0.1 ppm
Lead	≤0.1 ppm
Arsenic	≤0.1 ppm

Source: GOED, 2012.

Table 11.5 Quality parameters of vegetable oils and shortenings

	Shortening	Salad oil
Lovibond red color, max.	1.5	3.5
Free fatty acid, % max.	0.15	0.05
Peroxide value, meq/kg max.	0.5	0.5
Moisture, % max.	0.05	0.05
Filterable impurities, max.	None	None
OSI, h min.	40	15

Source: O'Brien, 1998.

For flaxseed oil, some companies use quality standards based on vegetable oils quality parameters, as shown in Table 11.5.

When fortifying foods with straight fish oils, it is recommended that, whenever possible, the omega-3 fat should be added as close to the end of the process as possible. This way, the oil comes into minimum contact with pro-oxidant conditions such as heat, light and oxygen. If there are other fat components in the formulation, it is advisable that the omega-3 oil be blended first with any other fats before adding to the process. This is especially useful when blending omega-3 oils with other oils that are more stable themselves, like more saturated oils such as olive, palm, canola, high oleic sunflower and partially hydrogenated oils. These blends have been reported to appreciably increase the overall stability of polyunsaturated fats (Frankel and Huang, 1994; Chapman *et al.*, 1998; Sundram *et al.*, 1999). Regarding processing environment and conditions, it is suggested that all equipment be free of metal ions such as copper and iron to reduce the chance of oxidation. Another important processing factor is to avoid any incorporation of air into the product. When mixing liquids, it is important to de-aerate the product and fill all tanks from the bottom as well as flushing tanks with nitrogen.

Plastic shortenings in baked goods are added to improve dough machinability, decrease rate of staling and improve bread texture and quality. Shortenings function as a barrier between dough components and serve as lubricants between the gluten strands. This results in a more pliable dough, improves loaf volume and tenderizes both the crumb and crust. The addition of omega-3 fats to the fat ingredient of the formulation may change the physical characteristics of the shortening blend and this may limit the amount of omega-3 fats that can be added. In some cases, other ingredients in bread formulations, such as surfactants and emulsifiers, can be included in the formulation to improve texture and quality of breads and thus facilitate the addition of omega-3 ingredients.

It is recommended that baked goods with omega-3s be refrigerated or frozen since they have a shorter shelf-life. They should also be packaged accordingly. In terms of handling, fish oil has to be stored frozen or refrigerated for long-term storage. Situations that may induce oxidation, such as extended mix times or long-term exposure to the atmosphere, should be avoided to protect product integrity. If vitamins and minerals have to be added to the baking mix, it is recommended that they be encapsulated to prevent triggering oxidation reactions, especially if these blends have pro-oxidant metals such as iron.

11.5 Analysis of omega-3 fatty acids

Omega-3s added are usually added in small amounts (mg per serving). This can easily result in the omega-3 fat becoming entrained with the rest of the food components. Therefore, appreciable differences can arise between the calculated levels of EPA and DHA in the products formulated and the experimental results from the lab.

There are two basic testing methods used to analyze for ALA, EPA and DHA, and fatty acids in general, in oils extracted from foods for analysis: area percent and weight percent. The area percent method calculates omega-3 fatty acids as a fraction of only the rest of fatty acids in the oil. This method does not take into account other non-fatty acid components naturally found in the oils, such as glycerol, cholesterol, phytosterols, alcohols, hydrocarbons, squalene. These other components can account for as much as 5–15 % of the total. The weight percent method takes into account the weight of the fatty acids plus glycerol plus the rest of unsaponifiable matter when calculating the EPA/DHA content. This method basically reports on the weight percent of each fatty acid as compared to the overall weight of the oil (mg/g). The type of analytical method used becomes important when formulating for fortified foods, and this is especially important for quality control and product validation. Analysis of EPA and DHA has been reported to be difficult in cases when the levels of fortification in foods are extremely low and the fat content of the product is also very low, as in the case of some fortified baked products. Some commercial breads can have a have as little as 15 mg of EPA and DHA in a serving (See Table 11.3). As the foods are cooked or baked, the omega-3 fatty acids become embedded in the matrix of the food, resulting in complexes of proteins, carbohydrates and other fats, making the analysis of EPA and DHA even more difficult.

A method commonly used for analysis of EPA and DHA is based on the American Oil Chemists Society Method, Ce 1b-89; here the fatty acids in the oil are converted first to methyl esters. This method normally provides % area distribution of all the fatty acids in the oil including EPA and DHA. An internal standard, usually a 23-carbon or 13-carbon fatty acid, can be used to allow for the calculation of % weight content of ALA, EPA or DHA content (Method AOCS Ce 1i-07). A common technique for recovery of the oil fraction from a food for analysis is by extraction with a solvent such as petroleum ether or hexane. However, this method may not be effective to extract the oil samples from some food matrices and acid or alkaline hydrolysis has to be performed before solvent extraction and derivatization for GC analysis. AOCS Official Method Ce 1k-09 offers the option for the preparation of fatty acid methyl esters directly from food matrices where the oil may be released from the matrix by *in situ* acid digestion, followed by alkali hydrolysis and methylation or by simultaneous alkali hydrolysis and methylation without prior digestion. Then the fatty acid methyl esters (FAMEs) are quantitatively determined by capillary GC. AOCS method Ce 1i-07 can be used for marine and PUFA-containing oils.

As mentioned above, the general quality of edible oils is assessed using methods such as listed in Table 11.6 and omega-3 fats such as flaxseed and marine oils use these as well. In addition, marine oil oils, coming from a source exposed to the environment for extended periods of time, have to be analyzed and closely monitored for harmful contaminants such as mercury, polychlorinated biphenyls (PCBs), dioxins and furans. The analysis of these compounds is more complicated and is usually done by specialized labs (Melanson *et al.*, 2005).

Table 11.6 Analytical methods for quality parameters of omega-3 oils

Parameter	Method
ALA/EPA/DHA	AOCS Ce 1i-07
Acid value	AOCS Cd 3d-63
Peroxide value (PV)	AOCS Cd 8–53
Anisidine value (AV)	AOCS Cd 18–90
TOTOX	AV + 2PV
Color	AOCS Cc 13e-92
Moisture	AOCS 2d-25
PCBs	US EPA Method 1668

Another issue in evaluating foods fortified with omega-3 is determining the absorption efficacy of omega-3s after ingestion. This is done through actual feed studies to determine if including a fortified food in a diet actually increases the level of omega-3s in the blood stream (Yep *et al.*, 2002). The analysis is done by taking blood samples from test subjects and analyzing the samples using techniques based on methods described above for extraction of lipid fraction, derivatization and GC analysis of omega-3 fatty acids.

11.6 Conclusion

Effective antioxidant and protection systems, such as emulsions and microencapsulation, are now available and allow for the fortification of baked goods and other foods with long chain omega-3s, without the development of fishy flavors. This has helped to satisfy the increasing demand for foods fortified with omega-3s. On the other hand, the demand for omega-3 supplements, with larger doses of EPA/DHA per serving, is increasing due to the growing awareness of the benefits of long chain omega-3s in cardiovascular protection, cognitive wellbeing, visual health and prevention of some inflammation-related diseases. As the lines between foods and supplements become blurred, it is evident that consumption of omega-3s will also increase through the introduction of new products in the areas of wellness nutrition and medical foods. Concerning bakery products, there are several products in the nutraceutical market that have been successfully introduced, such as omega-3 nutrition bars. These are also being sold as complete meals and convenient delivery systems of other supplemental nutrients.

11.7 References

ALIANI M, RYLAND D and PIERCE GN (2011) 'Effect of flax addition on the flavor profile of muffins and snack bars', *Food Res Int*, 44, 2489–2496.

ALIANI M, RYLAND D and PIERCE GN (2012) 'Effect of flax addition on the flavor profile and acceptability of bagels', *J Food Sci*, 71, S62–S70.

ARTERBURN LM, OKEN HA, HOFFMAN JP, BAILEY-HALL E, CHUNG G, ROM D, HAMERSLEY J and MCCARTHY D (2007) 'Bioequivalence of docosahexaenoic acid from different algal oils in capsules and in a DHA-fortified food', *Lipids*, 42, 1011–1024.

BRAZEL CS (1999) 'Microencapsulation: offering solutions for the food industry', *Cereal Foods World*, 44, 388–393.

CARLSON SE, WERKMAN SH, RHODES PG and TOLLEY EA (1993) 'Visual-acuity development in healthy preterm infants: effect of marine-oil supplementation', *Am J Clin Nutr*, 58(1), 35–42.

CARTER JF (1993) 'Potential of flaxseed and flaxseed oil in baked goods and other products in human nutrition', 38, *Cereal Foods World*, 38, 753–759.

CHANG SS, BAO Y and PELURA TJ (1991) *Fish Oil Antioxidants*, US Patent 5,023,100.

CHAPMAN KW, SAGI I, REGENSTEIN JM, BIMBO T, CROWTHER JB and STAUFFER CE (1998) 'Oxidative stability of hydrogenated menhaden oil shortening blends in cookies, crackers, and snacks', *J Am Oil Chem Soc*, 73, 167–172.

CHEATHAM, CL, COLOMBO J and CARLSON SE (2006) 'n-3 Fatty acids and cognitive and visual acuity development: methodologic and conceptual considerations', *Am J Clin Nutr*, 83, 1458S–1466S.

CHEN ZY, RATNAYAKE WMN and CUNNANE SC (1992) 'Stability of flaxseed during baking', *J Am Oil Chem Soc*, 71, 629–632.

CIFTCI ON, PRZYBYLSKI R and RUDZINSKA M (2012) 'Lipid components of flax, perilla, and chia seeds', *Eur J Lipid Sci Technol*, 114, 794–800.

COSTA DE CONTO L, PORTO-OLIVEIRA RS, PEREIRA-MARTIN LG, CHANG YK and STEEL CJ (2012) 'Effects of the addition of microencapsulated omega-3 and rosemary extract on the technological and sensory quality of white pan bread', *LWT – Food Sci Technol*, 45, 103–109.

DE AGUIAR AC, BOROSKI M, GIRIBONI-MONTEIRO AR, DE SOUZA NE and VISENTAINER JV (2011) 'Enrichment of whole wheat bread with flaxseed oil', *J Food Process Preserv*, 35, 605–609.

DROVER J, HOFFMAN DR, CASTANEDA YS, MORALE SE and BIRCH EE (2009) 'Three randomized controlled trials of early long-chain polyunsaturated fatty acid supplementation on means–end problem solving in 9-month-olds', *Child Dev*, 80, 1376–1384.

DUBOIS V, BRETON S, LINDER M, FANNI J and PARMENTIER M (2007) 'Fatty acid profiles of 80 vegetable oils with regard to their nutritional potential', *Eur J Lipid Sci Technol*, 109, 710–732.

DUPONT J (1996) 'Fatty acid-related functions', *Am J Clin Nutr*, 63, 991S–993S.

EGERT S, WOLFFRAM S, SCHULZE B, LANGGUTH P, HUBBERMANN EM, SCHWARZ K, ADOLPHI B, BOSY-WESTPHAL A, RIMBACH G and MULLER MJ (2012) 'Enriched cereal bars are more effective in increasing plasma quercetin compared with quercetin from powder-filled hard capsules', *Br J Nutr*, 107, 539–546.

ERICKSON DR (1995) *Practical Handbook of Soybean and Utilization*. Champaign, Il: AOCS Press.

FRANKEL EN and HUANG SW (1994) 'Improving the oxidative stability of polyunsaturated vegetables oils by blending with high-oleic sunflower oil', *J Am Oil Chem Soc*, 71, 255–259.

FRANKEL EN, HUANG SW, PRIOR E and AESCHBACH R (1996) 'Evaluation of antioxidant activity of rosemary extracts, carnosol and carnosic acid in bulk vegetable oils and fish oil and their emulsions', *J Agric Food Chem*, 72, 201–208.

FROST and SULLIVAN (2010) *2010 US Consumers' Choice: Omega-3 Nutrient Products*, August.

GOED (2012) GOED *Voluntary Monograph (v. 4). Omega-3 EPA, Omega-3 DHA, Omega-3 EPA & DHA*. Salt Lake City, UT: Global Organization for EPA and DHA Omega-3, available at: http://www.goedomega3.com/images/stories/files/goedmonograph.pdf [accessed February 2013].

GÖKMEN V, MOGOL BA, BARONE-LUMAGA R, FOGLIANO V, KAPLUN Z and SHIMONI E (2011) 'Development of functional bread containing nanoencapsulated omega-3 fatty acids', *J Food Eng*, 105, 585–591.

HALLUND J, BUGEL S, THOLSTRUP T, FERRARI M, TALBOT D, HALL WL, REIMANN M, WILLIAMS CM and WIINBERG N (2006) 'Soya isoflavone-enriched cereal bars affect markers of endothelial function in postmenopausal women', *Br J Nutr*, 95, 1120–1126.

HAYTA M and OZUGUR G (2011) 'Phytochemical fortification of flour and bread', in PREEDY VR, WATSON RR and PATEL B (eds), *Flour and Breads and Their Fortification in Health and Disease Prevention*. London: Academic Press, 293–300.

HERNANDEZ E (2005) 'Production, processing and refining of oils', in AKOH C and LAI OM (eds), *Healthful Lipids*, Champaign, Il. AOCS Press, 48–64.

HORN AF, NIELSEN NS and JACOBSEN C (2009) Additions of caffeic acid, ascorbyl palmitate or γ-tocopherol to fish oil-enriched energy bars affect lipid oxidation differently, *Food Chem*, 112, 412–420.

INDARTI E, MAJIDB MIA, HASHIMA R and CHONG A (2005) 'Direct FAME synthesis for rapid total lipid analysis from fish oil and cod liver oil', *J Food Compos Anal*, 18, 161–170.

JENAB E, REZAEI K and EMAM-DJOMEH Z (2006) 'Canola oil extracted by supercritical carbon dioxide and a commercial organic solvent', *Eur J Lipid Sci Technol*, 108, 488–492.

JENSEN CL, MAUDE M, ANDERSON RE and HEIRD WC (2000) 'Effect of docosahexaenoic acid supplementation of lactating women on the fatty acid composition of breast milk lipids and maternal and infant plasma phospholipids', *Am J Clin Nutr*, 71, 292S–299S.

JÓNSDÓTTIR R, BRAGADÓTTIR M, ARNARSON GO (2005) 'Oxidatively derived volatile compounds in micro-encapsulated fish oil monitored by solid-phase micro-extraction', *J Food Sci*, 70, 433–440.

KINSELLA JE (1988) 'Food lipids and fatty acids: importance in food quality, nutrition, and health', *Food Technol*, 42(10), 124–142.

KOCA AF and ANIL M (2007) 'Short communication. Effect of flaxseed and wheat flour blends on dough rheology and bread quality', *J Sci Food Agric*, 87, 1172–1175.

KOLANOWSKI W, SWIDERSKI F and BERGER S (2002) 'Possibilities of fish oil application for food products enrichment with omega-3 PUFA', *Int J Food Sci Nutr*, 50, 39–49.

KOLANOWSKI W, JAWORSKA D, WEISSBRODT J and KUNZ B (2007) 'Sensory assessment of microencapsulated fish oil powder', *J Am Oil Chem Soc*, 84, 37–45.

KORIYAMA T, WONGO S, WATANABE K and ABE H (2002) 'Fatty acid compositions of oil species affect the 5 basic taste perceptions', *J Food Sci*, 67, 868–873.

LIU M, WALLIN R and SALDEEN T (2001) 'Effect of bread containing stable fish oil on plasma phospholipid fatty acids, triglycerides, HDL-cholesterol, and malondialdehyde in subjects with hyperlipidemia', *Nutr Res*, 21, 1403–1410.

LU FSH and NORZIAH MH (2010) 'Stability of docosahexaenoic acid and eicosapentaenoic acid in breads after baking and upon storage', *Int J Food Sci Technol*, 45, 821–827.

MCGILL AS and MOFFAT CF (1992) 'A study of the composition of fish liver and body oil triglycerides', *Lipids*, 27, 360–370.

MELANSON SF, LEWANDROWSKI EL, FLOOD JG and LEWANDROWSKI KB (2005) 'Measurement of organochlorines in commercial over-the-counter fish oil preparations: implications for dietary and therapeutic recommendations for omega-3 fatty acids and a review of the literature, *Arch Pathol Lab Med*, 129, 74–77.

MASSRIEH W (2008) 'Health benefits of omega-3 fatty acids from Neptune krill oil', *Lipid Technol*, 20, 108–111.

MILLER CK, GABBAY RA, DILLON J, APGAR J and MILLER D (2006) 'The effect of three snack bars on glycemic response in healthy adults', *J Am Diet Assoc*, 106, 745–748.

NIELSEN H (1992) '*n-3* Polyunsaturated fish fatty acids in a fish-oil-supplemented bread', *J Sci Food Agric*, 59, 559–562.

NIELSEN NS and JACOBSEN C (2009) 'Methods for reducing lipid oxidation in fish-oil-enriched energy bars', *Int J Food Sci Technol*, 44, 1536–1546.

O'BRIEN RD (1998) *Fats and Oils.* Lancaster, PA: Technomic.

PACKAGED FACTS (2012) *Food Bars in the U.S.: Trends in Cereal/Granola Bars and Energy/Nutrition Bars.* Rockville, MD: Packaged Facts, available at: http://www.packagedfacts.com/Food-Bars-Cereal-6576315/ [accessed February 2013].

POHJANHEIMO TA, HKALA MA, TAHVONEN R, SALMINEN SJ and KALLIO HP (2006) 'Flaxseed in breadmaking: effects on sensory quality, aging, and composition of bakery products', *J Food Sci*, S343–S348.

PURDY RH (1986) 'High oleic sunflower: physical and chemical characteristics', *J Am Oil Chem Soc*, 63(8), 1062–1066.

SERNA-SALDIVAR S and ABRIL R (2011) 'Production and nutraceutical properties of breads fortified with DHA- and omega-3-containing oils', in PREEDY VR, WATSON RR and PATEL VB (eds), *Flour and Breads and their Fortification in Health and Disease Prevention.* London: Academic Press, 313–323.

SERNA-SALDIVAR S, ZORRILLA R, DE LA PARRA C, STAGNITTI G and ABRIL R (2006) 'Effect of DHA containing oils and powders on baking performance and quality of white pan bread', *Plant Foods Hum Nutr,* 61, 121–129.

SHAHIDI F (2011) 'Omega-3 fatty acids in health and disease', in HERNANDEZ E and HOSOKOWA H (eds), *Omega 3 Oils: Applications in Functional Foods*. Urbana, Il: AOCS Press, 1–29.

SHAHIDI F and ZHONG Y (2010) 'Novel antioxidants in food quality preservation and health promotion', Eur *J Lipid Sci Technol*, 112, 930–940.

SHEARER AEH and DAVIES CGA (2005) 'Physicochemical properties of freshly baked and stored whole-wheat muffins with and without flaxseed meal', *J Food Qual*, 28, 137–153.

SIMOPOULOS AP (1997) 'Essential fatty acids in health and chronic disease', *Food Revi Int*, 13(4), 623–631.

STANDAL IB, RAINUZZO J, AXELSON DE, VALDERSNES S, JULSHAMN K and AURSAND M (2012) 'Classification of geographical origin by PNN analysis of fatty acid data and level of contaminants in oils from Peruvian anchovy', *J Am Oil Chem Soc*, 89, 1173–1182.

SUNDRAM K, PERLMAN D and HAYES K (1999) *Blends of palm fat and corn oil provide oxidation-resistant shortenings for baking and frying*. US Patent 5,874,117.

VENKATESHWARLU G, LET MB, MEYER AS and JACOBSEN C (2004) 'Modeling the sensory impact of defined combinations of volatile lipid oxidation products on fishy and metallic off-flavors', *J Agric Food Chem*, 52, 311–317.

XIN F and SHUN W (1993) 'Enhancing the antioxidant effect of α-tocopherol with rosemary in inhibiting catalyzed oxidation caused by iron (II) and hemoprotein', *Food Res Int,* 26, 405–411.

YEP YL, LI D, MANN NJ, BOD O and SINCLAIR AJ (2002) 'Bread enriched with microencapsulated tuna oil increases plasma docosahexaenoic acid and total omega-3 fatty acids in humans', *Asia Pacific J Clin Nutr,* 11, 285–291.

12

Enrichment of emulsified foods with omega-3 fatty acids

C. Jacobsen, A. F. Horn and N. S. Nielsen, Technical University of Denmark, Denmark

DOI: 10.1533/9780857098863.3.336

Abstract: There is an increasing interest in adding omega-3 polyunsaturated fatty acids (PUFA) to foods. Due to the highly polyunsaturated nature of omega-3 fatty acids, avoiding lipid oxidation in omega-3 enriched foods remains a major challenge for food producers. This chapter describes the consequences of lipid oxidation in food products with respect to off-flavour formation. Moreover, the most important factors, such as oil quality, pH, choice of ingredients, processing conditions, etc., affecting lipid oxidation in a range of different products (e.g. milk, mayonnaise, dairy products) are summarized. Strategies to avoid lipid oxidation (apart from antioxidant addition) are also discussed.

Key words: off-flavour formation, emulsified food, mayonnaise, dairy products, omega-3 fatty acids.

12.1 Introduction

With the increasing consumer awareness of the health beneficial effects of long-chain marine omega-3 polyunsaturated fatty acids (PUFA), an increasing number of foods enriched with PUFA are entering the marketplace. Many of these foods are emulsion based, such as milk and other dairy products, mayonnaise, dressings, spreads, etc. Unfortunately, the high degree of polyunsaturation that contributes to making the two most important marine omega-3 PUFA – eicosapentaenoic acid (EPA) and docosahexaenoic acid (DHA) – so healthy also makes them highly susceptible to lipid oxidation. As described in Chapter 4, lipid oxidation will result in formation of lipid hydroperoxides and a myriad of volatile oxidation products such as ketones and aldehydes. Some of these oxidation products may have serious detrimental health effects that may counteract the positive health effects of omega-3 PUFA, and some of the volatile oxidation products will also give rise to undesirable fishy and rancid off-flavours as will be illustrated in this chapter. This chapter will also focus on factors important for lipid oxidation in emulsified foods and will discuss precautions that can be taken to prevent oxidation in such foods apart from adding antioxidants. The effect of antioxidant addition in emulsified foods is dealt with in Chapter 4.

12.2 Volatile oxidation products and off-flavour formation in omega-3 enriched food emulsions – using milk as an example

As previously mentioned, lipid oxidation of omega-3 fatty acids will give rise to a wide range of volatile oxidation products, but it is not an easy task to find markers for oxidation of omega-3 fatty acids, which are linked to the undesirable fishy, rancid and sometimes metallic off-flavours encountered in oxidized omega-3 enriched foods. The first step in doing so is to analyze the volatile oxidation products, and this can be done by gas chromatography–mass spectrometry (GC–MS). Different techniques, such as static headspace, dynamic headspace or solid-phase microextraction, can be used to extract the volatiles from the emulsified foods prior to analysis by GC–MS.

In our lab, we have used dynamic headspace GC–MS to determine the profile of volatiles in milk with or without fish oil after storage at 2 °C for 14 days (Venkateshwarlu *et al.*, 2004a). A total of 16 volatiles were identified in conventional milk, whereas 62 volatiles were identified in fish oil enriched milk. Most of the compounds isolated from pure milk by using this method were ketones, especially methyl ketones, which are known to be present in high levels in pasteurized milk. In addition, straight-chain aldehydes and n-alcohols were found. The volatiles identified in fish oil enriched milk encompassed alkenals, alkadienals, alkatrienals and vinyl ketones. Following the identification of these volatiles, we used GC–olfactometry to identify the odour associated with them. The data suggested that 1-penten-3-one, 4-*cis*-heptenal, 1-octen-3-one, 1,5-octadien-3-one, 2,4-*trans,trans*-heptadienal and 2,6-*trans,cis*-nonadienal were the most potent volatiles. Despite their potency, none of these individual volatiles gave rise to the same fishy or metallic odours that could be observed in oxidized fish oil enriched milk and it was therefore suggested that the fishy and metallic odours were due to a combination of several volatiles (Venkateshwarlu *et al.*, 2004a).

On the basis of these findings as well as other data from the literature, 1-penten-3-one, 4-*cis*-heptenal, 2,4-*trans,trans*-heptadienal and 2,6-*trans,cis*-nonadienal were selected for further study, which aimed at investigating whether these four compounds were responsible for the fishy and metallic off-odour and off-flavours in fish oil enriched milk. To obtain this aim, a sensory panel evaluated the sensory properties of conventional milk to which different combinations, and concentrations of these four volatiles had been added (Venkateshwarlu *et al.*, 2004b). Subsequently, partial least square regression was used to build a mathematical model that could describe the relationship between the concentration of the four volatiles and the intensity of fishy and metallic off-odour and off-flavours. Interestingly, the model only revealed significant main effects of 2,6-*trans,cis*-nonadienal and 1-penten-3-one, whereas the main effects of the other two volatiles (2,4-*trans,trans*-heptadienal and 4-*cis*-heptenal) were not significant. This suggests that particularly 2,6-*trans,cis*-nonadienal and 1-penten-3-one could be useful markers for fishy and metallic off-flavours in omega-3 enriched milk and perhaps also in other omega-3 enriched foods. Response surface plots revealed a curvature effect of 2,6-*trans,cis*-nonadienal, compensatory effect of 4-*cis*-heptenal and 2,4-*trans,trans*-heptadienal and synergistic effect of 2,6-*trans,cis*-nonadienal and 4-*cis*-heptenal with respect to the development of fishy off-flavours (Venkateshwarlu *et al.*, 2004b). Importantly, these four volatiles have also been identified in other omega-3 enriched emulsions such as mayonnaise and dressing (Hartvigsen *et al.*, 2000; Let *et al.*, 2007a).

12.3 Factors affecting lipid oxidation in emulsified omega-3 enriched foods

Importantly, lipid oxidation generally occurs faster in emulsions than in neat oils (Frankel *et al.*, 2002), and it may therefore also be expected to occur faster in most emulsified omega-3 enriched foods than in neat oils. This is partly due to the mechanical processing that is required for emulsification which, in some cases, also includes the use of high temperature and intensive agitation which introduces a significant amount of air into the emulsion. However, as will be discussed later, a high temperature during emulsification will not always lead to increased lipid oxidation. In many cases, the oil is exposed to air (oxygen) during processing, and this can also lead to oxidation. The increased oxidation rate of emulsions may also be due to an increased interfacial area as lipid oxidation is an interfacial phenomenon, although it also takes place inside of the emulsion droplets as well. Even after refining and deodorization, most omega-3 oils will contain trace levels of peroxides and several food ingredients contain trace levels of transition metal ions. Therefore, metal-catalyzed decomposition of peroxides is regarded as the most important driving force for lipid oxidation in many food products (see also Chapter 4). In the following, the different factors important for lipid oxidation will be discussed and examples on how to deal with these factors to reduce lipid oxidation are given.

12.3.1 The influence of the omega-3 oil quality

The oil quality (i.e. oxidative status of the omega-3 PUFA oil) may significantly influence the oxidative stability of the final omega-3 enriched emulsified food and should therefore be evaluated before the oil is used. The peroxide value (PV) has traditionally been used as a measure of oil quality. It measures the level of the primary oxidation products (lipid hydroperoxides). We have shown that in fish oil enriched milk the fish oil quality will have a great impact on oxidative flavour deterioration and that this impact was more important than the fatty acid composition and tocopherol level of the fish oils used in this study (Let *et al.*, 2004, 2005a). Thus, pasteurised milk emulsions based on cod liver oil with a slightly elevated PV of 1.5 meq/kg oxidized significantly faster than a similar emulsion containing with a low PV of 0.1 meq/kg despite the fact that the tuna oil was more unsaturated than the cod liver oil. It was suggested that the slightly elevated level of lipid hydroperoxides in the cod liver oil in combination with trace metals present in the milk were responsible for the rapid oxidative flavour deterioration of the milk enriched with this oil due to the ability of trace metals to decompose lipid hydroperoxides. Subsequently, it was shown that a sensory panel was able to distinguish milk emulsions produced with fish oil with a PV of 0.1 meq/kg as being less fishy and rancid as compared to milk produced with a fish oil with the same fatty acid composition and tocopherol level but with a PV of 0.5 meq/kg already after one day of storage (Let *et al.*, 2005a). Further studies in our laboratory have shown that the quality of the fish oil seems to be less important in yoghurt-like products than in pasteurized milk emulsions (Let *et al.*, 2007a). This is most likely due to the fact that peptides formed during the fermentation of milk to yoghurt have antioxidative properties that makes fish oil enriched yoghurt more oxidatively stable than fish oil enriched milk as will be further elaborated upon later (Farvin *et al.*, 2010a, b).

12.3.2 The influence of emulsifiers and pH

The pH has been observed to have a significant effect on lipid oxidation in fish oil enriched mayonnaise. Thus, lipid oxidation increased when pH was decreased from 6.0 to 3.8, which is the usual pH of mayonnaise (Jacobsen *et al.*, 1999, 2001). The following explanation was suggested for this phenomenon. In mayonnaise, egg yolk is used as an emulsifier and egg yolk contains large amounts of iron, which is bound to the protein phosvitin. At the natural pH of egg yolk (pH 6.0), the iron forms cation bridges between phosvitin and other components in egg yolk, namely low-density lipoproteins (LDL) and lipovitellin (Jacobsen *et al.*, 1999). These components are located at the oil–water (o/w) interface in mayonnaise. It is suggested that when pH decreases to around 4.0, the cation bridges between the aforementioned egg yolk components break whereby iron becomes dissociated from LDL and lipovitellin. Thereby, iron becomes more active as a catalyst of oxidation (Jacobsen *et al.*, 1999, 2001). Hence, the low pH in combination with the iron-rich egg yolk is the most important driving force for the rapid oxidation processes in fish oil enriched mayonnaise and it was therefore suggested that substitution of egg yolk with a less iron rich emulsifier such as milk protein could reduce oxidation.

Sørensen *et al.* (2010a) recently investigated this hypothesis in a fish oil enriched light mayonnaise, but they could not confirm that substitution of egg yolk with milk protein-based emulsifier could reduce lipid oxidation. The main reason for the lack of effect of this substitution was suggested to be the low quality of the milk protein-based emulsifier, which had a 50 times higher lipid hydroperoxide content than the egg yolk. Therefore, it was concluded that not only the iron content, but also the initial oxidative quality of the emulsifier is crucial for the oxidative stability of fish oil enriched mayonnaise. Further studies are therefore needed to investigate whether the use of a high-quality milk protein will increase the oxidative stability of fish oil enriched mayonnaise.

12.3.3 Choice of ingredients other than emulsifier

Recently, the effect on lipid oxidation of the different ingredients used to prepare fish oil enriched mayonnaise-based shrimp and tuna salad was reported (Sørensen *et al.*, 2010b). Interestingly, the ingredients and the salad type had a greater influence on lipid oxidation than substitution of 10 % of the soya oil with fish oil. A sensory panel could not significantly distinguish the intensity of rancid off-flavour in salads without fish oil from that in salads with fish oil throughout the storage period (57 days) for both salad types, except for tuna salads for which the panel could only descriminate between the salads with or without fish oil after 57 days of storage. The results of the sensory evaluation of the shrimp salads are shown in Fig. 12.1. These results thus indicated that it was possible to add fish oil to these two salad types without compromising the sensory properties if the labeled shelf-life was kept below 57 days. The tuna salads oxidized faster than the shrimp salads and this was suggested to be due to the heme content in tuna. For the shrimp salads, the presence of shrimp promoted lipid oxidation, whereas asparagus in brine had an antioxidative effect, which was able to counteract the pro-oxidative effect of the shrimps in this type of salad. For the tuna salad, the influence of ingredients herein seemed more complex and it was not possible to draw clear conclusions on the effect of the ingredients. The finding that the effect of the ingredients was not clear could be due to that the ingredients themselves had a high content of the same volatiles that were used as important parameters for evaluating oxidation. Therefore, small reductions in the concentration of volatiles due to possible antioxidative effects of the ingredients were most likely masked (Sørensen *et al.*, 2010b).

12.3.4 The effect of the emulsification conditions and oil droplet size

Production of omega-3 enriched food emulsions should be done under optimal conditions, which aim at minimizing lipid oxidation. This includes

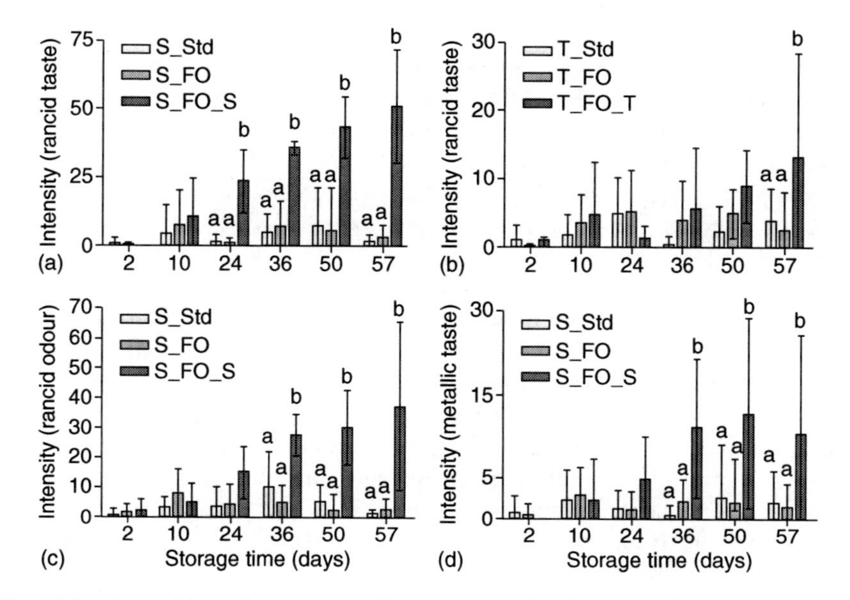

Fig. 12.1 Intensities of sensory attributes determined by descriptive profiling in mayonnaise-based shrimp salads. (a) Rancid taste in shrimp salads, (b) rancid taste in tuna salads, (c) rancid odour in shrimp salads, and (d) metallic taste in shrimp salad. The bars indicate the SD from all the panelists within each session. *S_Std* standard shrimp salad without fish oil. *S_FO* shrimp salad with fish oil, *S_FO_S* shrimp salad with fish oil but without asparagus, *T_Std* standard tuna salad without fish oil, *T_FO* tuna salad with fish oil, *T_FO_T* tuna salad with fish oil, tuna and onion but without the rest of the ingredients. Reprinted from: Sørensen, A.D.M., Nielsen, N.S., Jacobsen, C. Oxidative stability of fish oil enriched mayonnaise based salads. *Eur. J. Lipid Sci. Technol.* 112, 476–487. Copyright (2012) with permission from Wiley-VCH.

exclusion of air/oxygen during the production process as this will retard lipid oxidation as shown by Genot *et al.* (2003). Processing under vacuum or in a nitrogen atmosphere will therefore reduce lipid oxidation. In the final product, exclusion of headspace oxygen can be obtained by packaging in an air-tight container impermeable to oxygen, and preferably under modified atmosphere.

In most cases, processing at low temperatures will reduce lipid oxidation, as oxidation rates increase with increasing temperature. However, there are exceptions to this general rule as illustrated in two studies with fish oil enriched milk by Let *et al.* (2007b) and Sørensen *et al.* (2007). In both studies, fish oil was incorporated into milk at different temperatures (50 and 72 °C) and pressures (5, 15 and 22.5 MPa). Surprisingly, the highest oxidative stability was obtained at high homogenization pressure (22.5 MPa) and temperature (72 °C), even though the droplet size was smallest under these conditions. An increased number of droplets and thereby a large interfacial area could be expected to lead to increased oxidation as also observed in mayonnaise (Jacobsen *et al.*, 2000). However, this was not the case for omega-3 enriched milk emulsions. In order to explain why neither a high temperature nor a large interfacial area increased oxidation in this food system, the authors isolated the o/w interface and analyzed its protein composition by sodium dodecyl sulfate polyacrylamide gel electrophoresis (SDS-PAGE). They found that when temperature was increased from 50 to 72 °C an increased amount of β-lactoglobulin was adsorbed at the o/w interface and that even more β-lactoglobulin was adsorbed when the pressure was increased from 5 to 22.5 MPa (Sørensen *et al.*, 2007). In addition, the level of free thiol groups was increased at the high temperature and pressure (72 °C and 22.5 MPa). SDS-PAGE as well as confocal laser scanning microscopy (CLSM) also showed that less casein was present at the o/w interface with increasing pressure, meaning that more casein would be present in the aqueous phase. It can therefore be hypothesized that a combination of more β-lactoglobulin at the o/w interface and more casein in the aqueous phase was responsible for the increased oxidative stability.

Interestingly, studies in our laboratory have shown that a similar oxidation stabilizing effect of increasing the homogenization pressure could be observed in simple o/w emulsions when a combination of β-lactoglobulin and casein in a ratio similar to that in milk was used as emulsifier (Horn *et al.*, 2013). In contrast, lipid oxidation did not decrease with increasing pressure when whey proteins alone were used as emulsifier. This may suggest that the most important effect of increasing the pressure in fish oil enriched milk was that β-lactoglobulin replaced casein at the interface, whereby casein partitioned into the water phase where it could chelate metal ions, as also observed by Gallaher *et al.* (2005) in algal oil-enriched milk. Such a conclusion would be in agreement with other studies suggesting that increasing the casein concentration in the aqueous phase in simple o/w emulsions will increase the oxidative stability (Faraji *et al.*, 2004; Berton *et al.*, 2011).

12.4 Delivery systems

In the years since 2000, the development and use of omega-3 PUFA emulsion delivery systems have received substantial attention. The idea is that if properly designed, such delivery systems will protect the omega-3 PUFA against oxidation both prior to and after incorporation into the food emulsion. Several commercial omega-3 PUFA delivery systems are available and they all have a relatively low oil content, typically around 20 %. However, in our laboratory we have prepared delivery systems with up to 70 % fish oil using different emulsifiers, such as whey protein, casein, mixtures of milk phospholipids and milk proteins or lecithin (Horn *et al.*, 2011, 2012a). A general conclusion from these studies as well as studies on delivery emulsions with lower oil content is that the use of milk proteins as emulsifiers provides good oxidative stability to the delivery emulsions (Djordjevic

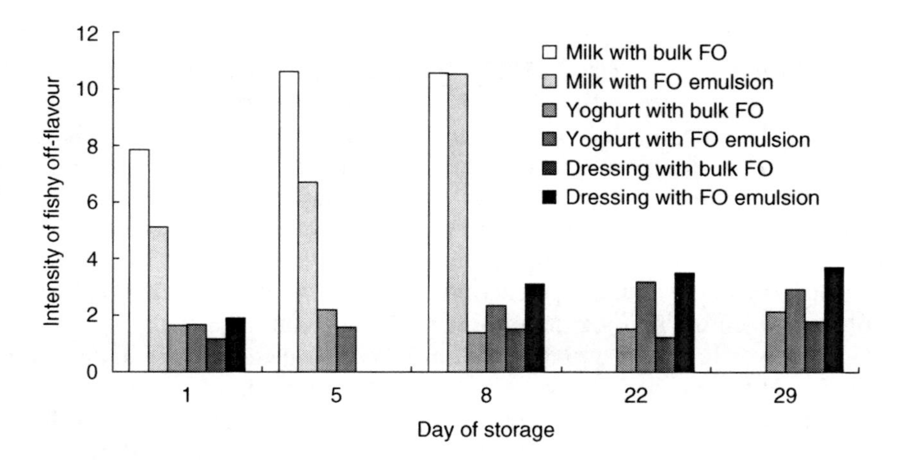

Fig. 12.2 Summarized intensity of fishy odour and flavour of milk, yoghurt and dressing enriched with either neat fish oil or fish o/w emulsion. Average standard deviations were 1.9, 1.3, and 1.4 for milk, yoghurt and dressing, respectively. Reprinted with permission from: Let, M.B., Jacobsen, C., Meyer, A.S. Lipid oxidation in milk, yoghurt and salad dressing enriched with neat fish oil or pre-emulsified fish oil. *J. Agric. Food Chem.* 55, 7802–7809. Copyright (2007) American Chemical Society.

et al., 2004; Horn *et al.*, 2011, 2012a). Whey proteins are often preferred in low pH delivery emulsions because they are easier to solubilize than caseins.

Only relatively few studies have aimed at comparing the effect on lipid oxidation of using omega-3 PUFA delivery emulsions or neat omega-3 oils in food emulsions. One of the few studies available investigated the effect on lipid oxidation of using a delivery system in milk, dressing and yoghurt (Fig. 12.2). Omega-3 PUFA were added either as neat oil or as an o/w emulsion (50 % oil) prepared with whey protein as an emulsifier (Let *et al.*, 2007a). Volatiles and sensory data indicated a better oxidative stability of dressing and yoghurt with neat fish oil compared to the corresponding products with the fish o/w emulsion. Hence, in these food systems the use of a delivery system did not improve the oxidative stability. This finding was explained by increased oxidation in the fish o/w emulsion itself, which was caused by the initial temperature increase (65 °C, 3 min) during homogenization of this emulsion. They also concluded that addition of antioxidants before homogenization of the pre-emulsion may be necessary to improve its oxidative stability. However, in the case of milk the use of a delivery system did improve the oxidative stability.

The effect of using a delivery emulsion with a lower oil content (10 %) in milk has also been investigated. In this study, the effect of using one of three different delivery emulsions prepared with either whey protein isolate, casein or pure β-lactoglobulin was investigated. Interestingly, both PV data and results for volatile secondary oxidation products revealed that the oxidative stability was better when fish oil was added as neat oil instead of as a delivery emulsion (Horn, 2012). Surprisingly, no clear differences were observed between the three milks with different delivery emulsions despite the fact that the delivery emulsions themselves had different oxidative stabilities. The differences in the oxidative stability of the delivery emulsions was attributed to the different protein composition at the o/w interface as well as in the aqueous phase. The lack of difference between the delivery emulsions when applied to milk could indicate that the protein components in the aqueous phase of the delivery emulsion did not play any role in preventing lipid oxidation when added to milk.

The lower oxidative stability of the milks to which delivery emulsions were added compared to that of the milk with neat oil added to it was in contrast to the study by Let *et al.* (2007a) mentioned above. These differences may be due to the different oil contents (10 vs 50 %) and physical structure of the delivery emulsions. The average oil droplet size was much smaller in milk prepared with 10 % o/w emulsions than in milk prepared with 50 % o/w emulsions. Since the homogenization of the milk with neat oil added was done at a similar pressure in the two studies (22.5 MPa), this resulted in the opposite relation between oil droplet sizes when prepared with neat oil or delivery emulsions in the two studies. Hence, milk with high-fat delivery emulsions had larger oil droplets than the milk prepared with neat oil, whereas the opposite was the case in the study with low-fat delivery emulsions. In this case, oil droplet size might therefore have influenced lipid oxidation rates, with the smaller oil droplets oxidizing more than the larger droplets in both studies, resulting in a lower oxidative stability of the milk with neat oil added in the study by Let *et al.* (2007a), and a lower oxidative stability of the milk with delivery emulsions added in the study by Horn (2012).

The effect of using three different types of delivery emulsions, prepared with either casein, whey protein isolate or a mixture of milk phospholipids and milk protein (MPL20), on lipid oxidation in cream cheese was recently investigated (Horn *et al.*, 2012b). In this study, a 70 % o/w emulsion was used as delivery emulsion. Results showed that cream cheese with fish oil added as delivery emulsions prepared with casein (CAS) or whey protein (WPI) oxidized the most during 20 weeks of storage, whereas cream cheese with fish oil added as neat oil or in a delivery emulsion prepared with MPL20 oxidized less, at least during the initial part of the storage period. Hence, in this type of food system the effect of using a delivery emulsion was dependent upon the type of emulsifier by which it was prepared, in contrast to the results for fish oil enriched milk. The macrostructure of the cream cheese was studied by CLSM, which revealed some interesting differences in the macrostructure of the cream cheeses. The cream cheese without fish oil and the cream cheese with neat fish oil had relatively large unprotected oil droplets, whereas the three cream cheeses with fish oil added as a delivery emulsion (MPL20, WPI and CAS) had far fewer unprotected lipid droplets. In particular, MPL20 could be distinguished from the other samples as more of the lipid (including the milk lipid) was hidden within the protein structure and this could probably explain why this cream cheese oxidized less than the other cream cheeses with fish oil. However, the better oxidative stability of the cream cheese with the MPL20 delivery emulsion compared to the WPI and CAS delivery emulsions could also be a result of the fact that MPL20 contained antioxidants, albeit in low amounts.

12.5 Antioxidative effects of other ingredients in emulsified omega-3 enriched foods

Let *et al.* (2004, 2005b) found that oxidative flavour deterioration in omega-3 enriched milk could be prevented by using a mixture of fish oil and rapeseed oil (1:1). The preventive effect of adding rapeseed oil to the fish oil was larger than what could be expected due to the dilution of the fish oil with a more oxidatively stable oil. The good oxidative stability obtained when using a mixture of rapeseed oil and fish oil was proposed to be due to the high content of γ-tocopherol in rapeseed oil.

As previously mentioned, Let *et al.* (2007a) found that fish oil enriched yoghurt had a better stability than fish oil enriched milk. This observation was confirmed by other studies (Chee *et al.*, 2005; Nielsen *et al.*, 2007). In the study by Chee *et al.* (2005) a yoghurt mix (2 g fat/100 g) was supplemented with an algae oil emulsion to provide 500 mg omega-3 PUFA per 272 g serving of yoghurt white mass. The emulsion was added to the yoghurt mix either before or after the homogenization step and prior to pasteurization. It was then flavoured with a strawberry fruit base and fermented and stored for up to three weeks. A trained sensory panel could distinguish a stronger fishy flavour in both of the supplemented yoghurts after 22 days storage, but a consumer panel rated both control and supplemented samples similarly, as 'moderately liked'. In the study by Nielsen *et al.* (2007) a drinking yoghurt, produced from commercial yoghurts (0.5 % fat, w/w) mixed with fish oil (1 %, w/w), flavour, sugar and stabilizer (pectin) also had a very high oxidative stability. The yoghurts were found to be stable for at least four weeks when stored at 2 °C. It was investigated whether one or more of the ingredients were responsible for the high oxidative stability of this product. However, due to a high stability even of plain yoghurt with fish oil added it was not possible to conclude on possible antioxidative effects of the added ingredients (Nielsen *et al.*, 2009).

As mentioned previously, it was hypothesized that peptides formed during fermentation of yoghurt could be responsible for the good oxidative stability of fish oil enriched yoghurt. To investigate this hypothesis, peptides from yoghurt were isolated and fractionated (Farvin *et al.*, 2010a). Subsequently, the antioxidant activity of the peptides was determined using different *in vitro* assays, including the 2,2-diphenyl-1-picrylhydrazyl (DPPH) radical scavenging activity, Fe^{2+} chelating activity, reducing power and inhibition of oxidation in liposome model system. Overall, the assays showed that the peptides of lower molecular weight had good metal-chelating and iron-reducing properties, whereas the higher molecular weight peptides were more efficient radical scavengers and exerted a better effect in the liposome model (Farvin *et al.*, 2010a). Further, the low molecular weight peptides were evaluated in fish oil enriched milk and they were shown to exert almost the same antioxidative effect as caseinophosphopeptides. Moreover, the oxidative stability of fish oil enriched milk with these peptides was significantly better than the control milk emulsion with fish oil but without the peptides (Fig. 12.3).

The peptide fractions were further characterized by liquid chromatography–mass spectroscopy (LC–MS). It was observed that the yoghurt contained a considerable amount of free amino acids such as His, Tyr, Thr and

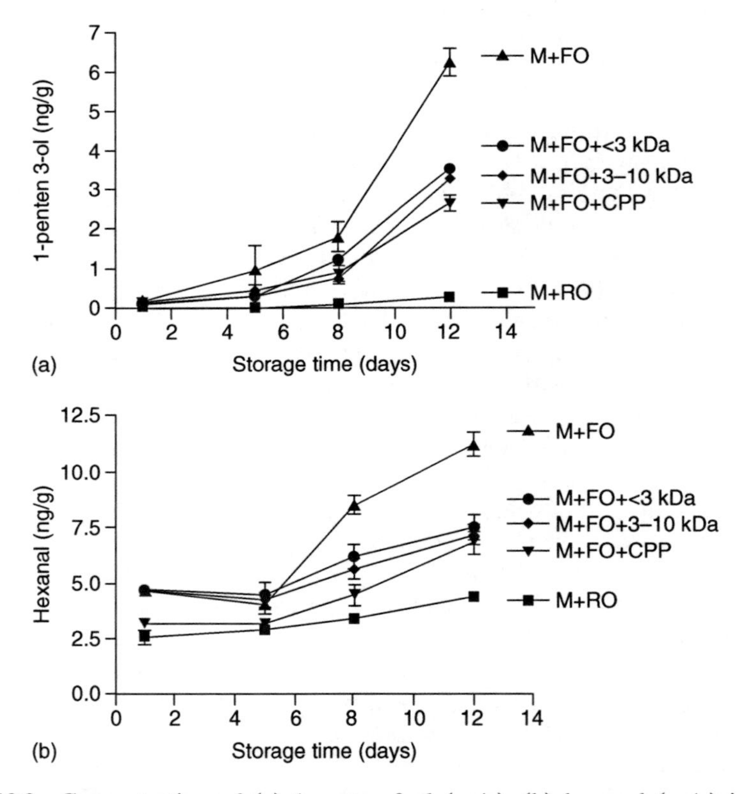

Fig. 12.3 Concentration of (a) 1-penten-3-ol (ng/g), (b) hexanal (ng/g) in milk emulisons during storage at 2 °C. M, milk; FO, fish oil; RO, rapeseed oil; CPP, caseinophosphopeptides. Results are the mean values of triplicate determinations on the same sample. Error bars indicate standard deviation. Reprinted from: Farvin, K.H.S., Baron, C.P., Nielsen, N.S., Jacobsen, C. (2010) Antioxidant activity of yoghurt peptides: Part 1 – *in vitro* assays and evaluation in ω-3 enriched milk. *Food Chemistry* 123, 1081–1089. Copyright (2010) Elsevier.

Lys, which have been reported to have antioxidant properties (Farvin *et al.*, 2010b). The identified peptides comprised a few N-terminal fragments of αs_1-CN, αs_2-CN, κ-CN and several fragments from β-CN. Almost all the peptides identified contained at least one proline residue. Some of the identified peptides included the hydrophobic amino acid residues Val or Leu at the N-terminus of the peptides and Pro, His or Tyr in the sequence which are the characteristic of antioxidant peptides (Farvin *et al.*, 2010b).

It was also speculated whether the bacteria used for fermenting yoghurt would lower the oxygen content and thereby decrease oxidation. Therefore, the oxygen content of the yoghurt and milk was compared and it was observed that the oxygen content was lowest in yoghurt (Farvin *et al.*, 2010a). It was therefore concluded that the higher oxidative stability of yoghurt might be due to the presence of antioxidant peptides and free amino acids formed during fermentation of the yoghurt and that the lower oxygen content of yoghurt, which subsequently reduces the oxidative stress of fish oil incorporated in the yoghurt, may also have contributed to the enhanced oxidative stability of fish oil enriched yoghurt compared to fish oil enriched milk.

From these studies it can thus be concluded that fish oil enriched yoghurt is a very suitable product for omega-3 enrichment from an oxidation point of view, and that no antioxidants are required to protect it from oxidation.

12.6 Other omega-3 enriched food emulsions

Apart from the above-mentioned studies on dairy products, mayonnaise and dressing, a few studies on other products have also been reported in the literature. In a study on low-calorie spreadable fats (soft margarine and a mix of butter and vegetable oil), it was concluded that spreads could be enriched with up to 1 % EPA and DHA without significantly affecting the sensory quality (Kolanowski *et al.*, 2001). The margarine spread may be stored up to six weeks and the spread based on butter and vegetable up to three weeks without significant decrease of quality. These spreads contained 55 % fat and no antioxidants were added.

Kolanowski and Weissbrodt (2007) investigated the sensory quality of yoghurts, cream, butter and different cheeses to which different levels of fish oil had been added. Table 12.1 shows the overall flavour score associated with different levels of fish oil as well as the upper tolerable level of fish oil that could be added to these products without significantly affecting the sensory quality. The results illustrate that the maximum tolerable level of fish oil that can be added varies significantly from product to product. This can be explained by the fact that volatile oxidation products will have different flavour threshold levels in different food products. The flavour threshold depends, amongst other factors, on how easily flavour compounds

Table 12.1 Overall flavour scores (expressed as sensory quality points*) for dairy products fortified with different amounts of fish oil

Fortified products	Amount of fish oil added (g kg^{-1})											
	0	1	2	3	5	10	15	20	30	40	60	80
Natural drinkable yoghurt	5.2	5.2	**4.7**	3.0	1.7	–	–	–	–	–	–	–
Yoghurt, drinkable, flavoured with strawberry	5.8	5.7	5.8	**4.6**	2.2	–	–	–	–	–	–	–
Cream, reduced fat	5.2	5.2	5.1	5.1	**4.0**	4.1	3.1	–	–	–	–	–
Cream, full fat	5.5	5.3	5.5	5.1	5.1	**4.9**	3.9	3.1	–	–	–	–
Processed fresh cheese (homogenized), not flavoured	5.5	5.4	5.5	**4.9**	3.0	1.2	–	–	–	–	–	–
Processed fresh cheese (homogenized), vanillin flavoured	5.8	5.8	5.5	**4.3**	2.9	1.4	–	–	–	–	–	–
Soft cheese (curd), reduced fat	5.4	5.4	5.1	**4.3**	2.4	0.7	–	–	–	–	–	–
Soft cheese (curd), full fat	5.4	5.4	5.4	5.1	**4.8**	2.4	1.7	–	–	–	–	–
Spreadable fresh cheese (Philadelphia type) not flavoured	5.2	5.0	5.1	5.2	5.2	5.1	**4.8**	4.0	3.5	–	–	–
Spreadable fresh cheese (Philadelphia type) with garlic	5.4	5.4	5.4	5.3	5.3	5.3	4.9	**4.5**	3,9	–	–	–
Processed cheese, not flavoured	5.4	5.3	5.5	5.3	5.3	5.4	5.5	5.4	5.2	**4.9**	3.4	3.3
Processed cheese with garlic	5.6	5.5	5.5	5.6	5.7	5.5	5.4	5.5	5.2	5.1	**4.7**	3.6
Butter	5.1	5.2	4.8	5.1	5.0	5.0	4.9	4.8	**4.7**	3.3	–	–

*Scaling method based on a 0–6 scale, with 0 indicating the lowest score and 6 the highest score, $p < 0.05$.
Note: Bold font reflects upper tolerable level of fish oil addition (threshold value).
Source: Kolanowski and Weissbrodt, Sensory quality of dairy products with fish oil. *Int. Dairy J.* 17 (2007), 1248–1253.

are released from the food product and on the presence of masking compounds.

Eidhin *et al.* (2003) compared the oxidative stability of camelina oil-based spreads with that of spreads based on sunflower oil. They found that the camelina oil-based spread had lower oxidative stability than the sunflower spread but maintained adequate sensory quality for 16 weeks of storage at 4 or 8 °C.

Song *et al.* (2011) studied the sensory properties and storage stability of chocolate ice cream, which was supplemented with both probiotics and omega-3 PUFA. The ice cream mix (40 % solids and 15 % fat) was supplemented with an omega-3 oil emulsion and 8 log CFU/g *Bificobacterium longum*. Ice creams without omega-3 PUFA were used as controls. Results showed that panelists detected the presence of omega-3 PUFA resulting in low acceptability scores, but they still indicated a willingness to purchase this kind of product as a source for omega-3 PUFA. The viability of probiotics was higher in the samples with omega-3 PUFA during frozen storage. Based on these results, the authors concluded that despite the fact that omega-3 PUFA addition resulted in lower sensory acceptability scores, ice cream can be used to deliver both probiotic cultures and omega-3 PUFA.

12.7 Future trends

The demand for new omega-3 enriched foods in the marketplace is expected to increase and to diversify. This will pose new challenges to food technologists. In order to obtain success, it is necessary for food technologists to understand which are the most important factors affecting lipid oxidation and sensory acceptability in their food products.

New and more advanced technologies to produce delivery systems will most likely emerge in the coming years. For example, electrospray was recently used to produce nanostructures with encapsulated omega-3 PUFA, which had a higher oxidative stability than the neat oil (Torres-Giner *et al.*, 2010), but these structures have not yet been evaluated in complex food emulsions. Also, the safety of using these structures in food products should be extensively studied as well.

12.8 Conclusion

As illustrated in this chapter, it is possible to produce oxidatively stable omega-3 enriched emulsified foods with acceptable sensory properties. However, there are many factors that can influence oxidative stability of such complex foods, and results obtained in one food system cannot be interpolated to another food system. Some of the most important factors to consider when optimizing the oxidative stability of omega-3 enriched food emulsions are the quality of the fish oil; composition and quality of the other ingredients, particularly the emulsifier; the emulsification conditions, including type of equipment used; and the use of a delivery emulsion. As discussed above, the same delivery system can have different effects in different food systems. Moreover, the oil content of the delivery system and in some cases also the emulsifier used in the delivery system can significantly affect oxidative stability of the resulting food emulsion. Hence, the composition of the delivery system must be optimized for each type of food system.

Among the food emulsions mentioned in this chapter, milk seems to be the most challenging food product with respect to obtaining a good oxidative stability. In contrast, it is much easier to obtain a good oxidative stability with fish oil enriched yoghurt or yoghurt drink no matter whether the product is flavoured or not. Further optimization of the oxidative stability can be obtained by antioxidant addition as discussed in Chapter 4.

12.9 References

BERTON, C., ROPERS, M. H., VIAU, M. and GENOT, C. (2011) 'Contribution of the interfacial layer to the protection of emulsified lipids against oxidation', *J. Agric. Food Chem.* **59**, 5052–5061.

CHEE, C. P., GALLAHER, J. J., DJORDJEVIC, D., FARAJI, H., MCCLEMENTS, D. J., DECKER, E. A., HOLLENDER, R., PETERSON, D. G., ROBERTS, R. F. and COUPLAND, J. N. (2005) 'Chemical and sensory analysis of strawberry flavoured yogurt supplemented with an algae oil emulsion', *J. Dairy Res.* **72**, 311–316.

DJORDJEVIC, D., MCCLEMENTS, D. J. and DECKER, E. A. (2004) 'Oxidative stability of whey protein-stabilized oil-in-water emulsions at pH 3: Potential omega-3 fatty acid delivery systems (Part B)', *J. Food Sci.* **69**, C356–C362.

EIDHIN, D. N., BURKE, J. and O'BEIRNE, D. (2003) 'Oxidative stability of ω3-rich camelina oil and camelina oil-based spread compared with plant and fish oils and sunflower spread', *J. Food Sci.* **68**, 345–353.

FARAJI, H., MCCLEMENTS, D. J. and DECKER, E. A. (2004) 'Role of continuous phase protein on the oxidative stability of fish oil-in-water emulsions', *J. Agric. Food Chem.* **52**, 4558–4564.

FARVIN, K. H. S., BARON, C. P., NIELSEN, N. S., OTTE, J. and JACOBSEN, C. (2010a) 'Antioxidant activity of yoghurt peptides: Part 1 – *in vitro* assays and evaluation in omega-3 enriched milk', *Food Chem.* **123**, 1081–1089,

FARVIN, K. H. S., BARON, C. P., NIELSEN, N. S., OTTE, J. and JACOBSEN, C. (2010b) 'Antioxidant activity of yoghurt peptides: Part 2 – Characterisation of peptide fractions', *Food Chem.* **123**, 1090–1097.

FRANKEL, E. N., SATUE-GRACIA, T., MEYER, A. S. and GERMAN, J. B. (2002) 'Oxidative stability of fish and algae oils containing long-chain polyunsaturated fatty acids in bulk and in oil-in-water emulsions', *J. Agric. Food Chem.* **50**, 2094–2099.

GALLAHER, J. J., HOLLENDER, R., PETERSON, D. G., ROBERTS, R. F. and COUPLAND, J. N. (2005) 'Effect of composition and antioxidants on the oxidative stability of fluid milk supplemented with an algae oil emulsion', *Int. Dairy J.* **15**, 333–341.

GENOT, C., MEYNIER, A. and RIAUBLANC, A. (2003) 'Lipid oxidation in emulsions', in KAMAL-ELDIN, A. (ed.), *Lipid Oxidation Pathways*, Champaign IL: AOCS Press, 190–244.

HARTVIGSEN, K., LUND, P., HANSEN, L. F. and HOLMER, G. (2000) 'Dynamic headspace gas chromatography/mass spectrometry characterization of volatiles produced in fish oil enriched mayonnaise during storage', *J. Agric. Food Chem.* **48**, 4858–4867.

HORN, A. F. (2012) 'Factors influencing the effect of milk-based emulsifiers on lipid oxidation in omega-3 emulsions', PhD Thesis. Technical University of Denmark, Denmark. ISBN: 978-87-92763-69-3.

HORN, A. F., NIELSEN, N. S., ANDERSEN, U., SØGAARD, L. H., HORSEWELL, A. and JACOBSEN, C. (2011) 'Oxidative stability of 70 % fish oil-in-water emulsions: Impact of emulsifiers and pH', *Eur. J. Lipid Sci. Technol.* **113**, 1243–1257.

HORN, A. F., NIELSEN, N. S. and JACOBSEN, C. (2012a) 'Iron-mediated lipid oxidation in 70 % fish oil-in-water emulsions: effect of emulsifier type and pH', *Int. J. Food Sci. Technol.* **47**, 1097–1108.

HORN, A. F., GREEN-PETERSEN, D., NIELSEN, N. S., ANDERSEN, U. and JACOBSEN, C. (2012b) 'Addition of fish oil to cream cheese affects lipid oxidation, sensory stability and macrostructure', *Agriculture*, **2**, 359–375.

HORN, A. F., BAROUH, N., NIELSEN, N. S., BARON, C. P. and JACOBSEN, C. (2013) 'Homogenization pressure and temperature affect composition of proteins in the aqueous phase and oxidative stability of fish-oil-in-water emulsions', *J. Am. Oil Chem. Soc. (submitted)*.

JACOBSEN, C., ADLER-NISSEN, J. and MEYER, A. S. (1999) 'Effect of ascorbic acid on iron release from the emulsifier interface and on the oxidative flavor deterioration in fish oil enriched mayonnaise', *J. Agric. Food Chem.* **47**, 4917–4926.

JACOBSEN, C., HARTVIGSEN, K., LUND, P., THOMSEN, M. K., SKIBSTED, L. H., ADLER-NISSEN, J., HOLMER, G. and MEYER, A. S. (2000) 'Oxidation in fish oil-enriched mayonnaise 3. Assessment of the influence of the emulsion structure on oxidation by discriminant partial least squares regression analysis', *Eur. Food Res. & Technol.* **211**, 86–98.

JACOBSEN, C., TIMM, M. and MEYER, A. S. (2001) 'Oxidation in fish oil enriched mayonnaise: Ascorbic acid and low pH increase oxidative deterioration', *J. Agric. Food Chem.* **49**, 3947–3956.

KOLANOWSKI, W and WEISSBRODT, J. (2007) 'Sensory quality of dairy products fortified with fish oil', *Int. Dairy J.* **17**, 1248–1253.

KOLANOWSKI, W., SWIDERSKI, F., LIS, E. *et al.* (2001) 'Enrichment of spreadable fats with polyunsaturated fatty acids omega-3 using fish oil', *Int. J. Food Sci. Nutr.* **52**, 469–476.

LET, M. B., JACOBSEN, C. and MEYER, A. S. (2004) 'Effects of fish oil type, lipid antioxidants and presence of rapeseed oil on oxidative flavour stability of fish oil enriched milk', *Eur. J. Lipid Sci. Technol.* **106**, 170–182.

LET, M. B., JACOBSEN, C. and MEYER, A. S. (2005a) 'Sensory stability and oxidation of fish oil enriched milk is affected by milk storage temperature and oil quality', *Int. Dairy J.* **15**, 173–182.

LET, M. B., JACOBSEN, C., PHAM, K. A. and MEYER, A. S. (2005b) 'Protection against oxidation of fish-oil-enriched milk emulsions through addition of rapeseed oil or antioxidants', *J. Agric. Food Chem.* **53**, 5429–5437.

LET, M. B., JACOBSEN, C. and MEYER, A. S. (2007a) 'Lipid oxidation in milk, yoghurt, and salad dressing enriched with neat fish oil or pre-emulsified fish oil', *J. Agric. Food Chem.* **55**, 7802–7809.

LET, M. B., JACOBSEN, C., SØRENSEN, A-D. M. and MEYER, A. S. (2007b) 'Homogenization conditions affects the oxidative stability of fish oil enriched milk emulsions: Lipid oxidation', *J. Agric. Food Chem.* **55**, 1773–1780.

NIELSEN, N. S., DEBNATH, D. and JACOBSEN, C. (2007) 'Oxidative stability of fish oil enriched drinking yoghurt'. *Int. Dairy J.* **17**, 1478–1485.

NIELSEN, N. S., KLEIN, V. and JACOBSEN, C (2009) 'Effect of ingredients on oxidative stability of fish oil-enriched drinking yoghurt', *Eur. J. Lipid Sci. Technol.* **111**, 337–345.

SONG, D., KHOURYIEH, H., ABUGHAZALEH, A. A., SALEM, M. M. E., HASSAN, O. and IBRAHIM, S. A. (2011) 'Sensory properties and viability of probiotic microorganisms in chocolate ice cream supplemented with omega-3 fatty acids', *Milchwissenschaft – Milk Science International* **66**, 172–175.

SØRENSEN, A-D. M., BARON, C. P., LET, M. B., BRÜGGEMANN, D., PEDERSEN, L. R. L. and JACOBSEN, C. (2007) 'Homogenization conditions affects the oxidative stability of fish oil enriched milk emulsions: Oxidation linked to changes in the protein composition at the oil–water interface', *J. Agric. Food Chem.* **55**, 1781–1789.

SØRENSEN, A-D. M., NIELSEN, N. S., HYLDIG, G. and JACOBSEN, C. (2010a) 'The influence of emulsifier type in fish oil enriched light mayonnaise', *Eur. J. Lipid Sci. Technol.* **112**, 1012–1023.

SØRENSEN, A-D. M., NIELSEN, N. S. and JACOBSEN, C. (2010b) 'Oxidative stability of fish oil-enriched mayonnaise-based salads', *Eur. J. Lipid Sci. Technol.* **112**, 476–487.

TORRES-GINER, S., MARTINEZ-ABAD, A., OCIO, M. J. and LAGARON, J. M. (2010) 'Stabilization of a nutraceutical omega-3 fatty acid by encapsulation in ultrathin electrosprayed zein prolamine', *J. Food Sci.* **75**, N69–N79.

VENKATESHWARLU, G., LET, M. B., MEYER, A. S. and JACOBSEN, C. (2004a) 'Chemical and olfactometric characterization of volatile flavor compounds in a fish oil enriched milk emulsion', *J. Agric. Food Chem.* **52**, 311–317.

VENKATESHWARLU, G., LET, M. B., MEYER, A. S. and JACOBSEN, C. (2004b) 'Modelling the sensory impact of defined combinations of volatile lipid oxidation products on fishy and metallic off-flavors', *J. Agric. Food Chem.* **52**, 1635–1641.

13

Enrichment of infant formula with omega-3 fatty acids

C. Kuratko, J. R. Abril, J. P. Hoffman and N. Salem, Jr, DSM Nutritional Products, USA

DOI: 10.1533/9780857098863.3.353

Abstract: The long-chain omega-3 fatty acid docosahexaenoic acid (DHA) and the long-chain omega-6 fatty acid arachidonic acid (ARA) are always found in breast milk and are recommended for addition to commercial infant formula. Use of these fatty acids is safe and supports growth along with providing support for the developing visual and neurological systems. Because of the multiple double bonds within DHA and ARA structures, they are highly susceptible to interaction with other nutrients and peroxidation. Special techniques are employed when incorporating DHA- and ARA-containing oils during the manufacturing process to preserve the integrity of these fatty acids for infant nutrition.

Key words: docosahexaenoic acid, arachidonic acid, infant formula, visual development, neurocognitive development, omega-3 fatty acids.

13.1 Introduction

There is compelling evidence regarding health benefits of n-3 fatty acids, particularly the long-chain polyunsaturated fatty acids (LC-PUFA), such as docosahexaenoic acid, 22:6 n3 (DHA) and eicosapentaenoic acid, 20:5 n3 (EPA). DHA in particular is highly recommended for use in infant formula along with the n-6 LC-PUFA, arachidonic acid, 20:4 n6 (ARA). DHA and ARA have been associated with beneficial effects on the development of the neural and visual systems of infants and, together, they support growth in babies during the first year of life (Kuratko *et al.*, 2010). Although mother's breast milk always contains these important fatty acids, the milk from cows does not inherently have DHA and ARA in significant amounts. Therefore, these LC-PUFA must be added from an additional source. DHA- and ARA-containing oils are now commercially available and are added to most infant formula products worldwide. Because of the multiple double bonds within DHA and ARA structures, they are highly susceptible to interaction with other nutrients and to peroxidation. Special techniques must, therefore, be used when incorporating DHA- and ARA-containing oils in the manufacture of infant formula. Over the years, nutrition research has led to the development of formulations and methods of manufacturing that preserve the integrity of these fatty acids for infant nutrition.

13.1.1 History of essential fats in infant formula

In humans, as in all mammals, breast milk from a well-nourished mother is the most nutritionally adequate and developmentally appropriate feeding. However, throughout history there has been a need to feed infants of mothers who cannot or choose not to breast feed (Stevens *et al.*, 2009; Castilho and Barros Filho, 2010). The feeding of artificial milk to infants has been recorded throughout history, but basic improvements in sanitation that occurred in the latter part of the 19th century allowed development of successful home and commercial methods for formula preparation and feeding (Fomon, 2001). Early, home-prepared formulas were based on modifications of whole cows' milk. Even in the early 1900s, the nutritional differences between human milk and cows' milk were known, and home-prepared formulas with modified cows' milk better reflected the composition of human milk. The problems of dehydration and poor digestibility associated with feeding cows' milk could be avoided by diluting it and also by adding a source of carbohydrate. It eventually became common practice to add vitamins and minerals to the formula or infant diet. The nutrients of early concern included vitamin C, vitamin D and iron due to their overt deficiency symptoms of scurvy, rickets and anemia; and, in most cases, the intake of essential fatty acids was low (Fomon, 2001).

Powdered commercial infant formula was available in the late 1800s. It was expensive, however, and not generally used. In 1951, commercial concentrated liquid formulas became generally available in the USA (Fomon, 2001). Compared to home-prepared formula, these liquid formulas provided a more consistent composition. They were convenient and their popularity increased. Ready-to-feed liquid formulas began to reach the market in the 1960s and 1970s. By the latter half of the 1960s, less than 10 % of infants in the USA received a home-prepared formula (Fomon, 2001).

These early liquid commercial formulas varied with regard to lipid source. One general type of formula was based on cows' milk and provided butterfat; a second type included vegetable oil rather than butterfat as the lipid source. According to the history by Fomon (2001), butterfat had an unpleasant odor and was commonly thought to cause constipation in the infant. Eventually, the use of liquid vegetable oils rather than butterfat became more commonplace.

Infant formula regulations for both safety and nutrient content had their beginnings in the mid-twentieth century. In 1971, the US Food and Drug Administration (FDA) published a list for required infant formula composition which included minimum levels for protein, fat, linoleic acid (LA 18:2 n-6) and 17 vitamins and minerals. However, there were no stated requirements for n-3 fatty acids (FDA, 1971).

Today, there continues to be an increased awareness of the benefits of producing infant formula which most closely mimics human milk. Even more important is providing formula which allows formula-fed infants to achieve the same nutritional status and meet the same developmental milestones as breastfed infants. Lipids function beyond the provision of calories and are known to contribute to infant development, particularly the long-chain n-3 and n-6 fatty acids. The LC-PUFA, including DHA and ARA, are bioactive forms of n-3 and n-6 fatty acids known to be important for the developing infant (Koletzko *et al.*, 2008). Included in infant formula at levels typically found in human milk, they are safe and provide a benefit to visual and cognitive development that continues longer term.

13.1.2 Omega-3 fatty acid deficiency in infants

Early descriptions of n-3 fatty acid deficiency in humans and animals included neural deficits and skin lesions (Innis, 1991; Lands, 1992; Cunnane, 2003). Studies showed that n-3 fatty acids were required in the diet for proper retinal and cognitive function (Innis, 1991).

Infants synthesize DHA from α-linolenic acid (ALA; 18:3 n-3) and obtain it from breast milk or DHA-supplemented infant formula. Likewise, ARA may be derived endogenously from linoleic acid (LA; 18:2 n-6) and is present in breast milk (Salem *et al.*, 1996) and also today in most DHA-supplemented infant formula. Endogenous synthesis of DHA from ALA is insufficient and numerous studies confirm that blood and tissue levels of DHA drop rapidly following birth unless the infant receives a dietary source from either human milk or a supplemented infant formula (Crawford, 1993; Salem *et al.*, 1996; Cunnane *et al.*, 2000). More specifically, plasma and red blood cell (RBC) levels of DHA are significantly lower in infants fed unsupplemented formula than in those who are breastfed or given supplemented formula (Koletzko *et al.*, 1989; Innis *et al.*, 1990; Clandinin *et al.*, 1997). Additionally, supplementation of formula with preformed DHA is required to achieve plasma and RBC levels equivalent to those of the breastfed infant (Koletzko *et al.*, 1989; Carlson *et al.*, 1993a; Hoffman *et al.*, 1993; Kohn *et al.*, 1994). Post-mortem analyses of brain tissue of young children revealed that DHA levels in phospholipids were significantly lower in infants fed unsupplemented formula compared to those who were breastfed (Farquharson *et al.*, 1992, 1995; Makrides *et al.*, 1994). Even with sufficient ALA in infant formula, blood and tissue levels of DHA decline if preformed DHA is not included. Therefore, it is clear that infant endogenous production of DHA is insufficient.

Full fat cow's milk, as used in early home-formula preparations, provided a small amount of ALA for the infant. However, with the introduction of vegetable oils as replacement for butterfat, formula ALA content became widely variable and the availability of n-3 fatty acids became questionable. The use of corn oil as the lipid source for formula provided very little ALA, while infant formulas containing soy oil generally provided ALA in amounts similar to human milk. However, the oxidative stability of ALA-containing oils proved to be a problem for manufacturers, and this was particularly true for powdered formulations. As a result, the very low ALA content of corn oil made it the choice of many manufacturers in the mid-twentieth century. Scientific and regulatory requirements for the inclusion of n-3 fatty acids in infant formula were not common at that time and their inclusion in formula was not consistent. It is important to note that, although the use of soy oil provided significant amounts of ALA in formula, neither it nor corn oil provide the long-chain n-3 fatty acid, DHA.

Today, DHA and ARA are widely accepted as important ingredients in infant formula and are considered the primary bioactive n-3 and n-6 fatty acids in the brain and retina. Providing adequate amounts of these fatty acids optimizes not only development in the short term, but also the long-term functioning of the visual, cognitive, cardiovascular and immune systems (Swanson *et al.*, 2012). Many scientific and regulatory bodies currently allow, and provide guidance for, the addition of DHA and ARA to infant formula. Table 13.1 shows recommendations from expert groups and regulatory agencies worldwide.

13.2 Importance of omega-3 fatty acids during infancy

13.2.1 Brain development

DHA and ARA are incorporated into all cell membrane structures and are particularly concentrated in certain cell types (Salem *et al.*, 1989). They are of particular interest because of their significant incorporation into membranes of the central and peripheral nervous system and retina (Salem *et al.*, 1989; Moriguchi *et al.*, 2001; Greiner *et al.*, 2003; Lim *et al.*, 2005). The period of late gestation up to age four is a time of rapid brain growth. It is a time of significant DHA accretion that is critical for neurodevelopment (Dobbing and Sands, 1973; Hadley *et al.*, 2009). During this time, brain mass increases approximately three-fold and the DHA content increases from approximately 2 to 4.5 g (Martinez, 1992).

DHA is highly enriched in synaptic regions of the white and gray matter of the brain. It is located predominantly in the sn-2 position of phosphatidylethanolamine and phosphatidylserine in biomembranes (O'Brien and Sampson, 1965; Svennerholm, 1968; Breckenridge *et al.*, 1972) where it

Table 13.1 Scientific recommendations / regulatory requirements regarding LC-PUFA content of term infant formula

Agency/group	n-3 LC-PUFA	n-6 LC-PUFA	Comments
US FDA (1980, 2001)	None stated	None stated	DHA and ARA from single-cell oils accepted as GRAS – May 2001
Commission of the European Communities (2006)	Optional EPA+DHA max of 1 % total fat	Max of 2 % of total fat for n-6 LC-PUFA Max of 1 % of total fat for ARA	EPA content shall not exceed that of DHA DHA content shall not exceed that of n-6 LC-PUFA No LC-PUFA claim possible if DHA less than 0.2 %
Codex Alimentarius Commission (2007)	Optional Guidance upper limit of 0.5 % total fat		ARA contents should reach at least the same concentration as DHA EPA content should not exceed the content of DHA
FSANZ (2007)	Optional		n-6: n-3 LC-PUFA ratio is not less than 1 DHA must be greater than EPA
ESPGHAN (Koletzko *et al.*, 2005)	Recommended DHA up to 0.5 % total fat		ARA ≥ DHA EPA ≤ DHA
WAPM and Child Health Foundation (Koletzko *et al.*, 2008)	Recommended DHA should be 0.2–0.5 % total fat		ARA ≥ DHA EPA ≤ DHA
FAO/WHO (2010)	0.20–0.36 % DHA total fat meets the AI for infants 0–6 months.	0.40–0.60 % ARA total fat meets the AI for infants 0–6 months.	
American Dietetic Association/Dietitians of Canada (Kris-Etherton and Innis, 2007)	DHA should be at least 0.2 % of total fat	ARA should not be lower than DHA	

AI = adequate intake; GRAS = generally recognized as safe.

provides a particularly fluid environment (Salem *et al.*, 1980; Feller *et al.*, 2002; Eldho *et al.*, 2003; Gawrisch and Soubia, 2008). DHA plays a role in the proliferation, size, connectivity and survivability of neuronal cells and, when released from the membrane, it serves as a precursor to other bioactive molecules (Ahmad *et al.*, 2002; Calderon and Kim, 2004; Akbar *et al.*, 2005; Stillwell *et al.*, 2005; Sang and Chen, 2006). Because of the important roles that DHA plays in nerve structure and function, it is not surprising that it also affects cognition and behavior. A decrease of DHA in the developing brain is associated with impairment in scores on tests of learning, memory and attention as well as visual function (Moriguchi and Salem, 2003; Fleith and Clandinin, 2005; Heird and Capillonne, 2005).

13.2.2 Retinal physiology

DHA is present at high levels in phospholipids of the retina, particularly the membrane structure of rod (and cone) outer segments. It can represent as much as half of total fatty acids present in these highly metabolically active structures (Hodge *et al.*, 2005). The more disordered and flexible environment that DHA creates in biomembranes allows visual pigments and transmembrane proteins and messengers to quickly change physical shape and position. This rapid change in conformation is required for visual activity (Niu *et al.*, 2004; Hodge *et al.*, 2005; Lien and Hammond, 2011). When levels of DHA are insufficient, these specialized retinal cells incorporate n-6 long-chain fatty acids, but visual acuity suffers (Galli *et al.*, 1970). For optimal function of cells in the retina, there is no effective substitute for DHA (Lim *et al.*, 2005; Greiner *et al.*, 2003).

In addition to providing structural and biophysical roles in membranes, DHA is also important for protective pathways in the eye. Recent reviews describe the mechanisms by which DHA provides protection for the retina and cornea (Liclican and Gronent, 2010; Bazan *et al.*, 2011; Querques *et al.*, 2011). DHA is a substrate for the production of resolvins and neuroprotectins, which limit inflammation, enhance wound healing, inhibit overproduction of blood vessels and provide neuroprotection against periods of ischemia and oxidative stress (Kremmyda *et al.*, 2011).

Although the eye has methods for conserving DHA, there is significant turnover and loss even during the normal visual cycle. Diet plays an important role in providing sufficient preformed DHA to replenish these losses, especially during rapid growth and development (Lien and Hammond, 2011). A number of studies in preterm and term infants demonstrate that inclusion of DHA in early feedings is needed for optimal visual development. Visual acuity is measurably better in infants and small children who receive DHA in their diets when compared to those who do not (Lien and Hammond, 2011).

Experts consider visual development an extension of brain development, with even small or transient changes in visual acuity reflecting overall central nervous system development (Birch *et al.*, 1998). In a 2003 publication, Hoffman stated that since both retina and brain tissues are derived embryologically from neuroectoderm, visual function provides a 'window to the brain' (Hoffman, 2003). It follows, therefore, that developmental maturation of both retina and brain can be monitored by assessment of visual function.

13.2.3 Breast milk

Omega-3 fatty acid composition of breast milk

DHA is transferred from the mother to the fetus during gestation via the placenta. DHA accretion in the central nervous system begins *in utero* and is especially rapid during the third trimester of gestation (Clandinin *et al.*, 1980a, b; Martinez and Mougan, 1998; Gil-Sanchez *et al.*, 2012). After birth, human milk supplies DHA to the infant (Koletzko *et al.*, 1992; Yuhas *et al.*, 2006; German, 2011).

Factors influencing composition of breast milk

The DHA content of breast milk is dependent on maternal DHA intake. The relationship is specific to DHA and not its precursor ALA (Makrides *et al.*, 1996). Francois *et al.* (2003) reported that supplementation of breastfeeding women with flax oil, as a source of ALA, successfully increased ALA, EPA and docosapentaenoic acid (DPA) n-3, but did not affect DHA levels in their milk. Breast milk DHA levels, therefore, vary widely depending on dietary intake of preformed DHA. Worldwide reports of breast milk DHA levels range from 0.1 to 1.4 % of total fatty acids (Innis, 1992; Brenna *et al.*, 2007). DHA levels in breast milk are important since higher levels of DHA result in higher DHA levels in breastfed infants. Gibson *et al.* (1997) reported this association in a double-blind, placebo-controlled study of 52 healthy term infants who were breastfed for a minimum of three months. In the study, mothers were supplemented with 0, 0.2, 0.4, 0.9 or 1.3 g DHA/d from day 5 through 12 weeks postpartum resulting in breast milk DHA levels which ranged from 0.1 to 1.7 % of total fatty acids. Incremental increases in DHA levels in infants were seen as breast milk DHA levels reached 0.8 % at which point infant RBC levels were reported to stabilize.

Effect of milk lipids on infant omega-3 status and development

Improving infant DHA status benefits infant visual and cognitive development (Hoffman *et al.*, 2009; Jensen and Lapillonne, 2009). Several observational studies of breastfeeding mothers and their infants report positive correlations of human milk DHA with better visual acuity in infants (Innis *et al.*, 2001, 2003; Jorgensen *et al.*, 2001).

Several clinical trials also reported that DHA supplementation in breastfeeding mothers improved infant DHA status and benefitted measures of neural development. In the study by Gibson *et al.* described above, measures of visual and cognitive outcomes were reported in breastfed infants of the DHA-supplemented mothers. While there was no significant relationship between milk DHA content and visual acuity at 12 or 16 weeks, there was a significant and positive relationship of infant erythrocyte DHA at 12 weeks and scores on the Mental Development Index (MDI) of the Bayley Scales of Infant Development (BSID) at 1 year (Gibson *et al.*, 1997). In another study, visual and cognitive outcomes were measured in breastfed infants of mothers supplemented with 620 mg EPA plus 799 mg DHA/d from fish oil. No vision benefits were reported at 2 or 4 months and no benefits in problem-solving ability were detectable at 9 months when comparing the supplemented group to placebo. However, the authors did report a significant positive correlation between infant blood DHA levels and visual acuity at 4 months of age. At 1 year of age, children from the supplemented group scored lower on a test of vocabulary comprehension, but there were no differences between the groups when tested again at 2 years (Lauritzen *et al.*, 2004, 2005). A later study by Helland, *et al.* reported higher scores on the Kaufmann Mental Processing Composite in 4-year olds initially breastfed by mothers who received a supplement of cod liver oil containing over 1 g DHA/d (Helland *et al.*, 2003). The benefit was no longer detected at 7 years (Helland *et al.*, 2008).

Study results from Jensen *et al.* (2005, 2010) included neurocognitive outcomes for breastfed infants of mothers supplemented with 200 mg DHA/d. Infants from DHA-supplemented mothers scored higher on the Psychomotor Development Index (PDI) of the BSID at 30 months of age and on the Sustained Attention Subtest of the Leiter International Performance Scale at 5 years of age. In the study, 200 mg DHA/d increased mean breast milk DHA content to 0.35 % as compared to 0.20 % in controls. Because of the neurocognitive benefits observed in infants consuming milk with 0.35 % DHA compared to those receiving 0.20 % DHA, the higher level is often determined as the most appropriate level for supplementation in infant formula.

13.3 Omega-3 fatty acid supplementation in infant formula

Expert recommendations for LC-PUFA supplementation of formula for term infants generally include a range of 0.2–0.4 % of total fatty acids as DHA and 0.35–0.7 % as ARA (Table 13.1). These recommendations approximate the levels of DHA and ARA commonly found in breast milk of well-nourished women. These levels of LC-PUFA have been used safely in clinical trials involving both term and preterm infants. They are considered to be levels needed for achieving benefits to fatty acid status and for development. Higher levels are safely used in clinical trials and may be particularly important for preterm infants.

13.3.1 Safety of DHA supplementation in infant formula

In most clinical trials, the source of DHA for addition to infant formula included either fish oil, egg phospholipid fractions, egg triglyceride fractions or algal oil. In general, adverse effects of any kind as the result of LC-PUFA supplementation are rare. However, problems of reduced growth parameters were reported from early clinical trials in preterm infants supplemented with high-EPA fish oil (Carlson *et al.*, 1992, 1996b; Ryan *et al.*, 1999). The reduction in growth was attributed to low blood levels of ARA which resulted from feeding formula containing high levels of EPA and no ARA. Normal growth is seen in term or preterm infants with the inclusion of ARA in the supplemented formula and a more balanced ratio of DHA/EPA.

Normal growth is consistently reported in trials where infants receive DHA plus ARA at ratios of 1:1 to 1:2, the range typically found in breast milk. Term infants are less likely than preterm infants to exhibit growth reduction in the absence of ARA. However, a review of the studies in term infants using formula supplemented with DHA alone showed that plasma ARA levels decreased an average of 25 % below control (Makrides *et al.*, 2005). While not severe enough to result in growth retardation, this decrease in ARA has a potential to compromise neurocognitive and immune function (Koletzko and Braun, 1991; Carlson *et al.*, 1993a; Harbige, 2003; Birch *et al.*, 2007). Therefore, recommendations for DHA-supplemented term infant formula also require the addition of ARA in a 1:1 or 1:2 ratio.

Since the addition of EPA to infant formula appears unnecessary, and in some cases is problematic, most authoritative groups do not recommend its addition to formula, but state that if added it should not exceed the amount of DHA in the formula (Koletzko *et al.*, 2008). A study by Clandinin *et al.* (2005) highlights the concern in preterm infants. In the study, preterm infants were provided unsupplemented formula or formula supplemented with either fish oil (EPA+DHA)+ARA or algal oil (DHA)+ARA. When comparing growth outcomes, only infants in the algal oil-supplemented group (DHA+ARA) grew at the same rate as did breastfed infants. There was no additional benefit for visual or neural function with inclusion of EPA in the infant formula supplementation.

In summary, today most recommendations for DHA-supplemented infant formula include the addition of ARA in an amount equal to or greater than the DHA; and EPA, if added, is in an amount no greater than DHA (Koletzko *et al.*, 2008). In their most recent edition of the *Pediatric Nutrition Handbook*, the American Academy of Pediatrics states that '... the amounts and the sources of LC-PUFA used in these studies are safe.' (AAP Committee of Nutrition, 2009).

13.3.2 DHA supplementation in preterm infant formula

Preterm infants are born prior to the major period of intrauterine LC-PUFA accretion, and their needs for DHA and ARA are therefore extremely high following birth. Preterm infants, as well as term infants, are not able to rely on endogenous DHA and ARA synthesis sufficient for their rapid growth and neurological development (Crawford, 1993). Many clinical trials have been designed to determine the impact of DHA supplementation on visual and neurocognitive development in preterm infants (Uauy *et al.*, 1990; Birch *et al.*, 1992, 1993; Carlson *et al.*, 1993b, 1996a; Hoffman *et al.*, 1993; Werkman and Carlson, 1996; Clandinin *et al.*, 2005; Henriksen *et al.*, 2008; Smithers *et al.*, 2008a, b; Makrides *et al.*, 2009). The studies include a wide variation in design and methods for measuring visual and behavioral outcomes. The significant optimization of visual and behavioral function as demonstrated in many of these studies emphasizes the importance of dietary DHA and ARA in order to prevent deficiency in preterm infants.

Visual development in DHA-supplemented preterm infants

Electrophysiological and behavioral methods are used in evaluating visual acuity in preterm infants. Many, but not all, clinical trials demonstrate that early visual development, as measured by one of those methods, is better in infants receiving LC-PUFA supplementation (Birch *et al.*, 1992, 1993; Carlson *et al.*, 1993b, 1996a, b; Smithers *et al.*, 2008b). A review and meta-analysis by SanGiovanni *et al.* (2000b) reported outcomes for four prospective randomized controlled trials (RCTs) involving a total of at least 265 preterm infants (Birch *et al.*, 1992, 1993; Carlson *et al.*, 1993b, 1996b). Their analysis of DHA-supplemented versus DHA-free formula showed significant benefit of supplementation for visual acuity at 2 and 4 months corrected age. A comprehensive systematic review and meta-analysis by Lewin *et al.* (2005) reported data from nine RCTs that examined visual acuity in infants fed either an LC-PUFA-supplemented formula or a control formula (O'Connor *et al.*, 2001; Birch *et al.*, 1992; Carlson *et al.*, 1992; Koletzko *et al.*, 1995; Carlson and Werkman, 1996; Faldella *et al.*, 1996; Bougle *et al.*, 1999; Innis *et al.*, 2002; van Wezel-Meijler *et al.*, 2002). The total number of enrolled infants, including reference non-randomized breastfed infants, across the nine trials was 1171. Five of the studies using visual evoked potential (VEP) reported better or faster maturation of visual function in LC-PUFA recipients.

A trial by Smithers *et al.* (2008a) was published following the meta-analysis by Lewin *et al.* The DINO study (DHA for the Improvement of Neurodevelopmental Outcome) compared outcomes in infants receiving high levels of DHA, approximately 1 % total fatty acids (from either infant formula or breast milk from DHA-supplemented mothers) to infants fed standard formula or breast milk. At 2 months corrected age, visual acuity of the high-DHA group did not differ from the control group. However, by 4 months, the high-DHA group demonstrated better visual acuity as measured by sweep VEP acuity and latency.

Neurocognitive development in DHA-supplemented preterm infants

Neurocognitive assessments are also reported in trials involving preterm infants, of which the MDI and PDI scores on the BSID are the most common. The review by Lewin *et al.* (2005) identified six RCTs which included a measure of neurocognitive development comparing LC-PUFA-supplemented to unsupplemented infants (Bougle *et al.*, 1999; O'Connor *et al.*, 2001; Clandinin, 2002; Fewtrell *et al.*, 2002, 2004; van Wezel-Meijler *et al.*, 2002). According to the authors, the diversity in study design and measurement outcome made it impossible to perform a valid meta-analysis with regard to neurological development.

Following the review by Lewin was another publication from the DINO trial that included measures of neurodevelopment (Makrides *et al.*, 2009). At 18 months of age, premature girls on a high DHA diet achieved a mean score approximately five points higher on the BSID MDI than girls receiving the standard DHA diet. The authors reported this as a 55 % reduction in mild mental delay and an 80 % reduction in significant mental delay, both statistically significant improvements versus the standard group. Male infants in the study, however, did not show improvement. A secondary publication in 2010 found no effect of DHA supplementation on measures of language development or behavior in this same cohort at 26 months corrected age (Smithers *et al.*, 2010).

13.3.3 DHA supplementation in term infant formula

Term infants also benefit from ARA and DHA supplementation. To date, more than 25 controlled clinical trials have been completed comparing LC-PUFA-supplemented formula with control formula. The literature consists of reports of both positive and null findings, with an almost complete absence of negative or adverse effects. In addition, many reviews of this literature have been published (Fleith and Clandinin, 2005; Heird and Lapillonne, 2005; AAP, 2009; Hoffman *et al.*, 2009; Simmer *et al.*, 2011).

Visual acuity in DHA-supplemented term infants

In term infants, as in preterm, DHA supplementation results in more mature retinal function as measured by electroretinography and VEP acuity compared to those not receiving DHA (Makrides *et al.*, 1995; Carlson *et al.*, 1996a; Birch *et al.*, 1998, 2002, 2005; Hoffman *et al.*, 2003). This improvement in visual acuity associated with DHA supplementation is often described as equivalent to 'one line on the eye chart' at one year of age (Birch *et al.*, 1998).

Several systematic reviews and meta-analyses of the literature support the beneficial effects of LC-PUFA supplementation in term infant formula, particularly for early visual development (Sangiovanni *et al.*, 2000a; Uauy *et al.*, 2003; Morale *et al.*, 2005). In 2003, Uauy *et al.* conducted a meta-regression analysis of 14 published trials of ALA and/or DHA supplementation in infant formula. The authors calculated a 'DHA-dose' based on the amount of preformed DHA plus a 10 % conversion factor from the amount of ALA present in the formula. Comparisons were then made with measures of visual acuity. The authors reported a significant relationship between 'DHA-dose' and visual acuity at 4 months. In a separate meta-analysis of four clinical trials comparing DHA/ARA supplemented formula to control, Sangiovanni *et al.* (2000b) reported significantly higher scores on tests of visual resolution at 2 and 4 months of age. In 2005, a meta-analysis by Morale *et al.* (2005) reported results from three studies showing that infants receiving sources of DHA (via formula or breast milk) throughout the first year scored higher on measures of visual acuity than those discontinuing supplemented formula or breast milk at an earlier time point.

The comprehensive systematic review by Lewin *et al.* (2005) reviewed 13 studies in term infants (sample size ranged from 33 to 274) which assessed visual acuity by VEP as well as Teller cards. The results of the 13 studies were mixed with regard to improvement on either of the tests. Further, due to large differences in dose and duration of supplementation, subject selection and the diversity and variability of primary outcomes, a meta-analysis was not possible. Similarly, the systematic review from the Cochrane Library (Simmer *et al.*, 2011) regarding LC-PUFA supplementation in term infants concluded that no clear long-term benefits or harms were demonstrated for term infants receiving LC-PUFA-supplemented formula. As with the review by Lewin, Simmer comments on the heterogeneity of the studies, noting that the study methods, dose and source of supplementation and fatty acid composition of the control formula varied between trials. Such heterogeneity makes meaningful meta-analyses difficult, and the results of such analyses should not be over interpreted.

Since the AHRQ Report by Lewin *et al.* (2005), two additional trial results have been published. First, the DIAMOND (DHA Intake and Measurement of Neural Development) study was a double-blind, randomized trial involving 343 healthy term infants and conducted at two US sites (Birch *et al.*, 2010). The infants were fed formula containing 0, 0.32, 0.64 or 0.96 % DHA. The DHA-formulas also contained 0.64 % ARA. At 12 months, visual acuity was measured by VEP. Infants fed the control formula had significantly poorer VEP at 12 months than those receiving any of the DHA-supplemented formula. Second, an important follow-up study of visual and neurocognitive development was published in 2007 (Birch *et al.*, 2007). Infants who previously enrolled in a single-center, double-blind, randomized clinical trial of DHA and ARA supplementation of infant formula were assessed for visual acuity during follow-up at 4 years of age. At follow-up, the control formula group had poorer visual acuity than the breastfed group while the LC-PUFA-supplement groups did not differ significantly from the breastfed group. These results support the benefit of

LC-PUFA formula as compared to control formula for visual acuity well beyond the period of supplementation into childhood.

Neurocognitive function in DHA-supplemented term infants

ARA and DHA play structural and biochemical roles in neural tissue contributing to optimal cognitive function and development during infancy (Martinez, 1992). Infants receiving both ARA and DHA supplementation demonstrate higher scores than controls on measures of sensory, cognitive and motor skills such as the BSID or the Brunet-Lezine test (Agostoni *et al.*, 1995, 1997; Birch *et al.*, 2000); tests of problem-solving ability and look duration to novel visual stimuli (Willatts *et al.*, 1998a, b); and task completions and goal-directed behaviors (Drover *et al.*, 2009). Meta-analyses of the data, however, as reported by Lewin *et al.* (2005) and Simmer *et al.* (2011) found no significant differences in measures of neuro-cognitive function between supplemented and unsupplemented infants. As with vision, both reports comment on the wide variation in study methodology.

Three recent publications, not included in the previous reviews, provide additional data regarding the effect of LC-PUFA on neurocognitive outcomes. First, The DIAMOND study cohort, as described in the previous section, measured cognitive function at 18 months in infants fed one of three levels of DHA-supplemented formula or a control formula. In a report of this cohort by Drover *et al.* (2011), there was a significant increase in BSID MDI scores of DHA-supplemented children as compared to controls at 18 months. In a second publication by Colombo *et al.* (2011), the DIAMOND investigators reported the results of a planned secondary analysis of infant behavioral and psychophysiological indices of attention. The investigators found that LC-PUFA-supplemented infants had lower heart rates than did unsupplemented infants. In addition, the infants supplemented with 0.32 or 0.64 % DHA plus 0.64 % ARA spent more time engaged in active stimulus-processing than infants fed the unsupplemented formula.

A second recent RCT included term infants fed a DHA-enriched fish oil supplement or placebo from birth to 6 months (Meldrum *et al.*, 2012). At an 18-month follow-up visit, neurodevelopment was assessed using a variety of tools, including the BSID-III and the Macarthur-Bates Communicative Development Inventory. Although there was no global increase in scores on the BSID-III, the mean scores for each subtest tended to be higher for the fish oil-supplemented group. In addition, erythrocyte DHA measurements at 6 months significantly predicted communication skills in the Adaptive Behaviour Questionnaire of the BSID-III. Children in the fish oil group performed significantly better in language assessments at 12 and 18 months of age, and they scored higher on both 'later developing gestures' and the 'total number of gestures' compared with those on placebo. These scores indicate benefit for development of vocabulary skills.

As with vision, studies demonstrate a long-term neurological benefit for providing DHA in the early diet. In two reports, supplementation with DHA+ARA positively affected mental skills, measured by the BSID, at 12 and 18 months of age and older (Birch *et al.*, 2000, 2007). Similarly, DHA+ARA supplementation increased cognitive function at 10 months and 6 years, as measured by tests of problem-solving and information-processing (Agostoni *et al.*, 1997; Willatts *et al.*, 1998b).

13.4 Adding omega-3 fatty acids to infant formula

DHA and ARA are highly unsaturated fatty acids containing six and four double bonds, respectively. These double bonds make them more susceptible to oxidation resulting in loss of sensory integrity and physiological activity (Aruoma, 1998). The chemistry of PUFA oxidation is well known, as described elsewhere in this book, and the beneficial effects of adding antioxidants to prevent or minimize oxidation are well understood (Kamal-Elidin and Yanishlieva, 2002; Schaich, 2005; Taneja and Zhu, 2006; Jacobsen, 2008). During the process of oxidation, relatively small amounts of volatile, chemical compounds (aldehydes, ketones and alcohols) are generated which produce off-flavors and aromas in foods, including infant formula (Ries, 2009). The oxidation process can be slowed, but not stopped. Therefore, steps for its prevention are the prime objective for retaining sensory and physiologic integrity of PUFA-containing oils (Eunok and David, 2009).

In principle, the main differences in the composition of infant formulas are represented by variations in protein, ratios of protein types (whey and casein), fats, carbohydrates and ash (Koletzko *et al.*, 2005). For many infant formulas, manufacturers use components from cows' milk for reformulation into a human-like milk product for infants.

Table 13.2 shows the complexity of a formulation containing the major required components. The precise formulation is driven by the nutritional requirements of the infant, as well as the regulatory constraints of the country in which the formula is sold. The ingredients also include components which are required for the growing infant, but are known to promote oxidation of DHA and ARA, such as trace or transition metals (LSRO, 1988).

In addition to the complexities of formulation, consideration must be given to the manufacturing steps needed in order to fortify the formula with LC-PUFA without causing oxidation, and to ensure sensory quality throughout the shelf-life of the formula. At the end of the formula's shelf-life, the quality and concentration of the LC-PUFA should be the same as they were initially. These steps are achievable as exemplified by the many commercial infant formula products now in the marketplace which exhibit a long shelf-life, a good flavor profile and excellent nutrient retention. In fact, most

Table 13.2 List of typical ingredients found in an infant formula

Non-fat milk powder	Long-chain PUFAs (DHA and ARA)
Vegetable oils	Calcium chloride
Whey powder (reduced minerals)	Choline chloride
Lactose	Potassium phosphate
Soy lecithin	Magnesium chloride
Sodium citrate	Sodium bicarbonate
Citric acid	Ferrous sulfate
Calcium hydroxide	Zinc sulfate
Nucleotides	Potassium citrate
Tocopherols	Ascorbyl palmitate
Vitamin E	Niacin
Vitamin A	Pantothenic acid
Copper sulfate	Vitamin B1
Vitamin D	Vitamin B6
Magnesium sulfate	Folic acid
Potassium iodide	Vitamin K
Vitamin B2	Vitamin B12

Source: modified from Teagasc Food Research Center, 2011.

commercially available infant formulas currently have a shelf-life of one year or more at room temperature. A list of the ingredients in a marketed infant formula for newborn infants is shown in Table 13.3.

13.4.1 Methods for adding omega-3 fatty acids to infant formula

Powdered infant formulas represent the main segment of the commercially made products and will be the focus of the following discussion. Powdered preparations are manufactured using three different approaches: (i) dry blending of ingredients; (ii) wet blending of ingredients, followed by spray drying; or (iii) a combination of wet and dry blending.

In the case of the dry blending process, all the main ingredients, both macro and micro, are sourced as powders from suppliers and blended in specific ratios to achieve the final formula composition. In terms of energy and capital investment, dry blending is generally recognized as a less expensive process than wet blending. The ingredients are blended using equipment such as ribbon blenders or continuous blenders to produce a homogeneous final product ready for packaging. When dry blending ingredients, care must be taken to ensure that the microbial load of all the ingredients is exceptionally low since there is no practical commercial process for sterilizing the final powder. Even the smallest amount of dry ingredients with a high microbial load will contaminate the entire batch and compromise the final product.

In the case of wet blending, both wet and dry ingredients are mixed to create a coarse, stable oil-in-water (o/w) emulsion (McClements, 2010)

Table 13.3 Nutrients in a marketed newborn infant formula (liquid and powder)

Nutrient* (normal dilution)	Per 100 cal (5 fl oz)	Per 100 g powder (510 cal)
Protein, g	2.1	10.8
Fat, g	5.3	27
Linoleic acid, mg	860	4400
Linolenic acid, mg	80	410
DHA, mg	17	87
ARA, mg	34	174
Carbohydrate, g	11.2	57
Water, g	133	2
Vitamins/other nutrients		
Vitamin A, IU	300	1540
Vitamin D, IU	75	380
Vitamin E, IU	2	10.3
Vitamin K, mcg	9	46
Thiamin (Vitamin B_1), mcg	80	410
Riboflavin (Vitamin B_2), mcg	140	720
Vitamin B_6, mcg	60	310
Vitamin B_{12}, mcg	0.3	1.54
Niacin, mcg	1000	5100
Folic acid (folacin), mcg	16	82
Pantothenic acid, mcg	500	2600
Biotin, mcg	3	15.4
Vitamin C (ascorbic acid), mg	12	62
Choline, mg	24	123
Inositol, mg	6	31
Carnitine, mg	2	10.3
Taurine, mg	6	31
Minerals		
Calcium, mg	78	400
Phosphorus, mg	43	220
Magnesium, mg	8	41
Iron, mg	1.8	9.2
Zinc, mg	1	5.1
Manganese, mcg	15	77
Copper, mcg	75	380
Iodine, mcg	15	77
Selenium, mcg	2.8	14.4
Sodium, mg	27	138
Potassium, mg	108	550
Chloride, mg	63	320
Molybdenum, mcg	NA	NA
Chromium, mcg	NA	NA

*Product nutrient values and ingredients are subject to change. Please see product label for current information.
NA = none added.
Source: taken from Enfamil Premium® Newborn on the following website accessed 6/12/12: http://www.mjn.com/app/iwp/hcp2/content2.do?dm=mj&id=/HCP_Home2/Product Information/hcpProducts/hcpNewborns&iwpst=HCP&ls=0&csred=1&r=3516983200

which is later pasteurized and homogenized. The emulsion can either be formulated as a solid, allowing it to be spray dried directly, or as a wet emulsion which is first passed through an evaporator prior to spray drying.

In some instances, a hybrid process is employed whereby some of the dry ingredients are added at the end of the spray drying. In most of these instances, the ingredients that are dry blended are heat-sensitive ingredients, such as vitamins, amino acids, probiotics and microencapsulated LC-PUFA. Since these ingredients are added at a moderate temperature at this stage, the microbial quality is of extreme importance in order to prevent contamination of the finished product. Also, in the case of microencapsulated LC-PUFA, care must be taken to minimize damage to the encapsulated outer shell and prevent exposure of oxygen to the oil inside. This damage can be due to mechanical shear or abrasion which occurs during the blending/mixing process of the other ingredients.

As an alternative to this hybrid process, a dry ingredient can be added by direct injection or with air pumped into the cooling zone of the spray dryer. As the dry powder droplets fall from the top of the spray dryer, other ingredients can be added. A slow and well-controlled rate of addition allows a homogeneous distribution and a proper concentration.

Of the different approaches for manufacturing powdered infant formula, the one offering the best solution for prevention of oxidation is the wet process. By adding the LC-PUFA oils directly into the fat fraction of the formulation to make the emulsion, followed by homogenization, pasteurization, evaporation and finally spray drying to complete the process (Fig. 13.1), it is possible to engineer the best possible methods to add thermally sensitive ingredients, such as the LC-PUFA oils, to the formulation. Compared to the numerous options of the wet process, the dry process is limited and offers only one alternative of adding the microencapsulated oils to a blending tank and packaging. Furthermore, with dry blending, it is sometimes overlooked that shear forces are constantly at work with all the other ingredients in the mix and these forces might possibly damage the fine structure of the oil microencapsulation, causing oxidation to the exposed oil. In the wet process, the LC-PUFA oils are typically added in with the other vegetable oils, creating a dilution and, to some extent, intrinsic antioxidants in the vegetable oil may offer protection for these unsaturated oils. The oil mixture is further combined with other ingredients including milk proteins (whey and casein) and homogenized to produce a physically stable emulsion, further protecting the oils. Finally, the process of spray drying dehydrates and, in essence, creates encapsulated oil, avoiding the need for dry mixing.

13.4.2 Preventing oxidation during processing

Throughout processing, it is important to examine alternatives for the addition of LC-PUFA in order to minimize oxidation of the oils. As discussed

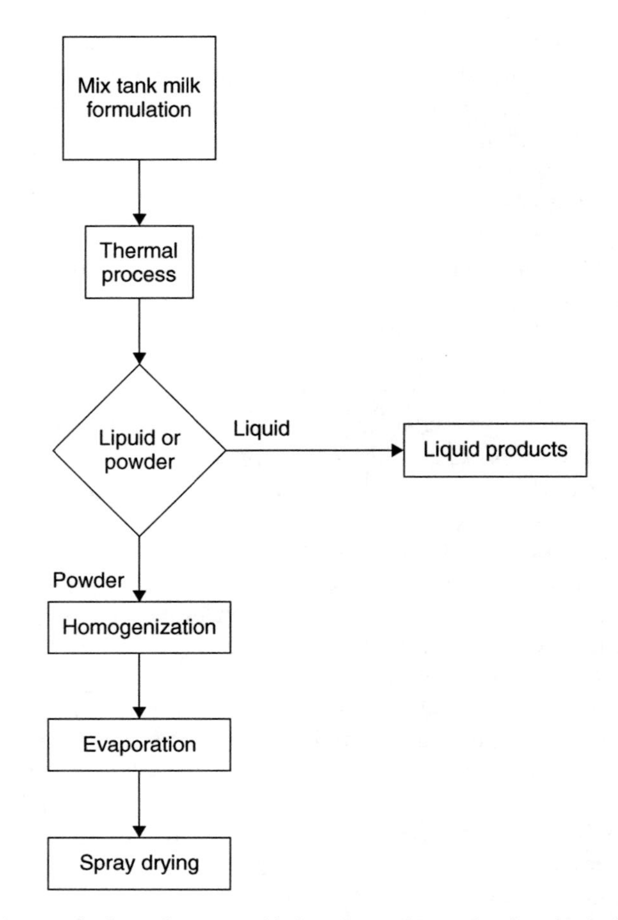

Fig. 13.1 A generic flow diagram of infant formula production, including the main unit operations in the manufacture of a powder product.

previously, premixing the LC-PUFA-containing oils with the larger fat blend of the formula is advantageous. Furthermore, to allow for proper homogenization and prevention of oxidation, it is beneficial to add polyunsaturated oils to the rest of the formulation, beginning in a small volume and diluting to a larger volume. This may be best achieved by adding the oils into balanced tanks holding the milk formulation, followed by the transfer to a larger holding tank or the final production tank. The oil blend can be efficiently delivered to the production tank by use of a medium-sized volume (500 L) liquefier/blender. A more elegant approach, as shown in Fig. 13.2, utilizes an in-line mixer to add the oils, thereby eliminating the evaporation step.

An extremely important consideration is the quality of the vegetable fat used in blending the LC-PUFA oils. In all cases, these oils represent a much greater volume than the ARA- and DHA-containing oils. Therefore, if the

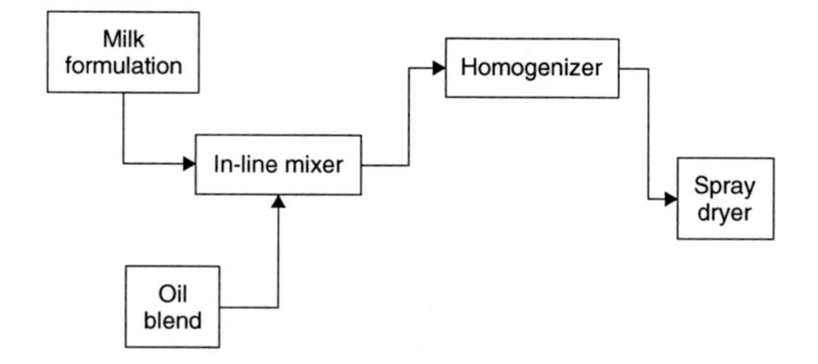

Fig. 13.2 Addition of a PUFA-containing oil blend using an in-line mixer before spray drying.

vegetable fat sources have already begun to oxidize, they will promote oxidation of the LC-PUFA. By maintaining a tight specification on these vegetable fats, the oxidative quality of the finished product will be protected. When calculated as a percentage from the data provided in Table 16.3, the overall fat contribution of a typical formula accounts for almost 24 % of the whole, whereas in a DHA- and ARA-supplemented formula, these two fatty acids will only represent approximately 1.0 % of the total fat. Therefore it is beneficial to dilute the sensitive oils into the more stable ones and, at the same time, allow for better distribution and homogeneity.

Another important consideration for manufacturing LC-PUFA supplemented formula is the need to exclude air/oxygen as much as possible. This may necessitate multiple modifications of operations which, at times, seem complicated, impractical or expensive. However, a careful study of plant and manufacturing procedures to determine critical points of oxygen entry is needed in order devise steps to eliminate its contact with the oils. Such steps can include the addition of nitrogen gas lines, minimization of mixing times or covering of open tanks.

To show the effects of oxygen in PUFA-oil, a simple experiment conducted by Abril and Wills (2009) used water-jacketed glass-reactor vessels to mimic the effects of the presence of air in a production tank. The vessels were held at 60 °C, with a blend of vegetable fats and ARA- and DHA-oils maintained at a ratio of 2:1. The oils were later used to produce an infant formula powder. In the experiment, the oil mixture was held in the tank and exposed to either atmospheric air or pure nitrogen for maximum of 48 h before emptying. The stability of the oil that was exposed to the air versus the oil that was exposed to nitrogen was measured and compared. Figure 13.3 shows the results of that experiment. The addition of nitrogen gas to exclude air in the headspace of the tank provided a significant positive effect on the oxidative stability of the oil mixture. In addition, the oil was held at 60 °C, an extreme condition for this length of time. The concentrations of ARA and DHA were 0.7 and 0.3 % (w/w), respectively. Over

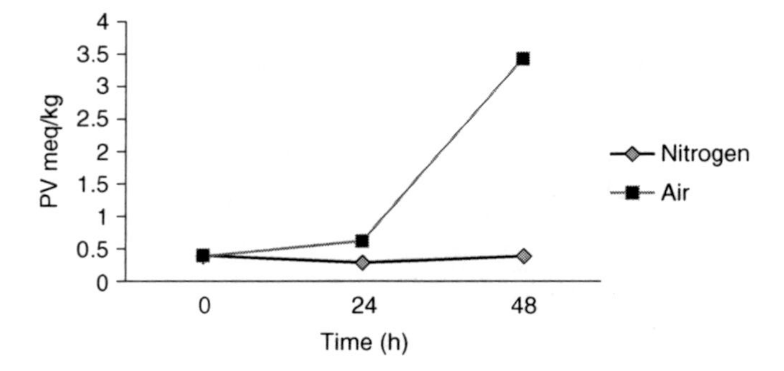

Fig. 13.3 Effect of air vs nitrogen in the head space of a reactor, showing the production of peroxides (PV). Mixture contained vegetable oil and ARA and DHA at 0.7 and 0.3 % (w/w), respectively. (Source: Abril and Wills, 2009)

the course of the experiment, the concentrations of the fatty acids remained stable. However, there was significant oxidation as measured by peroxide values in the oil without nitrogen in the headspace. This resulted in a change in the flavor profile of the oil blend. Off-notes, described as 'fishy', were detected as early as 24 h and by 48 h were significantly increased. If used in the production of a powder for addition to infant formula, the sensory characteristics of the final product would be impacted. Therefore, identifying techniques for excluding air and adding nitrogen in the headspace of containers used for mixing or holding is important for preventing oxidation. This is a practice employed by most companies for ensuring the integrity of their finished product.

During lipid oxidation, which occurs mostly in thermal processing, hydroperoxides are produced by the decomposition of the unsaturated fatty acids which, in turn, decompose into, most importantly, aldehydes, ketones and alcohols, but also alkanes and alkenes. These secondary products of oxidation are responsible for many of the off-flavors in the final product, and they potentially affect its nutritional value and shelf-life (Garcia-Llatas *et al.*, 2006). In addition to heat, other nutrients such as iron or zinc may promote the oxidation of oils. These metals have important nutritional value and are commonly used to fortify infant formulas and many other foods. They already possess inherent sensory characteristics such as salty, bitter or astringent, all of which are usually considered undesirable (Murphy *et al.*, 1981). Still, a larger concern when formulating infant formulas containing these metals is their strong pro-oxidant characteristics. These metals will not only impact the stability of fats, but can lead to protein and vitamin deterioration (Galdi *et al.*, 1989).

In essence, fortification of infant formula products can be done with success, allowing for a wholesome product with acceptable chemical and sensorial qualities, if considerations such as the ones mentioned above are followed. The quality of the oils, how the oils containing the PUFAs are handled as well as how and when the oils are added will greatly influence the quality of the finished product and its stability over a long shelf-life. In addition, using the correct product containers and modified atmospheres will have a definite positive effect in the protection of these sensitive fatty acids.

13.5 Sensory characteristics of omega-3 enriched infant formula

An area of concern in the production of infant formula is the sensory quality of the finished product. For example, powdered milk can be categorized as whole milk powder, partially skimmed milk powder, skim milk powder or fat-free powder. It is possible that infant formula powders may contain one or all of these milk powders in their final formulation, and milk-fat plays a significant role in the flavor profile of the powder. Many other oils, as well as the process used for their addition, also affect flavor characteristics of the end product. The addition of LC-PUFA may further intensify the complex sensory qualities of the mixture, particularly if the oils are not safe-guarded against peroxidation throughout the entire formula making process. Therefore, in order to achieve a satisfactory product that will retain a high sensorial quality throughout its entire shelf-life, it is necessary to ensure proper handling and processing of the LC-PUFA oils.

There are multiple sensory evaluation methods that can be used to evaluate infant formula powders. However, there is little agreement among manufacturers regarding their use. Numerous resources are available which discuss various methods (Bodyfelt *et al.*, 1988; Meilgaard *et al.*, 1999, Clark *et al.*, 2009). However, there continues to be a disparity in the 'sensory languages and terminologies' most commonly used. For example, the grading for the industrial production of milk powders has been used for years to evaluate sensory quality. However, the grading system is based on the presence of flavor defects, without recognizing that milk has a clean and pleasant taste. There is no common descriptive language to evaluate milk powders and dried dairy ingredients (Drake *et al.*, 2003). Milk flavors are graded using a score of 1 to 10, with the higher score being considered better. Table 13.4 describes a typical scoring table based on defects. Interestingly, a few of these descriptors and criticisms could be used to grade or evaluate infant formula powders as well as the dairy products.

To obtain a descriptive flavor analysis of infant formula powders, the powders are reconstituted in water at a concentration of 0.1 g/ml, and presented to a taste panel at room temperature. Panels are provided with positive and negative descriptors for odor and flavor, and they must use a structured scale to rate the intensity of each flavor. Some examples of positive odor and flavor descriptors can be: milky, cooked, fatty and creamy, buttery and sweet; whereas, examples of negative terms can be phenolic,

Table 13.4 Suggested flavor scores used for grading milk

Flavor criticisms	Intensity of defect*		
	Slight	Definite	Pronounced
Astringent	8	7	5
Barny	7	5	3
Bitter	7	5	3
Cooked	9	8	6
Cowy	6	4	1
Feed	9	7	5
Flat	9	8	7
Foreign	5	3	0
Garlic/onion	5	3	1
High acid	3	1	0
Bacterial	5	3	0
Lacks freshness	7	5	3
Malty	7	5	3
Oxidized	7	5	3
Rancid	7	5	3
Salty	8	6	4
Unclean	7	5	3

*Milk flavors are graded using a score of 1 to 10, with the higher score being considered better as described in: *Dairy Science and Technology*, characterization of Flavour Defects–ASDA. http://www.uoguelph.ca/foodscience/dairy-science-and-technology/milk-grading-and-defects/characterization-flavour-defects-asda.

musty and rancid for odor; and beany, burnt and sour for flavor. Depending on the composition of the product being evaluated and the volatility of flavor compounds including oxidation products, flavor may make a better tool for the evaluation than odor (Anupama *et al.*, 1999). It is well established that both volatile and non-volatile compounds that are released from the food are responsible for the perception of flavor. Their release will be influenced by the structure of the food as well as their physical and chemical characteristics (Ross, 2009).

When fortifying infant formula powders with PUFAs, in order to minimize or prevent the oxidation of these fats, one must be cognizant of the large contribution that PUFAs play in the overall sensory quality of the powder or liquid. Since the sensory evaluation methodologies vary, there may be disagreements on the results of the same product but, in the end, the consumer will ultimately determine the quality of the product. In addition, with some restrictions because of the nature of the products, the presence of natural antioxidants can be considered to provide added protection to fortified infant formula products. As noted, the regulatory constraints are a big factor, but still compounds such as tocopherols (mixed isomers) and ascorbic acid are two widely accepted compounds that can be considered to protect the integrity of PUFAs.

13.6 Future trends

Interest in the importance of fatty acids in infant health and development will continue to grow. There will be a need to assure sources of these lipids which are of high quality, sustainable and affordable in a worldwide market.

The effect that inclusion of LC-PUFA in early life has on long-term development will continue to be investigated. It is apparent that fetal and infant nutrition impacts health and development in the long-term for many biological processes (Singhal *et al.*, 2001; Demmelmair *et al.*, 2006; Plagemann *et al.*, 2006). Researchers will explore the subtle changes in infant nutrition that not only impact normal development, but also impact risk for disease in later life. Future work will need to determine more closely the optimal levels of DHA and ARA required for achieving these long-term benefits.

The outcomes currently thought to be related to early programming include cardiovascular development and energy metabolism. Pivik *et al.* (2009) and others identify infant cardiovascular development as a progressive maturation of the autonomic nervous system (Singhal and Lucas, 2004). Early inclusion of DHA in the infant diet is marked by declines in heart rate and increases in heart rate variability, both signs of cardiovascular maturation.

Identifying early risk factors associated with metabolic syndrome including obesity and insulin sensitivity will also be of interest in future studies of infant nutrition. While results from most trials of LC-PUFA supplementation in infant formula show no differences in weight, length or head circumference as the result of supplementation (Lewin *et al.*, 2005), future studies will define how LC-PUFA supplementation in early life may provide benefits for body composition, insulin sensitivity and energy utilization.

13.7 Conclusion

The rationale for adding the LC-PUFA, DHA and ARA, to infant formula is clear. Both fatty acids are found at high levels in cell membranes of the brain and retina among many other tissues and organs and both are always found in breast milk. There is a rapid increase in brain weight during the early months and years of life. Infants are not able to produce sufficient DHA endogenously from ALA for optimal development; therefore, preformed sources either from breast milk or from infant formula are required. Without dietary sources of DHA, blood DHA levels decline rapidly after birth. As a result, brain tissue levels drop as well. Since human milk always contains both DHA and ARA, and their inclusion in infant formula is known to be safe, virtually all infant formula companies in the USA offer them. Studies show that infants who are not breastfed or are not given

DHA/ARA supplemented formula score lower on tests of vision, cognition and neural development than do their LC-PUFA-supplemented peers.

As structural components of the brain and retina, both DHA and ARA are required for normal cognitive and behavioral infant development. Similarly, DHA, as a component in retinal membranes, plays a vital role in optimal visual development. Most important, the developmental benefits of DHA and ARA supplementation to improve vision and cognition extend beyond changes observed in the first few months of life. Long-term follow-up studies now confirm sustained benefits in visual, cognitive and vascular function extending throughout the first year, and into early childhood as the result of DHA and ARA formula supplementation. Studies now also confirm a need for continued dietary sources of DHA and ARA throughout the first year for optimal growth, cognitive and visual development.

In conclusion, it is helpful to recall that adding DHA and ARA into infant formula was based initially on their presence in breast milk. Although the addition of LC-PUFAs to infant formula remains optional, a sizeable body of peer-reviewed scientific evidence supports their addition to infant formula. The studies described in this chapter highlight the optimization of visual and neurocognitive functions associated with including DHA in infant formula. ARA is added to DHA at 1:1 to 2:1 ratio. Various experts, authoritative panels and regulatory agencies support the addition of DHA and ARA to infant formula and also state that these LC-PUFA are safe for use in infant formula.

13.8 Sources of further information and advice

The nutrition and health of infants is important to a wide range of agencies and organizations. Therefore, there are organizational communities in nutrition and health, lipid science, infant formula manufacturing and government which continually provide information on the topic. Below are descriptions of just a few such organizations.

The Global Organization for EPA and DHA Omega-3 (GOED–1 http://www.goedomega3.com) is an association of members from manufacturing, marketing and other areas of product development, research and support of EPA and DHA omega-3 fatty acids. As a group, they work to educate consumers and work with government groups and the healthcare community regarding EPA and DHA. They also strive to set high ethical and quality standards for the industry. GOED has offices in Salt Lake City, Utah, and maintains a website with links to industry news, events and current research.

Another source of information regarding the omega-3 fatty acids is the International Society for the Study of Fatty Acids and Lipids (ISSFAL) (http://www.issfal.org). This organization of corporate and individual members regularly sponsors meetings and publications with a focused interest in lipid science and nutrition. ISSFAL members include researchers carrying out studies on the health effects of omega-3 and omega-6 fatty acids in addition to other nutritional lipids.

Pediatric health and nutrition professionals in organizations such as the American Academy of Pediatrics, the European Society of Pediatric Gastroenterology, Hepatology, and Nutrition, the Academy of Nutrition and Dietetics, Dietitians of Canada and their related international organizations maintain high interest in the composition of infant formula. Many of their policy and consensus statements have been included earlier in this chapter.

The American Oil Chemists Society (AOCS) and related international groups include members with interest in pediatric nutrition. Through publication of books and annual meetings, members and the public can be kept current on n-3 nutrition in infants (http://www.aocs.org).

13.9 References

AAP COMMITTEE ON NUTRITION (2009) *Pediatric Nutrition Handbook* (6th edn). Elk Grove Village, IL: American Academics of Pediatrics.

ABRIL, J. and WILLS, T. (2009) Unpublished data.

AGOSTONI, C., TROJAN, S., BELLU, R., RIVA, E. and GIOVANNINI, M. (1995) Neurodevelopmental quotient of healthy term infants at 4 months and feeding practice: the role of long-chain polyunsaturated fatty acids. *Pediatr Res*, 38, 262–6.

AGOSTONI, C., TROJAN, S., BELLU, R., RIVA, E., BRUZZESE, M. G. and GIOVANNINI, M. (1997) Developmental quotient at 24 months and fatty acid composition of diet in early infancy: a follow up study. *Arch Dis Child*, 76, 421–4.

AHMAD, A., MORIGUCHI, T. and SALEM JR, N. (2002) Decrease in neuron size in docosahexaenoic acid-deficient brain. *Pediatr Neurol* 26, 210–8.

AKBAR, M., CALDERON, F., ZHIMING W. and KIM, H. (2005) Docosahexaenoic acid: a positive modulator of Akt signaling in neuronal survival. *Proc Natl Acad Sci USA*, 102, 10858–63.

ANUPAMA, K., RAVI, R. and RAJALAKSHIM, D. (1999) Sensory profiling and positioning of commercial samples of milk powder. *J Sens Stud*, 14, 303–19.

ARUOMA, O. I. (1998) Free radicals, oxidative stress, and antioxidants in human health and disease. *J Am Oil Chem Soc*, 75, 199–212.

BAZAN, N. G., MOLINA, M. F. and GORDON, W. C. (2011) Docosahexaenoic acid signalolipidomics in nutrition: significance in aging, neuroinflammation, macular degeneration, Alzheimer's, and other neurodegenerative diseases. *Annu Rev Nutr*, 31, 321–51.

BIRCH, E. E., BIRCH, D. G., HOFFMAN, D. R. and UAUY, R. (1992) Dietary essential fatty acid supply and visual acuity development. *Invest Ophthalmol Vis Sci*, 33, 3242–53.

BIRCH, E., BIRCH, D., HOFFMAN, D., HALE, L., EVERETT, M. and UAUY, R. (1993) Breastfeeding and optimal visual development. *J Pediatr Ophthalmol Strabismus*, 30, 33–8.

BIRCH, E. E., HOFFMAN, D. R., UAUY, R., BIRCH, D. G. and PRESTIDGE, C. (1998) Visual acuity and the essentiality of docosahexaenoic acid and arachidonic acid in the diet of term infants. *Pediatr Res*, 44, 201–9.

BIRCH, E. E., GARFIELD, S., HOFFMAN, D. R., UAUY, R. and BIRCH, D. G. (2000) A randomized controlled trial of early dietary supply of long-chain polyunsaturated fatty acids and mental development in term infants. *Dev Med Child Neurol*, 42, 174–81.

BIRCH, E. E., HOFFMAN, D. R., CASTANEDA, Y. S., FAWCETT, S. L., BIRCH, D. G. and UAUY, R. D. (2002) A randomized controlled trial of long-chain polyunsaturated fatty acid supplementation of formula in term infants after weaning at 6 wk of age. *Am J Clin Nutr*, 75, 570–80.

BIRCH, E. E., CASTANEDA, Y. S., WHEATON, D. H., BIRCH, D. G., UAUY, R. D. and HOFFMAN, D. R. (2005) Visual maturation of term infants fed long-chain polyunsaturated fatty acid-supplemented or control formula for 12 mo. *Am J Clin Nutr*, 81, 871–9.

BIRCH, E. E., GARFIELD, S., CASTANEDA, Y., HUGHBANKS-WHEATON, D., UAUY, R. and HOFFMAN, D. (2007) Visual acuity and cognitive outcomes at 4 years of age in a double-blind, randomized trial of long-chain polyunsaturated fatty acid-supplemented infant formula. *Early Hum Dev*, 83, 279–84.

BIRCH, E. E., CARLSON, S. E., HOFFMAN, D. R., FITZGERALD-GUSTAFSON, K. M., FU, V. L., DROVER, J. R., CASTANEDA, Y. S., MINNS, L., WHEATON, D. K., MUNDY, D., MARUNYCZ, J. and DIERSEN-SCHADE, D. A. (2010) The DIAMOND (DHA Intake And Measurement Of Neural Development) Study: a double-masked, randomized controlled clinical trial of the maturation of infant visual acuity as a function of the dietary level of docosahexaenoic acid. *Am J Clin Nutr*, 91, 848–59.

BODYFELT, F., TOBIAS W. and TROUT G. (1998) *The Sensory Evaluation of Dairy Products*. Westport, CT: AVI.

BOUGLE, D., DENISE, P., VIMARD, F., NOUVELOT, A., PENNEILLO, M. J. and GUILLOIS, B. (1999) Early neurological and neuropsychological development of the preterm infant and polyunsaturated fatty acids supply. *Clin Neurophysiol*, 110, 1363–70.

BRECKENRIDGE, W. C., GOMBOS, G. and MORGAN, I. G. (1972) The lipid composition of adult rat brain synaptosomal plasma membranes. *Biochim Biophys Acta*, 266, 695–707.

BRENNA, J. T., VARAMINI, B., JENSEN, R. G., DIERSEN-SCHADE, D. A., BOETTCHER, J. A. and ARTERBURN, L. M. (2007) Docosahexaenoic and arachidonic acid concentrations in human breast milk worldwide. *Am J Clin Nutr*, 85, 1457–64.

CALDERON, F. and KIM, H. Y. (2004) Docosahexaenoic acid promotes neurite growth in hippocampal neurons. *J Neurochem*, 90, 979–88.

CARLSON, S. E. and WERKMAN, S. H. (1996) A randomized trial of visual attention of preterm infants fed docosahexaenoic acid until two months. *Lipids*, 31, 85–90.

CARLSON, S. E., COOKE, R. J., WERKMAN, S. H. and TOLLEY, E. A. (1992) First year growth of preterm infants fed standard compared to marine oil n-3 supplemented formula. *Lipids*, 27, 901–7.

CARLSON, S. E., WERKMAN, S. H., PEEPLES, J. M., COOKE, R. J. and TOLLEY, E. A. (1993a) Arachidonic acid status correlates with first year growth in preterm infants. *Proc Natl Acad Sci USA*, 90, 1073–7.

CARLSON, S. E., WERKMAN, S. H., RHODES, P. G. and TOLLEY, E. A. (1993b) Visual-acuity development in healthy preterm infants: effect of marine-oil supplementation. *Am J Clin Nutr*, 58, 35–42.

CARLSON, S. E., FORD, A. J., WERKMAN, S. H., PEEPLES, J. M. and KOO, W. W. (1996a) Visual acuity and fatty acid status of term infants fed human milk and formulas with and without docosahexaenoate and arachidonate from egg yolk lecithin. *Pediatr Res*, 39, 882–8.

CARLSON, S. E., WERKMAN, S. H. and TOLLEY, E. A. (1996b) Effect of long-chain n-3 fatty acid supplementation on visual acuity and growth of preterm infants with and without bronchopulmonary dysplasia. *Am J Clin Nutr*, 63, 687–97.

CASTILHO, S. D. and BARROS FILHO, A. A. (2010) The history of infant nutrition. *J Pediatr (Rio J)*, 86, 179–88.

CLANDININ, M. T. V. (2002) Growth and development of very-low-birth-weight infants (VLBW) is enhanced by formulas supplemented with docosahexaenoic acid (DHA) and arachidonic acid (ARA). *J Pediatr Gastroenterol Nutr*, 34, 479–85.

CLANDININ, M. T., CHAPPELL, J. E., LEONG, S., HEIM, T., SWYER, P. R. and CHANCE, G. W. (1980a) Intrauterine fatty acid accretion rates in human brain: implications for fatty acid requirements. *Early Hum Dev*, 4, 121–9.

CLANDININ, M. T., CHAPPELL, J. E., LEONG, S., HEIM, T., SWYER, P. R. and CHANCE, G. W. (1980b) Extrauterine fatty acid accretion in infant brain: implications for fatty acid requirements. *Early Hum Dev*, 4, 131–8.

CLANDININ, M. T., VAN AERDE, J. E., PARROTT, A., FIELD, C. J., EULER, A. R. and LIEN, E. L. (1997) Assessment of the efficacious dose of arachidonic and docosahexaenoic acids in preterm infant formulas: fatty acid composition of erythrocyte membrane lipids. *Pediatr Res*, 42, 819–25.

CLANDININ, M. T., VAN AERDE, J. E., MERKEL, K. L., HARRIS, C. L., SPRINGER, M. A., HANSEN, J. W. and DIERSEN-SCHADE, D. A. (2005) Growth and development of preterm infants fed infant formulas containing docosahexaenoic acid and arachidonic acid. *J Pediatr*, 146, 461–8.

CLARK, S., COSTELLO, M., DRAKE, M. and BODYFELT, F. (2009) *Sensory Evaluation of Dairy Products* (2nd edn). New York: Springer.

CODEX ALIMENTARIUS COMMISSION (2007) *Standard for infant formula and formulas for special medical purposes intended for infants*. CODEX STAN 72–1981, revised 2007, available at: http://www.codexalimentarius.net/download/standards/288/CXS_072e.pdf [accessed February 2013].

COLOMBO, J., CARLSON S. E., CHEATHAM, C., FITZGERALD-GUSTAFSON, K., KEPLER, A. and DOTY, T. (2011) Long-chain polyunsaturated fatty acid supplementation in infancy reduces heart rate and positively affects distribution of attention. *Pediatr Res*, 70, 406–10.

Commission Directive 2006/141/EC of 22 December 2006 on infant formulae and amending Directive 1999/21/EC. *OJ*, L401/1401/33.

CRAWFORD, M. A. (1993) The role of essential fatty acids in neural development: implications for perinatal nutrition. *Am J Clin Nutr*, 57, 703S–709S; discussion 709S–710S.

CUNNANE, S. C. (2003) Problems with essential fatty acids: time for a new paradigm? *Prog Lipid Res*, 42, 544–68.

CUNNANE, S. C., FRANCESCUTTI, V., BRENNA, J. T. and CRAWFORD, M. A. (2000) Breast-fed infants achieve a higher rate of brain and whole body docosahexaenoate accumulation than formula-fed infants not consuming dietary docosahexaenoate. *Lipids*, 35, 105–11.

DEMMELMAIR, H., VON ROSEN, J. and KOLETZKO, B. (2006) Long-term consequences of early nutrition. *Early Hum Dev*, 82, 567–74.

DOBBING, J. and SANDS, J. (1973) Quantitative growth and development of human brain. *Arch Dis Child*, 48, 757–67.

DRAKE, M. A., KARAGUL-YUCEER, Y., CADWALLADER, K. R., CIVILLE, C. V. and TONG, P. S. (2003) Determination of the sensory attributes of dried milk powders and dairy ingredients. *J Sens Stud*, 18, 199–216.

DROVER, J., HOFFMAN, D. R., CASTAÑEDA, Y. S., MORALE, S. E. and BIRCH, E. E. (2009) Three randomized controlled trials of early long-chain polyunsaturated fatty acid supplementation on means-end problem solving in 9-month-olds. *Child Dev*, 80(5), 1376–84.

DROVER, J. R., HOFFMAN, D. R., CASTAÑEDA, Y. S., MORALE, S. E., GARFIELD, S., WHEATON, D. H. and BIRCH, E. E. (2011) Cognitive function in 18-month-old term infants of the DIAMOND study: a randomized, controlled clinical trial with multiple dietary levels of docosahexaenoic acid. *Early Hum Dev*, 87, 223–30.

ELDHO, N., FELLER, S., TRISTRAM-NAGLE, S., POLOZOV, I. and GAWRISCH, K. (2003) Polyunsaturated docosahexaenoic vs docosapentaenoic acid – differences in lipid matrix properties from the loss of one double bond. *J Am Chem Soc*, 125, 6409–21.

EUNOK, C. and DAVID, B. M. (2009) Mechanisms of antioxidants in the oxidation of foods. *Comp Rev in Food Sci Food Safety*, 8, 345–58.

FALDELLA, G., GOVONI, M., ALESSANDRONI, R., MARCHIANI, E., SALVIOLI, G. P., BIAGI, P. L. and SPANO, C. (1996) Visual evoked potentials and dietary long chain polyunsaturated fatty acids in preterm infants. *Arch Dis Child Fetal Neonatal Ed*, 75, F108–12.

FAO/WHO (2010) *Fats and fatty acids in human nutrition: report of an expert consultation*, FAO Food and Nutrition Paper 91. Rome: Food and Agriculture Organization of the United Nations.

FARQUHARSON, J., COCKBURN, F., PATRICK, W. A., JAMIESON, E. C. and LOGAN, R. W. (1992) Infant cerebral cortex phospholipid fatty-acid composition and diet. *Lancet*, 340, 810–13.

FARQUHARSON, J., JAMIESON, E. C., ABBASI, K. A., PATRICK, W. J., LOGAN, R. W. and COCKBURN, F. (1995) Effect of diet on the fatty acid composition of the major phospholipids of infant cerebral cortex. *Arch Dis Child*, 72, 198–203.

FELLER, S., GAWRISCH, K. and MACKERELL JR, A. (2002) Polyunsaturated fatty acids in lipid bilayers: intrinsic and environmental contributions to their unique physical properties. *J Am Chem Soc*, 124, 318–26.

FEWTRELL, M. S., MORLEY, R., ABBOTT, R. A., SINGHAL, A., ISAACS, E. B., STEPHENSON, T., MACFADYEN, U. and LUCAS, A. (2002) Double-blind, randomized trial of long-chain polyunsaturated fatty acid supplementation in formula fed to preterm infants. *Pediatrics*, 110, 73–82.

FEWTRELL, M. S., ABBOTT, R. A., KENNEDY, K., SINGHAL, A., MORLEY, R., CAINE, E., JAMIESON, C., COCKBURN, F. and LUCAS, A. (2004) Randomized, double-blind trial of long-chain polyunsaturated fatty acid supplementation with fish oil and borage oil in preterm infants. *J Pediatr*, 144, 471–9.

FLEITH, M. and CLANDININ, M. T. (2005) Dietary PUFA for preterm and term infants: review of clinical studies. *Crit Rev Food Sci Nutr*, 45, 205–29.

FOMON, S. (2001) Infant feeding in the 20th century: formula and beikost. *J Nutr*, 131, 409S–20S.

FRANCOIS, C. A., CONNOR, S. L., BOLEWICZ, L. C. and CONNOR, W. E. (2003) Supplementing lactating women with flaxseed oil does not increase docosahexaenoic acid in their milk. *Am J Clin Nutr*, 77, 226–33.

FSANZ (2007) *Australia New Zealand Food Standards Code* – Amendment No. 95, Gazette No. FSC 37, 13 December. Canberra: Food Standards Australia New Zealand, available at: http://www.foodstandards.gov.au/_srcfiles/Gazette_Notice_Amendment_No_95.pdf [accessed February 2013].

GALDI, M., CARBONE, N. and VALENCIA, M. E. (1989) Comparison of ferric glycinate to ferrous sulfate in model infant formulas: kinetics of vitamin losses. *J of Food Sci*, 54, 1530–39.

GALLI, C., TRZECIAK, H. I. and PAOLETTI, R. (1971) Effects of dietary fatty acids on the fatty acid composition of brain ethanolamine phosphoglyceride: Reciprocal replacement on n-6 and n-3 polyunsaturated fatty acids. *Biochim Biophys Acta Neurol Scand*, 248, 449–54.

GARCIA-LLATAS, G., LAGARDA, M. J., CLEMENTE, G. and FARRE, R. (2006) Monitoring of headspace volatiles in milk-cereal-based liquid infant foods during storage. *Eur J Lipid Sci*, 108, 1028–36.

GAWRISCH, K. and SOUBIA, O. (2008) Structure and dynamics of polyunsaturated hydrocarbon chains in lipid bilayers-significance for GPCR function. *Chem Phys Lipids*, 153, 64–75.

GERMAN, J. B. (2011) Dietary lipids from an evolutionary perspective: sources, structures and functions. *Matern Child Nutr,* 7 Suppl 2, 2–16.

GIBSON, R. A., NEUMANN, M. A. and MAKRIDES, M. (1997) Effect of increasing breast milk docosahexaenoic acid on plasma and erythrocyte phospholipid fatty acids and neural indices of exclusively breast fed infants. *Eur J Clin Nutr*, 51, 578–84.

GIL-SANCHEZ, A., KOLETZKO, B. and LARQUÉ, E. (2012) Current understanding of placental fatty acid transport. *Curr Opin Clin Nutr Metab Care*, 15, 265–72.

GREINER, R. S., CATALAN, J. N., MORIGUCHI, T. and SALEM, N., JR (2003) Docosapentaenoic acid does not completely replace DHA in n-3 FA-deficient rats during early development. *Lipids*, 38, 431–5.

HADLEY, K. B., RYAN, A. S., NELSON, E. B. and SALEM, N. (2009) An assessment of dietary docosahexaenoic acid requirements for brain accretion and turnover during early childhood. *World Rev Nutr Diet*, 99, 97–104.

HARBIGE, L. S. (2003) Fatty acids, the immune response, and autoimmunity: a question of n-6 essentiality and the balance between n-6 and n-3. *Lipids*, 38, 323–41.

HEIRD, W. C. and LAPILLONNE, A. (2005) The role of essential fatty acids in development. *Annu Rev Nutr*, 25, 549–71.

HELLAND, I. B., SMITH, L., SAAREM, K., SAUGSTAD, O. D. and DREVON, C. A. (2003) Maternal supplementation with very-long-chain n-3 fatty acids during pregnancy and lactation augments children's IQ at 4 years of age. *Pediatrics*, 111, e39–44.

HELLAND, I. B., SMITH, L., BLOMEN, B., SAAREM, K., SAUGSTAD, O. D. and DREVON, C. A. (2008) Effect of supplementing pregnant and lactating mothers with n-3 very-long-chain fatty acids on children's IQ and body mass index at 7 years of age. *Pediatrics*, 122, e472–9.

HENRIKSEN, C., HAUGHOLT, K., LINDGREN, M., AURVAG, A. K., RONNESTAD, A., GRONN, M., SOLBERG, R., MOEN, A., NAKSTAD, B., BERGE, R. K., SMITH, L., IVERSEN, P. O. and DREVON, C. A. (2008) Improved cognitive development among preterm infants attributable to early supplementation of human milk with docosahexaenoic acid and arachidonic acid. *Pediatrics*, 121, 1137–45.

HODGE, C. W., BARNES, D., SCHACHTER, H., PAN, Y., LOWCOCK, E., ZHANG, L., SAMPSON, M., MORRISON, A., TRAN, K., MIGUELEZ, M. and LEWIN, G. (2005) *Effects of omega-3 fatty acids on eye health*. Evidence Report/Technology Assessment No. 117, AHRQ Publication No. 05-E008–2. Rockeville, MN: Agency for Healthcare Research and Quality.

HOFFMAN, D. R. (2003) LCPUFA levels for breastfeeding and weaning infants: visual acuity outcomes. *Pediatr Perspect*, 2, 1.

HOFFMAN, D. R., BIRCH, E. E., BIRCH, D. G. and UAUY, R. D. (1993) Effects of supplementation with omega 3 long-chain polyunsaturated fatty acids on retinal and cortical development in premature infants. *Am J Clin Nutr*, 57, 807S–12S.

HOFFMAN, D. R., BIRCH, E. E., CASTANEDA, Y. S., FAWCETT, S. L., WHEATON, D. H., BIRCH, D. G. and UAUY, R. (2003) Visual function in breast-fed term infants weaned to formula with or without long-chain polyunsaturates at 4 to 6 months: a randomized clinical trial. *J Pediatr*, 142, 669–77.

HOFFMAN, D. R., BOETTCHER, J. A. and DIERSEN-SCHADE, D. A. (2009) Toward optimizing vision and cognition in term infants by dietary docosahexaenoic and arachidonic acid supplementation: a review of randomized controlled trials. *Prostaglandins Leukot Essent Fatty Acids*, 81, 151–8.

INNIS, S. M. (1991) Essential fatty acids in growth and development. *Prog Lipid Res*, 30, 39–103.

INNIS, S. M. (1992) Human milk and formula fatty acids. *J Pediatr*, 120, S56–61.

INNIS, S. M., GILLEY, J. and WERKER, J. (2001) Are human milk long-chain polyunsaturated fatty acids related to visual and neural development in breast-fed term infants? *J Pediatr*, 139, 532–8.

INNIS, S. M., FOOTE, K. D., MACKINNON, M. J. and KING, D. J. (1990) Plasma and red blood cell fatty acids of low-birth-weight infants fed their mother's expressed breast milk or preterm-infant formula. *Am J Clin Nutr*, 51, 994–1000.

INNIS, S. M., ADAMKIN, D. H., HALL, R. T., KALHAN, S. C., LAIR, C., LIM, M., STEVENS, D. C., TWIST, P. F., DIERSEN-SCHADE, D. A., HARRIS, C. L., MERKEL, K. L. and HANSEN, J. W. (2002)

Docosahexaenoic acid and arachidonic acid enhance growth with no adverse effects in preterm infants fed formula. *J Pediatr*, 140, 547–54.

INNIS, S. M., DAVIDSON, A. G., CHEN, A., DYER, R., MELNYK, S. and JAMES, S. J. (2003) Increased plasma homocysteine and S-adenosylhomocysteine and decreased methionine is associated with altered phosphatidylcholine and phosphatidylethanolamine in cystic fibrosis. *J Pediatr*, 143, 351–6.

JACOBSEN, C. (2008) Omega-3's in food emulsions: overview and case studies. *Agro Food Ind Hi-Tech*, 19, 9–12.

JENSEN, C. L. and LAPILLONNE, A. (2009) Docosahexaenoic acid and lactation. *Prostaglandins Leukot Essent Fatty Acids*, 81, 175–8.

JENSEN, C. L., VOIGT, R. G., PRAGER, T. C., ZOU, Y. L., FRALEY, J. K., ROZELLE, J. C., TURCICH, M. R. LLORENTE, A. M., ANDERSON, R. E. and HEIRD, W. C. (2005) Effects of maternal docosahexaenoic acid intake on visual function and neurodevelopment in breastfed term infants. *Am J Clin Nutr*, 82, 125–32.

JENSEN, C. L., VOIGT, R. G., LLORENTE, A. M., PETERS, S. U., PRAGER, T. C., ZOU, Y. L., ROZELLE, J. C., TURCICH, M. R., FRALEY, J. K., ANDERSON, R. E. and HEIRD, W. C. (2010) Effects of early maternal docosahexaenoic acid intake on neuropsychological status and visual acuity at five years of age of breast-fed term infants. *J Pediatr*, 157, 900–905.

JORGENSEN, M. H., HERNELL, O., HUGHES, E. and MICHAELSEN, K. F. (2001) Is there a relation between docosahexaenoic acid concentration in mothers' milk and visual development in term infants? *J Pediatr Gastroenterol Nutr*, 32, 293–6.

KAMAL-ELDIN, A. and YANISHLIEVA, N. V. (2002) N-3 fatty acids for human nutrition: Stability considerations, *Eur J Lipid Sci Technol*, 104, 825–36.

KOHN, G., SAWATZKI, G., VAN BIERVLIET, J. P. and ROSSENEU, M. (1994) Diet and the essential fatty acid status of term infants. *Acta Paediatr Suppl*, 402, 69–74.

KOLETZKO, B. and BRAUN, M. (1991) Arachidonic acid and early human growth: is there a relation? *Ann Nutr Metab*, 35, 128–31.

KOLETZKO, B., SCHMIDT, E., BREMER, H. J., HAUG, M. and HARZER, G. (1989) Effects of dietary long-chain polyunsaturated fatty acids on the essential fatty acid status of premature infants. *Eur J Pediatr*, 148, 669–75.

KOLETZKO, B., THIEL, I. and ABIODUN, P. O. (1992) The fatty acid composition of human milk in Europe and Africa. *J Pediatr*, 120, S62–70.

KOLETZKO, B., EDENHOFER, S., LIPOWSKY, G. and REINHARDT, D. (1995) Effects of a low birthweight infant formula containing human milk levels of docosahexaenoic and arachidonic acids. *J Pediatr Gastroenterol Nutr*, 21, 200–208.

KOLETZKO, B., BAKER, S., CLEGHORN, G., NETO, U. F., GOPALAN, S., HERNELL, O., HOCK, Q. S., JIRAPINYO, P., LONNERDAL, B., PENCHARZ, P., PZYREMBEL, H., RAMIREZ-MAYANS, J., SHAMIR, R., TURCK, D., YAMASHIRO, Y. and SONG-YI, D. (2005) Global standard for the composition of infant formula: recommendations of an ESPGHAN coordinated international expert group. *J Pediatr Gastroent Nutr*, 41, 584–99.

KOLETZKO, B., LIEN, E., AGOSTONI, C., BOHLES, H., CAMPOY, C., CETIN, I., DECSI, T., DUDENHAUSEN, J. W., DUPONT, C., FORSYTH, S., HOESLI, I., HOLZGREVE, W., LAPILLONNE, A., PUTET, G., SECHER, N. J., SYMONDS, M., SZAJEWSKA, H., WILLATTS, P. and UAUY, R. (2008) The roles of long-chain polyunsaturated fatty acids in pregnancy, lactation and infancy: review of current knowledge and consensus recommendations. *J Perinat Med*, 36, 5–14.

KREMMYDA, L. S., TVRZICKA, E., STANKOVA, B. and ZAK, A. (2011) Fatty acids as biocompounds: their role in human metabolism, health and disease: a review. Part 2: fatty acid physiological roles and applications in human health and disease. *Biomed Pap Med Fac Univ Palacky Olomouc Czech Repub*, 155(3), 195–218.

KRIS-ETHERTON, P. M., INNIS, S., AMERICAN DIETETIC ASSOCIATION and DIETITIANS OF CANADA (2007) Position of the American Dietetic Association and Dietitians of Canada: dietary fatty acids. *J Am Diet Assoc*, 107, 1599–611.

KURATKO, C. N., HOFFMAN, J. P., VAN ELSWYK, M. E. and SALEM, JR, N. (2010) Recent developments in the human nutrition of polyunsaturated fatty acids from single cell oils, in: COHEN, Z. and RATLEDGE, C. (eds), *Single Cell Oils, Microbial and Algal Oils* (2nd edn). Chicago IL: AOCS Press, 369–87.

LANDS, W. E. (1992) Biochemistry and physiology of n-3 fatty acids. *FASEB J*, 6, 2530–36.

LAURITZEN, L., JORGENSEN, M. H., MIKKELSEN, T. B., SKOVGAARD, M., STRAARUP, E. M., OLSEN, S. F., HOY, C. E. and MICHAELSEN, K. F. (2004) Maternal fish oil supplementation in lactation: effect on visual acuity and n-3 fatty acid content of infant erythrocytes. *Lipids*, 39, 195–206.

LAURITZEN, L., JORGENSEN, M. H., OLSEN, S. F., STRAARUP, E. M. and MICHAELSEN, K. F. (2005) Maternal fish oil supplementation in lactation: effect on developmental outcome in breast-fed infants, *Reprod Nutr Dev*, 45, 535–47.

LEWIN, G. A., SCHACHTER, H. M., YUEN, D., MERCHANT, P., MAMALADZE, V. and TSERTSVADZE, A. (2005) Effects of omega-3 fatty acids on child and maternal health. *Evid Rep Technol Assess (Summ)*, 1–11.

LICLICAN, E. L. and GRONERT, K. (2010) Molecular circuits of resolution in the eye. *Scientific World Journal*, 10, 1029–47.

LIEN, E. L. and HAMMOND, B. R. (2011) Nutritional influences on visual development and function. *Prog Retin Eye Res*, 30, 188–203.

LIFE SCIENCES RESEARCH OFFICE (1988) American Societies for Nutritional Sciences. Assessments of nutritional requirements for infant formulas, *J Nutr*, 128, 2059S–2298S.

LIM, S. Y., HOSHIBA, J. and SALEM, N., JR (2005) An extraordinary degree of structural specificity is required in neural phospholipids for optimal brain function: n-6 docosapentaenoic acid substitution for docosahexaenoic acid leads to a loss in spatial task performance. *J Neurochem*, 95, 848–57.

MAKRIDES, M., NEUMANN, M. A., BYARD, R. W., SIMMER, K. and GIBSON, R. A. (1994) Fatty acid composition of brain, retina, and erythrocytes in breast- and formula-fed infants. *Am J Clin Nutr*, 60, 189–94.

MAKRIDES, M., NEUMANN, M., SIMMER, K., PATER, J. and GIBSON, R. (1995) Are long-chain polyunsaturated fatty acids essential nutrients in infancy? *Lancet*, 345, 1463–8.

MAKRIDES, M., NEUMANN, M. A. and GIBSON, R. A. (1996) Effect of maternal docosahexaenoic acid (DHA) supplementation on breast milk composition. *Eur J Clin Nutr*, 50, 352–7.

MAKRIDES, M., GIBSON, R. A., UDELL, T. and RIED, K. (2005) Supplementation of infant formula with long-chain polyunsaturated fatty acids does not influence the growth of term infants. *Am J Clin Nutr*, 81, 1094–101.

MAKRIDES, M., GIBSON, R. A., MCPHEE, A. J., COLLINS, C. T., DAVIS, P. G., DOYLE, L. W., SIMMER, K., COLDITZ, P. B., MORRIS, S., SMITHERS, L. G., WILLSON, K. and RYAN, P. (2009) Neurodevelopmental outcomes of preterm infants fed high-dose docosahexaenoic acid: a randomized controlled trial. *JAMA*, 301, 175–82.

MARTINEZ, M. (1992) Tissue levels of polyunsaturated fatty acids during early human development. *J Pediatr*, 120, S129–38.

MARTINEZ, M. and MOUGAN, I. (1998) Fatty acid composition of human brain phospholipids during normal development. *J Neurochem*, 71, 2528–33.

MCCLEMENTS, D. J. (2010) Emulsion design to improve the delivery of functional lipophilic components. *Annu Rev Food Sci Technol*, 1, 241–269.

MEILGAARD, M., CIVILLE, G.V. and CARR, B. T. (1999) *Sensory Evaluation Techniques* (3rd edn). Boca Raton, FL, London, New York, Washington, DC: CRC Press.

MELDRUM, S. J., D'VAZ, N., SIMMER, K., DUNSTAN, J. A., HIRD, K. and PRESCOTT, S. L. (2012) Effects of high-dose fish oil supplementation during early infancy on neurodevelopment and language: a randomised controlled trial. *Br J Nutr*, 108, 1443–54.

MORALE, S. E., HOFFMAN, D. R., CASTANEDA, Y. S., WHEATON, D. H., BURNS, R. A. and BIRCH, E. E. (2005) Duration of long-chain polyunsaturated fatty acids availability in the diet and visual acuity. *Early Hum Dev*, 81, 197–203.

MORIGUCHI, T. and SALEM, N., JR (2003) Recovery of brain docosahexaenoate leads to recovery of spatial task performance, *J Neurochem*, 87, 297–309.

MORIGUCHI, T., LOEWKE, J., GARRISON, M., CATALAN, J. N. and SALEM, N., JR (2001) Reversal of docosahexaenoic acid deficiency in the rat brain, retina, liver, and serum. *J Lipid Res*, 42, 419–27.

MURPHY, C. L., CARDELLO, A. V. and BRAND, J. G. (1981) Taste of fifteen halide salts following water and NaCl: Anion and cation effects, *Physiol Behav*, 26, 1083–95.

NIU, S. L., MITCHELL, D. C., LIM, S. Y., WEN, Z. M., KIM, H. Y., SALEM, N., JR and LITMAN, B. J. (2004) Reduced G protein-coupled signaling efficiency in retinal rod outer segments in response to n-3 fatty acid deficiency. *J Biol Chem*, 279, 31098–104.

O'BRIEN, J. S. and SAMPSON, E. L. (1965) Fatty acid and fatty aldehyde composition of the major brain lipids in normal human gray matter, white matter, and myelin. *J Lipid Res*, 6, 545–51.

O'CONNOR, D. L., HALL, R., ADAMKIN, D., AUESTAD, N., CASTILLO, M., CONNOR, W. E., CONNOR, S. L., FITZGERALD, K., GROH-WARGO, S., HARTMANN, E. E., JACOBS, J., JANOWSKY, J., LUCAS, A., MARGESON, D., MENA, P., NEURINGER, M., NESIN, M., SINGER, L., STEPHENSON, T., SZABO, J. and ZEMON, V. (2001) Growth and development in preterm infants fed long-chain polyunsaturated fatty acids: a prospective, randomized controlled trial. *Pediatrics*, 108, 359–71.

PIVIK, R. T., DYKMAN, R. A., JING, H., GILCHRIST, J. M. and BADGER, T. M. (2009) Early infant diet and the omega 3 fatty acid DHA: effects on resting cardiovascular activity and behavioral development during the first half-year of life. *Dev Neuropsychol*, 34, 139–58.

PLAGEMANN, A., DAVIDOWA, H., HARDER, T. and DUDENHAUSEN, J. W. (2006) Developmental programming of the hypothalamus: a matter of insulin. A comment on: Horvath, T. L., Bruning, J. C.: Developmental programming of the hypothalamus: a matter of fat. *Nat Med*, 12, 52–53.

QUERQUES, G., AVELLIS, F. O., QUERQUES, L., BANDELLO, F. and SOUIED, E. H. (2011) Age-related macular degeneration. *Clin Ophthalmol*, 5, 593–601.

RIES, D. (2009) *Studies on the antioxidant activity of milk proteins in model oil-in-water emulsions*. PhD thesis, Massey University, New Zealand.

ROSS, C. (2009) Physiology of sensory perception, in CLARK, S., COSTELLO, M., DRAKE, M. and BODYFELT, F. (eds). *Sensory Evaluation of Dairy Products* (2nd edn). New York: Springer, 17–42.

RYAN, A. S., MONTALTO, M. B., GROH-WARGO, S., MIMOUNI, F., SENTIPAL-WALERIUS, J., DOYLE, J., SIEGMAN, J. S. and THOMAS, A. J. (1999) Effect of DHA-containing formula on growth of preterm infants to 59 weeks postmenstrual age. *Am J Hum Biol*, 11, 457–67.

SALEM, N., JR, SERPENTINO, P., PUSKIN, J. and ABOOD L. (1980) Preparation and spectroscopic characterization of molecular species of brain phosphatidylserines. *Chem Phys Lipids*, 27, 289–304.

SALEM, N., JR, HULLIN, F., YOFFE, A. M., KARANIAN, J. W. and KIM, H. Y. (1989) Fatty acid and phospholipid species composition of rat tissues after a fish oil diet. *Adv Prostaglandin Thromboxane Leukot Res*, 19, 618–22.

SALEM, N., JR, WEGHER, B., MENA, P. and UAUY, R. (1996) Arachidonic and docosahexaenoic acids are biosynthesized from their 18-carbon precursors in human infants. *Proc Natl Acad Sci U S A*, 93, 49–54.

SANG, N. and CHEN, C. (2006) Lipid signaling and synaptic plasticity. *Neuroscientist*, 12, 425–34.

SANGIOVANNI, J. P., BERKEY, C. S., DWYER, J. T. and COLDITZ, G. A. (2000a) Dietary essential fatty acids, long-chain polyunsaturated fatty acids, and visual resolution acuity in healthy fullterm infants: a systematic review. *Early Hum Dev*, 57, 165–88.

SANGIOVANNI, J. P., PARRA-CABRERA, S., COLDITZ, G. A., BERKEY, C. S. and DWYER, J. T. (2000b) Meta-analysis of dietary essential fatty acids and long-chain polyunsaturated fatty acids as they relate to visual resolution acuity in healthy preterm infants. *Pediatrics*, 105, 1292–8.

SCHAICH, K. (2005) Lipid oxidation theoretical aspects, in SHAHIDI, F. (ed.), *Baileys' Industrial Oil and Fat Products* (6th edn). Hoboken, NJ: 269–355.

SIMMER, K., PATOLE, S. K. and RAO, S. C. (2011) Longchain polyunsaturated fatty acid supplementation in infants born at term. *Cochrane Database Syst Rev*, CD000376.

SINGHAL, A. and LUCAS, A. (2004) Early origins of cardiovascular disease: is there a unifying hypothesis? *Lancet*, 363, 1642–5.

SINGHAL, A., KATTENHORN, M., COLE, T. J., DEANFIELD, J. and LUCAS, A. (2001) Preterm birth, vascular function, and risk factors for atherosclerosis, *Lancet*, 358, 1159–60.

SMITHERS, L. G., GIBSON, R. A., MCPHEE, A. and MAKRIDES, M. (2008a) Higher dose of docosahexaenoic acid in the neonatal period improves visual acuity of preterm infants: results of a randomized controlled trial. *Am J Clin Nutr*, 88, 1049–56.

SMITHERS, L. G., GIBSON, R. A., MCPHEE, A. and MAKRIDES, M. (2008b) Effect of long-chain polyunsaturated fatty acid supplementation of preterm infants on disease risk and neurodevelopment: a systematic review of randomized controlled trials. *Am J Clin Nutr*, 87, 912–20.

SMITHERS, L. G., COLLINS, C. T., SIMMONDS, L. A., GIBSON, R. A., MCPHEE, A. and MAKRIDES, M. (2010) Feeding preterm infants milk with a higher dose of docosahexaenoic acid than that used in current practice does not influence language or behavior in early childhood: a follow-up study of a randomized controlled trial. *Am J Clin Nutr*, 91, 628–34.

STEVENS, E. E., PATRICK, T. E. and PICKLER, R. (2009) A history of infant feeding. *J Perinat Educ*, 18, 32–9.

STILLWELL, W., SHAIKH, S. R., ZEROUGA, M., SIDDIQUI, R. and WASSALL, S. R. (2005) Docosahexaenoic acid affects cell signaling by altering lipid rafts. *Reprod Nutr Dev*, 45, 559–79.

SVENNERHOLM, L. (1968) Distribution and fatty acid composition of phosphoglycerides in normal human brain. *J Lipid Res*, 9, 570–9.

SWANSON, D., BLOCK, R. and MOUSA, S. A. (2012) Omega-3 fatty acids EPA and DHA: health benefits throughout life. *Adv Nutr*, 3(1), 1–7.

TANEJA, A. and ZHU, X. (2006) The trouble with omega-3 oils. *Funct Ingred*, Sept, 16–18.

TEAGASC FOOD RESEARCH CENTER (2011) *Workshop: Nutrient stability during infant formula manufacture and storage*, September 21–22.

UAUY, R. D., BIRCH, D. G., BIRCH, E. E., TYSON, J. E. and HOFFMAN, D. R. (1990) Effect of dietary omega-3 fatty acids on retinal function of very-low-birth-weight neonates. *Pediatr Res*, 28, 485–92.

UAUY, R., HOFFMAN, D. R., MENA, P., LLANOS, A. and BIRCH, E. E. (2003) Term infant studies of DHA and ARA supplementation on neurodevelopment: results of randomized controlled trials. *J Pediatr*, 143, S17–25.

US FDA (1971) Rules and regulations: Label statements concerning dietary properties of food purporting to be or represented for specific dietary uses. *Federal Register*, 36, 23553–6.

US FDA (1980) The Infant Formula Act of 1980. Public Law No. 96–359, 94 Stat. 1190 [codified at 21 U.S.C.§350(a), 301, 321 (aa), 331, 374(a)]. September 26, 1980.

US FDA (2001) Agency Response Letter GRAS Notice No. GRN 000041, available at: http://www.fda.gov/Food/FoodIngredientsPackaging/GenerallyRecognizedasSafeGRAS/GRASListings/ucm154126.htm [accessed January 2013].

VAN WEZEL-MEIJLER, G., VAN DER KNAAP, M. S., HUISMAN, J., JONKMAN, E. J., VALK, J. and LAFEBER, H. N. (2002) Dietary supplementation of long-chain polyunsaturated fatty acids in preterm infants: effects on cerebral maturation. *Acta Paediatr*, 91, 942–50.

WERKMAN, S. H. and CARLSON, S. E. (1996) A randomized trial of visual attention of preterm infants fed docosahexaenoic acid until nine months. *Lipids*, 31, 91–7.

WHO (1986) Thirty-ninth world health assembly. *Guidelines concerning the main health and socioeconomic circumstances in which infants have to be fed on breast-milk substitutes*, Ed A39/8 Add. 1:1986. Geneva: World Health Organization.

WILLATTS, P., FORSYTH, J. S., DIMODUGNO, M. K., VARMA, S. and COLVIN, M. (1998a) Influence of long-chain polyunsaturated fatty acids on infant cognitive function. *Lipids*, 33, 973–80.

WILLATTS, P., FORSYTH, J. S., DIMODUGNO, M. K., VARMA, S. and COLVIN, M. (1998b) Effect of long-chain polyunsaturated fatty acids in infant formula on problem solving at 10 months of age. *Lancet*, 352, 688–91.

YUHAS, R., PRAMUK, K. and LIEN, E. L. (2006) Human milk fatty acid composition from nine countries varies most in DHA. *Lipids*, 41, 851–8.

Part IV

New directions

14

Algal oil as a source of omega-3 fatty acids

R. J. Winwood, DSM Nutritional Products, UK

DOI: 10.1533/9780857098863.4.389

Abstract: Certain marine algae are primary sources of the long chain polyunsaturated fatty acids (LC-PUFA) docosahexaenoic acid (DHA) and eicosapentaenoic acid (EPA) found in fish and other seafood products. An algal oil, rich in DHA and EPA, can be extracted from algal biomass grown in contained fermention vessels. Some of the reasons why an algal oil could be preferred to fish oil are: improved taste properties, sustainability, avoidance of contaminants currently found in ocean waters and complete suitability for a vegetarian diet. Products of Martek Biosciences, life'sDHA and DHASCO as discussed in detail.

Key words: algal oil, PUFA, DHA, EPA, omega-3 fatty acids, Martek Biosciences, DHASCO, life'sDHA.

14.1 Introduction

The long-chain omega-3 fatty acids docosahexaenoic acid (DHA) and eicosapentaenoic acid (EPA) essentially benefit human health by supporting a healthy heart and blood circulation and supporting healthy immune responses. However, DHA specifically is an essential structural component of the eye, brain and heart; facilitates and regulates electronic signalling; and helps facilitate neurogenesis in the foetus.

Certain marine algae are the primary source of the long-chain polyunsaturated fatty acids (LC-PUFA) DHA and EPA that are found in fish and other seafood. In the oceans, marine algae are consumed by small fish, crustaceans (e.g. krill) and other small marine creatures that are then consumed by carnivorous fish (e.g. salmon, tuna), from many of which we extract oil containing DHA and EPA. Figure 14.1 shows the usual routes by which the marine omega-3 fatty acids DHA and EPA are introduced into the diet.

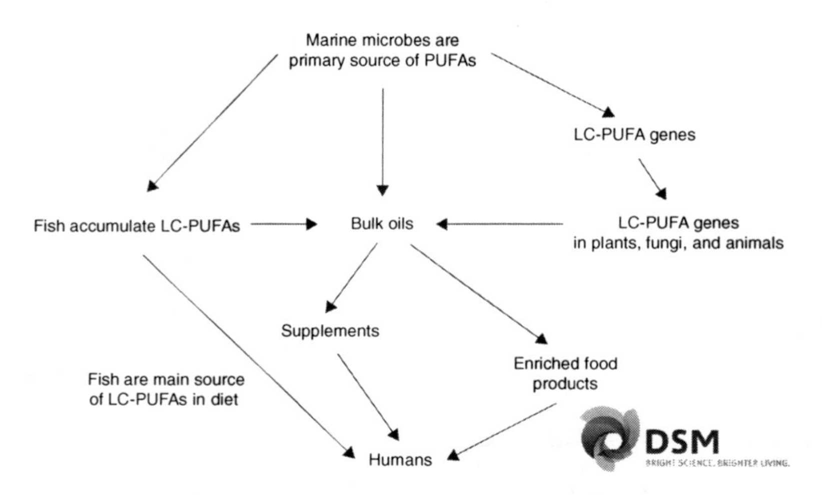

Fig. 14.1 Where do we get our LC-PUFAs?

We are familiar with the use of bacterial and fungal fermentation for the production of a wide range of complex biochemicals, but fermentation with microalgae is much more difficult. The process is expensive, slow and often produces a low yield. Special care is given to the illumination, nutrient source and handling (due to the delicate nature of algal cell walls). Most microalgae are autotrophic, which means they require a light source for growth. In practice, providing an efficient light source in a large fermenter is a complex matter and provides a limitation to the size of the fermentation vessel. The use of heterotrophic algae eliminates the light problem.

Algal-sourced DHA and EPA is more expensive on a weight-for-weight basis than when obtained from fish oils (although currently, very highly purified fish oils now approach a similar price). There are important advantages for using an algal source versus a fish source. There is a guaranteed freedom from ocean-borne contaminants, since the algae are grown in large tanks with fresh water. The finished oil has superior organoleptic properties (largely due to clean production conditions and the reduced time from production to delivery) and the algal product is suitable for vegetarian diets. Additionally, the ratio of DHA to EPA is generally constant, unlike fish, which varies considerably depending on the type of fish, their nutrient source and the location in which they are caught.

For these, and other reasons, the largest interest in algal DHA applications has been for the infant formula market. It is added to infant formula to emulate the DHA that is naturally found in human breast milk (see Chapter 13 for more details).

To date, the algal infant formula DHA market has been led by Martek Biosciences Corporation (Martek). Martek is a wholly-owned subsidiary of DSM, having been purchased by DSM in 2011. Martek has historically focused on solving the yield problems of microalgal fermentation, which led to them publishing a large quantity of intellectual property in the area. However, today there are a number of other algal DHA producers, particularly in China.

14.1.1 The evolutionary origins of DHA

Three billion years ago, dinoflagellates and certain microalgae evolved metabolic pathways to convert α-linolenic acid (ALA) to DHA using the enzyme Δ^4-desaturase. These phytoplankton remain the source of DHA for all aquatic life. Six hundred million years ago, complex life began in the so-called 'Cambrian explosion', fueled by oxygen and specialised lipids enabling cell differentiation, including the development of neurones. An unrestricted supply of DHA allowed the formation of complex neural systems in larger vertebrates in the oceans (Lassek and Gaulin, 2011). DHA was the dominant fatty acid in the cell membranes of new photoreceptors that converted photons from light into electrical impulses (Crawford *et al.*, 2008).

14.2 Using microalgae to produce food ingredients

14.2.1 Reasons for making marine-sourced omega-3 LC PUFA (DHA/EPA/DPA omega-3) from algae

Marine algae are the primary source of the LC-PUFA DHA and EPA in the human diet. Fish contain these LC-PUFAs from their consumption of algae. Eggs and organ meats also contain DHA and EPA (albeit at much lower levels), and changes in farming practices, particularly the feeding of corn (maize) oil (almost no LC-PUFA) instead of grass feeding (an ALA-containing feed), have greatly reduced the amount of n-3 LC-PUFA in the food supply. The most important sources of DHA and EPA in the diet are the preformed sources such as fatty fish. Farmed fish may not even be a good source, due to the increasing trend of feeding of corn (maize) and other grain products instead of fish meal. Individuals who cannot, or will not, eat fish may be at particular risk for LC-PUFA deficiency.

Sustainability of a clean fish supply is, unfortunately becoming a problem. The planet also faces a situation where fish stocks are in decline and unlikely to recover. In short, a viable alternative is required, and the extraction of LC-PUFA from the oil of microalgae can provide a solution.

The term microalgae encompasses all microscopic algae, both unicellular and filamentous. The value of commercial products produced from microalgae in 2011 is estimated at €600 million per annum, with the human nutrition sector representing 74 % of the market value (Tramoy, 2011). There are two basic types of commercial microalgae:

- *autotrophic*: which require a light source for growth;
- *heterotropic*: which utilise organic compounds as nutrients.

14.2.2 Reasons for using microalgae to produce food ingredients

Microalgae have a higher growth rate and higher biomass density in comparison to land-based crops. They are a source of rare, key bioactive nutrients normally only found in the marine environment and provide an alternative to extraction from fish. The fermentation substrates used in microalgal fermentation are readily available and derived from renewable resources. (Glucose syrup is a popular choice as the major constituent!) Microalgal fermentations have other environmental benefits too, in that they do not compete for land space and can be used to fix carbon dioxide.

Numerous phototrophic algae are able to adapt their metabolism to heterotrophic conditions – indeed that is the only way they can function when the sun's rays are not available! They simply metabolise a glucose source to produce energy when they are unable to use photosynthesis.

14.2.3 Lipids from microalgae

Microalgae produce between 1 and 70 % of their cell weight as lipids. However, under certain, specialised conditions, this lipid yield can be increased to over 90 %. Table 14.1 gives some examples of various fatty acids that can be produced by algal fermentation. However, it is the ability of microalgae to produce EPA and DHA which is of particular interest. These long-chain fatty acids can also be produced using yeasts and bacteria that have been subjected to recombinant gene technology, but the yields are low.

The production of long-chain fatty acids by the fermentation of algae is technically challenging. The fermentation is slow and the extraction process complex. However, the technology allows the production of a sustainable vegetarian source of omega-3 fatty acids, free from contamination with polychlorinated biphenyls (PCBs) and heavy metals.

Table 14.1 Fatty acid yields from various microalgal fermentations

Micro-organism	Oil (%)	Fatty acids in oil (%)	Extraction method
Crypthecodinium cohnii	25.9	DHA 39.3	Ultrasonic
Spirulina platensis	77.9	GLA 20.2	SC-CO_2
Phaedodactylum tricornutum	96.1	EPA 23.7	Solvent
Botryococcus braunii	12.1	Oleic 65.3 Linolenic 19	Solvent

GLA: γ-linolenic acid, SC-CO_2: Supercritical carbon dioxide.
Source: data extracted from Mercer and Armenta, 2011.

14.2.4 How to select suitable microalgae for industrial production of algal oils

The most popular microalgae used in commercial LC-PUFA enriched oil and biomass are from the marine members of the families *Thraustochytriacea* and *Crythecodiniacea*. The *Thraustochytrids* include the genii Schizochytrium and Ulkenia, whereas Crythecodinium is a genus of the family *Crythecodiniacea*. In each genus, there are a large variety of species, which are diversely dispersed in the oceans of the world. Microbiologists have collected literally thousands of different species, and these are now held in extensive culture collections by both industry and academia. *Thraustochytrids* have the advantage of growing under heterotrophic conditions. Autotrophic algae require a source of light, using the light of the sun to drive their metabolism. This seriously limits the design of the fermenter, particularly the size which, in turn, limits the yield. However, microbiologists have been able to isolate strains of some autotrophic microalgae that grow well under heterotrophic conditions without resorting to genetic modification technology. This has facilitated the use of normal large fermenters (that have no light source), which can have a capacity in excess of 100 000 L.

14.2.5 Industrial production of oils from microalgae

Starting with a pure, axenic culture of a microalgae, growing conditions are optimised to enable maximum biomass production. In some cases, the biomass is dried (by spray or roller drying). The next stages involve disruption of the algal cells and separation of the oil from the cell debris using a centrifuge. Solvents, including hexane, are often used to increase the yields. Table 14.2 gives some examples of extraction techniques that can be used with algal biomass. The extraction stage is fraught with

Table 14.2 Microalgal oil extraction methods

Extraction method	Advantage	Limitation
Pressing	Simple, no solvents	Slow Poor yields
Solvent extraction	Solvents are inexpensive Yields improved and reproducible	Most suitable solvents are flammable Toxicity Recovery is expensive
Supercritical fluid	Safe, non-toxic solvents, simple	Expensive Complex scale-up
Ultrasonic assisted	Reduced solvent consumption and extraction time	High power consumption Complex scale-up

Source: derived from Mercer and Armenta, 2011.

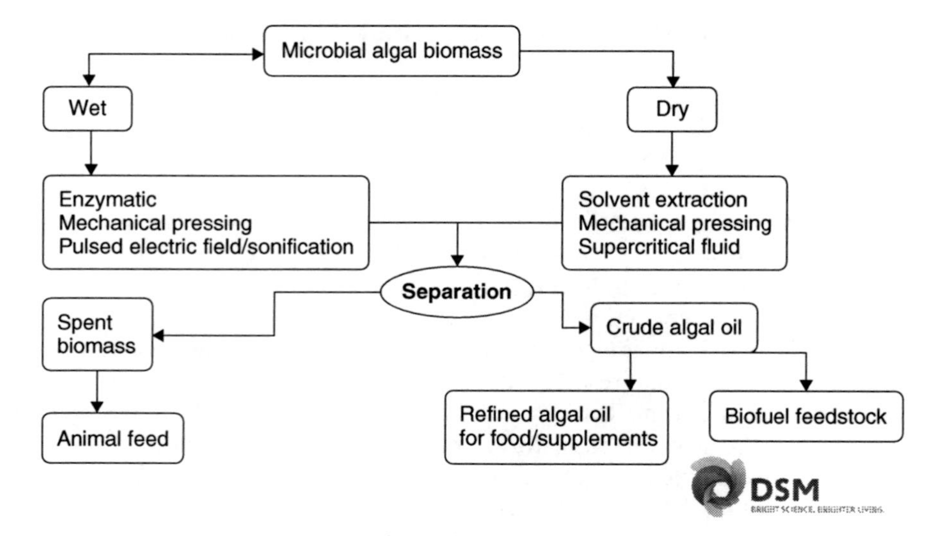

Fig. 14.2 Extraction/downstream processing of microbial oils. Derived from: Mercer and Armenta, 2011, *Eur J Lipid Sci Technol*, 113: 539–547.

difficulty because the protection offered to the LC-PUFA from the natural antioxidants present within the microalgae is not effective once the cell is ruptured. Hence, it is very important to minimise exposure to air at this stage. A variety of techniques can be used to enhance oil recovery (see Fig. 14.2), including enzyme pretreatment, ultrasonics and supercritical fluid extraction (usually with carbon dioxide). However, the most cost-effective procedure involves extraction with the solvent hexane, which can be accompanied by mechanical pressing. The spent, de-oiled biomass can generally be used for animal feed. The crude oil is then subject to standard food oil refining techniques. Waste or oxidised oil can be diverted to biofuel production.

Martek has used two heterotrophic algae to make two DHA-rich oils. The DHASCO™ oil is aimed at the infant formula market as it has been designed to minimise the EPA content. It utilises the fermentation of the microalgae *Crypthecodinium cohnii*. The oil is pale yellow to dark orange in colour. The DHA content of the oil is 40–45 % w/w. The next most common fatty acid is oleic acid (C18:1) which can be as high as 40 %. The life'sDHA™ oil, which also contains low levels of EPA (<2 %), is aimed at the food, beverage and supplement industries. It uses the microalgae *Schizochytrium* which has around 50 % of cell weight as triglycerides. The fatty acid composition of life'sDHA™ is standardised at 35 % or 40 % DHA (w/w) with a carefully selected vegetable oil. The commercial oil is pale yellow in colour and has a neutral flavour. The microalgae *Ulkenia* sp are also used for commercial DHA production.

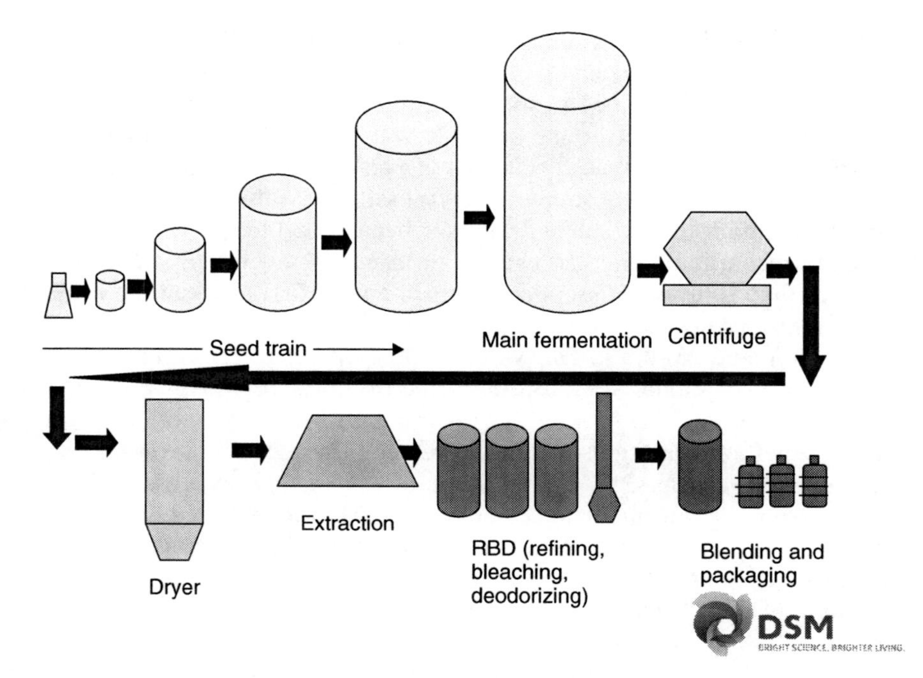

Fig. 14.3 DHA oil production process for infant formula (some steps are optional depending on the source material).

14.3 Typical production of docosahexaenoic acid (DHA) algal oils

14.3.1 Fermentation: the seed train from shake flask to main fermentation vessel

A typical production process for algal oils is shown in Fig. 14.3. Any commercial algal oil fermentation unit needs to have a sterile area that houses a microbiology laboratory and seed production area. It is critical to prevent cross-contamination of the main culture, as this can lead to a complete main batch fermentation being abandoned and follow-up cleandown being required which, in effect, leads to the fermenter being out of service for many weeks at a time. The microbiology laboratory on an algal oil production site will have a reference culture of the microalgae it uses, usually kept in a deep frozen condition. From this culture, the microalgae are grown in shake flasks, typically 0.2–1 L. The flasks are prefilled with a suitable culture medium under aseptic conditions. The inoculated flasks are then incubated at a suitable growing temperature. Again, a check should be made that the fermentation broth is axenic, and without contamination.

The verified flasks are then moved to the 'seed' production area (which is usually directly connected to the microbiology laboratory). Here, the contents of the shake flask are added aseptically to the first vessel of the 'seed train'. This initial seed vessel is typically 5–25 L and of glass construction. It will be sterilised before use and fitted with an agitator, pH control and facilities for sterile air/gas input. It will be precharged with sterile growth medium, which typically consists of a glucose base (typically glucose syrup) with added protein sources, mineral salts and other micronutrients. Once the contents of the shake flask have been added to the primary seed vessel, fermentation is then allowed to proceed for several days. The contents are then transferred aseptically (again having first checked the broth is axenic) to a sterilised intermediate seed vessel, usually of stainless steel construction and 25–100 L. This will have been precharged with a growth medium of very similar composition to the primary vessel. Again the fermentation is allowed to proceed for several days with close monitoring of the fermentation conditions within the vessel. (There can be several intermediate seed transfers.) The final stage of the seed train is the aseptic transfer from the intermediate vessel to the sterilised final seed fermenter. This, larger seed vessel is designed to be removed from the confines of the seed production area to the top of the main fermenter in the main production area. A final check is made of the contents of the final seed vessel for contamination and growth/reproduction rate.

The main fermenters have a very large capacity, typically 200 000 L or more. The main fermenters are sterilised and precharged with sterilised fermentation media in exactly the same way as the earlier stages in the seed train, though the growth medium itself may be simplified. The main fermentation tank is fitted with a means of agitation, pH control, air/gas input and precise temperature control. The tank should also have observation ports and sampling points. The aseptic transfer from the final seed vessel to the main fermenter is the critical point of the whole algal biomass production process. Any contamination at this stage will prove extremely costly as the whole batch would need to be abandoned. This final fermentation is longer than seed train stages, typically 7–14 days or even longer. This means expensive production capacity is tied up and helps explain the high cost of products made from algal fermentation.

14.3.2 Extraction: rupturing the algal cell and separation of the oil

Extraction of algal oil for the production of DHA and EPA is difficult because, as soon as the algal cell walls are ruptured, these LC-PUFA are exposed to potential oxidation. Once these highly unsaturated fatty acids have reacted with oxidised radicals, an unstoppable chain reaction begins which leads to the production of rancid, highly odourous oil which is unsuitable for human consumption. Hence, so far as possible, all sources of materials that can initiate the oxidation process (e.g. copper, ferrous metal) should be eliminated from the extraction and oil storage areas. A variety of extraction methods can be used, though all involve rupturing of the cell wall with some form of milling (often assisted with enzymes, sonification, etc.) followed by extraction with solvent. Classically, hexane, as used in most vegetable oil production, was used as solvent but, more recently, solventless extraction processes have been developed. In any event, careful checks are made to ensure that no residual solvent remains in the oil. The residual, spent biomass will still contain small amounts of omega-3 fatty acids and thus can be sold for use in animal feed. The crude algal oil is kept cool, usually under a nitrogen blanket, ready for refining.

14.3.3 Purification: refining, bleaching and removing odour from algal oils

Crude vegetable oils, including algal oils, require refining to improve colour, clarity and odour, and remove any particulate material and chemical contaminants. There are a wide range of impurities in the crude oil that can be removed by the refining process, including: free fatty acids, phospholipids (i.e. lecithin), pigments (i.e. carotenoids, chlorophyll), trace metals, sterols (i.e. cholesterol), waxes, monoacyl- and diacylglycerides (MAGs and DAGs), oxidation products and trace contaminants. Free fatty acids (FFAs) are usually removed by chemical refining where the FFAs are neutralised with caustic soda then easily removed as a soap. Physical refining is less suitable for algal oils because of the high temperatures involved. The neutralisation step is usually preceded by a degumming process where water is added to remove phosphatides, sterols, etc. Removal of the soap is achieved by washing the oil with water followed by physical separation of aqueous phase and drying under vacuum (which also helps remove any dissolved oxygen).

The next stage is bleaching, where typically absorbent clay or activated carbon is added to remove colour pigments, oxidation products and trace metals. The bleaching aid is then removed by filtration. Additional recovery processes may be used to recover any residue in the spent filter aid before it is sent for landfill. The bleached oil is then sent to the deodoriser which can be thought of as a steam cleaner. High-pressure steam is added to the oil under high vacuum to remove any remaining oil components that contribute to taste, odour and colour including any produced in the refining process up to this stage. The oil is then cooled.

Finally, the oil may be dewaxed to improve its clarity. Dewaxing (also known as winterisation) removes the high-melting waxes which otherwise will give the oil a cloudy appearance. Dewaxing can be carried out both before and after the deodorisation stage. This process involves chilling the oil to allow the wax crystals to develop and grow. The wax crystals are then removed by filtration and/or centrifugation. The resulting product is refined, algal oil.

The final refined algal oil should be clear, bright and pale in colour. It should have a bland flavour and have minimal odour. The algal oil should have good oxidative stability and meet all legal limits for trace contaminants.

14.3.4 Storage conditions for the refined algal oil

In order to maintain the oxidative stability of the algal oil, it is usual to add one or more antioxidants. Typically, a synergistic blend of several antioxidants is used. Preference is given to naturally derived antioxidants, such as rosemary oil (active constituent: carnosic acid) and tocopherols, but others, such as ascorbyl palmitate, may also be added. As the addition levels are very low, it is best to make an oil preblend, before adding to the total bulk of algal oil, to ensure homogeneous distribution. Typically, this blending is done warm, but exposure to air must continue to be avoided. Also if the algal oil is to be standardised to a particular DHA or EPA content, then the batch concerned can be blended with other batches of algal oil and a suitable, standardising vegetable oil (e.g. high oleic sunflower oil). Once blending is complete, the oil should be packed into clean suitable size containers, frozen and then kept frozen for storage and distribution.

High-quality DHA and EPA oils can be made in a food-grade plant operating Good Manufacturing Practice (GMP) and globally recognised quality systems. This complex production process needs to be closely monitored by a suitably qualified quality control team throughout the process. It is possible to produce algal oils that meet the requirements of certifying kosher and halal organisations.

14.4 DSM DHA intellectual property

DSM (through its acquisition of Martek Biosciences Corporation) has an extensive portfolio of granted patents and pending applications covering its DHA compositions, production processes and methods of use in the USA and Europe, as well as other countries. Martek had built additional layers of protection around its DHA technologies.

Some of the earliest DHA patents, filed by Martek over 20 years ago, have begun to expire. These patents covered early production processes and use of the resulting DHA oils in food applications. However, these early inventions have now been improved on with more efficient techniques and improved compositions that are protected by newer patents with much later expiration dates. DSM has also in-licensed numerous complementary patents and applications that help strengthen protection of its DHA technologies.

14.5 Regulatory approval of algal oil

14.5.1 European Union

Martek's life'sDHA™-S algal oil is approved for use as a novel food ingredient in specific food categories and dietary supplements under Commission Decisions of 5 June 2003 and 22 October 2009. This algal oil must be labeled 'DHA rich oil from the microalga *Schizochytrium* sp.' under these regulations.

The DHA algal oil DHASCO® has been approved for use in infant formula in the European Union under Commission Directive 2006/141/EC. When added, 1 % of the total fat content should consist of n-3 LC-PUFA and 2 % of the fat content should be n-6 LC-PUFA of which 1 % is arachidonic acid (ARA). So, in practice DHA can only be used if ARA is also added. DHASCO® is also considered food in the EU (i.e., not a novel food) based on a 'significant degree of use' prior to 1997.

With regard to health claims, the following Article 14 claims have been authorised and published in the *Official Journal of the European Union* [Commission Regulation (EU) No 440/2011 of 6th May 2011].

- 'DHA intake contributes to the normal visual development of infants up to 12 months of age'
- 'DHA maternal intake contributes to the normal development of the eye of the foetus and breastfed infants'
- 'DHA maternal intake contributes to the normal brain development of the foetus and breastfed infants'

With regard to article 13.1 claims, the final approved claims appeared in *Official Journal of the European Union*, 25.5.12, Commission regulation (EU) 432/2012 of 16th May 2012. In this, the following claims appear for DHA alone: 'Maintenance of normal brain function' and 'Maintenance of normal vision', whilst for EPA and DHA, a claim of 'maintenance of normal cardiac function' appears. The accompanying conditions of use for all three claims are a recommended total daily intake of 250 mg per day for the general population.

14.5.2 USA

In the USA, the Martek algal DHA oil, life'sDHA™-S, has generally recognised as safe (GRAS) status for use in a variety of foods (USA FDA, 2004). Maximum use levels depend on application, but are not to exceed 1.5 g/day. It is permitted for use as a new dietary ingredient (supplements) up to 1 g DHA oil per day. The DHASCO® Algal DHA Oil has GRAS status for use in infant formulas and foods (US FDA, 2001). It can be used in infant formulas at a level up to 1.25 % each of total dietary fat and at a ratio of DHA to ARA of 1:1 to 1:2. (Note this ratio applies to formula and foods intended for infants only.) Also it is permitted for use as a dietary supplement based on prior history of use.

14.6 A case study: the story of the development of Martek Biosciences Corporation

The story of algal DHA (Behrens, 2011) is principally one of Martek Biosciences Corporation. Martek became a wholly-owned subsidiary of DSM in the spring of 2011. The founders of Martek (five bioscientists and three technicians) originally worked for the biosciences division of Martin Marietta Corporation, based at Bethesda in Maryland, USA. In 1985, this company decided to dispose of its peripheral business and concentrate on material for aeronautics; in 1995 it merged with the Lockheed Corporation, and today is very well known under its current name of Lockheed Martin. The founders of Martek were specialists in algal fermentation. This was a relatively unexplored branch of fermentation science with little in the way of intellectual property to curtail exploration. However, algae grow slowly and usually under conditions not suited to industrial production (i.e. need light and/or saline). The photosynthetic abilities of most algae mean they possess metabolic pathways not found in other micro-organisms. Essentially, they can produce organic molecules from inorganic substrates.

In the early years, despite a plethora of ideas and enthusiasm, the Martek scientists failed to find a commercially viable product from their microalgae. They then used phototrophic microalgae, in relatively small-scale fermentation (ca 100–200 L) to produce stable isotopes for medical diagnostics. The algae could be grown using C_{13} or deuterium labelled heavy water. The resulting, labelled carbon dioxide or fatty acids/sugars, respectively, could be used in metabolic laboratory test materials. This developed into a multimillion dollar business, but was limited in further growth by the available production capacity.

This success enabled Martek to build up what is believed to be the largest collection of microalgae specimens in the world. This culture collection was first used to produce interesting natural biochemical candidates for anti-cancer/AIDS activity for the National Cancer Institute. Martek then extended this activity into private companies in the pharmaceutical sector. However, the advent of the production of biochemical candidates from combinatorial chemistry in the mid-1990s drastically reduced the use of naturally derived candidates and Martek had to look for alternative cash generating products if they were to survive.

Back in the days of Martin Marietta, the Martek founders had worked with NASA to use algae to produce oxygen and purify the air (by fixing carbon dioxide) in long-distance space flight. The idea was born of using the algae produced as a food source. Analysis of the nutrients produced by the algae threw up a little known fatty acid called DHA. The interest in

DHA had been maintained at a low level during the early days of Martek, but literature searches did reveal its importance for the development and maintenance of human neural function. As other business avenues were narrowing, a decision was made in the mid-1990s to investigate the potential for commercial production of DHA from microalgae.

The algae that produced the most DHA was *Crypthecodinium*. This was a member of the dinoflagellates, some of which are toxic – so extensive safety screening was necessary. The next problem was to select a strain that would grow in the low saline environment of large-scale fermenters. (*Crypthecodinium* is found in seawater!) Another constraint was that *Crypthecodinium* grew very slowly, but it did have the advantage of being heterotrophic which meant it was not necessary to have a light source (a factor that severely limits the dimensions of a fermenter).

It was known that DHA was present in human breast milk, but not present at the time in infant formula, so Martek opened up a dialogue with infant formula manufacturers. By approaching this market, Martek knew they would not be able to use GM technology in strain development – something that became an advantage in future years. Infant formula itself is a high-cost food material, and seen at the time as one of the few human food areas that could bear the high cost of algal oil. Initially, the response was lukewarm but, with time, the industry saw that DHA was key to ensuring proper cognitive and visual development in neonates, but they would not commit to adding it to their products unless Martek could guarantee supply. So the Martek company had to make a paradigm shift from being purely a research company to becoming a large-scale manufacturing company. They became a public company in 1993 so that the necessary funds could be obtained for expansion and purchased the former Coors brewery fermentation plant at Winchester, Kentucky (which had most recently been used for riboflavin production). A strain of *Crypthecodinium* was found that tolerated low-sodium conditions. Years of work then followed to improve the yields and production process. At each stage they protected their developments with suitable intellectual property.

The first DHA products were targeted at aquaculture, where it maximised growth and survival of the fish as well as increasing the levels of DHA in the fish tissues. However, in 2001, the decision was made to concentrate solely on producing an algal oil suitable for infant formula. In 2002, Martek acquired Omegatech of Boulder, Colorado for USD 50 million in shares. Omegatech were the only other significant company working in the same area at the time (Nutraingredients, 2002). Omegatech had developed algal oils rich in DHA from Thraustrochytrids, and conducted toll fermentations at the Monsanto (formerly Kelco International) fermentation facility in San Diego, California (Abril, 2011). Due to the intellectual property position, Omegatech had concentrated on the animal nutrition market. The new, combined company rapidly developed and in 2003 earned a profit for the first time in its history. This was due to infant formula companies finally incorporating algal oils into their product ranges, and discovering that the increased production cost was rewarded with significantly increased sales. Indeed, the demand became such that there was a serious risk that Martek would run out of capacity. Therefore in September 2003, Martek enabled a major expansion of production by buying FermPro for USD 10 million. This gave access to a large, easily expandable, specialist fermentation site at Kingstree, South Carolina. The Kingstree site had formerly been part of the Dutch company Gist Brocades. Production capacity at the site has increased year-on-year until the present day.

14.7 Future trends

It is possible to produce EPA-rich algal oil as some species of algae can produce useful amounts of EPA; however, it should be remembered that around 10–15 % of DHA retro-converts to EPA in the human body and also that EPA does not contribute to structural cell membranes in the brain or eyes, but it is a useful source of anti-inflammatory eicosanoids.

DSM now produces a DHA and EPA-rich algal oil called life'sDHA and EPA™ produced using *Schizochytrium* sp. The oil is specified as having a minimum 22.5 % DHA and 10 % EPA (with palmitic acid being the other major fatty acid) and thus contains a similar DHA:EPA ratio to many fish oils. In April 2011, an application in the UK from Martek Biosciences Corporation for the authorisation of DHA and EPA-rich algal oil (under the name DHA-O) was made under the European Novel Food Regulation (EC) 258/97. The UK issued a positive opinion in December 2011 (FSA, 2011).

Processes at lab scale for the production of an EPA-rich oil from the microalgae *Phaedodactylum tricornutum*, *Nannochloropsis* and the diatom *Nitzchia* have been previously described in the literature, but not operated commercially (Milledge, 2012).

The production costs of microalgal oils will continue to fall as process efficiencies are made. One way of reducing costs is using alternative fermentation substrates. Zhiyou Wen of Iowa State University has recently reported that it is possible to produce DHA (using *Schizochytrium limacinum*) and EPA (using *Pythium irregular*) with a feedstock of glycerol derived from biodiesel production (Eisberg, 2011).

The range of LC-PUFA produced in this way will be extended. Commercial production of docosapentaenoic acid (DPA) n-3 is an interesting proposition.

As existing process patents expire, it can be expected that many more companies will consider production of DHA and EPA by microalgal fermentation. Existing producers in China and the India subcontinent are likely to significantly improve the quality of their production.

However, the fact that 2011 marked the peak possible production of fish oil means that microalgal fermentation provides the production method of choice to meet the considerable shortfall in the world's requirement for the conditionally essential LC-PUFA DHA and EPA, especially as Europe and many other parts of the world are reluctant to embrace the gene recombinant technologies that would enable them to source these LC-PUFA from cereal crops.

14.8 Sources of further information and advice

- GOED Omega-3, the Global Organization for EPA and DHA Omega-3 1075 Hollywood Avenue, Salt Lake City, UT 84105, USA. Tel: +1-801-746-1413 www.goedomega3.com
- ISSFAL, International Society for the Study of Fatty Acids. www.issfal.org
- National Algae Association, 4747 Research Forest Dr., Suite 180, The Woodlands, TX 77381, USA. Tel: +1-936-321-1125. www.nationalalgaeassociation.com
- NUTRI-FACTS, a website that is a useful source of scientific information on essential micronutrients. www.nutri-facts.org
- 'Oils and Fats – Production Properties and Uses' training course, held annually at the Leatherhead Food Research (see www.leatherheadfood.com for details).

14.9 Acknowledgements

I thank the following for recounting their long careers with algal DHA with me.

- Dr Paul Behrens (DSM Nutritional Products and a founder member of Martek Biosciences)
- Dr Ruben Abril (DSM Nutritional Products and long-serving employee of Omegatech and Martek Biosciences).
- I would also like to thank the following colleagues for reviewing and making suggestions for the early drafts of this chapter: Dr Ed Nelson, Connye Kuratko, John Rutten and Lauren Israelow.

14.10 References

ABRIL R. (2011) personal communication (telephone discussion with author dated 8th December 2011).

BEHRENS P. (2011) personal communication (telephone discussion with author dated 14th December 2011).

Commission Decision of 5 June 2003 authorising the placing on the market of oil rich in DHA (docosahexaenoic acid) from the microalgae *Schizochytrium sp.* as a novel food ingredient under Regulation (EC) No 258/97 of the European Parliament and of the Council, *OJ*, L44/13.

Commission Decision of 22 October 2009 concerning the extension of uses of algal oil from the micro-algae *Schizochytrium sp.* as a novel food ingredient under Regulation (EC) No 258/97 of the European Parliament and of the Council, *OJ*, L278/56.

Commission Directive 2006/141/EC of 22 December 2006 on infant formulae and follow-on formulae and amending Directive 1999/21/EC, *OJ*, L401/1.

Commission Regulation (EU) No 258/97 of the European Parliament and of the Council of 27 January 1997 concerning novel foods and novel food ingredients, *OJ*, L43/1.

Commission Regulation (EU) No 440/2011 of 6 May 2011 on the authorisation and refusal of authorisation of certain health claims made on foods and referring to children's development and health, *OJ*, L119/4.

Commission Regulation (EU) No 432/2012 of 16 May 2012 establishing a list of permitted health claims made on foods, other than those referring to the reduction of disease risk and to children's development and health, *OJ*, L136/1.

CRAWFORD M.A., BROADHURST C.L., GHEBREMESKEL K., HOLMSEN H., SAUGSTAD L.F., SCHMIDT W.F., SINCLAIR A.J. and CUNNANE S.C. (2008) 'The role of docosahexaenoic and arachidonic acids as determinants of evolution and hominid brain development', in TSUKAMOTO K., KAWAMURA T., TAKEUCHI T., BEARD T.D. JR and KAISER M.J. (eds), *Fisheries for Global Welfare and Environment: Memorial Book of the 5th World Fisheries Congress*. Tokyo: Terrapub, 57–76.

EISBERG N. (2011) 'Bio-based chemicals broaden their scope', *Chem. Ind.*, 7th November.

FSA (2011) Initial opinion: A DHA and EPA rich oil from the microalgae schitzochytrium. London: Food Standards Agency, available at: http://www.food.gov.uk/multimedia/pdfs/inopdhamartek.pdf [accessed February 2013].

LASSEK W.D. and GAULIN S.J.C. (2011) 'Sex differences in the relationship of dietary fatty acids to cognitive measures in American children', *Front. Evol. Neurosci.*, 3(5):1–8.

MERCER P. and ARMENTA R.E. (2011) 'Developments in oil extraction from microalgae', *Eur. J. Lipid Sci. Technol.*, 113: 539–547.

MILLEDGE J.J. (2012) 'Microalgae – commercial potential for fuel, food and feed', *Food Sci. Technol.* 26(1): 28–30.

Nutraingredients.com (2002) 'Martek completes OmegaTech acquisition', 26th April, available at: http://www.nutraingredients.com/Industry/Martek-completes-OmegaTech-acquisition [accessed January 2013].

TRAMOY P. (2011) 'Microalgae Market and Application Outlook' , CBDMT market and Business Intelligence, available from: www.cbdmt.com/index.php?id=7&raport=23 [accessed January 2013].

US FDA (2001) Agency Response Letter GRAS Notice No. GRN 000041. Silver Spring, MD: US Food and Drug Administration, available at: http://www.fda.gov/Food/FoodIngredientsPackaging/GenerallyRecognizedasSafeGRAS/GRASListings/ucm154126.htm [accessed January 2013].

US FDA (2004) Agency Response Letter GRAS Notice No. GRN 000137. Silver Spring, MD: US Food and Drug Administration, available at: http://www.fda.gov/Food/FoodIngredientsPackaging/GenerallyRecognizedasSafeGRAS/GRASListings/ucm153961.htm [accessed January 2013].

15

Labelling and claims in foods containing omega-3 fatty acids

E. M. Hernandez, Omega Protein Inc., USA

DOI: 10.1533/9780857098863.3.405

Abstract: The European Food Safety Authority (EFSA) has released a series of scientific opinions on health claims for omega-3s for a variety of health conditions, and has proposed a specific daily recommended intake for omega-3 fatty acids of 250 mg/day as the labelling reference intake value. In the USA, adequate intakes (AI) have been set only for short-chain omega 3 ALA. No daily intake recommendations or adequate intakes have been set up for EPA or DHA. Australia's National Health and Medical Research Council (NHMRC) has issued recommended daily allowances of EPA and DHA to help reduce the risk of cardiovascular disease. This chapter discusses labelling and regulatory guidelines for foods and supplements fortified with omega-3s, including information that can be included on packaging labels regarding nutrient content and health claims.

Key words: omega-3 fatty acids, food labelling health claims, nutrient content claims, recommended daily allowances.

15.1 Introduction

As omega-3 fatty acids become commonly used functional ingredients in both supplements and food products, issues have arisen around effective ways to provide useful information to the consumer regarding nutrition facts and to the manufacturer on health claims and appropriate labelling. Globally, there is no uniform agreement regarding omega-3 health claims and no consensus on issues such as recommended daily allowances (RDA) for EPA and DHA. Regulatory authorities in Europe, North America and other countries in Asia have issued a variety of recommendations for intake levels of EPA and DHA and have allowed certain claims to be included in food and supplements labels but, in general, these claims differ widely from region to region.

15.2 Status of omega-3 health and nutrition claims in Europe

The European Food Safety Authority (EFSA) has released a series of scientific opinions pursuant to Articles 13 and 14 regarding health claims for omega-3s, including three that address EPA and/or DHA claims for a variety of health conditions (Commission Regulation (EC) No. 1924/2006). 'General function' claims under Article 13.1 refer to the role of a nutrient or substance in growth, development and body functions; psychological and behavioral functions; slimming and weight control, satiety or reduction of available energy from the diet (EFSA, 2010). Claims that address reduction of disease risk and claims referring to children's development and health are addressed by EFSA pursuant to Article 14 (EFSA, 2012b).

Specifically in relation to omega-3 fatty acids, a review from EFSA (2009) on proposed labelling for reference intake values for omega-3 and omega-6 polyunsaturated fatty acids (PUFA) included typical recommended daily allowances of omega-3 fatty acids that include α-linolenic acid (ALA) and the long-chain omega-3 PUFA (mainly EPA and DHA). These values can be used in food labelling by the consumer as a reference for omega-3 content in foods as well as by the retailer in making PUFA-related health claims. The intake recommendations for ALA based on considerations of cardiovascular health and neurodevelopment are 2–3 g ALA/day for energy intakes of 1800–2700 kcal/day and the proposed labelling reference intake value for the short-chain omega-3 fatty acid ALA is 2 g. This opinion was based on the upper end of the range of average intakes observed in adults in some European countries (0.7–2.3 g/day).

Concerning the long-chain omega-3 PUFA, EPA and DHA, the EFSA Panel proposed 250 mg/day as the labelling reference intake value. This was based on evidence showing that the intake of EPA+DHA is negatively related to cardiovascular risk in doses up to about 250 mg/day (or one to two servings of oily fish per week) in healthy populations. The observed average intakes of EPA+DHA in adults in some European countries varied between 80 and 420 mg/day.

EFSA also released a scientific opinion pursuant to Article 13 of EC 1924/2006 on 'general function' health claims for long-chain PUFA. EPA and DHA received positive opinions for three claims: (i) maintenance of normal cardiac function; (ii) maintenance of normal blood pressure; (iii) maintenance of normal (fasting) blood concentrations of triglycerides. DHA, added by itself, received positive opinions for three claims: (i) maintenance of normal (fasting) blood concentrations of triglycerides; (ii) maintenance of normal brain function; (iii) maintenance of normal vision. The claim 'Maintenance of normal blood concentrations of triglycerides' requires the of use 2 g/day of DHA in one or more servings, and the target population is adult men and women. The claim 'Maintenance of normal brain function' requires the use of foods that contain 250 mg/day of DHA in one or more servings and is targeted to the general population; the claim 'Maintenance of normal vision' requires foods to contain 250 mg/day of DHA in one or more servings and is also targeted at the general population (EFSA, 2012a).

Regarding claims pursuant to Article 14, EFSA first issued a positive opinion linking omega-3 from ALA with brain and nerve tissue development in children up to three years. The claim may state: 'Alpha-linolenic acid, an essential fatty acid, contributes to brain and nerve tissue development'. Long-chain omega-3s were also approved for three Article 14 claims: (i) DHA intake contributes to the normal visual development of infants up to 12 months of age (100 mg/day of DHA); (ii) DHA maternal intake contributes to the normal development of the eye of the fetus and breastfed infants (200 mg/day of DHA in addition to the recommended intake for omega-3 fatty acids for adults, i.e. 250 mg of EPA+DHA); (iii) DHA maternal intake contributes to the normal brain development of the fetus and breastfed infants (200 mg/day of DHA in addition to the recommended intake for omega-3 fatty acids for adults, i.e. 250 mg of EPA+DHA) (EFSA, 2012b).

With regard to nutrition labels, a claim that a food is a 'source of omega-3 fatty acids' can be made if the product contains at least 0.3 g ALA per 100 g and per 100 kcal, or at least 40 mg of the sum of EPA+DHA per 100 g and per 100 kcal. The label claim 'high in omega-3 fatty acids' may be made when the product contains at least 0.6 g ALA per 100 g and per 100 kcal, or at least 80 mg of EPA+DHA per 100 g and per 100 kcal (Commission Regulation (EC) No. 1924/2006).

More recently, EFSA issued a scientific opinion on the tolerable upper intake level (UL) of long-chain EPA/DHA of 5 g/day at which the long-chain PUFA do not appear to increase the risk of spontaneous bleeding episodes or bleeding complications, or affect glucose homeostasis immune function or lipid peroxidation, provided the oxidative stability of the PUFA is guaranteed. Also it was stated in this scientific opinion that supplemental intakes of EPA and DHA combined at doses up to 5 g/day, and supplemental intakes of EPA alone up to 1.8 g/day, do not raise safety concerns for adults. Supplemental intakes of DHA alone up to about 1 g/day do not raise safety concerns for the general population (EFSA, 2012c).

The EFSA panel also issued an opinion on omega-6 PUFA, including linolenic acid (LA) and arachidonic acid (ARA). They proposed a labelling reference intake value of 6 g/day of omega-6 PUFA. The intakes observed in Europe were between 7 and 19 g/day (EFSA, 2009).

15.3 Status of omega-3 health and nutrition claims in North America

In the USA, claims that can be used on food and dietary supplement labels fall into three categories: health claims, nutrient content claims and structure/function claims. The responsibility for ensuring the validity of these claims rests with the manufacturer, FDA (Food and Drug Administration) and, in the case of advertising, with the Federal Trade Commission (FDA, 2003).

In the USA, only qualified health claims are allowed for omega-3s; in other words, a health claim made on the label is expressed by implication only, as opposed to 'Authorized health claims' that include 'significant scientific agreement'. A qualified health claim, on the one hand, does not require a high level of scientific support but, on the other hand, does not have the advantage of being backed by the factual scientific evidence that would be needed to underpin, for example, a recommended daily allowance (RDA). The qualified health claim for omega-3s states: Supportive but not conclusive research shows that consumption of EPA and DHA omega-3 fatty acids may reduce the risk of coronary heart disease. One serving of [Name of the food] provides [x] gram of EPA and DHA omega-3 fatty acids (FDA/CFSAN, 2004a).

Food labels can also include nutrient content claims, such as 'Excellent Source of EPA & DHA Omega-3s' or 'Rich in EPA & DHA Omega-3s' as long as content in the food exceeds 32 mg of EPA and DHA per serving. The 'excellent source' claim is based on the AI (adequate intake) level of 160 mg/day for adult males established for linolenic acid by the US Institutes of Medicine (IOM, 2002). This follows the same principle for all other nutrient content claims in the USA, namely that a product can claim to be an 'excellent source' of a nutrient if it contains 20 % of the average daily requirement levels of the nutrient.

Considered more tentative and less precise, 'structure/function' claims can also be included in some labels. This type of claim basically describes the role of a nutrient or functional component in affecting or maintaining normal body structure or function or general wellbeing. However, the claim cannot describe or imply that a nutrient or functional component affects a disease or health-related condition via diagnosis, cure, mitigation, treatment or prevention. For omega-3s such as EPA and DHA, structure/function claims may include: 'may contribute to maintenance of heart health' and 'may contribute to maintenance of mental and visual function'. Table 15.1 shows examples of claims that can be included in food products fortified with omega-3s.

For foods in general, the FDA recommends that consumers do not exceed an intake of 3 g/day of combined EPA and DHA fatty acids. For dietary supplements, there is a labelling precondition that a label should not recommend/suggest a daily intake exceeding 2 g/day of EPA and DHA. Other conditions for dietary supplements include that total fat content in dietary supplements that weigh more than 5 g per RACC (reference amount customarily consumed) must not exceed the total fat disqualifying level (13.0 g per RACC). For saturated fat content, dietary supplements must meet the criterion for low saturated fat with regard to the saturated fat

Table 15.1 Examples of omega-3 health claims in baked foods

Claim	Message on label
Qualified health claim	'Supportive but not conclusive research shows that consumption of EPA and DHA omega-3 fatty acids may reduce the risk of coronary heart disease. One serving of [name of food] provides [x] grams of EPA and DHA omega-3 fatty acids. [See nutrition information for total fat, saturated fat and cholesterol content.]'
Nutrient content claim	'Excellent source of EPA & DHA omega-3s' 'Rich in EPA & DHA omega-3s'
Structure function claim	'May contribute to maintenance of heart health' 'May contribute to maintenance of mental and visual function'
Content claims	'Contains 30 mg of EPA & DHA Omega-3s'

content (≤1 g per RACC). Also, fish may not exceed the saturated fat disqualifying level of 4.0 g per RACC (or 4.0 g per 50 g if the reference amount is ≤30 g or ≤2 tbsp). Conventional foods other than fish must meet the criteria for low saturated fat (≤1 g per RACC and no more than 15 % of calories from saturated fat for individual foods). Dietary supplements that weigh more than 5 g per RACC must also meet the criterion for low cholesterol (≤20 mg per 50 g). All conventional foods and dietary supplements must meet the sodium disqualifying level (≤480 mg per RACC). Also, all conventional foods must meet the 10 % minimum nutrient requirement (vitamin A 500 IU, vitamin C 6 mg, iron 1.8 mg, calcium 100 mg, protein 5 g, fiber 2.5 g per RACC), prior to any nutrient addition. The 10 % minimum nutrient requirement does not apply to dietary supplements (21 CFR 101.14(e)(6). Table 15.1 shows examples of claims that can be included in food products fortified with omega-3s (FDA/CFSAN, 2004a, b).

Although the USA does not have intake recommendations for EPA and DHA, it does have recommendations for adequate intakes (AI) of omega-3 as ALA and omega-6 as linoleic acid (LA) (IOM, 2002). AI is defined as nutrient intake estimate observed in healthy individuals where sufficient scientific data is not available to suggest a RDA (recommended daily allowance). The AIs set for LA were 17 and 12 g/day for men and women, respectively, aged 19–50 years. The AIs for ALA were 1.6 and 1.1 g/day for men and women, respectively, aged 19–70 years (IOM, 2002) (see Table 15.2). The nutrition recommendations of the US National Academy of Sciences (IOM, 2002) are used by both USA and Canada.

For patients with documented heart disease, the American Heart Association (AHA) recommends an intake of about 1 g/day of EPA+DHA. For people who need to lower their blood triglycerides, the recommended intake is 2–4 g/day of EPA+DHA under a physician's care. They also recommend that patients without documented coronary heart disease get

Table 15.2 Adequate intake (AI) for omega-3 fatty acids

Life stage	Age	Source	Males (g/day)	Females (g/day)
Infants	0–6 months	ALA, EPA, DHA	0.5	0.5
Infants	7–12 months	ALA, EPA, DHA	0.5	0.5
Children	1–3 years	ALA	0.7	0.7
Children	4–8 years	ALA	0.9	0.9
Children	9–13 years	ALA	1.2	1.0
Adolescents	14–18 years	ALA	1.6	1.1
Adults	19 years and older	ALA	1.6	1.1
Pregnancy	All ages	ALA	–	1.4
Breastfeeding	All ages	ALA	–	1.3

Source: IOM, 2002.

omega-3s through the consumption of a variety of fish (preferably fatty fish) at least twice a week and include oils rich in ALA (flaxseed, canola soybean oils and walnut oils) in their diet (AHA, 2013).

15.4 Status of omega-3 health and nutrition claims in Asia and Australia

China adopted a national standard for mandatory nutrition labelling effective 1 January 2013. The standard Nutrition Labelling of Pre-packaged Food Regulation establishes the general principle and labelling requirements and reporting components of nutrition in the food label for direct use by the consumer. Mandatory labelling requirements were set for energy and core nutrients (protein, fat, carbohydrates and sodium). Other nutrients such as vitamins and minerals are required only when a nutrition claim is being made; otherwise labelling is voluntary. These labelling guidelines will be used by food manufacturers to validate any nutritional claims and nutrient functions.

Australia and New Zealand use Food Standards Australia New Zealand (FSANZ) to regulate nutrition labelling and health claims. Nutrition content and function claims are allowed in some cases, but references to curing disease and/or weight reduction are not. More recently, FSANZ regulations on nutrition and health claims allowed a wider variety of claims that can be made, including reduction of disease risk claims. These allowed claims are divided into 'general' and 'high level' according to the extent of the identified benefit to consumer. General level claims include nutrient content claims, nutrient function claims describing a constituent and its function in the body; and claims that refer to the maintenance of good health. High level claims are those that refer to the potential for a food or constituent to assist in controlling a serious disease or condition by either reducing risk factors or improving health (FSANZ, 2013).

With regard to omega-3 fatty acids, the allowed claims fall under the general claims category. After review of the published literature on the health benefits of omega-3s, a scientific committee for FSANZ concluded that further evidence was needed to establish an omega-3 intake requirement for reduction in risk of cardiovascular disease (CVD). FSANZ considers that the evidence for a benefit of long-chain omega-3 fatty acids EPA and DHA on CVD morbidity and mortality can be rated as 'probable' but cannot be rated as 'convincing'. Therefore, FSANZ issued an opinion that there is sufficient evidence to support a 'general' level health claim based on the diet–disease relationship between long-chain omega-3 fatty acids and cardiovascular health (FSANZ, 2013). Australia's government National Health and Medical Research Council (NHMRC), on the other hand, recommends 430–570 mg/day from foods, as an amount which might be expected to reduce the risk of CVD in the ANZ population (NHMRC, 2006). Japan's Ministry of Health Labor and Welfare recommends an intake of 1.8–2.4 g of total omega-3 fatty acids per day (NIH, 2005).

15.5 Implications of omega-3 nutrition and health claims for the global food industry

The growing consumer interest in the nutrition content of foods and supplements has resulted in the introduction of a wide variety of more health-oriented products with more specialized bioactive compounds. As a result, the information about nutrition and health provided in packaging can be complex and difficult to understand. This information has become increasingly important as both the general population and health institutions become more interested in areas such as children's nutrition, heart, digestive, cognitive and immune health, obesity, and healthy aging. The demand for health-oriented foods has also spurred manufacturers to market food products with healthier connotations, such as low in saturated fats, non-trans fats, low in cholesterol, higher protein content, lower in carbohydrates, higher in fiber. This has led manufacturers to introduce supplements and fortified foods with ingredients that have disease prevention and, in some cases, pharmaceutic-like properties. Omega-3 fatty acids are considered ingredients that have disease prevention properties and, as mentioned before, their use as an ingredient in foods and supplements has grown appreciably in the last few years.

15.6 Conclusion and future trends

The demand for fortified foods with bioactive compounds will continue to grow and the distinction between some fortified foods and supplements will become less apparent. This new generation of health-oriented food products will require more accurate and better explanatory information to be included in the labels. This will also require involvement of official institutions to set labelling guidelines for nutrition or health claims, for example: identifying allowable claims, and implementation and enforcement mechanisms for compliance.

Technological advances have enabled manufacturers to overcome formulation challenges with omega-3s in regard to shelf-life enhancement and product stability. The widely recognized health benefits of omega-3s have translated into these fatty acids becoming integrated not just through supplements but also into the general diet through new products in the areas of wellness nutrition and medical foods. New labelling guidelines for omega-3 fatty acids in foods and supplements will allow the consumer to become better informed on the health benefits of omega-3s and help distinguish between food and therapeutic-type dietary supplements.

15.7 References

AHA (2013) *Frequently Asked Questions About Fish*. Dallas, TX: American Heart Association, available at: http://www.heart.org/HEARTORG/General/Frequently-Asked-Questions-About-Fish_UCM_306451_Article.jsp [accessed February 2013].

COMMISSION REGULATION (EC) No. 1924/2006 of the European Parliament and of the Council of 20 December 2006 on nutrition and health claims made on foods, *OJ*, L404, 9–25.

EFSA (2009) Labelling reference intake values for n-3 and n-6 polyunsaturated fatty acids, *EFSA Journal*, 1176, 1–11.

EFSA (2010) 'Scientific opinion on the substantiation of health claims related to eicosapentaenoic acid (EPA), docosahexaenoic acid (DHA), docosapentaenoic acid (DPA) and maintenance of normal cardiac function', *EFSA Journal*, 8(10): 1796.

EFSA (2012a) *'General function' health claims under article 13*. Parma: European Food Safety Authority, available at: http://www.efsa.europa.eu/en/topics/topic/article13.htm [accessed February 2013].

EFSA (2012b) *Claims on disease risk reduction and child development or health under Article 14*. Parma: European Food Safety Authority, available at: http://www.efsa.europa.eu/en/topics/topic/article14.htm [accessed February 2013].

EFSA (2012c) 'Scientific opinion on the tolerable upper intake level of eicosapentaenoic acid (EPA), docosahexaenoic acid (DHA) and docosapentaenoic acid (DPA)', *EFSA Journal*, 10(7), 2815.

FDA (2003) Claims That Can Be Made for Conventional Foods and Dietary Supplements. http://www.fda.gov/Food/LabelingNutrition/LabelClaims/ucm111447.htm [accesed 7/9/2012].

FDA/CFSAN (2004a) Letter Responding to Health Claim Petition dated June 23, 2003 (Wellness petition): Omega-3 Fatty Acids and Reduced Risk of Coronary Heart Disease (Docket No. 2003Q-0401), available at: http://www.fda.gov/Food/LabelingNutrition/LabelClaims/QualifiedHealthClaims/ucm072936.htm [accessed February 2013].

FDA/CFSAN (2004b) Letter Responding to Health Claim Petition dated November 3, 2003 (Martek Petition): Omega-3 Fatty Acids and Reduced Risk of Coronary Heart Disease (Docket No. 2003Q-0401), available at: http://www.fda.gov/Food/LabelingNutrition/LabelClaims/QualifiedHealthClaims/ucm072932.htm [accessed February 2013].

FSANZ (2013) *Long chain omega-3 fatty acids and cardiovascular disease – FSANZ consideration of a commissioned review*. Food Standards Australia New Zealand, available at: http://www.foodstandards.gov.au/_srcfiles/FSANZ%20consideration%20of%20omega-3%20review1.pdf [accessed February 2013].

IOM (Institutes of Medicine) (2002) *Dietary Reference Intakes for Energy, Carbohydrate, Fiber, Fat, Fatty Acids, Cholesterol, Protein, and Amino Acids*. Washington DC: National Academies Press.

NIH (2005) *Dietary Reference Intakes for Japanese*. Tokyo: Ministry of Health, Labour and Welfare, available at: http://www0.nih.go.jp/eiken/english/research/pdf/dris2005_eng.pdf [accessed February 2013].

Index

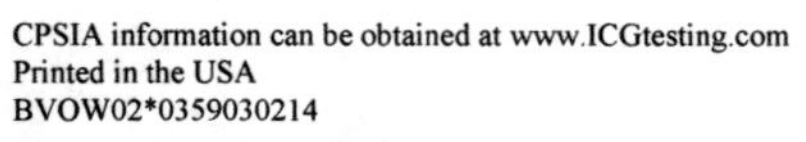
CPSIA information can be obtained at www.ICGtesting.com
Printed in the USA
BVOW02*0359030214

343683BV00006B/169/P